NEUROPSYCHOLOGICAL ASSESSMENT AND INTERVENTION FOR CHILDHOOD AND ADOLESCENT DISORDERS

NEUROPSYCHOLOGICAL ASSESSMENT AND INTERVENTION FOR CHILDHOOD AND ADOLESCENT DISORDERS

Cynthia A. Riccio
Jeremy R. Sullivan
Morris J. Cohen

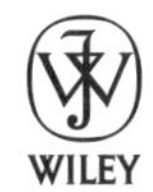

John Wiley & Sons, Inc.

This book is printed on acid-free paper. ♾

Published by John Wiley & Sons, Inc., Hoboken, New Jersey.
Published simultaneously in Canada.

For general information on our other products and services please contact our Customer Care Department within the U.S. at (800) 762-2974, outside the United States at (317) 572-3993 or fax (317) 572-4002.

Wiley also publishes its books in a variety of electronic formats. Some content that appears in print may not be available in electronic books. For more information about Wiley products, visit our web site at www.wiley.com.

Library of Congress Cataloging-in-Publication Data:

Riccio, Cynthia A.

Neuropsychological assessment and intervention for childhood and adolescent disorders / Cynthia A. Riccio, Jeremy R. Sullivan, Morris J. Cohen.

p. ; cm.

Includes bibliographical references and indexes.

ISBN 978-0-470-18413-4 (cloth : alk. paper)

1. Pediatric neuropsychology. I. Sullivan, Jeremy R. II. Cohen, Morris J., 1953- III. Title.

[DNLM: 1. Brain Diseases—diagnosis. 2. Adolescent. 3. Child. 4. Mental Disorders Diagnosed in Childhood. WL 141 R493n 2010]

RJ486.5.R53 2010

618.92'8—dc22

2009027782

Printed in the United States of America.

10 9 8 7 6 5 4 3 2 1

In appreciation of my husband's patience and support as this project unfolded and took on a life of its own, and my coauthors, who tolerated my nagging.

—CAR

Thanks to my family and friends, for listening patiently as I talked about this book over the last several years. Also, thanks to my coauthors for the opportunity to collaborate on this project.

—JRS

Dedicated to my loving and supportive family and to the children and their families who make this book necessary.

—MJC

Contents

Foreword

> The structural variation of the higher mental functions at different stages of ontogenetic (and in some cases functional) development means that their cortical organization likewise does not remain unchanged and that at different stages of development they are carried out by different constellations of cortical zones....[Thus]...the character of the intercentral relationships does not remain the same at different stages of development of a function and...the effects of a lesion of a particular part of the brain will differ at different stages of functional development.
>
> —Luria, 1980, pp. 34–35

Some 30 years ago, I drove to Santa Fe, New Mexico, in a blinding snowstorm to attend one of the early meetings of the International Neuropsychological Society. At that meeting, most of the presentations focused on the neuropsychological effects of stroke or closed-head injury in adults. Only a few presentations, those I was particularly interested in, dealt with disorders affecting children and adolescents. Most of the presentations relative to children and adolescents addressed the neuropsychological basis of learning disabilities, especially developmental reading disorders. Clinical assessment of children with disorders of presumed neurodevelopmental origin was limited to instruments assessing expressive and receptive language, visual-motor functioning, and perhaps a few experimental measures with generally poor or nonexisting psychometric qualities.

Reflecting how much our research has contributed to our clinical practice since those early days in the history of neuropsychology, this volume accomplishes two things simultaneously. First, the authors have undertaken the task of providing neuropsychologists with a much-needed integration of research on disorders impacting children and adolescents while at the same time illustrating how a much more comprehensive and research-based clinical neuropsychological assessment can inform evidence-based intervention or rehabilitation. Clearly, what is now considered a comprehensive neuropsychological assessment has changed greatly since the early days of our profession.

Second, the range of clinical syndromes addressed in this volume represents how much the field of clinical child/pediatric neuropsychology has grown in respect and practice in the past 30 or so years. While neurodevelopmental disorders such as dyslexia, dyscalculia, and specific language impairment are still of theoretical and clinical interest, neuropsychological research clearly has informed us greatly in our clinical practice with children and adolescents who may suffer the entire range of disorders addressed in this important volume.

The range of disorders now seen by clinical neuropsychologists also reflects in part the appreciation by medical professionals of the importance of the clinical neuropsychological assessment in patient diagnosis and management. No longer are referrals to clinical child/pediatric neuropsychologists coming exclusively from neurologists or psychiatrists; now oncologists, pediatricians, and physicians with expertise in other medical specializations often refer patients for neuropsychological evaluation.

As can be seen, our theoretical understanding of neurodevelopmental, genetic, traumatic, and disorders linked to disease or environmental causes has been greatly informed by the results of experimental and clinical assessments. Importantly, the quality of our clinical neuropsychological assessments not only informs those who must treat children and adolescents but, through studies, the characteristics and quality of our clinical neuropsychological evaluations improve as we increase our understanding of the cognitive and behavioral outcomes of neurodevelopmental disorders and disease processes. Thus, there is a synergy between our evolving understanding of how brain-behavior relations are impacted by variations in brain ontogeny or disease and how we conceptualize and consequently organize our clinical evaluations.

The practice of clinical child/pediatric neuropsychology is in some regards more complicated than that which focuses on disorders impacting adults. While the evaluation of neuropsychological status of adults with traumatic or degenerative disease processes has its own constellation of challenges, the practice of neuropsychology with children and adolescents is influenced significantly by the often-complicated interplay between rapid physical and cognitive development and the behavioral outcomes of developmental disorders or disease.

While neuropsychological assessment instruments today typically have adequate psychometric qualities, unlike decades past, the behavioral outcome of alterations in the structure or functioning of the brain in children or adolescents may manifest differentially at different stages of development. Further, the long-term behavioral and cognitive impact may depend to some extent on the timing of the insult or first clinical manifestation and the quality and extent of the intervention or rehabilitation.

Years of clinical experience with children and adolescents who manifest disorders resulting from disturbed brain processes prepare clinicians well for the referral of children and adolescents with disorders outside of their typical caseload. One of the important aspects of this volume is that it presents exemplars of clinical assessments of children and adolescents with a wide range of disorders. For referrals outside the clinician's typical caseload, this volume presents an excellent overview of the particular disorder and integrates the approach to clinical assessment with evidence-based interventions.

The chapters in this book provide a solid basis for clinicians who need to craft their approach to clinical neuropsychological assessment in a way that respects and reflects current research and exceeds the standard of practice. It is for precisely this reason that this book will become the most cited reference for what constitutes a research-based, best practice guide for clinical neuropsychological assessment and intervention for children and adolescents.

George W. Hynd

Foundation Professor
Senior Vice Provost, Dean, and Director
Mary Lou Fulton Institute and Graduate School of Education
Arizona State University

Preface

There are any number of texts and reference books related to clinical neuropsychology, child/pediatric neuropsychology, neuropsychological assessment, and rehabilitation. The intent in writing *this* book was to describe various disorders as they manifest in children and youth from a neuropsychological perspective. While summarizing the research on the neurological and etiological components of disorders, the focus is on assessment and what is established with regard to evidence-based practices for children with these disorders. Finally, to emphasize the practical aspects of neuropsychological practice, each chapter includes one or more case studies, including detailed background information, assessment results, and recommendations based on assessment data. The case studies are used to personalize the effects of various disorders as well as to demonstrate the usefulness of neuropsychological information in treatment/intervention planning, especially within children's educational and social contexts. We hope the case studies complement the content of each chapter by illustrating how the assessment process can inform intervention efforts for children with a range of disorders.

Cynthia A. Riccio
Jeremy R. Sullivan
Morris J. Cohen

Acknowledgments

Clearly, a book such as this is a major undertaking. It would not have been possible without the contributions of case study and other materials from fellow colleagues:

Christine Castillo, Ph.D., Children's Medical Center—Dallas

J. Brad Hale, Ph.D., Philadelphia College of Osteopathic Medicine

Kelly Pizzitola Jarratt, Ph.D., Assistant Professor/Pediatric Neuropsychologist, Department of Pediatrics, UAMS College of Medicine, Arkansas Children's Hospital

Michelle Y. Kibby, Ph.D., Assistant Professor, Department of Psychology, Southern Illinois University

Mary C. Kral, Ph.D., Assistant Professor of Pediatrics, Division of Genetics and Developmental Pediatrics, Medical University of South Carolina

Sarika U. Peters, Ph.D., Pediatric Neuropsychologist, Department of Pediatrics, Baylor College of Medicine

Suzanne Strickland, M.D., Assistant Professor, Section of Child Neurology, Department of Neurology, Medical College of Georgia

About the Authors

Cynthia A. Riccio, Ph.D., is a Professor, Director of Training for the School Psychology Program, and a Professor of the Faculty of Neuroscience, at Texas A & M University.

Jeremy R. Sullivan, Ph.D., is an Assistant Professor in the Department of Educational Psychology at the University of Texas at San Antonio.

Morris J. Cohen, Ed.D., is a Professor of Neurology, Pediatrics & Psychiatry, and Director of the Pediatric Neuropsychology Service at the Medical College of Georgia. Dr. Cohen also holds adjunct faculty status in the School Psychology Program, at the University of Georgia.

NEUROPSYCHOLOGICAL ASSESSMENT AND INTERVENTION FOR CHILDHOOD AND ADOLESCENT DISORDERS

Chapter 1

INTRODUCTION TO PEDIATRIC NEUROPSYCHOLOGY

WHAT IS PEDIATRIC NEUROPSYCHOLOGY?

Neuropsychology has its roots in behavioral neurology. Behavioral neurology, which can be traced back to ancient Greece and Egypt (Zillmer, Spiers, & Culbertson, 2008), is a branch of neurology that deals with disorders of higher cognitive functioning (e.g., language, cognition, visual perception). Aristotle referred to the brain, and Herophilus described hydrocephaly and the ventricles of the brain. Behavioral neurology posits that behavior, at least to some extent, is dependent on the functioning of the central nervous system. Neuropsychology is the clinical application of the understanding of brain-behavior relations as derived from behavioral neurology (Stuss & Levine, 2002); pediatric neuropsychology applies this understanding within the developmental context of children, particularly those with neurodevelopmental disorders. Research in pediatric neuropsychology has not reached its full potential, and research and practice continue to expand (Baron, 2008). Pediatric neuropsychology has applications across neurology, neurosurgery, psychology, psychiatry, family medicine, nursing, and education (Witsken, D'Amato, & Hartlage, 2008).

Children with neurodevelopmental disorders are those who have, or who are at risk for, limitations in some or all life activities as a result of impairments in the central nervous system (Mudrick, 2002; Spreen, Risser, & Edgell, 1995). The possible consequences and limitations range from mild to severe cognitive, sensory, motor, educational, and behavioral/psychological impairments (Mendola, Selevan, Gutter, & Rice, 2002). The major premise of neuropsychological assessment is that the information obtained reflects the integrity of the central nervous system (Stuss & Levine, 2002). Neuropsychologists use their knowledge and understanding of brain-behavior relations in the conceptualization of an individual's functioning in a variety of domains including: cognition ("g"), auditory-linguistic, problem-solving, learning and memory, visual-spatial and constructional areas, academic achievement, and interpersonal/behavioral. Neuropsychologists engage in "hypothesis-driven" assessment that involves integration of all the information obtained in the context of neurodevelopmental systems (Berkelhammer, 2008). The goal of this integration is the generation of recommendations for habilitation, accommodations, or modifications.

Neuropsychology incorporates knowledge of behavioral neurology gained through research in clinical contexts; what is known about brain-behavior relations has changed over time as medical technology has increased. Current perspectives incorporate principles of both equipotentiality and pluripotentiality. The concept of equipotentiality embodies the idea that if sufficient cortical material is intact, this intact material will subsume the functions of the damaged tissue; thus, the size of the injury and not the location determines the effect on brain functioning (Zillmer et al., 2008). Alternatively, the idea of pluripotentiality is that any given area of the brain can be involved in multiple behaviors to varying degrees (Luria, 1980). The principles of equipotentiality and pluripotentiality, as well as plasticity, give rise to the connection between knowledge of brain-behavior relations, assessment of neurocognitive functioning, and rehabilitation/habilitation.

In the interpretation of individual behavior, sometimes inferences are made that seem to draw from localization theory; unfortunately, evidence suggests that brain-behavior relations are not that simplistic; rather, behavior is the result of complex functional systems or networks within the brain (Luria, 1980). Medical findings continue to support and validate localization to some extent while also supporting the widely distributed functional systems of Alexander Luria for more complex behavior. The 20th century saw continued advancement in technology and the ability to examine brain structures through multiple methods. Current technology provides greater insight and information through various functional imaging methods; with this increased technology, understanding of brain behavior relations will continue to improve rapidly. This is the research component to neuropsychology and the means by which neuropsychology seeks to advance the understanding of the effects of neurodevelopmental and genetic disorders (Berkelhammer, 2008).

It is important to remember, however, that overall functioning is not only the result of the integrity of brain function but that brain function is influenced by (and influences) environmental contexts; hence, the context in which the individual functions is also of importance. The invariance hypothesis dictates that brain functions are asymmetrically located in the cerebral hemispheres and that hemispheric dominance is genetically determined, but that each hemisphere has the potential for acquiring various functions. Research suggests that deprivation of stimulation can result in impaired or absent development (e.g., binocular and monocular deprivation in animal studies can result in blindness or optical deficits). The idea of the deprived area being deficient or stimulation relating to increased function is one possible explanation for the inability of humans to perceive certain sounds in languages unfamiliar to us and why children are much better bilingual learners than adults. In effect, the genetic contributions may serve as a predisposition or diathesis that can be altered or modified for better or worse by environmental stimulation or exposure (Asbury, Wachs, & Plomin, 2005; Pennington et al., 2009; Schmidt, Polak, & Spooner, 2005).

Related to diathesis, maturation theory posits that functional asymmetry of the hemispheres develops with age, beginning at conception, and is influenced by environmental events and stimulation. From the time of conception, an interruption in normal development or abnormal development for any of one area of the brain for any reason leads to associated abnormalities at levels of functioning and can potentially affect multiple systems (Zillmer et al., 2008). Neural development does not stop at birth; rather, fine tuning of neural functioning continues throughout the life span and is continuously affected by environmental contexts. From a developmental perspective, notions related to equipotentiality, pluripotentiality, and plasticity serve as the foundation of many early intervention programs. While neuropsychology embraces the idea that the neurological hardware of the individual determines their behavior, there is evidence that failure to stimulate particular areas of the brain will impact on functioning; alternatively, there are indications that stimulation or intervention can result in changes in brain function (Zillmer et al., 2008).

Early intervention efforts are targeting the potential effects of increased stimulation; similarly, many of the rehabilitation efforts for stroke and traumatic brain injury (TBI) are based on the premise that the brain can be "retrained" to some degree.

NEUROPSYCHOLOGICAL ASSESSMENT

When an individual is referred for a neuropsychological assessment, often the primary purpose is to identify (or rule out) pathology. The neuropsychological approach to case conceptualization incorporates information related to various behavioral domains believed to reflect functional neurological systems (Luria, 1980; Riccio & Reynolds, 1998). A major premise of neuropsychological assessment is that different behaviors involve differing neurological structures or functional systems (Luria, 1980); as such, neuropsychological assessment is intended to be sufficiently comprehensive to address all functional systems.

The pathology in question is generally considered to be in the central nervous system or the peripheral nervous system. Typically, the neurologist assesses functioning by looking at what are referred to as "soft signs." These include reflexes (e.g., tapping on knee), balance (e.g., walking a straight line), short-term memory (e.g., recall of digits or unrelated words), mental status (e.g., awareness of time and place), coordination (e.g., touching nose with eyes closed), visual tracking (e.g., following a pencil), verbal skills (e.g., in conversation), and cognitive flexibility (e.g., counting backward by 3s). Neurologists also will verify the functioning of cranial nerves to the extent feasible through observation of the associated behaviors (Zillmer et al., 2008). Neurologists will look at head circumference, height, weight, gait (e.g., toe walking, heel-toe walking), and right versus left differences (e.g., in hand strength). Neuropsychological assessment may include similar tasks but also samples behaviors known to depend on the integrity of the central nervous system through the use of various measures that correlate with cognitive, sensorimotor, and emotional functioning (R. S. Dean & Gray, 1990).

The assessment process is hypothesis driven (Berkelhammer, 2008), to the extent that the methods and measures are selected based on hypotheses regarding the underlying pathology due to the reason for referral, medical history, and developmental information obtained in advance. The assessment incorporates components of a typical psychoeducational or psychological evaluation but extends the scope to other areas of functioning. Neuropsychological assessment includes measures of cognitive ability, achievement, and personality/behavior. It also involves more extensive measures of language, visual spatial perception, visual motor construction, learning and memory of new material (e.g., list learning tasks), fine motor functioning, tactile perception, attention, executive function (problem-solving, abstract reasoning, planning, and organization), and working memory (Riccio & Reynolds, 1998).

Many clinicians use a predetermined battery of tests for neuropsychological assessment of children (Riccio, 2008); this is often referred to as the fixed battery or nomethetic approach. Specific neuropsychological batteries, such as the Halstead-Reitan Neuropsychological Battery (HRNB) (Reitan & Davison, 1974; Reitan & Wolfson, 1985), the Reitan-Indiana Neuropsychological Battery (RINB) (Reitan, 1969), the Luria Nebraska Neuropsychological Battery—Children's Revision (LNNB-CR) (Golden, 1984; Golden, Freshwater, & Vayalakkara, 2000), the Kaplan Baycrest Neurocognitive Assessment (Leach, Kaplan, Rewilak, Richards, & Proulx, 2000), or the Neuropsychological Assessment-Second Edition (NEPSY-2) (Korkman, Kirk, & Kemp, 2007) are often used in neuropsychological assessment in conjunction with intelligence tests, achievement tests, and measures of behavior and personality. These neuropsychological batteries provide a sampling of sensory and motor functions as well as additional information relating to left/right–hemisphere differences and anterior/posterior differences. Of these, the HRNB continues to be one of the most widely used neuropsychological test batteries but may require some updating if it is going to continue to be useful in clinical practice (Sinco, D'Amato, & Davis, 2008).

Alternatively, neuropsychologists may adopt a more idiographic approach and tailor the selection of measures based on the child's presenting problems, with others added based on the child's performance on initial measures (Berkelhammer, 2008; Christensen, 1975; Luria, 1973). This type of approach, often referred to as a deficit approach, is intended to isolate those mechanisms that are contributing to a specific, identified problem as part of hypothesis testing. The deficit-only model may be more cost effective; the emphasis is clearly on understanding deficit systems and not identifying intact functional systems—hypotheses related to intact systems are not addressed. Further, the more idiographic approach may fail to assess domains that are of importance and subsequently impact on rehabilitation efforts (Riccio & Reynolds, 1998).

Traditionally, neuropsychological assessment has focused more on analysis of the functional systems and overall integrity of the central nervous system (CNS) than on the identification of a single neurological disorder (Riccio & Reynolds, 1998). In assessing CNS integrity, it is important to ensure that the results obtained allow for evaluation of the four major quadrants of the neocortex (left, right, anterior, posterior). Therefore, it is important that the assessment sample the relative efficiency of the right and left hemispheres. Similarly, the anterior region of the brain generally is viewed as being associated with different functions (e.g., regulatory) as opposed to the posterior region of the brain (receptivity). Just as lateralization of dysfunction is important, anterior-posterior comparisons can provide important information for treatment planning. The cumulative performances of the individual on neuropsychological measures are seen as behavioral indicators of brain function (Fennell & Bauer, 1997; Stuss & Levine, 2002).

There is no single method to select measures to be included in a neuropsychological assessment that is used across settings or individuals; in fact, the range of measures and methods available is continuously expanding and allows for assessment of a wider range of behaviors. Whether the approach is a fixed battery or a flexible battery, the assessment may or may not include naturalistic observation and informal assessment (Reynolds, 1997). In addition, the approach may be standardized or incorporate a process orientation (Kaplan, 1988, 1990; Milberg & Hebben, 2006). Although some may choose to rely on actuarial or quantitative methods, reliance on qualitative methods is not recommended. Many clinicians prefer a combination of quantitative and qualitative measures to balance the strengths and weaknesses of both approaches. In particular, reliance on a qualitative approach does not allow for verification of diagnostic accuracy and does not allow for formal evaluation of treatment methods; further, it is not easily replicated, and interdiagnostician agreement may be compromised (Poreh, 2006). Regardless of the approach, the influences of child psychology, school psychology, and education are evident in the composition of neuropsychological assessment batteries, procedures, and measures used with children; the variety of perspectives contribute to the variations in methods used (Batchelor, 1996). Various methods that typically are used to evaluate the domains comprising the neuropsychological assessment of children and adolescents are provided in Table 1.1; this table is not, however, intended to be an exhaustive list. Given the variability in test selection possible, the case studies provided in the chapters to

Table 1.1 Possible Components to Pediatric Neuropsychological Assessment

Domain of Functioning	Possible Measure (Battery, if Part of a Battery)
Cognition	Bayley Scales of Infant Development, Second Edition Differential Ability Scales, Second Edition (DAS-II) Kaufman Assessment Battery for Children, Second Edition (KABC-2) Leiter—Revised Ravens Standard Progressive Matrices Stanford-Binet Intelligence Scale, Fifth Edition (SB5) Universal Nonverbal Intelligence Test (UNIT) Wechsler Intelligence Scale for Children, Fourth Edition (WISC-IV) Wechsler Adult Intelligence Scale, Fourth Edition (WAIS-IV) Wechsler Preschool and Primary Scale of Intelligence, Third Edition (WPPSI-III) Wechsler Nonverbal Scale of Intelligence (WNV) Woodcock Johnson Tests of Cognitive Ability, Third Edition (WJ III)
Auditory-Linguistic/Language Function	Aphasia Screening Test from Halstead Reitan Neuropsychological Battery (HRNB) Auditory Attention and Response Set from Neuropsychological Assessment, Second Edition (NEPSY-2) Boston Naming Test California Verbal Learning Test—Children's Version (CVLT-C) Clinical Evaluation of Language Fundamentals, Fourth Edition (CELF-IV) Comprehensive Assessment of Speech and Language (CASL) Comprehensive Receptive and Expressive Vocabulary Test, Second Edition Comprehensive Test of Phonological Processing Comprehension of Instructions (NEPSY-2) Controlled Oral Word Association Test (COWAT) Dichotic Listening Tasks Expressive One-Word Picture Vocabulary Test Expressive Vocabulary Test, Second Edition FAS or other Verbal Fluency Test (e.g., on NEPSY-2) Revised Token Test Peabody Picture Vocabulary Test, Fourth Edition (PPVT-IV) Phonological Processing (NEPSY-2) Pitch Pattern Sequence Test Receptive One-Word Picture Vocabulary Test Speech Perceptions Test (HRNB) Test of Early Language Development (TELD) Test of Adolescent and Adult Language, Third Edition (TAAL-3) Test for Auditory Comprehension of Language, Third Edition (TACL-3) Test of Auditory Perceptual Skills (TAPS) Test of Pragmatic Language, Second Edition (TOPL-2) Vocabulary, Similarities, and Comprehension Subtests of Wechsler Scales
Visual-Perception and Constructional Praxis	Arrows (NEPSY-2) Beery Developmental Test of Visual Motor Integration, Fifth Edition Benton Visual Form Discrimination Test Block Construction (NEPSY-2) Block Design, Matrix Reasoning of Wechsler Scales

(continued)

Table 1.1 *(Continued)*

Domain of Functioning	Possible Measure (Battery, if Part of a Battery)
	Clock Face Drawing Test Design Copy (NEPSY-2) Rey-Osterreith Complex Figure Test Route Finding (NEPSY-2) Scotopic Form Discrimination
Perceptual/ Sensory Perception	Finger Discrimination (NEPSY-2) Finger Number Writing (HRNB) Sensory Perceptual Examination (HNRB) Tactual Performance Test (HRNB) Tactile Form Recognition (HRNB) Lateral Preference from Dean Woodcock Neuropsychological Battery (DWNB) Palm Writing (DWNB) Finger Identification (DWNB)
Learning and Memory	Benton Visual Retention Test, Fifth Edition Digit Span Forward from Children's Memory Scale (CMS), Wechsler Scales, Test of Memory and Learning –Second Edition (TOMAL-2) List Learning from CMS, CVLT-C, NEPSY-2, Wide Range Assessment of Memory and Learning, Second Edition (WRAML-2, TOMAL-2) Memory for Faces (CMS, NEPSY-2, TOMAL-2) Memory for Names (NEPSY-2) Paired Associate Recall (CMS, TOMAL-2) Rey Auditory Verbal Learning Test Sentence Repetition (NEPSY-2) Serial Digit Learning Spatial Span Forward Story Recall (CMS, WJIII, NEPSY-2, WRAML-2, TOMAL-2) Spatial Location (CMS Dot Locations, TOMAL-2) Tactual Performance Test (HRNB) Complex Figure Recall Tasks n-Back Tasks Digit Span Backward (Wechsler Scales, CMS, TOMAL-2) Letter Number Sequencing Spatial Span Backward Working Memory Battery from Cambridge Neuropsychological Testing Automated Battery (CANTAB)
Processing Speed/ Tracking	Cancellation Tasks Digit Symbol/Coding Rapid Naming Stroop Color Word Test Symbol Search
Executive Function	Behavior Rating Inventory of Executive Function (BRIEF) Card Sorting Tasks Category Test (HRNB) Matching Familiar Figures Test Planning Battery of the CANTAB Tower Tasks (Tower of Hanoi, Tower of London, Tower Task from D-KEFS) Trails (HRNB, Comprehensive Trail Making Test, Color Trails Test)

Domain of Functioning	Possible Measure (Battery, if Part of a Battery)
Attention/ Concentration	Auditory Attention and Response Set (NEPSY-2)
	Cancellation Tasks
	Children's Embedded Figures Test
	Children's Auditory Verbal Learning Test
	Children's Memory Scale (Attention/Concentration Scale)
	Continuous Performance Tests
	Digit Span Tasks
	Dual Task Paradigms
	Fluency (Figural, Verbal, COWAT)
	Matching Familiar Figures Task
	Stroop Color Word Test
	Trails (HRNB, Comprehensive Trail Making Test, Color Trails Test)
	Visual Attention (NEPSY-2)
	Test of Everyday Attention for Children (TEA-Ch)
Motor Function	Design Copy (NEPSY-2)
	Finger Oscillation Test (HRNB) or Finger Tapping Test (NEPSY-2; DWNB)
	Grip Strength Test (HRNB)
	Grooved Pegboard Test
	Imitating Hand Positions (NEPSY-2)
	Manual Motor Sequences (NEPSY-2)
	Motor Impersistence Test
	Oromotor Sequences (NEPSY-2)
	Reaction Time Tasks
	Beery Developmental Test of Visual Motor Integration, Fifth Edition
	Visuomotor Precision (NEPSY-2)
	Bender Visual Motor Gestalt Test II
	Gait and Station (DWNB)
	Romberg (DWNB)
	Construction Test (DWNB)
	Hand Movements (KABC-2)
Achievement/ Academic Skills	Woodcock Johnson Tests of Achievement, Third Edition
	Wechsler Individual Achievement Test, Second Edition (WIAT-II)
	Kaufman Test of Educational Achievement, Second Edition (KTEA-II)
	Gray Oral Reading Test, Fourth Edition (GORT-4)
	Test of Written Language, Third Edition (TOWL-3)
	Wide Range Achievement Test, Fourth Edition (WRAT-4)
	Curriculum Based Assessment
	Criterion Referenced Assessment
	Basic Achievement Skills Inventory
Emotional/ Behavioral Functioning	Achenbach System of Empirically Based Assessment (ASEBA)
	ADHD Rating Scale, Fourth Edition
	Behavior Assessment System for Children, Second Edition (BASC-2)
	Conners' Rating Scales, Third Edition
	DSM-IV ADHD Checklist
	Minnesota Multiphasic Personality Inventory—Adolescent Version
	Personality Assessment Inventory—Adolescent
	Children's Depression Inventory
	Vineland Adaptive Behavior Scales

(continued)

Table 1.1 *(Continued)*

Domain of Functioning	Possible Measure (Battery, if Part of a Battery)
	Adaptive Behavior Assessment Scale, Second Edition (ABAS-2) Social Skills Rating Scale Social Responsiveness Scale ADHD Rating Scale for Adults Personality Inventory for Children, Second Edition Various Structured Diagnostic Interviews (e.g., Diagnostic Interview for Children and Adolescents, Fourth Edition; Diagnostic Interview Schedule for Children, Fourth Edition; Children's Interview for Psychiatric Syndromes [ChIPS] Direct Observation)

Note: This table is not intended to be exhaustive but rather to provide a representative sampling of possible measures.

come do not represent any single perspective but rather provide a sampling of what might be seen in a neuropsychological assessment.

Although there is much variation in neuropsychological assessment, it is important to attend to the psychometric properties and limitations of available measures (Reynolds & Mason, 2009). Historically, neuropsychology has been criticized for its failure to incorporate psychometric advances in test use and construction (Cicchetti, 1994; Reynolds, 1986a; M. D. Ris & Noll, 1994). A second concern has been that neuropsychologists overlook the psychometric concepts of reliability and validity, making interpretations based on the "clinical" nature of the tasks. The need for the establishment of reliability and validity of scores as well as their interpretation related to neuropsychological test performance has been an important issue in the literature (Reynolds, 1982; Riccio & Reynolds, 1998). In particular, reliability is a key component not only in that it is related directly to inter- and intraindividual differences, but also as it serves as the foundation on which validity is founded (Reynolds, 1986b). More recently, there has been greater attention to the psychometrics of measures as well as the reliability and validity for use of these measures across cultures (J. G. Harris, Wagner, & Cullum, 2007; Llorente, 2008; P. Smith, Lane, & Llorente, 2008). Application of the theoretical bases for understanding brain-behavior relations (e.g., the Lurian model) across cultures is also being considered with more and more individuals being seen who come from a variety of cultures and linguistic backgrounds (Kotik-Friedgut, 2006).

Because of the need for adequate normative data, some clinicians advocate the interpretation of traditional measures of cognitive ability (e.g., the Wechsler scales) from a neuropsychological perspective (D'Amato, Rothlisberg, & Rhodes, 1997). Concerns and criticisms of the recategorization of subtests from standardized measures that were not developed based on neuropsychological theory and have not been validated for this purpose are evident in the literature (Kamphaus, Petoskey, & Rowe, 2000; Lezak, 1995; Lezak, Howieson, & Loring, 2004). Finally, it has been suggested that measures used in the neuropsychological assessment process need to vary along a continuum of difficulty, include both rote and novel tasks, and include variations with regard to processing and response requirements within modalities (Rourke, 1994, 2005). These varying concerns and issues have resulted in the development of a number of standardized measures.

INTERPRETATION

Results are interpreted based on functional neuroanatomy and brain development in order to approximate the extent and nature of brain damage or dysfunction; at the same time, context needs to be considered (Berkelhammer, 2008). Inference, or the process of reaching a conclusion by reasoning based on evidence/data, also plays a part in the interpretation process (Fennell & Bauer, 1997). Rules specify what kind of evidence can be used for making inferences, the kind of conclusions that can be reached given the type of evidence, and the set of logical connections between evidence and the conclusions or inferences. The inferential process involves initial development of hypotheses as well as the validation of those hypotheses (Fennell & Bauer, 1997); hence, the hypothesis-driven conceptualization of the assessment process (Berkelhammer, 2008). This inferential process needs to consider not only the type of functional system(s) and the number of systems impaired, but also the characteristics of the impairments (Reynolds & Mayfield, 1999; Riccio & Reynolds, 1998). In neuropsychology, additional assumptions dictate that the measures used as a basis for inference provide valid information (i.e., have demonstrated construct validity) and provide meaningful information on aspects of the individual's functioning (have ecological validity). Based on all of the data generated in the evaluation process and inferences, hypotheses are generated regarding how and why the individual processes information; hypotheses are also offered as to what areas of functioning are likely to be affected (Berkelhammer, 2008; D'Amato et al., 1997; R. S. Dean, 1986). Information on strengths and weaknesses then is used to generate an appropriate rehabilitation or habilitation plan.

The first inference made is a general conclusion about integrity of brain function. This conclusion may be based on overall performance level across tasks (Reitan, 1986, 1987). For example, one method is the use of criterion or cut-off scores such that scores above (or below) criterion are considered indicative of brain damage or impaired function. With increased emphasis on psychometric methods, use of normative data and measures that provide valid and reliable results are emphasized in the contemporary literature; this is particularly critical when working with individuals from diverse backgrounds and those who were not part of the sampling process (Llorente, 2008). With the actuarial or normative model, conclusions are reached based on comparison of the child's overall level of performance to normative data. There are multiple problems with this model, including the variability among typically developing children, insensitivity for individuals with higher cognitive abilities, and a tendency to yield a high number of false positives due to the potential impact of fatigue and motivation on test performance (Nussbaum & Bigler, 1997; Reitan & Wolfson, 1985).

Another model examines performance patterns across tasks (Reitan, 1986, 1987) as a means of differentiating functional from dysfunctional neural systems; this model may incorporate examination of intra-individual differences or asymmetry (i.e., lateralization of function; Reitan, 1986, 1987). Examination of intra-individual differences allows for identification of strengths as well as weaknesses; emphasis on a strength model for intervention planning is viewed as more efficacious than focusing only on deficits (Reynolds, Kamphaus, Rosenthal, & Hiemenz, 1997). Again, this examination usually is addressed in terms of anterior-posterior differences or left-right differences rather than consideration of single scores. Another model of interpretation involves looking for, or identifying, "pathognomonic," or clear, signs of brain damage of some kind (Kaplan, 1988; Lezak et al., 2004; Reitan, 1986, 1987; Spreen et al., 1995). While this method has been used reliably with adult populations, its reliability with children has not been demonstrated (Batchelor, 1996). Similarly, the reliability of profile analysis has not been consistently demonstrated (Iverson, Brooks, & Holdnack, 2008; Reynolds, 2007; M. W. Watkins, Glutting, & Youngstrom, 2005); however, some argue for the usefulness of profile analysis (Gioia, Isquith, Kenworthy, & Barton, 2002; Livingston, Pritchard, Moses, & Haak, 1997). In practice, clinicians use any one or some combination of these features (Reitan, 1986, 1987; Riccio & Reynolds, 1998) in the interpretation process, including clinical judgment. The theoretical model should lead to accurate predictions about the individual's ability to function in multiple contexts and inform intervention planning (Reynolds et al., 1997; Riccio & Reynolds, 1998). This is one of the core assumptions of the Cognitive Hypothesis Testing model (Hale & Fiorello, 2004; Hale, Fiorello, Bertin, & Sherman, 2003).

WHY NEUROPSYCHOLOGICAL ASSESSMENT?

Anyone who works with children with disabilities will likely, at some point, work with a child who is identified as having a "neurological impairment," "traumatic brain injury," "other health impairment," or is identified with a neurodevelopmental or genetic disorder. Understanding how neurology relates to higher cognitive function is important in appreciating the neurocognitive and behavioral impairments of individuals with brain-based disorders (Berkelhammer, 2008). One of the major purposes of both neurological and neuropsychological evaluation is to document the impact of brain abnormality, damage, or dysfunction. The wider range of behavioral domains sampled facilitates differential diagnosis among disorders with similar symptom presentations (Reynolds & Mayfield, 1999; Riccio & Reynolds, 1998), and neuropsychological perspectives provide a foundation for better integration of behavioral data that ultimately leads to a more unified or holistic picture of a child's functioning (Riccio & Reynolds, 1998). Neuropsychological assessment may be appropriate to establish initial functioning as well as to track progress; it may serve to clarify intervention needs and result in referrals to other specialists (Berkelhammer, 2008).

A key concept is the link between the neuropsychological assessment and intervention. Enhanced understanding of the neurological correlates of various skills, in conjunction with knowledge of instructional methods, can assist in the formulation of hypotheses regarding potential instructional methods/materials for a particular child (Reynolds & Mayfield, 1999). To inform intervention efforts, results are integrated with information regarding the type and number of functional system(s) that are impaired as well as the nature and characteristics of the functional systems that remain intact. Identifying deficits in working memory, for example, may necessitate specific compensatory skills or accommodations in school settings; further, these accommodations or compensations will continue to be needed as the child develops and contextual demands increase. Thus, inferences are made not only regarding specific behaviors that are assessed but also, through the use of information about how various skills correlate in the developmental process, about skills that have not been evaluated. Ultimately, data generated from the neuropsychological assessment process are used to develop recommendations regarding whether the individual would profit from compensatory strategies, remedial instruction, or a combination (Gaddes & D. Edgell, 1994; Riccio & Reynolds, 1998).

With a medical model and emphasis on pathology, historically, there has been a tendency to focus on identifying deficits. More recently, however, it is seen as imperative to the development of effective treatment programs that the child's strengths and intact systems also be identified. Identifying both strengths and weaknesses provides a more in-depth understanding of the types of accommodations or modifications that may be appropriate. Identification of intact functional systems enables rehabilitation and remediation programs that are based on individual strengths to be implemented (Reynolds, 1986b; Silver et al., 2006). The intact systems that have been identified can be used to develop compensatory behaviors as part of the rehabilitation program; for example, an individual who has difficulty with manipulating information mentally, but who has good visual memory, may be able to use visual imagery to support memory function. Finally, identification of intact systems suggests a more positive outcome and increases the likelihood of motivated support systems (home and school) for the child (Riccio & Reynolds, 1998).

LINKING ASSESSMENT TO INTERVENTION

Neuropsychological assessment is generally considered appropriate whenever a child is suspected of having a neurological disorder or when it is believed that the integrity of the central nervous system has been compromised. In general, indications are that parents are satisfied with the diagnostic or assessment component but may not be as satisfied with information on next steps or treatment approaches to address the difficulties identified (Bodin, Beetar, Yeates, Boyer, & Colvin, 2007). As previously stated, the intent should not be for diagnostic purposes alone but for identification of individual strengths and weaknesses with the intent to inform rehabilitation efforts. The ultimate goal of the assessment should be to develop an intervention or rehabilitation plan. One component of developing the intervention plan is the determination of target areas.

The second component to intervention or rehabilitation planning is the selection of evidence-based practices to address those target areas. Generally speaking, evidence-based decision making takes into account research evidence, clinical expertise, and client preference (Chambliss & Ollendick, 2001; Simpson, 2005b; Spirito, 1999). More and more, from both a forensic and an ethical perspective, it is important to critically examine the research evidence as it relates to a given treatment component or program. Levels of evidence range from randomized clinical trials (Level I) to case studies and anecdotal evidence (Level IV) with multiple subcategories. Different terms and labels for the current state of evidence are used in the research; in some cases, no comprehensive review of an intervention may exist as yet, and evidence is limited to the available published literature. The various definitions and levels of evidence can be subdivided in multiple ways. (See Table 1.2 for the descriptors that will be used in this volume.)

Interventions must be considered separately for each target area. For example, one intervention for autism may be effective for interpersonal skills but not in reducing stereotypy. Similarly, what is effective as an intervention may vary depending on the strengths and weaknesses of the individual child. For each chapter, to the extent feasible, the research base relating to interventions by domain and disorder is summarized. Unfortunately, there exists minimal evidence bases or empirical support specific to neurodevelopmental and genetic disorders (Gingras, Santosh, & Baird, 2006). Providing an evidence base for programs across disorders is an area clearly in need of additional

Table 1.2 Descriptors for Evidence-Based Practice

Term Used	Alternate Terms	How Determined/Criteria Applied
Positive practice	Scientifically based, empirically supported, well-established	Significant empirical efficacy and support as in randomized clinical trials; treatment manuals; comparison to placebo or alternative treatment
Promising practice	Probably efficacious, possibly efficacious, established	Evidence for efficacy and utility as compared to placebo or alternative but further replication and objective verification needed
Emerging		Insufficient studies or replication; small samples
Inconclusive		Results are equivocal or methodological flaws prevent conclusions from being drawn
Ineffective	Not recommended	No available evidence to support use; some evidence that intervention did not have any effect
Adverse effects	Not recommended	Evidence suggests that intervention has potential to be harmful

research; the intent here is to synthesize the available research based on existing reviews or studies identified in the existing research base.

CONCLUDING COMMENTS

A major premise of neuropsychological assessment and the resulting case conceptualization is that not only is information gained related to the individual's functioning at a given point in time but that, based on the knowledge base (i.e., the neuroscience), programs can be developed and implemented to address the anticipated problems associated with a given disorder (Nilsson & Bradford, 1999; Riccio & Reynolds, 1998). With variability in test selection, administration, approach to interpretation, and approaches to intervention or treatment planning, ethical issues are likely to arise and need to be considered (T. M. Wong, 2006). At the same time that there are concerns with the measurement aspect of neuropsychological assessment (Reynolds & Mason, 2009), there are concerns that there is a lack of agreement on what constitutes the standards of practice (T. M. Wong, 2006). These concerns go beyond the issues of release of raw data (Rapp, Ferber, & Bush, 2008) and confidentiality (Bush & Martin, 2008) to determination of what should or should not be included in a neuropsychological setting. Questions have been raised, for example, with regard to how to consider culture or ethnicity/race (Brickman, Cabo, & Manly, 2006), but no standard means for accomplishing this has been determined. Specific methods for training may be helpful in establishing standards of practice as well as for determining level of competence in neuropsychology (Boake, 2008; Hannay et al., 1998; Moberg & Kniele, 2006).

A second issue of importance is the extent to which the components of neuropsychological assessment reflect brain function. Several studies have investigated the research behind the use of specific measures (Riccio & Hynd, 2000; Riccio, Reynolds, Lowe, & Moore, 2002). At the same time, there are concerns that even if the measures reflect integrity of brain function (or atypicality in brain function), the information obtained may not reflect the individual's day-to-day functioning, or what has been referred to as *ecological validity* (Rabin, Burton, & Barr, 2007; Ready, Stierman, & Paulsen, 2001; Sbordone, 2008). These issues will continue to be discussed and new measures will be developed as standards for measurement, the need for real-world outcomes, and standards for practice collide with the evidence-based practice movement in the 21st century. In part, the next chapters provide a review of the scientific literature as a foundation along with the review of research on the clinical implications and evidence-based practices to foster the bridging of science and practice. The case studies in the chapters highlight some of the differences that exist in the field, in part driven by philosophical or theoretical perspectives and in part dictated by the developmental and real-world nature of the individuals with neurodevelopmental and genetic disorders.

Chapter 2

LEARNING DISABILITIES: READING DISABILITY/DYSLEXIA

DEFINITION

Learning disability has been conceptualized as the presence of a *processing deficit* that manifests itself as a discrepancy between ability and academic achievement, in the absence of other conditions that might produce the same delay, or an unexpected underachievement (Fletcher, Lyon, Fuchs, & Barnes, 2007). How learning disabilities are defined operationally continues to be controversial (Fletcher et al., 2007; S. E. Shaywitz, Morris, & Shaywitz, 2008); one area of consensus, however, is that there is heterogeneity when discussing specific learning disabilities, particularly in relation to reading or mathematics (Lerner, 1989; Riccio & Hynd, 1996; Stanovich, 1993). Some have argued that learning disability and learning difficulty are the same, while others argue that what is unique to the individual with a learning disability is the presence of a deficit, not a more global delay (D. J. Francis, Shaywitz, Stuebing, Shaywitz, & Fletcher, 1996). Available evidence suggests that learning disability is "specific" to one or more academic components but is not unitary (Fletcher et al., 2007); individual differences also need to be considered (Hale et al., 2008). Learning disabilities collectively are considered high-incidence disabilities and constitute a large proportion of the children struggling in schools and receiving services in special education (Lerner, 1989).

Of the learning disabilities, reading disability or dyslexia is the one most often identified and researched; it is estimated that for 80% of those identified with a learning disability, reading is a deficit area (S. E. Shaywitz & Shaywitz, 2006). Historically, reading disability was differentiated from other explanations for poor reading skills in part based on "soft signs" consistent with a conceptualization of minimal brain dysfunction. These soft signs included forming a circle in a "clockwise" direction beyond the age of 7 years, reversals in reading or writing, and physical anomalies such as dimples or attached ear lobes (Brookes & Stirling, 2005; Wolff & Melngailis, 1996). Diagnosis and definition of reading disability requires more standardized data and, in practice, may be defined by some difference between IQ ("g") and achievement (American Psychiatric Association [APA], 2000), a pattern of strengths and weaknesses, or a lack of response to intervention (Individuals with Disabilities Education Improvement Act [IDEIA], 2004). Reading, however, is not a singular process; as such, reading disability is not a homogenous disorder and may manifest differently across the life span depending on a variety of factors. Individuals with dyslexia tend to evidence a range of cognitive and visual-motor deficits. These deficits may include phonological awareness, automaticity of retrieval, processing speed, motor skills, and balance (R. I. Nicolson, Fawcett, & Dean, 2001), as well as memory and language (Kibby, in press; Kibby & Cohen, 2008; Kibby et al., 2004).

Subtypes of Reading Disability

In educational contexts—according to the Individuals with Disabilities Education Improvement Act (IDEIA)—three types of reading skills are considered:

1. Basic reading skills, including word recognition and word attack
2. Reading comprehension
3. Reading fluency or the automaticity of the reading process

Alternatively, phenotypic studies suggest subtypes with (a) word recognition and subsequent reading comprehension problems; and (b) reading comprehension and listening comprehension deficits (Keenan, Betjemann, Wadsworth, DeFries, & Olson, 2006).

Others consider whether it is the visual spatial, morphological, or phonological components of decoding that are impaired in determining subtypes (Hynd & Cohen, 1983; Richards, Aylward, Field et al., 2006). The more frequently discussed subtype is the phonological deficit or auditory/linguistic subtype with delayed language and difficulty in naming. This subtype tends to be associated with left-hemisphere anomalies similar to those with specific language impairment (see Chapter 4). At the morphological level, the difficulty is more with the conveyance of meaning and grammar. It is believed that those with phonological deficits have trouble applying the "alphabetic principle" when reading unfamiliar words (Torgesen & Mathes, 1999). Alternatively, some individuals have difficulty with the processing of the orthographic features of print (Stanovich, 1993). This may be related to the visual/spatial aspects of reading and is characterized by poor eye-hand coordination, clumsiness, and problems with directionality. This subtype is more likely to have variation in the right hemisphere and cerebellum but may also have anomalies in prefrontal (motor) areas. The visual/spatial subtype is most often associated with toxemia during pregnancy. In deference to the fluency component and the automaticity of reading that comes with skill acquisition, some have added processing speed as a contributing component to reading comprehension (Joshi & Aaron, 2000). Often these associated problems occur in concert, but they may occur in isolation. For example, hyperlexia is characterized by the comprehension difficulties with strengths in word recognition and decoding skills (M. J. Cohen, Hall, & Riccio, 1997).

Hyperlexia is the term used to describe children who read words at levels beyond expected for their ability and oral communication skills (Silberberg & Silberberg, 1967). This is most common in conjunction with specific language impairment (see Chapter 4) but also has been noted among children with autism (Nation, Clarke, Wright, & Williams, 2006). Characteristics of hyperlexia include advanced word recognition skills, often without explicit reading instruction, in combination with reading comprehension that is more consistent with impaired language (M. J. Cohen, Campbell, & Gelardo, 1987; Glosser, Friedman, & Roeltgen, 1996; Glosser, Grugan, & Friedman, 1997; Huttenlocher & Huttenlocher, 1973; C. M. Temple, 1990). Based on one population-based study, hyperlexia occurs in 2.2 per 10,000 children (Yeargin-Allsopp et al., 2003); less is known about the frequency of hyperlexia in children who are not English speakers, but the same mechanisms appear to be in effect (Talero-Gutierrez, 2006). The combination of strengths and weaknesses suggests that visual pattern recognition is a key component to the presentation of hyperlexia in children with specific language impairment (M. J. Cohen et al., 1997). Others have proposed a strength in declarative as opposed to procedural memory (T. E. Goldberg, 1987) or a reliance on orthographic memory (R. L. Sparks, 1995). Notably, with hyperlexia, covert reading is associated with increased activation of the left inferior frontal and superior temporal cortices as well as increased activation of the right inferior temporal sulcus (Turkeltaub, Gareau, Flowers, Zeffiro, & Eden, 2004). This suggests that hyperlexia is the result of both right (orthographic or visual) and left (phonological) systems.

Prevalence/Incidence

Dyslexia, or reading disability, is the most common of the learning disabilities (Lerner, 1989). It is estimated that 10% to 36% of school-age children have reading difficulties, depending on how the extent of difficulty is defined (Grigg, Donahue, & Dion, 2007); this difficulty is severe enough to be identified as a reading disability in about 3% to 12% of the population, again depending on the criteria employed (APA, 2000; Riccio & Hynd, 1996; Schumacher, Hoffmann, Schmäl, Schulte-Körne, & Nöthen, 2007). Historically, more males than females have been identified as having reading disabilities; epidemiological studies, however, indicate that similar proportions of males and females exhibit reading disabilities (Flynn & Rahbar, 1994; L. S. Siegel & Smythe, 2005). In the related area of written expression, there is continued evidence, in children and adults, of males evidencing more difficulties than females (Berninger, Nielsen, Abbott, Wijsman, & Raskind, 2008a). There is also a high rate of comorbidity of reading disability and math disability (Kovas et al., 2007). Dyslexia occurs across ethnic groups, geographic areas, and for both alphabetic and orthographic languages (S. E. Shaywitz et al., 2008). There is a consistent and convincing body of evidence that dyslexia (or reading disability) is associated with and is causally related to juvenile delinquency; in effect, the reading levels of a majority of children and youth involved with the judicial system are well below expectancy (Shelley-Tremblay, O'Brien, & Langhinrichsen-Rohling, 2007).

ETIOLOGY

Genetic Influences

There is considerable evidence of a familial basis to reading disability (Cardon et al., 1994; S. E. Fisher & DeFries, 2002; Olson, 2004; B. F. Pennington et al., 1991). Studies have yielded concordance rates of 47% to 71% for monozygotic twins and up to 49% for dizygotic twins (Kovas et al., 2007; Lewitter, DeFries, & Elston, 1980). In a similar study of 64 pairs of identical twins and 55 pairs of fraternal twins, in which at least one member of the pair had a reading disability, evidence was found for a significant genetic etiology (DeFries, Fulker, & Labuda, 1987). Further, it was found that 40% of the variance in word recognition is genetic, with a genetic correlation of .67 with math disability, suggesting that reading disability and math disability are largely affected by the same genetic influences (Kovas et al., 2007). Indications of heritable forms of learning disability would support a neurobiological etiology (B. F. Pennington et al., 1991). Genetic studies further suggest continuity between children and adults with reading disabilities, particularly as related to phonological deficits (Kovas et al., 2007; Tiu, Wadsworth, Olson, & DeFries, 2004).

Reading disability is believed to be autosomal dominant; it has been suggested that the genetic mechanism is the same as for reading ability (Meaburn, Harlaar, Craig, Schalkwyk, & Plomin, 2008). Although reading disability affects more males than females, reading disability is not believed to be sex linked but involves multiple genes as well as environmental factors (S. E. Fisher & DeFries, 2002; Raskind, 2004). Notably, the group heritability for females was found to be higher than for males, but this difference was not significant (Hawke, Wadsworth, & Defries, 2006). At least nine possible genetic sites have been identified as contributing to reading and spelling processes (Schumacher et al., 2007). Linkage 15 is believed to be associated with visual-spatial abilities that may be related to reading disabilities (Chapman et al., 2004; D. W. Morris et al., 2004), while linkage and locus on 2q relates to speed of processing phonological information (Raskind, 2004). Other chromosomes have also been identified as potentially involved in the heritability of reading disability. Grigorenko and colleagues identified two reading-related phenotypes, both of which are linked to two different chromosomal regions (15 and 16) and reflect differing reading skills. For example, correlation coefficients of chromosomal markers and reading skills had differing levels of significance for tasks involving phonological awareness and decoding, rapid naming, and single-word reading (Grigorenko et al., 1997). More recently, twin studies have concluded that approximately half of the deficits in accuracy, speed of word recognition (automaticity), and phonological decoding were due to genetic influences; in contrast, genetics were not found to account for the same variance in orthographic coding and phonemic awareness (Gayan & Olson, 2001).

Environmental Influences

In utero exposure to various teratogens has been indicated as a factor in reading disability, with particular attention to high intrauterine testosterone concentrations indicated as a risk factor (James, 2008). Alternatively, there is some agreement that many specific learning disabilities, particularly in areas of reading and written expression, are secondary to specific language impairment (Wiig, 2005). Regardless of genetic predisposition and intrauterine effects, exposure to language and print are necessary conditions for awareness of morphemes, graphemes, and phonemes (Mann, 1991). The role of the environment has not been completely examined, but there is evidence of change in the activation patterns of children with reading disabilities as a result of various interventions (Richards, Aylward, Field et al., 2006). The component model of reading (P. G. Aaron, Joshi, Gooden, & Kentum, 2008) includes home variables, culture, and parental involvement in the ecological component.

A number of home influences that affect early language and literacy development have been identified (Tabors, Beals, & Weizman, 2001). Environmental influences include the value placed on reading in the home, parent responsiveness to children's interest in reading, availability of reading material in the home, and extent to which parents read with or to their children (Dickinson & Tabors, 1991; Tabors et al., 2001). Further, the quality of parent-child verbal interaction has an effect on vocabulary development and subsequent literacy (Zaslow et al., 2006). The extent to which the individual engages in reading activities over time, across the life span, also has an effect (Stanovich, 1986). Notably, with little environmental overlap in math and reading disabilities, it has been suggested that when the two disorders do not occur together, this may be the result of independent environmental influences (Kovas et al., 2007).

Neurological Substrates

Traditionally, dyslexia is believed to be neurologically based, with the neurological dysfunction manifesting as a learning disability; more recently, there has been increased behavioral evidence of the association between brain morphology and function in relation to reading (B. A. Shaywitz, Lyon, & Shaywitz, 2006). It was initially believed that understanding of the damage and recovery of function from acquired reading disability (alexia) would help in the understanding of developmental reading disorders; this is no longer believed to be the case. Instead, it is believed that there are differences in developmental and acquired reading problems such that there are deficits in underlying processes that relate to the development of reading skills (Schulte-Körne et al., 2007). In most cases, neurological evaluation does not suggest gross abnormality. In resting states and nondemanding tasks, no differences have been found between normal readers and those with dyslexia on regional cerebral blood flow (rCBF) or electroencephalography (Rumsey et al., 1987; Yingling, Galin, Fein, Peltzmann, & Davenport, 1986). The abnormality is believed to be more subtle and to involve the frontal, the temporal-parietal, and occipital-temporal regions (S. Shaywitz & Shaywitz, 2003). Sentence reading in children with dyslexia resulted in decreased activation of the left-lateralized language system as compared to normals; semantic processing was also centered in the left hemisphere with decreased activation of the inferior parietal regions (Schulz et al., 2008). Schulz et al. concluded that the problems with semantic processing modulated the sentence reading activation, particularly in the inferior parietal regions. Studies of nonimpaired readers indicate that many of the processes involved with reading, such as perception of single sounds and retrieval of phonemes from memory (Bradley & Bryant, 1983; Torgesen, Wagner, & Rashotte, 1994; R. K. Wagner et al., 1997), have specific neural substrates (Cao, Bitan, Chou, Burman, & Booth, 2006; Dufour, Serniclaes, Sprenger-Charolles, & Démonet, 2007; Richards, Aylward, Field et al., 2006). These substrates are summarized in Table 2.1.

Similarly, research consistently indicates patterns of structural anomalies and functional differences in children and adults with dyslexia. For example, both adults and children with dyslexia consistently have been found to have smaller regions in language areas (e.g., left planum, bilateral insular regions, and right anterior region), resulting in exaggerated asymmetry (C. M. Leonard et al., 2002; Paré-Blagoev, 2007). Also, for children with dyslexia, there is a positive correlation between performance on working memory tasks and activation of the prefrontal regions that was not evident in controls; this supports the idea of functional differences in those cortical regions associated not only with language processing but also with executive function (Vasic, Lohr, Steinbrink, Martin, & Wolf, 2008). At the same time, it is clear that no single or unitary neurological factor but rather a combination of structural or functional differences accounts for dyslexia (Kibby, Fancher, Markanen, & Hynd, 2008; Riccio & Hynd, 1996; Semrud-Clikeman, Hynd, Novey, & Eliopulos, 1991). Differences in activation patterns are evident in preschool children, with those children with lower prereading skills activating multiple regions of the brain (frontal, parietal, and occipital), while higher-achieving children evidenced more focused activation of the occipital lobe (D. L. Molfese et al., 2008). Magnetic resonance imaging (MRI) studies of individuals with dyslexia and age- and sex-matched controls further indicated that those with dyslexia have decreased cerebral volume as well as decreased gyrification (Casanova, Araque, Giedd, & Rumsey, 2004). The number of differing possible structures involved in dyslexia is consistent with the somewhat heterogeneous group when referring to individuals with reading disabilities.

Table 2.1 Neural Substrates to Components of Reading Ability and Implicated in Reading Disability

Component of Reading	Brain Region
Across components	Left middle frontal gyrus, left posterior parietal regions, right lingual (Richards, Aylward, Berninger et al., 2006) Inferior frontal gyrus (Broca's area) (Haller, Klarhoefer, Schwarzbach, Radue, & Indefrey, 2007; M. Hampson et al., 2006)
Phonological	Left inferior temporal gyrus, left middle temporal gyrus (Cao et al., 2006; Richards, Aylward, Berninger et al., 2006; Stanberry et al., 2006) Left superior temporal and inferior lateral frontal cortex (Dufour et al., 2007) Left inferior frontal gyrus (Dufour et al., 2007; Stanberry et al., 2006) Left inferior parietal lobe (Cao et al., 2006; Dufour et al., 2007)
Morphological	Left cerebellum, bilateral striatal and occipital regions, right posterior parietal (Richards, Aylward, Berninger et al., 2006) Inferior parietal regions (Schulz et al., 2008) Middle temporal gyrus (Roux et al., 2004) Occipital temporal regions (B. A. Shaywitz et al., 2006)
Orthographic	Left superior temporal gyrus (Richards, Aylward, Berninger et al., 2006) Left fusiform gyrus (McCandliss, Beck, Sandak, & Perfetti, 2003)
Automaticity/Fluency	Left occipital-temporal region (McCandliss et al., 2003) Cerebellum (Fawcett, Nicolson, & Dean, 1996; Fawcett, Nicolson, & Maclagan, 2001; R. I. Nicolson et al., 2001)

The variation in processes and structures best supports a conceptualization of reading as involving a widely distributed functional system, with any impairment or developmental deficit in the system resulting in distinct patterns of reading failure (Duffy, Denckla, Bartels, & Sandini, 1980).

Corpus Callosum

Using evoked potentials and focusing on callosal function, adults with dyslexia demonstrated significantly slower interhemispheric transfer times than controls, particularly for P1 and N1 wave forms (Markee, Moore, Brown, & Theberge, 1994). Event-related potentials (ERPs) were found to be absent or slowed in response to low-contrast, pattern-reversal stimuli (Livingstone, Rosen, Drislane, & Galaburda, 1991). Very few studies have been completed that focused on the corpus callosum in reading. There are some early indications that larger midsagittal areas of the corpus callosum are associated with better reading; however, corpus callosum volume was not correlated to reading (J. G. Fine, Semrud-Clikeman, Keith, Stapleton, & Hynd, 2007).

Cerebral Asymmetry and Dyslexia

Variations in cerebral asymmetry have been reported for adults with dyslexia (Galaburda & Kemper, 1979; Galaburda, Sherman, Rosen, Aboitiz, & Geschwind, 1985). Both computed tomography and postmortem studies document that about 66% of normal brains are asymmetric (left [L] > right [R]), favoring the left planum temporale.

In a typical individual, the anterior portion of the brain is R > L and posterior portion is L > R; with reading disability, the posterior asymmetry is reversed (R > L) or absent (R = L). In contrast, only about 10% of adults with dyslexia evidence the LR posterior asymmetry (Duara et al., 1991). Similarly, normal asymmetry (L > R) also has been found in the anterior speech region, auditory cortex, and posterior thalamus. Most recently, based on MRI, the structures involved (larger structures or smaller structures) that demonstrate differences in asymmetry appear to predict the type of deficits (e.g., written language, phonological deficits) for adults with compensated dyslexia (C. M. Leonard & Eckert, 2008).

Taken together, extensive research implicates the structures of the parietal operculum (e.g., planum temporale, supramarginal gyrus, and angular gyrus) in reading (Craggs, Sanchez, Kibby, Gilger, & Hynd, 2006). Further, it has been found that while normal readers activate the extrastriate area with speeded reading, individuals with dyslexia rely on the operculum and Broca's area on speeded reading; notably, groups did not differ in brain regions activated for "slow" reading (Karni et al., 2005). Moreover, results of dichotic listening (ear advantage) parallel the differences in planum asymmetry (L. M. Foster, Hynd, Morgan, & Hugdahl, 2002; C. J. Miller, Sanchez, & Hynd, 2003). The difference in asymmetry is due to a greater right planum (as opposed to smaller left planum) when the surface areas are compared (Galaburda et al., 1985; C. M. Leonard, Voeller, Lombardino, Morris, Hynd, Alexander, Andersen et al., 1993; Wood, Flowers, Buchsbaum, & Tallal, 1991). Similar differences in asymmetry are evident in the angular gyrus, an association area that provides cross-modal integration, such as writing and reading. In normal controls, the angular gyrus tends to be symmetrical; however, with dyslexia, right greater than left asymmetry is more likely to be found (Duara et al., 1991). Leftward asymmetry of the temporal bank of the planum temporale was related to better encoding and storage of phonological stimuli (Kibby et al., 2004). Further, the presence of an extra gyrus in the parietal region was associated with reduced working memory for phonological input.

Differences in cerebral asymmetry are evident not only from morphology but in activation patterns. Both right and left hemispheres are involved in the normal reading process, with increased activation of left hemisphere regions in normal readers. Using positron emission tomography (PET) and rCBF on serial word reading, indications are that adults with dyslexia who demonstrate significant deficits in word recognition, evidenced less activation in the right posterior cortex as compared to normals; adults with dyslexia who evidence deficits in phonological processing exhibited less activation bilaterally as compared to normals (Hynd, Hynd, Sullivan, & Kingsbury, 1987). More recently, using PET, it was found that adults with dyslexia had decreased activation in both frontal and parietal regions of the left hemisphere, resulting in decreased asymmetry in activation (Dufour et al., 2007). Using transcranial magnetic stimulation, it was found that stimulation of the right hemisphere disrupted oral reading while stimulation of the left hemisphere resulted in impaired word recognition (Skarratt & Lavidor, 2006; Tomasino, Fink, Sparing, Dafotakis, & Weiss, 2008). In the prefrontal region, normal readers tend toward higher right than left prefrontal activity on oral reading, but adults with dyslexia demonstrate equivalent left/right activity (Gross-Glenn et al., 1991). Adults with dyslexia failed to activate the left temporoparietal region on the rhyming task; normals demonstrated activation in the left parietal region near the angular gyrus, the left middle temporal region (e.g., Wernicke's area), the left posterior frontal region, the right middle temporal, and the right parietal area (Rumsey et al., 1992). Left temporal blood flow significantly, positively correlated with single-word and paragraph reading, spelling, nonword reading, and rapid naming; angular gyrus flow was found to be significantly but negatively correlated with oral and silent reading comprehension (Flowers, 1993). Additional studies have compared individuals with dyslexia to normal readers with evidence of decreased left-hemisphere activation specific to the left inferior parietal lobe and in the areas of the left inferior frontal gyrus, left temporal/fusiform gyrus, and left middle temporal gyrus (Cao et al., 2006; Dufour et al., 2007).

Insular Region

The left insular region historically has been associated with language impairment. As such, it is not surprising that this region is also implicated in dyslexia. Adults with reading disability demonstrate decreased levels of regional cerebral glucose mechanism in the insular region bilaterally. In normal children, the insular region is almost symmetric and elongated; in adults with dyslexia, the insular region is asymmetric with left side longer than right, and overall shorter than either children with Attention-Deficit/Hyperactivity Disorder (ADHD) or normal individuals (Gross-Glenn et al., 1986).

Parietal and Posterior Structures

Differences in several other areas have been implicated as well, with some indications that reading disability is due to posterior dysfunction. Multiple studies have suggested that there is decreased activation in the posterior regions associated with reading in individuals with dyslexia (Brambati et al., 2006; C. J. Price & Mechelli, 2005; B. A. Shaywitz et al., 2002; Turkeltaub et al., 2003). These areas may be related to the ability to connect the stored visual word form with the associated sounds and meanings and are involved not only in reading but in the attachment of meaning to any visual stimulus (J. T. Devlin, Jamison, Gonnerman, & Matthews, 2006). Using PET, metabolism in the left caudate for individuals with dyslexia was not highly or uniformly correlated with other brain regions as found with normals; linkage in the individuals with dyslexia appeared to be with the left inferior parietal lobe, while in normal individuals the left caudate metabolism correlated best with the left temporal lobe (Wood et al., 1991). With single-word reading, there is evidence of asymmetry of metabolic activity in the occipital lobe favoring the left hemisphere in normals, whereas with dyslexia there is no asymmetry of activation or favored right occipital lobe reported (Gross-Glenn et al., 1991). On letter matching, while normal readers evidence activation to the visual (extrastriate) cortex, the same activation is not evident for individuals with dyslexia (E. Temple et al., 2001). Alternatively, rhyme tasks were associated with increased activation of the left temporoparietal cortex in normal readers but not in those with dyslexia (E. Temple et al., 2001). Even on morphemic tasks, individuals with dyslexia evidenced decreased activation in the left medial frontal gyrus, right superior parietal, and fusiform/occipital region as compared to normal readers (E. H. Aylward et al., 2003). Across studies with phonological tasks, the involvement of the left temporoparietal lobe is implicated (Paulesu et al., 1996; Sandak, Mencl, Frost, & Pugh, 2004; B. A. Shaywitz et al., 2006; E. Temple et al., 2001).

In a study of 144 children, those with dyslexia demonstrated decreased activation of the posterior regions involved in reading (B. A. Shaywitz et al., 2002). Shaywitz and colleagues found that reading skill best correlated with activation of the left occipitotemporal region. Notably, differences in anterior activation were found in relation to age, such that older children with dyslexia exhibited greater activation bilaterally of the inferior frontal gyri. Related to automaticity and fluency of reading, individuals with dyslexia showed reduced activation of the left occipitotemporal region for both word reading and picture naming, suggesting that this brain region may be involved in the integration of phonology and orthography (McCrory, Mechelli, Frith, & Price, 2005; Ramus, 2004). Even among compensated readers, there continues to be evidence of relative underactivation of the posterior regions, particularly the parietotemporal and occipitotemporal areas (S. E. Shaywitz et al., 2003).

Cerebellum

The relation between the cerebellum and verbal working memory underlies the hypothesized link between cerebellar dysfunction and developmental dyslexia (Fawcett et al., 1996; Kibby et al., 2008; R. I. Nicolson et al., 2001). One recent study examined cerebellar volume and phonological processing and phonological short-term memory in groups of children with and without dyslexia (Kibby et al., 2008). Morphometrically, while no significant differences emerged for volume, children without dyslexia evidenced greater rightward cerebellar asymmetry. Further, volumetric measurement was significantly correlated with phonological measures for children without dyslexia but not for children with dyslexia (Kibby et al., 2008). This cerebellar dysfunction is consistent with observations that children with dyslexia often evidence impaired balance, coordination, and temporal processing (Fawcett et al., 1996, 2001; R. I. Nicolson et al., 2001). Based on a case study with posterior fossa tumor, an association was found between clumsiness, coordination problems, and reading problems (Fabbro, Moretti, & Bava, 2000). It has been argued that, based on cases such as this, integrity of cerebellar function may be necessary for adequate phonological processing.

Cytoarchitectonic Studies

Autopsy studies identified the presence of disproportionate clustering of cellular abnormalities (focal dysplasias) in the left planum and the left inferior frontal and right frontal regions (Galaburda et al., 1985). Further, a higher incidence of cerebral anomalies, such as missing or duplicated gyri bilaterally in the planum and parietal operculum, have been identified (C. M. Leonard et al., 1993). Similarly, there is evidence of disorganization of subcortical pathways specific to the lateral geniculate nucleus of the thalamus (Livingstone et al., 1991). It has been hypothesized that these focal, cellular differences may be the result of differences in cell migration during the fifth to seventh months of gestation. It is believed that the location and distribution of clusters may result in variation or subtypes of reading disabilities (Galaburda, 1994; Galaburda et al., 1985). Differences with regard to minicolumns have also been identified (Casanova, Buxhoeveden, Cohen, Switala, & Roy, 2002). Minicolumns arise from germinal cell divisions and are involved in processing and perception of language. With dyslexia, case study data indicate that the minicolumns may be larger but of similar number in comparison to what typically is found. Additional research in specific to effects of differences in neuronal migration and the relation between these differences and the genes identified is needed (Schumacher et al., 2007).

COURSE AND PROGNOSIS

In any discussion of the course and prognosis for reading disability, it is important to understand that the task demands of reading vary over the course of development (Klingner, Vaughn, & Boardman, 2007). In early stages, often more emphasis is placed on phonological skills and the decoding process; over time, the emphasis shifts to fluency and comprehension. While decoding and comprehension are highly correlated in early stages of literacy, the level of association declines as children progress through school (M. E. Curtis, 1980). This shift parallels the shift from "learning to read" to "reading to learn" that generally occurs in third to fourth grade (H. W. Catts, Hogan, & Adlof, 2005; Scarborough, 2005). Although there is some evidence that decoding problems and resulting poor fluency can contribute to poor comprehension, in many cases the comprehension problems are not restricted to reading and affect all aspects of reading except decoding (Keenan et al., 2006; Perfetti, Landi, & Oakhill, 2005; Scarborough, 2005).

Reading difficulties do not disappear or remit over time; even those individuals who learn the necessary basic skills do not attain the same level as their peers (D. J. Francis et al., 1996; Gross-Glenn et al., 1986; S. E. Shaywitz et al., 2003). In effect, individuals with reading difficulties avoid reading and do not gain the same level of automaticity. Further, over time, the effects seem to be cumulative. This is related to what Stanovich called the "Matthew effect" in that because of the difficulty with reading, individuals with dyslexia are not exposed to the same range of general knowledge and vocabulary as readers are (Stanovich, 1986). The lack of reading and subsequent decreased exposure results in an increased disparity in overall cognitive ability and general knowledge over time as compared to readers. A related area that is often overlooked or deemphasized is the extent to which individuals with developmental dyslexia also evidence difficulties in written expression (Berninger, Nielsen, Abbott, Wijsman, & Raskind, 2008b). In a sample of 122 children, various causal models were examined and a significant pathway was identified from automatic letter writing and verbal fluency to spelling, and from spelling to composition for both children and their parents with dyslexia (Berninger, Nielsen et al., 2008b).

Neuropsychological Correlates

Children with deficits in basic reading skills (i.e., phonological deficits) evidence weaknesses on vocabulary and other verbal measures; the extent to which verbal deficits are the cause or the effect of the reading problem is indeterminable, and probably reciprocal (Mann, 1991; Stanovich, 1993). Depending on the subtype, individuals with reading disability may evidence difficulty in phonemic/auditory processing, visual-spatial processing, or automatization (Katzir, Kim, Wolf, Morris, & Lovett, 2008; Liberman & Liberman, 1990; Stanovich, 1993). In a study of familial dyslexia, associated impairments were evidenced in short-term memory, phonological awareness, and automatization abilities in conjunction with decreased activation of posterior reading areas (Brambati et al., 2006). The role of working memory in dyslexia has also been explored with some variations found depending on genetic code (Berninger, Raskind, Richards, Abbott, & Stock, 2008).

The role of executive function and reading has been explored across a number of studies, in part because of the high comorbidity of reading disability and ADHD (Seidman, Biederman, Monuteaux, Doyle, & Faraone, 2001; Willcutt, Pennington, Olson, Chhabildas, & Hulslander, 2005). Using hierarchical linear modeling of growth trajectories for inhibition, rapid automatized switching, and combined inhibition/switching in typical readers and children with dyslexia, it was determined that these three tasks predicted literacy at grade 4 (Altemeier, Abbott, & Berninger, in press). While inhibition and switching contributed uniquely to literacy levels for typical readers, they were found to contribute less to literacy levels in children with dyslexia.

Social-Emotional Correlates

It is estimated that approximately 40% of individuals with reading disabilities also have co-occurring emotional/behavioral or psychiatric disorders (Taggart, Cousins, & Milner, 2007). It is not clear, however, if having a reading disability places individuals at risk for social emotional difficulties, or vice versa. In a recent study, for example, results indicated that children with dyslexia were not at elevated risk for behaviors related to anxiety, depression, and somatization; in fact, even at the lowest end of the distribution, children with reading difficulties were no more likely to have significant internalizing symptoms than children with better reading abilities (C. J. Miller, Hynd, & Miller, 2005). Alternatively, for psychiatric samples, the incidence of reading disabilities alone, or in conjunction with learning disabilities in written expression or reading, is much higher than in the general population, suggesting that psychiatric problems may impact on acquisition of reading skills (Mayes & Calhoun, 2006). Further, there is a high rate of reading disability (40%) among adjudicated adolescents (Shelley-Tremblay et al., 2007). These comorbid conditions contribute to the perception of less than positive outcomes for children and adults with reading disability but do not consider which is the cause and which is the effect.

Assessment Considerations

The current emphasis on response to intervention (RtI) and curriculum-based measurement tends to focus on early reading skills (e.g., phonological awareness, word decoding, word recognition, fluency). These provide indicators of specific aspects of reading but may not be sufficient to ensure that a child learns to read. Given the extensive research to suggest that in many instances, auditory/linguistic deficits underlie reading disability, it may be appropriate to ensure that this domain is assessed early on. This is one component (Ga) of the Cross-Battery Approach (Flanagan, Ortiz, & Alfonso, 2007) that could be examined using various subtests from the Differential Ability Scales, Second Edition (DAS-II) or Woodcock Johnson Tests of Cognitive Ability, Third Edition (WJ III) to assess both analysis and synthesis of single sounds. Automaticity or fluency of naming is also considered important in reading fluency; in the Cross-Battery Approach, this is part of the Glr and also can be assessed through subtests of the DAS-II or WJ III. Although some areas of language are tapped by cognitive measures, none adequately addresses potential deficits in language comprehension, and particularly pragramatic language, that may affect comprehension skills. Specific language measures were identified in Chapter 1. More in-depth assessment of language may be appropriate when reading difficulties are present and suggest additional avenues for intervention, particularly if specific language impairment (see Chapter 4) is identified. Additional perspectives on how neuropsychological assessment can be aligned with RtI have been offered as well (Fletcher-Janzen & Reynolds, 2008).

EVIDENCE-BASED INTERVENTIONS

A variety of interventions have been used with children and adults with reading disabilities (see Table 2.2); however, these interventions are specific to only one domain of the Component Model of Reading (P. G. Aaron et al., 2008). Results of meta-analysis indicate that systematic phonics instruction in grades kindergarten through 6 has significant

Table 2.2 Evidence-based Interventions for Reading Disabilities

Intervention	Skill Targeted	Level of Support/Studies
Explicit phonics instruction (e.g., analogy, analytic, embedded, synthetic)	Phonemic awareness	Promising practice (Berninger, Raskind et al., 2008; NICHD, 2000; Schneider, Ennemoser, Roth, & Küspert, 1999)
Orton-Gillingham	Phonemic awareness	Promising practice (Vickery et al., 1987)
Lindamood-Bell Reading/ Lindamood Phonemic Sequencing® (LiPS)	Phonemic awareness	Promising practice (Institute of Educational Sciences, 2007; Pokorni, Worthington, & Jamison, 2004)
Earobics®	Phonemic awareness	Promising practice (Pokorni et al., 2004)
Fast ForWord®	Phonemic awareness	Emerging (Gillam et al., 2008a; Hook, Macaruso, & Jones, 2001; Pokorni et al., 2004; Tallal, Merzenich, Miller, & Jenkins, 1998)
Reading Recovery Program	Phonological core deficits, Alphabetic skills, fluency	Promising to positive practice depending on target skill (Institute of Educational Sciences, 2007)
Stepping Stones to Reading	Alphabetic skills	Positive practice (Institute of Educational Sciences, 2007)
Ladders to Literacy	Alphabetic skills, fluency	Promising practice (Institute of Educational Sciences, 2007)
Daisy Quest®	Alphabetic skills	Positive practice (Institute of Educational Sciences, 2007)
DISSECT: Word identification strategy	Decoding	Promising practice (Lenz & Hughes, 1990; Rathvon, 2008)
Paired reading	Decoding	Promising practice (Fiala & Sheridan, 2003; Rathvon, 2008)
Word building	Decoding	Promising practice (McCandliss et al., 2003; Rathvon, 2008)
Graphosyllabic Analysis	Decoding	Promising practice (Bhattacharya & Ehri, 2004; Rathvon, 2008)
Peer Assisted Learning Strategies in Reading (PALS)	Fluency, vocabulary	Promising practice (Institute of Educational Sciences, 2007; Rathvon, 2008)
Oral repeated reading	Fluency	Promising practice (NICHD, 2000)
Cover-copy-compare	Vocabulary	Promising practice (Institute of Educational Sciences, 2007; Rathvon, 2008)
Story mapping	Comprehension	Positive practice (Rathvon, 2008)
Silent independent reading	Fluency, comprehension	Inconclusive (NICHD, 2000)
Strategy instruction (e.g., comprehension monitoring, question generation and answering, summarization, story mapping)	Comprehension	Promising practice (B. Y. L. Wong, Harris, Graham, & Butler, 2003)
Reciprocal teaching	Comprehension	Promising practice (A. L. Brown, Palincsar, & Armbruster, 1994)

benefits (National Institute of Child Health and Human Development [NICHD], 2000). The intent of early intervention during the emergent and early literacy stages is to lower a child's risk for reading difficulties; in contrast, approaches that focus on those identified with a reading disability tend to be more reactive than proactive in that the difficulties are already evident. Notably, systematic synthetic phonics (i.e., teaching students explicitly to convert letters to sounds and then blend sounds to form words) yielded small but significant gains for children with reading disabilities. Students from low socioeconomic status also evidenced increases in alphabetic knowledge and word reading skills with this synthetic approach. There is some disagreement, however, when and for how long phonics instruction is appropriate; it is also not clear how intense (time/phonemes per session) is most appropriate. While phonics instruction often is indicated, this approach is only one component of total reading and is not sufficient by itself (NICHD, 2000).

The Orton-Gillingham method is one program that has been used for many years (Vickery, Reynolds, & Cochran, 1987). The multisensory methodology uses phonetics and emphasizes visual, auditory, and kinesthetic learning styles. Instruction begins by focusing on the structure of language and gradually moves toward reading. The program provides students with immediate feedback and a predictable sequence that integrates reading, writing, and spelling. The Orton-Gillingham approach is a language-based, multisensory, structured, sequential, cumulative, cognitive, and flexible program that dates back to the 1930s. It is intended to be diagnostic-prescriptive such that the teacher identifies how the child best learns to read through various activities. The Orton-Gillingham approach addresses phonology, vocabulary, sentence structure, composition, and reading comprehension. It incorporates frequent review to foster automaticity. The extensive research base is limited predominantly to case studies (Perlo & Rak, 1971; Post, 2003; Vickery et al., 1987).

Another programmatic intervention with a long history is the Lindamood Phoneme Sequencing (LiPS®), or what was previously known as the Auditory Discrimination in Depth (ADD) program. The focus is on phonological awareness in conjunction with increased awareness of mouth position and actions in conjunction with sounds produced. There is a limited research base, again, predominantly limited to case studies or small group studies (A. Alexander, Anderson, Heilman, Voeller, & Torgesen, 1991; Conway et al., 1998; Pokorni et al., 2004; Torgesen et al., 1999). Related to the LiPS® program is the Lindamood Visualizing and Verbalizing program (VV®). Only one large-scale study has been conducted with the LiPS program (Sadoski & Willson, 2006). This program focuses on development of the gestalt (grasping the whole rather than parts); there is less research on this program (Bell, 1991). Limited research evidence is available for the VV® program (Burke, Howard, & Evangelou, 2005; Johnson-Glenberg, 2000).

Phonemic skills, in part, are assessed by examining the fluency with which the individual reads a passage. Guided oral reading and repeated reading with guidance have been found to have significant positive effects on reading fluency across grades, but there are no multiyear studies available (NICHD, 2000). Fluency is also a contributing factor to reading comprehension. Comprehension is a complex process, and few studies on vocabulary development meet the methodological rigor to demonstrate effectiveness of interventions; more address fluency as a means of affecting comprehension (Duff et al., 2008; Vadasy & Sanders, 2008). Some strategies have been indicated as possibly having positive effects (NICHD, 2000). These include preteaching new vocabulary words prior to seeing them in text and repeated exposure to the same vocabulary in various contexts. Results of the meta-analyses suggest that vocabulary needs to be taught both directly and indirectly; dependence on single vocabulary instruction is insufficient. Results further indicate that for text comprehension, a combination of approaches may be most effective. These approaches include explicit strategy instruction (Houtveen & van de Grift, 2007; B. Y. L. Wong et al., 2003). Specifically, teaching comprehension monitoring, use of graphic and semantic organizers (e.g., story maps), question answering and generating, examination of story structure, and summarization are recommended. Notably, independent silent reading (i.e., programs geared toward increasing student independent silent reading) has not been shown to be predictive of reading achievement, in part due to insufficient data.

It has been suggested that some intensive evidence-based reading interventions alter the neural functioning of the individual, in some instances with brain activation patterns on postintervention scans approximating nonimpaired subjects (E. H. Aylward et al., 2003; Richards, Aylward, Berninger et al., 2006; B. A. Shaywitz et al., 2006). In particular, those that focus on phonological awareness have been shown to result in increased activation bilaterally of the inferior frontal gyrus with resulting L > R asymmetry consistent with that found in controls. Alternatively, following intensive intervention, changes have included increased activity in the left temporoparietal region as well as a change in the timing of activity in the temporoparietal and frontal regions (Simos et al., 2006). Increased activation of the occipitotemporal, temporoparietal, and inferior frontal areas was found in response to a simple phonologic task following intervention with the Fast ForWord program (E. Temple et al., 2003). Others have found that with orthographic training, there is normalization of activation to the right inferior frontal gyrus and right posterior parietal gyrus (Richards, Aylward, Berninger et al., 2006). Based on a number of studies, it has been suggested that although orthographic training results in the most changes to brain activation, phonological, morphological, and orthographic processes all need to be assessed and taught (Richards et al., 2005). Similarly, the same approaches may not have the same effects depending on dyslexia subtype (Rowse & Wilshire, 2007). Finally, with differing definitions of learning disability/dyslexia as opposed to "garden-variety poor readers" (Stanovich, 1986), methodology in selection of subjects may have had an effect on the results.

CASE STUDY: CORD—DYSLEXIA

The following report is from a hospital-based clinic. Identifying information, such as child and family name, teacher or physician name, and school information, has been altered or fictionalized to protect confidentiality.

Reason for Referral

Cord Calhoun is a 13-year 9-month-old adolescent who was reevaluated by the pediatric neuropsychology service at the request of his parents, who have been homeschooling Cord due to his history of developmental dyslexia (learning disability in reading). As a result, neuropsychological reevaluation was undertaken in order to monitor higher cortical functioning and make appropriate recommendations regarding Cord's school program and the need for supportive therapies.

Assessment Procedures

Wechsler Intelligence Scale for Children, Fourth Edition (WISC-IV)
Wisconsin Card Sorting Test (WCST)

Peabody Picture Vocabulary Test, Fourth Edition (PPVT-IV)
Boston Naming Test (BNT)
Delis-Kaplan Executive Function Scales (D-KEFS; selected subtests)
Clinical Evaluation of Language Fundamentals, Fourth Edition (CELF-IV; selected subtests)
Kaufman Assessment Battery for Children, Second Edition (KABC-2; selected subtests)
Developmental Test of Visual-Motor Integration (DTVMI-V)
Clock Face Drawing Test
Rey Complex Figure Test
Finger Tapping Test
Children's Memory Scales (CMS)
Gray Oral Reading Test, Fourth Edition (GORT-4)
Wechsler Individual Achievement Test, Second Edition (WIAT-II)
DSM-IV ADHD Checklist
Behavior Assessment Scale for Children, Second Edition (BASC-2; Parent and Teacher Rating Scale, Adolescent Form)

Background Information

Home

Cord resides in the southeastern region of the United States with his parents, Dr. Carl and Sandra Calhoun. Dr. Calhoun is on the faculty at a nearby university; he is in good health. Although he has attained a high level of education, he repeated the second grade due to difficulty with reading. Mrs. Calhoun has two master's degrees and is currently on leave from her position as pastor of a local church. She too is in good health. The family history is significant for a paternal male cousin who is described as being "hyperactive" and a paternal female cousin with undiagnosed reading difficulty. The history is otherwise negative for neurologic and psychiatric disorder, including intellectual disability.

Developmental/Medical

Review of Cord's developmental and medical history indicates that he is the product of a normal 36-week gestation pregnancy and difficult delivery requiring the use of forceps and vacuum extraction. Birth weight was reported to be 9 pounds 10 ounces. Cord did well as a newborn, going home with his mother from the hospital on schedule. The parents were unable to recall Cord's exact developmental motor and language milestones; however, Mrs. Calhoun felt that Cord was late talking and walking. Toilet training was fully accomplished at 2 to 3 years of age without difficulty. Aside from the usual childhood illnesses, Cord's past medical history is significant for frequent ear infections throughout the first six years of life and allergy to milk, cheese, eggs, nuts, dogs/cats, dust, and grasses, for which he has been followed by a pediatric allergist. Cord's history is negative for head injury or seizure disorder. At present, Cord exhibits a good appetite and does not exhibit any sleep difficulty.

Educational

Review of academic history indicates that at 4 years of age, Cord attended a prekindergarten program two mornings a week. Mrs. Calhoun describes this program as focusing on structured play and socialization. Cord did well in this setting with no behavior problems noted; however, he tended play by himself. At 5 years of age, Cord attended a kindergarten program five mornings a week. Early on in the school year, Cord demonstrated difficulty learning his letters and numbers, reversed letters and numbers, and had difficulty learning letter sounds and performing writing activities. In addition, he exhibited fine motor difficulty with activities that involved cutting and coloring as well as tying his shoes. Midway through the school year, his parents initiated private tutoring for Cord. Even with the initiation of tutoring, Cord continued to exhibit academic difficulty, and, as a result, he was evaluated by a private psychologist. Results of intellectual screening with the Slosson Intelligence Test—Revised indicated that Cord was functioning in the high average to superior range; however, academic assessment with the Wechsler Individual Achievement Test revealed that he was significantly underachieving in the areas of basic reading and spelling. His performance in the area of mathematics and listening comprehension were at expectancy level. Behavior rating scales completed by Mrs. Calhoun and Cord's teacher were not consistent with ADHD. Based on the results of this evaluation and Cord's poor academic progress, it was recommended that he repeat kindergarten.

That summer, Cord's parents had Cord evaluated at a private reading center. As part of this assessment, Cord was administered the Wechsler Intelligence Scale for Children, Third Edition, on which he was found to be functioning in the superior range. Specifically, Cord obtained a full-scale IQ of 126, which was comprised of a verbal IQ of 123 and a performance IQ of 125. Additional testing revealed deficits in the areas of auditory processing and visual discrimination in conjunction with significant underachievement in the areas of reading and written expression. Based on these results, the parents initiated tutoring sessions at the center two times a week in order to continue working on Cord's reading skill development. In addition, they continued private tutoring.

Cord repeated kindergarten with continuation of his program at the reading center and tutoring. By the end of the year, Cord's teacher felt that he had made enough progress for promotion to first grade; however, his parents were still concerned given his superior intellectual ability and the significant amount of tutoring that Cord was receiving. They continued tutoring during the summer. Cord began attending first grade. Tutoring sessions were stopped at the recommendation of his teacher; however, Cord continued to struggle with mastery of phonetic word attack skills as well as in his sight word vocabulary. As a result, the parents requested psychological evaluation by the county school system. At that time, Cord was readministered the Wechsler Intelligence Scale for Children, Third Edition (WISC-III), and obtained a full-scale IQ of 121, which was comprised of a verbal IQ of 114 and a performance IQ of 123. Additional achievement testing indicated that Cord continued to exhibit significant discrepancies in the areas of basic reading and reading comprehension. Further, Cord demonstrated declines in his performance on tests of numerical calculation. Written expression was not formally assessed. Based on the results of this evaluation, a Special Education Eligibility/Individualized Education Program meeting was held at which time Cord was deemed eligible for special education services under the category of specific learning disability. It was recommended that Cord receive one hour of learning disability resource services daily. This was initiated in April of that year. During the summer, Cord was tutored three times a week with a combination of the Orton-Gillingham and Lindamood-Bell Reading Programs, with good success reported by the parents.

That summer, Cord underwent initial neuropsychological evaluation by this service. The results of the evaluation indicated that Cord continued to function within the superior range of intellectual ability. He demonstrated relative strengths in areas of sequential planning/reasoning; receptive and expressive vocabulary development; visual-spatial perception/construction (when not using paper and pencil); fine motor functioning; sustained attention; verbal memory for organized, meaningful material; and visual memory for spatial location. These were contrasted by relative weaknesses in auditory working memory; auditory discrimination; phonological processing; motor planning; verbal learning and memory for rote, unorganized material; and visual memory for content (i.e., what he sees, such as pictured human faces). Academically, Cord demonstrated relative strengths in math reasoning and calculation contrasted by relative weaknesses in basic reading, reading comprehension, and spelling. Behaviorally, Cord exhibited mild problems with attention span, likely secondary to his academic difficulties. He was also somewhat socially withdrawn and immature. Taken together, this pattern of neuropsychological test performance was felt to be consistent with a diagnosis of Developmental Dyslexia, Mixed Type (auditory linguistic/dysphonetic and visual spatial/dyseidetic). Further, Cord was thought to be at significant risk for development of a learning disability in written expression, given his reading difficulties and his weak spelling skills. Based on these findings, it was recommended that Cord continue to receive special education services for children with learning disabilities either through the public school system or through a private school program. Continuation of tutoring specific to reading disability via a multisensory approach was also recommended along with classroom accommodations and the use of compensatory strategies, such as textbooks on tape and a word processor.

Cord attended a private school for second grade with continuation of the tutoring sessions. He underwent further evaluation as part of a National Institutes of Health research grant on dyslexia, which included neuropsychological assessment and a structural MRI scan. Based on the results of that evaluation, the diagnosis of Developmental Dyslexia was supported. Analysis of Cord's MRI scan revealed atypical posterior perisylvian morphology in the left hemisphere, with presence of an extra gyrus between the post-central sulcus and the supramarginal gyrus (see Figure 2.1). Presence of an extra gyrus in this location is associated with the presence of dyslexia (C. M. Leonard, Eckert, Given, Berninger, & Eden, 2006) and reduced verbal working memory (Kibby et al., 2004). When focusing on the anterior perisylvian region, his left pars triangularis is of typical structure (V-shape, which is better seen on more medial slices), but his right pars triangularis is I/J-shaped, indicative of a poorly formed anterior horizontal ramus (see Figure 2.2). Atypical morphology in this region is associated with slower rapid naming ability (Kibby, Kroese, Krebbs, Hill, & Hynd, in press) which, in turn, is associated with slower reading rate. In order to assess asymmetry of the planum temporale, temporal and parietal banks, this region was traced using the software package Analyze (see Figure 2.2). The planum was measured throughout its entirety bilaterally, despite Figure 2.2 showing only one slice on either side. Cord's temporal bank has the typical leftward asymmetry that is associated with good learning and memory for stories; however, his parietal bank also has leftward asymmetry, despite the parietal bank typically having rightward asymmetry. Atypical asymmetry in the planum parietal bank is associated with reduced rapid naming and learning of rote verbal material (Kibby et al., 2004).

The following summer, Cord and his mother went to a school specializing in dyslexia, where he was enrolled in a tutorial program. At the same time, Mrs. Calhoun took a course on instructional strategies for students with dyslexia. With the beginning of third grade, Mrs. Calhoun began homeschooling Cord. This has continued to the present.

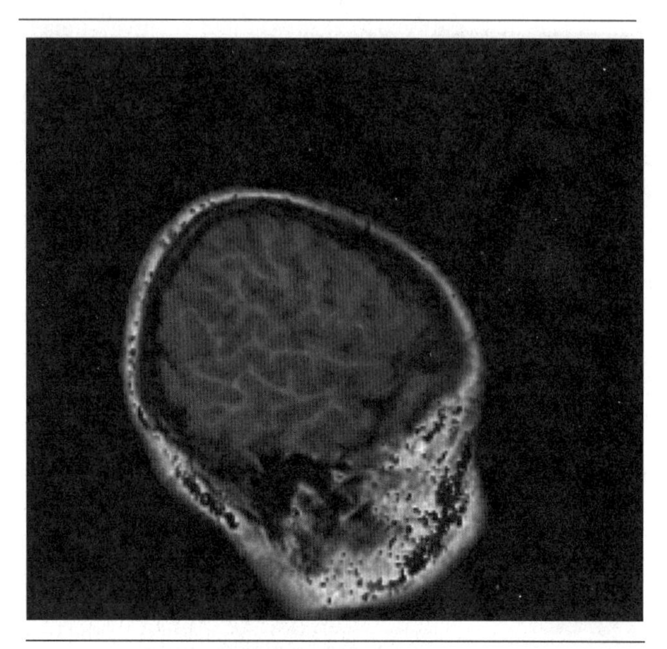

Figure 2.1 Left hemisphere slice showing the extra gyrus between the post-central sulcus and the supramarginal gyrus.

Behavioral Observations

Cord presented himself for testing as a tall, neatly groomed adolescent with blue eyes and brown hair who was casually dressed in a white shirt, black jeans, and a black vest. He separated appropriately from his father and accompanied the examiners to the testing room without difficulty. Cord was oriented and related appropriately toward the examiners with good eye contact and manners noted. In response to direct questions as well as when conversation was spontaneous, Cord's use of language was fluent and prosodic, with good comprehension of task demands evident. Throughout the evaluation, which consisted of two sessions separated by a lunch break, Cord's attention span and activity level were felt to be age appropriate. On more challenging tasks, Cord demonstrated good task persistence, and his frustration tolerance was excellent. Lateral dominance was firmly established in the right hand for paper-and-pencil manipulations. Vision and hearing were formally screened and found to be functioning within normal limits.

Assessment Results and Interpretation

The results of neuropsychological evaluation indicate that Cord continues to function in the superior range of intellectual ability as measured by the Wechsler Intelligence Scale for Children, Fourth Edition (WISC-IV), with fairly good consolidation noted between the Verbal Comprehension and Perceptual Reasoning Index scores. In contrast, his performance on the Working Memory Index was in the low average range and a continued area of weakness (see Table 2.3). Additional assessment indicates that Cord demonstrated

(a)

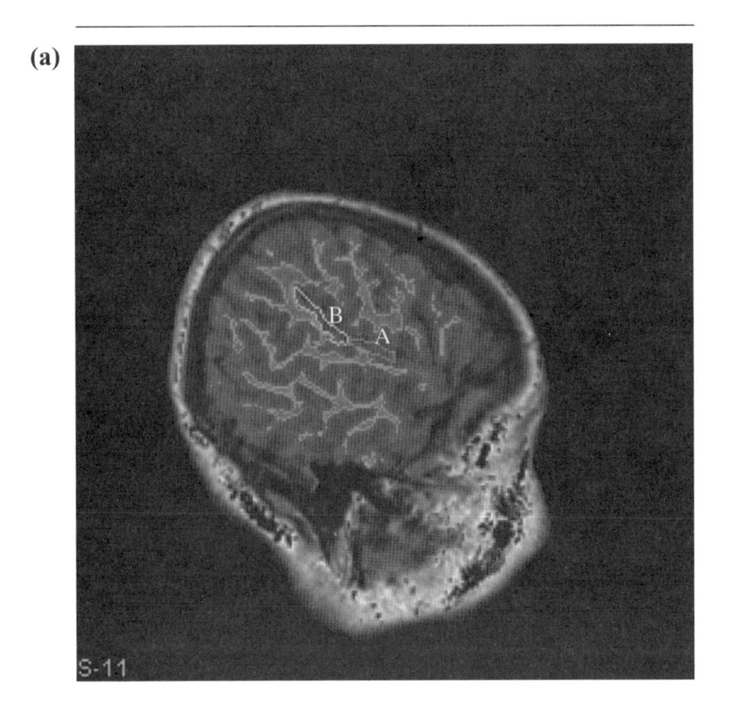

(b)

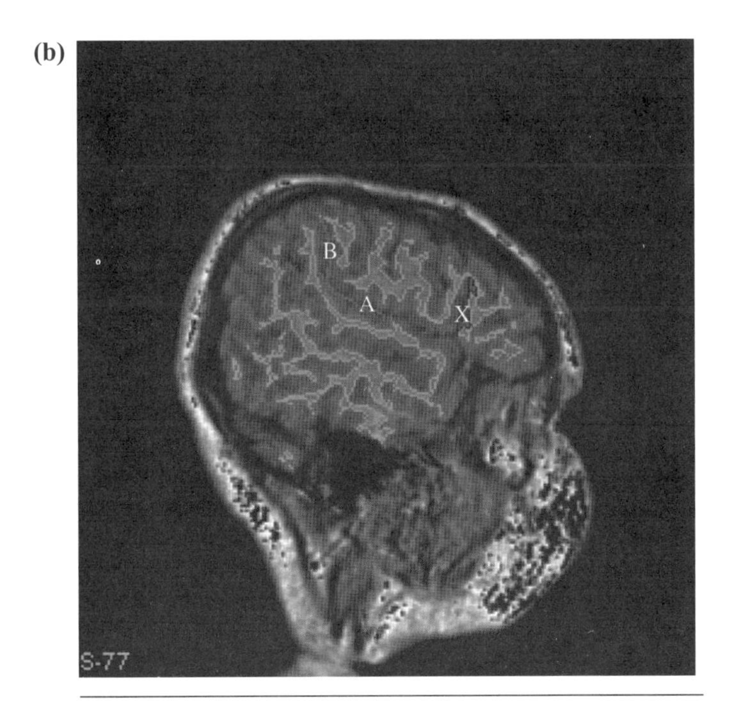

Figure 2.2 (a) Left hemisphere. Planum temporale, A: temporal bank; B: parietal bank. (b) Right hemisphere. Planum temporale, A: temporal bank; B: parietal bank; X: ascending ramus of the pars. The horizontal ramus is poorly formed and not traced.

Table 2.3 Psychometric Summary for Cord

	Scaled Scores	Standard Scores
Wechsler Intelligence Scale for Children, Fourth Edition (WISC-IV)		
Full Scale IQ		120
General Ability Index		132
Verbal Comprehension Index		126
Similarities	13	
Vocabulary	13	
Comprehension	17	
Perceptual Reasoning Index		129
Block Design	19	
Picture Concepts	13	
Matrix Reasoning	12	
Working Memory Index		86
Digit Span	7	
Letter-Number Sequencing	8	
Processing Speed Index		112
Coding	10	
Symbol Search	14	
Wisconsin Card Sorting Test (WCST)		
Categories Achieved		117
Perseverative Errors		135
Failure to Maintain Set		119
Peabody Picture Vocabulary Test, Fourth Edition (PPVT-IV)		119
Boston Naming Test (BNT)		92
Verbal Fluency from Delis-Kaplan Executive Function Scale (D-KEFS)	9	
Formulated Sentences from Clinical Evaluations of Language Fundamentals-Fourth Edition (CELF-IV)	11	
Gestalt Closure from Kaufman Assessment Battery for Children-Second Edition (KABC-2)	11	
Developmental Test of Visual-Motor Integration-Fifth Edition (DTVMI-V)		106
Rey Complex Figure Test (copy)		102
Clock Face Drawing Test		
Form		75
Time (10:20)		106
Finger Tapping Test		
Right (dominant) Hand 46.3 Taps/10 seconds		110
Left (nondominant) Hand 40.0 Taps/10 seconds		103

Table 2.3 (*Continued*)

	Scaled Scores	Standard Scores
Children's Memory Scale (CMS)		
Attention/Concentration Index		78
Numbers	9	
Sequences	8	
Picture Locations (supplemental)	13	
General Memory Index		90
Verbal Immediate Index		82
Stories	12	
Word Pairs	2	
Visual Immediate Index		106
Dot Locations	14	
Faces	8	
Verbal Delayed Index		82
Stories	12	
Word Pairs	2	
Visual Delayed Index		103
Dot Locations	13	
Faces	8	
Delayed Recognition Index		115
Stories	14	
Word Pairs	11	
Learning Index		88
Word Pairs	2	
Dot Locations	14	
Gray Oral Reading Test, Fourth Edition (GORT-4)		
Fluency		90
Comprehension		100
Wechsler Individual Achievement Test, Second Edition (WIAT-II)		
Word Reading		84
Pseudoword Decoding		82
Written Expression		83
Mathematical Reasoning		115
Numerical Operations		117
Behavior Assessment System for Children, Second Edition (BASC-2)		

	T-Scores	
	Parent Rating Scale (Dad)	Teacher Rating Scale (Mom)
Clinical Scales		
Hyperactivity	38	46
Aggression	42	48
Conduct	41	43
Anxiety	30	53
Depression	45	48

(continued)

Table 2.3 (*Continued*)

	T-Scores	
	Parent Rating Scale (Dad)	Teacher Rating Scale (Mom)
Somatization	41	43
Atypical	51	47
Withdrawal	54	49
Attention	43	41
Learning Problems	NA	62
Adaptive Scales		
Adaptability	50	62
Social Skills	49	70
Leadership	51	65
Study Skills	NA	56
Activities of Daily Living	56	NA
Functional Communication	51	53
DSM-IV ADHD Checklist	**Raw Scores**	
Inattention	12/27	7/27
Hyperactivity/Impulsivity	6/27	2/27

Note. NA = Not applicable.

above-average (maximum possible score) problem-solving capability and mental flexibility on the Wisconsin Card Sorting Test consistent with intellectual expectancy.

Cord's performance on tests of expressive and receptive language was generally in the average to high-average range contrasted by low-average to average word finding/retrieval capability. He exhibited average visual-spatial perception. His visual-motor integration/ constructional ability were also average when motor planning requirements were emphasized. This is contrasted by superior constructional ability when Cord is allowed to self-correct (Block Design). Thus, motor planning is an area of weakness for Cord. His fine motor tapping was found to be within normal limits bilaterally as measured by the Finger Oscillation Test.

Analysis of Cord's ability to learn and remember new material indicates that at the present time, he exhibits borderline to low-average ability to hold auditory/verbal material in immediate working memory contrasted by above-average visual working memory. Within the verbal modality, Cord demonstrated above-average ability to learn and recall (30 minutes later) stories that were read to him, contrasted by significant difficulty learning (over three highly structured learning trials) and recalling a list of rote word pairs. It should be noted that Cord's recall performance was significantly aided by the use of a recognition recall paradigm (cued recall), which is indicative of information retrieval difficulty. Within the visual domain, Cord exhibited superior ability to learn and recall the spatial location of an array of dots (where) contrasted by average ability to recall a series of pictured human faces (what he sees). This pattern of performance is generally consistent with that obtained on initial assessment by this service.

Academic Functioning

Academically, Cord performed in the high-average range on tasks assessing mathematical reasoning and calculation. Reading comprehension was found to be in the average range, and word recognition, pseudoword decoding, reading fluency, and written expression were all in the low-average range. Thus, Cord continues to demonstrate deficits in word recognition, reading fluency, and reading comprehension that are of learning disability proportion. It should be noted that Cord's written expression capability is now of learning disability proportion as well.

Social-Emotional and Behavioral Functioning

Behaviorally, analysis of rating scales completed by Cord's parents indicates that they are not endorsing any significant emotional or behavioral difficulty at the present time. Cord is very active in his church youth group. He takes a tae kwon do class and volunteers one day a week at the local science center.

Summary and Diagnostic Impressions

Cord is a 13-year 9-month-old adolescent who is currently homeschooled. He has a history of difficulty with reading. He is of above-average to superior cognitive ability with relative weaknesses in auditory working memory and verbal fluency/word retrieval, motor planning, rote verbal learning and information retrieval, and recall of visual content (what he sees). Taken together, this pattern of neuropsychological test performance continues to be consistent with a diagnosis of dyslexia (learning disability in the area of reading). In addition, Cord now meets diagnostic criteria for learning disability in the area of written expression.

Recommendations

As a result, it is felt that Cord will require resource/inclusion special education services designed for students with learning disabilities under the eligibility category of "Specific Learning Disability," should his parents elect to educate him within a public or private school setting. Resource placement should be utilized for further development of reading and written expression skills with inclusion services provided for other academics that emphasize reading and writing skills as a prerequisite.

- Given Cord's pattern of strengths and weaknesses, it is recommended that academic instruction in reading and writing expression emphasize multisensory approaches.
- In order to enhance Cord's learning/retention, new material should be presented in an organized format that is meaningful to him. The material to be learned should be pretaught and broken down into smaller components/steps.
- Presentations should be highly structured, and Cord should be provided with frequent repetition to facilitate new learning.
- Instruction should be supplemented with visual aids, demonstrations, and experiential/procedural learning.
- Cord would benefit greatly from being taught how to use mnemonic strategies when learning new material and studying for tests. These include but are not limited to four areas:
  1. Rehearsal—showing Cord how to repeat information verbally, to write it, and look at it a finite number of times
  2. Transformation—showing Cord how to convert difficult information into simpler components that can be remembered more easily
  3. Elaboration—instructing Cord in how to identify key elements of new information and to create relationships or associations with previously learned material

4. Imagery—showing Cord how to visualize and make a "mental picture" of information to be learned

- When studying for tests or doing multiple homework assignments on the same day, similar subject material should be aggregated in order to lessen interference.
- Finally, Cord should be provided with periodic review of previously learned material in order to enhance long-term retention.

Accommodations will be necessary to enhance Cord's ability to succeed in the classroom; these include:

- Cord should have preferential seating in close proximity to the teacher so that he or she can monitor Cord's progress.
- He should have additional time to complete written assignments.
- He should be tested in multiple-choice/matching/short answer formats instead of essay format and tests should be administered individually/orally, with additional time provided when necessary.
- Finally, Cord should be allowed and encouraged to use various compensatory devices, such as textbooks on tape/reading pen and a computer with word processing capability. Most word processing programs are equipped with spell checks and cut and paste and can be adapted for voice dictation if necessary.

Additional suggestions:

- Cord would also benefit from study skills training emphasizing such techniques as the appropriate outlining of lecture notes and how to study for tests. He will benefit from being taught how to take notes on text material and plan written reports using an outlining method as well.
- Training in word processing is strongly encouraged.
- Cord also may require instruction on how to organize and plan his approach to his studies. In addition, direct instruction in basic organizational strategies will assist Cord in knowing what to do, when to do it, and how to do it. Specifically, he should be guided in the use of checklists and other organizational aids, such as a daily planner.
- Cord should undergo neuropsychological reevaluation in preparation for postsecondary education.

Further Discussion of Case Study

What is most notable about Cord is the pattern of strengths and weaknesses, with working memory, particularly related to auditory information, emerging as the most consistent weakness. For Cord, this is most evident on recall of unrelated items (digits, words) and less evident for semantically related information (story). Consistent with this, he has more difficulty with decoding or recognizing words in isolation as compared to his reading comprehension; expressive skills at a semantic or syntactic level appear to be better developed than his word retrieval (naming, fluency); finally, he now evidences difficulty in written expression, which is consistent with the patterns of developmental progression often seen in children with dyslexia/reading disability. Also of note, and not consistent with the rest of his profile, Cord does evidence some difficulty with clock face drawing (motor planning) and recall of visual content. Taken together, this combination of relative weaknesses continues to be consistent with a picture of mixed developmental dyslexia (auditory linguistic/dysphonetic and visual spatial/dyseidetic). Further, it is of note that this pattern of performance has persisted across the multiple evaluations, with continual supports and interventions, with no indication of decreased overall language skills or "Matthew effect."

CONCLUDING COMMENTS

There is an extensive and still-growing knowledge base with regard to dyslexia/reading disability; reading difficulties are the most common of the academic problems identified in the general population, in psychiatric populations, and in incarcerated populations. Reading is not a unitary process but a complex one; it involves multiple functional systems. There is no single or unitary neurological factor or single gene that is responsible for reading ability but rather a combination of structural or functional differences, some of which may be genetically determined that accounts for individual differences. As noted earlier, the variation in etiology, processes, and structures best supports a conceptualization of reading as involving a widely distributed functional system, with any impairment or developmental deficit in the system resulting in a distinct pattern of reading failure (Duffy et al., 1980). The number of differing structures and genetic as well as environmental influences that come into play in dyslexia portend a somewhat heterogeneous group when referring to individuals with reading disabilities. In the current age of response to intervention, it is important to keep in mind the heterogeneity of these individuals and the need to consider the neurocognitive strengths of the individual in intervention planning. With the emergence of brain activation and neuroimaging changes as a result of specific reading interventions, there should be renewed awareness of the need for neuropsychological perspectives in the identification of specific learning disabilities and appropriate interventions (Kaufman, 2008).

Chapter 3

LEARNING DISABILITIES: DYSCALCULIA/MATH DISABILITY

DEFINITION

Mathematical abilities are important cognitive skills, often included as a component of many measures of cognitive ability. Mathematics skills are also considered in the area of achievement, when included as part of psychoeducational and neuropsychological assessment; mathematic skills are even considered in the context of determining mental status (i.e., counting backward by threes). Math abilities are distributed across the population with educational level having a robust effect on math abilities. The neuropsychological and neurological literature uses the term *dyscalculia* when deficits in math are identified and these deficits represent a developmental delay or deviance in the acquisition of one or more of mathematical functions; when the deficits are the result of brain injury or cerebral pathology, the result is referred to as *acalculia* (Ardila & Rosselli, 2002; Mazzocco, 2007). The American Psychiatric Association identifies the comparable disorder as mathematics disability, defined as mathematical ability that is below expected for chronological age, measured cognitive ability, and age-appropriate education; it is included in the section of disorders that arise in childhood, thus presuming a deviance or delay in the developmental process of math concept and skill acquisition (American Psychiatric Association, 2000). Regardless of when or how it occurs, there is consensus that there is a neurological basis to the math difficulties (von Aster & Shalev, 2007). In educational contexts, there is no differentiation of math disability as developmental or acquired. There remains, however, the issue of differentiating math disability from math difficulty (Mazzocco, 2007). In addition, there is the need to consider the extent to which the math disability occurs alone or in the context of intact language, reading, and writing abilities (Strang & Rourke, 1985).

Regardless of the terminology, whether the math disability is specific or generalized, or the presumed underlying mechanism, it is important to consider the type of math tasks involved and the developmental progression of the understanding of mathematics. Three different types of math tasks have been considered: arithmetic, algorithmic computation, and word problems (Geary, 1993). In educational settings, math skills often are broken down into math calculation skills and math reasoning (Flanagan, Ortiz, Alfonso, & Mascolo, 2002). *Math calculation* refers to the application of computation skills and basic algorithms with accuracy, while *math reasoning* requires problem solving and understanding of math operations and algorithms in conjunction with quantitative reasoning (Proctor, Floyd, & Shaver, 2005). Much in the same way as automaticity or fluency is considered in reading, automaticity can be considered in relation to basic calculation skills. Hécaen et al. created the first classification system for different types of acalculia in 1961 (as cited in Rourke & Conway, 1997). Type I is the inability to read and write numbers; Type II is the inability to organize numbers spatially, called spatial acalculia; and Type III is the inability to carry out mathematical processes, called anarithmetria. Researchers have further divided Type I into two concepts: the inability to read numbers is called number alexia or alexic acalculia, and the ability to write numbers is called number agraphia or agraphic acalculia.

Kosc (1974) was the first major researcher to look into a developmental form of math disability. He described six subtypes of dyscalculia that elaborated on Hécaen's work:

1. Verbal dyscalculia, the inability to name mathematical terms
2. Lexical dyscalculia, the inability to recognize numbers
3. Graphical dyslexia, the inability to write numbers or mathematical symbols
4. Operational dyscalculia, the inability to perform math operations
5. Practognostic dyscalculia, the inability to manipulate objects for mathematical purposes
6. Ideognostic dyscalculia, the inability to understand mathematical concepts

Other literature on adults with dyscalculia or math disability indicates three basic groups:

1. Dyscalculia in conjunction with aphasia
2. Dyscalculia due to visual-perceptual deficits
3. Dyscalculia that is specific to math calculation (Hécaen, Angelergues, & Houiller, 1961)

In contrast, other classification systems look at the processes involved (Grunau & Low, 1987; Kosc, 1974) and discovered six groups:

1. Operational dyscalculia (difficulty with actual calculation)
2. Primary or ideognostical dyscalculia (inability to grasp concepts involved in mathematics)
3. Practognostic dyscalculia (inability to apply math skills)
4. Verbal dyscalculia (difficulty with naming mathematical amounts, numerals, terms, symbols)
5. Lexical dyscalculia (inability to read math symbols)
6. Graphical dyscalculia (inability to write/produce math symbols)

Some researchers have reported on individuals who could read and write the numbers but evidenced severe difficulty in retrieval of math facts (number-fact dyscalculia of memory subtype) or those who have a good grasp of the basic operations but are unable to apply basic arithmetic procedures (procedural dyscalculia) (Barnes, Fletcher, & Ewing-Cobbs, 2007). In one case there was a report of an 11-year-old boy who was unable to read or write dictated Arabic numbers but had age-appropriate reading and spelling skills (C. Temple, 1991). This would be consistent with the visual-spatial subtype.

Another disability that is closely linked to dyscalculia is nonverbal learning disability (NVLD). Rourke (1989) identified two subtypes of math disability—the RS subtype, or those with math, reading, and spelling problems, and the A subtype or nonverbal learning disability (NVLD) subtype, who perform poorly only in math. The RS group is characterized by good performance on visual-spatial tasks and tactile tasks but deficits in auditory-linguistic processing, verbal attention, and verbal memory (Rourke, 1989). In contrast, the A or NVLD group is characterized by deficits on visual-spatial and tactile tasks as well as psychomotor deficits. It is hypothesized that the difficulty in math is due to deficits in nonverbal concept formation. NVLD also is associated with primary deficits in novel situations, tactile and visual perception, and with problems with problem solving, concept formation, and memory. In addition to impaired math abilities, NVLD is associated with deficits in the understanding of pragmatic language (the social and emotional components of the message) as well as in understanding of nonverbal behaviors or cues and in the communication of emotion through nonverbal cues (Rourke, 1989). Rourke concluded that this group had a deficit in right-hemisphere functioning. Further evidence of right-hemisphere deficits were demonstrated by difficulties on motor, psychomotor, and tactile-perceptual tasks, particularly those involving the left hand.

Also related to dyscalculia, and worthy of note, is Gerstmann syndrome. Gerstmann syndrome manifests as acalculia, finger agnosia, right/left disorientation, and dysgraphia. A similar syndrome (termed *developmental Gerstmann syndrome*) has been proposed to occur in children with or without co-occurring language dysfunction. It was postulated that these children had additional difficulties in constructional praxis and were likely to evidence nonverbal rather than verbal deficits (Kinsbourne, 1968; Kinsbourne & Warrington, 1963). Children with developmental Gerstmann syndrome present with intact language skills; reading is generally at expectancy (PeBenito, Fisch, & Fisch, 1988). The deficits Gerstmann observed were bilateral finger agnosia, right-left confusion, dysgraphia, and dyscalculia. He initially concluded that this syndrome was caused by a lesion in the left angular gyrus. Further research showed that while a lesion may not exist in the left angular gyrus, the majority of cases had a lesion somewhere in the left parietal lobe that may or may not cross over into the occipital lobe (Lebrun, 2005). Some neuropsychologists question whether Gerstmann syndrome is actually a clinical concept or a mistake of observations. The combination of symptoms are related to multiple other neurodevelopmental disorders, which suggests that it is not a unique disorder (C. J. Miller & Hynd, 2004). Its value lies in that it was the first time dyscalculia was considered in neuropsychology research, and the work on Gerstmann's syndrome has had a positive influence on subsequent research.

Prevalence and Incidence

Although less often studied than dyslexia, dyscalculia, or learning disability in math (Ardila & Rosselli, 2002; Gersten, Clarke, & Mazzocco, 2007; Gersten, Jordan, & Flojo, 2005), is said to occur in 5% to 8% of children (Geary, Hoard, Byrd-Craven, & DeSoto, 2004; Gross-Tur, Manor, & Shalev, 1996; Shalev, 2004; Shalev, Auerbach, Manor, & Gross-Tsur, 2000). Research studies suggest relatively equal numbers of girls and boys to be affected by math disabilities (Gross-Tur et al., 1996; C. Lewis, Hitch, & Walker, 1994). The manifestation of dyscalculia varies by age; younger children show difficulties in basic number concepts, while older children show difficulties in understanding algorithms and learning facts. At the same time, daily functioning, success in school, and many forms of employment require at least minimal competency in math (Geary & Hoard, 2001; Light &

DeFries, 1995). Despite the significance of math difficulties, less attention is paid to difficulties in math. This is attributed to the decreased social stigma attached to dyscalculia (O'Hare, Brown, & Aitken, 1991); the decreased attention and research also affects what is known about the etiology of dyscalculia.

Of those individuals with math disability, approximately 17% of the children with math disability also evidence reading disability (Kovas et al., 2007), 25% evidence symptoms associated with Attention-Deficit/Hyperactivity Disorder (ADHD) (Gross-Tur et al., 1996). There is evidence across studies, based on bivariate heritability estimates, that the comorbidity of math and reading disabilities is genetically influenced (Knopik, Alarcón, & DeFries, 1997; Light & DeFries, 1995). One study found that 53% of children with a reading disability also had a math disability, while 46% of children with a math disability also had a reading disability (Knopik et al., 1997); the correlation between the two disabilities is 0.53, implying a similar genetic origin. In addition, there is a higher than expected prevalence of math disability associated with epilepsy and in girls with sex chromosome deficits such as Turner syndrome (Gross-Tur et al., 1996). Finally, there is some evidence that girls with fragile X syndrome (see Chapter 15) are at risk for math learning disability but may demonstrate average rote math skills, similar to hyperlexia in reading (M. M. Murphy & Mazzocco, 2008). Other than association with specific X-linked disorders, there is little evidence of gender effects on math ability in the literature (Hyde, 2005).

ETIOLOGY

Acalculia is generally considered the loss of the ability to perform some combination of computation skills as a result of identified cerebral pathology (D. Loring, 1999). Although there is not necessarily a known underlying cerebral pathology, it is presumed that there is a neurological underpinning to math learning disabilities or dyscalculia. This neurological basis may be the result of genetic or nongenetic factors.

Genetic

Research has shown that dyscalculia is a familial disorder. Shalev and his colleagues (2001) studied the families of children with developmental dyscalculia to determine the heredity of the disorder; in their sample, 66% of mothers, 44% of fathers, 53% of siblings, and 44% of second-degree relatives also were determined to have developmental dyscalculia, with a prevalence almost 10 times higher within families than in the general population. Twin studies have shown that monozygotic twins of those with dyscalculia are 12 times more likely to have the disorder while dizygotic twins are 8 times more likely (Alarcón, DeFries, & Pennington, 1997; Alarcón, Knopik, & DeFries, 2000; Shalev, 2004).

Two genetic disorders that have dyscalculia as a manifestation often are discussed together in neuropsychology to better understand the math component of the disorders. Turner syndrome is a genetic anomaly in which one of the two X chromosomes is missing in females (see Chapter 15). These girls tend to have average intelligence but low mathematical abilities (M. M. Murphy & Mazzocco, 2008). Their math difficulties have been shown to be caused by abnormalities in the right intraparietal sulcus, which has an abnormal length, shape, and depth. Imaging showed that in girls with Turner syndrome, the right intraparietal sulcus does not appropriately respond to number size changes in math problems (Molko et al., 2003). The inferior parietal sulcus is also abnormal in patients with fragile X syndrome (see Chapter 15). Fragile X is an abnormality in the X chromosome that usually causes mental retardation in males; in females, it is more likely to present as a learning disability (Mazzocco, 2001). Williams syndrome (see Chapter 15) also has been associated with specific deficits in mathematical skill acquisition (O'Hearn & Landau, 2007; Paterson, Girelli, Butterworth, & Karmiloff-Smith, 2006).

Environmental

In addition to genotype, ecological variables of the home (Jordan, Kaplan, & Hanich, 2002; Mullis, Dossey, Owen, & Phillips, 1991) may affect acquisition of math skills. As with reading disability, children from low-income families are more likely to evidence math difficulties by the end of second grade and demonstrated lower performance and slower rate of growth (Jordan et al., 2002). These environmental influences further contribute to the covariance of reading and math deficits (Light & DeFries, 1995). Math knowledge is largely acquired through schooling, so it is important to understand whether a child truly has a disability or whether a problem with curriculum, teaching, or educational opportunity is present. Even preschool curricula have been found to affect later math skills (Booth & Siegler, 2008; Griffin, 2004).

It is also important to examine anxiety issues in children who are struggling in math to determine if the anxiety is causing the struggles, or if it is a reflection of a deeper problem. Math anxiety is a related condition or concern that may be related to deficits in math skill (Ashcraft, Krause, & Hopko, 2007). Ashcraft et al. defined math anxiety as "the negative emotional reaction some people experience when placed in situations that require mathematical reasoning or problem solving" (p. 329). It may be as mild as apprehension or dislike or as severe as a phobic reaction. There is relatively little empirical research on how math anxiety is defined, but much discussion has ensued related to the presence of math anxiety and its effects on math performance and learning. It is fairly well documented that the relationship between math anxiety and intellectual ability is minimal. Alternatively, there is some indication that math anxiety will result in avoidance of math-related activities and poor self-esteem with math skills, subsequently resulting in decreased math performance (Ashcraft et al., 2007). Stereotype threat among females and minority groups also may affect math performance (Beilock, Rydell, & McConnell, 2007).

Neurological Substrates

Functional imaging studies indicate that multiple areas are involved in math skills and dyscalculia (von Aster & Shalev, 2007). A problem in studying the neurological substrates of math is that the actual processes involved in mathematics tend to vary depending on the actual math task (Geary, Hoard, & Hamson, 1999) as well as with age (Xuan et al., 2007). In a study of adolescents and using voxel-based morphometry, there is evidence that respondents with calculation difficulties had less gray matter in the left parietal lobe than those with average abilities, particularly in the left intraparietal sulcus, supporting previous research (Isaacs, Edmonds, Lucas, & Gadian, 2001). With adults, brain activity during different number-related tasks varies depending on the task requirement (Dehaene, Spelke, Pinel, Stanescu, & Tsivkin, 1999). Tasks requiring estimation or approximation or number comparison were associated with a pattern of cortical activation with maximum activation in the inferior parietal regions of both hemispheres; this was conceptualized as the analog internal number line representation. Tasks requiring exact calculation and counting were associated with maximum activity in the left inferior prefrontal cortex; this was conceptualized as representing the verbal word frame. In the triple-code model, a third module for number-related tasks related to multidigit operations in which the numbers are represented by their number code (visual Arabic number form). Number functions involve the parietal areas and tend to be underactivated in children with dyscalculia. These three components constitute the number processing and calculation system; these components are interconnected yet independent (von Aster & Shalev, 2007).

Using modern technology, such as positron emission tomography (PET) and functional magnetic resonance imaging (fMRI) scans, neuropsychologists have been able to determine the parts of the brain involved in mathematical processes (Delazer et al., 2003; Krueger et al., 2008). The parietal lobe, which is responsible for visual-spatial functioning, is dominant in many activities. The intraparietal sulcus also is activated by mental calculations and numerical comparisons. It is more active when addition and multiplication are performed; this is theorized to be true because addition and multiplication facts are more often memorized and are consequently more language-dependent than subtraction and division, which require more calculation. The intraparietal sulcus is also used when numbers are presented as words, either visual or spoken. In fact, the horizontal segment of the bilateral intraparietal sulcus (HIPS) seems to be the most important region in basic number processing; it is activated in the presence of numbers, no matter how they are presented (Dehaene, Molko, Cohen, & Wilson, 2004). Further, the right inferior parietal lobule, left precuneus, and left superior parietal gyrus are important for doing subtraction, while the bilateral medial frontal/cingulate cortex is important in processing the complexity of a problem (Kong et al., 2005). The left inferior intraparietal sulcus, left inferior frontal gyrus, and bilateral cingulate were activated as math problems became more difficult (Krueger et al., 2008).

Dehaene et al. (1999) compared brain activation in calculation tasks and estimation or approximation tasks. Two parietal areas, the horizontal segment of the intraparietal sulcus and the posterior superior parietal sulcus, become active in estimation and approximation tasks; other areas that are activated include the right precuneus, left and right precentral sulci, left dorsolateral prefrontal cortex, left superior prefrontal gyrus, left cerebellum, and left and right thalamus. In contrast, for exact calculations, activation is seen in the left inferior frontal lobe, with lower level of activation in the left cingulate gyrus, left precuneus, right parieto-occipital sulcus, bilateral angular gyri, and right middle temporal gyrus. Thus, the areas activated in calculation are similar to those activated for language processing, once again demonstrating the connection between memorized facts and language (Dehaene et al., 1999).

The extent to which one or the other hemisphere is involved in dyscalculia has been debated, yet this is key to the NVLD conceptualization of dyslexia. For example, it has been argued that the memory subtype and procedural subtype are associated with left-hemisphere dysfunction, while the visual-spatial subtype was related to right-hemisphere dysfunction (Geary, 1994). Support for right-hemisphere involvement has been found in electroencephalography study of children with dyslexia, dyscalculia, and controls while they were engaged in solving verbal and nonverbal tasks (A. J. Mattson, Sheer, & Fletcher, 1992). Results indicated that children with reading problems had less left-hemisphere activity while performing verbal tasks relative to the other groups. In contrast, children with math problems had less right-hemisphere activity while performing nonverbal tasks relative to the other groups. Replication has not supported the NVLD/

right-hemisphere hypothesis consistently; the pattern was found in about 50% of children in one study, but it did not follow for the other 50% (von Aster, 1994).

One theoretical perspective on the mental representation of math facts relies on cognitive components, wherein a central semantic system is used for all calculation regardless of how presented; the nature of this semantic system is related to the abstract representation of the magnitude (McCloskey, Aliminosa, & Sokol, 1991). A multicomponent system model (C. Temple, 1991) has been suggested as well. Under this model, primary acalculia (conceptual understanding) is associated with dysfunction of the parietal, occipital, and/or temporal lobes specific to the dominant (left) hemisphere. Specifically, the temporal lobe is implicated in the use of subvocalization and internal speech for problem solving, memory for the series of steps and basic facts, and any reading required. Frontal lobes are hypothesized to be the centers for quick calculation and abstract conceptualization, sequencing as well as problem solving, oral responding, and written performance (Gaddes & Edgell, 1994; Luria, 1966). The parietal lobes are responsible for some arithmetic functions (Xuan et al., 2007). Finally, the occipital lobe is implicated in the visual discrimination of written math symbols, geometry, and routine calculations (Gaddes & Edgell, 1994). This conceptualization is supported by evidence from focal brain pathology (Grafman, Kampen, Rosenberg, Salazar, & Boller, 1989; Rosselli & Ardila, 1989). Dehaene and Changeux (1993) proposed a model of basic number ability at the neural level. In the numerosity detection system, numerical information, visual or auditory, is presented on an input map, or "retina," placed on a set of neurons that form a topographical map of object locations and a map of numerosity detectors that adds up all of the output from the location map. This information is then sent to a motor output system (Dehaene, Cohen, & Changeux, 1998).

When dyscalculia occurs in conjunction with dyslexia and/or dysgraphia for numbers, the dysfunction may be localized to the dominant hemisphere or it may be bilateral. In contrast, when dyscalculia is associated with visual-spatial deficits, the dysfunction either is localized to the parietal lobe of the nondominant (right) hemisphere or is bilateral. Thus, this model explains the equivocal support for the NVLD pattern. Subcortical structures also have been implicated in that studies suggest a correlation between dyscalculia and visual discrimination, memory, spatial visualization, visual coordination, visual sequencing, and logical reasoning abilities (Grunau & Low, 1987; S. C. Larsen & Hammill, 1975; McLeod & Crump, 1978). Geary (1993) examined the processes involved in both disorders as well as information from acquired forms of the disorders and theorized that both disorders involve the posterior regions of the left hemisphere. Differences in these left posterior regions could manifest as difficulty retrieving semantic information from long-term memory, whether the information is encoded as words or numbers. Robinson, Menchetti, and Torgensen (2002) proposed a theory of dyscalculia that incorporates reading ability. Their theory hypothesizes that the difficulty in learning math facts can be caused by a weakness in the phonological loop related to working memory in Baddeley's model (2007). In people with this form of math disability, the auditory and phonological features of numbers and facts are weakened. Because the brain does not have a solid representation of the math facts, math facts are not processed well enough, and this makes it more difficult for retrieval (Robinson et al., 2002).

Gerstmann syndrome is associated with circumscribed left-hemisphere lesions in the area of the angular gyrus and parietal lobe when presenting with deficits in language processing. Neuroimaging studies have confirmed a relation between Gerstmann syndrome and left posterior parietal damage (Mazzoni, Pardossi, Cantini, Giornetti, & Arena,

1990). Alternatively, it was further hypothesized that the syndrome without language processing deficits is restricted to the right hemisphere. There are some indications that developmental Gerstmann syndrome is associated with specific chromosomal disorders, including fragile X (J. P. Grigsby, Kemper, & Hagerman, 1987) and other disorders.

COURSE AND PROGNOSIS

From the perspective that mathematical competencies (i.e., number sense) are core modular attributes (Butterworth, 2005) and develop in a trajectory, early identification and intervention with children experiencing math difficulties is important. Even in third grade, it is evident that children with math disabilities lag behind their peers in their ability to use approximation and are not able to identify implausible solutions (Rousselle & Noël, 2008). Longitudinal studies suggest that a vast majority (95%) of children with math disability in grade 5 will continue to evidence achievement below the 25th percentile in 11th grade (Shalev, Manor, & Gross-Tsur, 2005). With the sequential nature of mathematics, and later skills dependent to some extent on earlier skills across calculation, procedures, and problem solving, it is not surprising that earlier difficulties predict later difficulties.

There is a paucity of research on the long-term prognosis of math disability, but it is believed that math disability or developmental dyscalculia is an enduring and persisting problem for at least half of the children who exhibit the difficulties (Shalev et al., 2000). Although no publications discuss an analogous Matthew effect in mathematics skills, the extent of literature related to math anxiety and the idea that the experience (or anticipation) of difficulty in math would result in avoidance and decreased exposure to mathematical skills and concepts over time would support such a phenomenon. Studies have demonstrated, for example, that math performance is positively correlated with self-perceived math ability and negatively correlated with math anxiety (Standing, 2006).

One longitudinal study of children with math disability suggested that persistence of the math disability was associated with the initial severity of the disorder at the time of diagnosis as well as the presence of others in the family with the same disorder (Shalev, Manor, Auerbach, & Gross-Tsur, 1998). In contrast, no effects of socioeconomic status, gender, or types of intervention were found. Children who continued to demonstrate math difficulties at follow-up were more likely to exhibit behavioral and emotional problems, particularly in areas of attention problems and anxiety/depression (Shalev et al., 1998). This study only followed the children through eighth grade. The longer-term consequences of math disability and math anxiety on employment, level of attained education, and overall psychological adjustment require further research (Shalev et al., 2000).

Neuropsychological Correlates

Mathematic skill development, like reading, increases in complexity and a range of component skills (Mazzocco, 2007). Taken together, these component mathematical tasks are believed to involve a variety of skills including verbal, spatial, memory, and executive skills (Ardila, Galeano, & Rosselli, 1998); see Table 3.1. Math learning disability, or dyscalculia, is conceptualized as involving deficits in computation skills (Bull & Johnston, 1997; Geary, Hamson, & Hoard, 2000), working memory (Geary, Brown, & Samaranayake, 1991; Hitch & McAuley, 1991; McLean & Hitch, 1999; Schuchardt, Maehler, & Hasselhorn, 2008; H. L. Swanson & Sachse-Lee, 2001), and conceptual

Table 3.1 Neuropsychological Domains and Math Difficulties

Neuropsychological Domain	Math Difficulties
Auditory-linguistic/ Language Function	Problems in verbal organization of numbers and procedures Difficulty with understanding of directions and word problems
Visual Perception and Constructional Praxis	Difficulty with reading the arithmetic signs Difficulty in reading numbers Difficulty in forming the appropriate numbers Difficulty copying the problems Difficulties in placing numbers in columns Consistently working right to left; following correct directionality for process Nonverbal ability predicts math skills in grade 1 but variance accounted for dissipates over time
Learning and Memory	Problems in recall of facts or procedures; fact retrieval Problems with verbal memory when problems, directions provided verbally Deficits in visual short-term memory and visual working memory Visual short-term memory and working memory predict math achievement
Executive Function	Omission or addition of a step in the procedure Problem in sequencing of steps in the procedure; attentional-sequential problems Application of procedure to the wrong type of problem Errors that imply impossible results; lack of application of reasoning skills Difficulty in understanding of mathematical ideas and concepts Difficulty in shifting between one operation and another Repetition of the same number

knowledge and problem solving (Hanich, Jordan, Kaplan, & Dick, 2001; Jordan & Hanich, 2000; Jordan & Montani, 1997). Conceptually, these areas involve the representation of quantity, understanding of the number line and the position of numbers within the system, understanding of relations between numbers, and understanding of various numerical symbols and their verbal representations (Tsvetkova, 1996). Most measures used in assessment do not directly measure the conceptual basis but rely on the application of these concepts. For example, arithmetic generally is restricted to retrieval of single-digit operations or basic facts with reliance on memory span. Problems in the execution of arithmetical procedures or algorithmic computation most likely are related to executive function due to the reliance on sequencing and problem solving as well as to long-term memory. There are also some indications that children demonstrate greater response interference than adults on number comparison tasks (Szucs, Soltész, Jármi, & Csépe, 2007). Word problems may incorporate both arithmetic and algorithmic computation, in conjunction with language ability (Geary, 1993). In older children with math learning disability, poor fact mastery and calculation fluency, as well as working memory, tend to be significantly different from age-matched peers (Mabbott & Bisanz, 2008).

Executive Function

Executive function is a category of higher-level functions that are either directly or indirectly developed in the frontal lobes. Types of executive functions include planning, problem solving, working memory, attention, inhibition, and self-monitoring of behavior (Zillmer et al., 2008). Numerous studies have explored a link between executive functioning and children's mathematical abilities (Bull & Scerif, 2001; S. E. Gathercole & Pickering, 2000; Lorsbach, Wilson, & Reimer, 1996; McLean & Hitch, 1999). This hypothesized relationship has been examined in a diverse range of populations. Specifically, preschool children (Espy et al., 2004; S. E. Gathercole & Pickering, 2000), school-age children (Bull & Scerif, 2001; Lehto, Juujarvi, Kooistra, & Pulkkinen, 2003), children with ADHD (Cornoldi, Barbieri, Gaiani, & Zocchi, 1999; Ozonoff & Jensen, 1999b), children with learning disabilities (Lorsbach et al., 1996), children with arithmetic learning difficulties (McLean & Hitch, 1999), children with Tourette syndrome (Ozonoff & Jensen, 1999b), children with autism (Ozonoff & Jensen, 1999b), and students with anxiety or mood disorder (Cirino, Morris, & Morris, 2002) have been considered. Collectively, these studies reveal that executive function is a promising predictor of arithmetic performance in children; however, the relation between different components of executive function (EF) to mathematics ability may vary with age. Additionally, some differences between populations have emerged. For example, children with ADHD exhibit difficulty with tasks requiring inhibition but not on those requiring flexibility. Conversely, children with autism experience difficulty with tasks requiring flexibility but do not experience problems on tasks requiring inhibition (Ozonoff & Jensen, 1999b).

Mathematical skills are related to aspects of EF in school-age children (S. E. Gathercole & Pickering, 2000; J. Holmes & Adams, 2006; Mazzocco & Kover, 2007; McLean & Hitch, 1999; Xuan et al., 2007) as well as adults (Cirino et al., 2002; Osmon, Smerz, Braun, & Plambeck, 2006). For example, Mazzocco and Kover found that scores obtained on executive function tasks at age 6 to 7 were associated with math skills at the same age as well as with math achievement over time through at least age 10 or 11. Various components of EF have been related to mathematical functioning as well (McLean & Hitch, 1999). McLean and Hitch (1999) reported that for 9-year-olds scoring below the 25th percentile on a standardized mathematics achievement test, arithmetic performance was correlated with amount of time taken to complete written, verbal, and color trail making tests; this finding is indicative of difficulty switching between retrieval plans. Others also have found that children with math difficulties had more difficulty switching between classification systems and had a lower ability to regulate their actions and select appropriate strategies (Bull, Johnston, & Roy, 1999). It has been suggested that inhibitory processes are deficient in children with dyscalculia (Bull & Scerif, 2001; Passolunghi & Siegel, 2004). In particular, Passolunghi and Siegel argued that in solving a math problem, information must be included or excluded before a calculation is performed, and if children cannot determine how to use the information provided, they will not be able to carry out the task. Espy et al. (2004) found that, when controlling for other EF measures, only measures assessing inhibitory control explained unique variance in scores of mathematical ability in preschool children. Others, however, have not found inhibition to be related to mathematical ability (Censabella & Noël, 2008). A follow-up study examined the broader concept of executive function in children with dyscalculia (Bull & Scerif, 2001). Using the Wisconsin Card Sorting Test (WCST), the Stroop task, and counting span tasks, the researchers showed that children with dyscalculia had significant difficulties with inhibitory tasks, whether inhibiting a learned strategy or switching to a new strategy. This finding supported the earlier study that many aspects of executive functioning are implicated in dyscalculia, although the exact brain origins still are being determined.

A recent study examined the relation between parent ratings of children's executive function and calculation, applied problems, and math fluency with 92 consecutive referrals (Barrois, Haynes, Riccio, & Haws, 2006). The children had a mean age of 11.76 years (standard deviation [SD] = 2.07); all had a Full Scale IQ above 80. The sample included predominantly males (67.39 %) and was predominantly white (80.43 %). Executive function was measured using the parent form of the Behavior Rating Inventory of Executive Function (BRIEF). The results of the Parent BRIEF significantly predicted Calculation on the Woodcock Johnson Tests of Achievement, Third Edition (WJ III) with the greatest variance accounted for by the Shift subscale ($r = -.32$; $p = .001$). Regression results were not significant for the BRIEF with Applied Problems; however, correlations between Applied Problems and multiple BRIEF subscales (Inhibit, Shift, Initiate, Working Memory) were significant. BRIEF subscales did not predict Math Fluency despite significant correlations with Initiate and Working Memory (Barrois et al., 2006).

Memory

Many researchers have proposed that dyscalculia is really a function of larger memory deficits. Geary has done many studies to determine the role of working memory in dyscalculia (Geary et al., 2004). For example, one study showed that children with dyscalculia do not understand basic counting concepts even in first and second grade, and the errors indicated that these children had difficulty when holding the counting sequence in working memory. A follow-up study showed that younger children with dyscalculia used finger counting more often than their peers, indicating an inability to retrieve basic facts from working memory (Geary et al., 2004). Other studies have examined working memory with similar conclusions (Hitch & McAuley, 1991).

In Baddeley's model of working memory, executive control represents the behaviors seen in executive functioning. The central executive, the element of Baddeley's model of working memory that is closely tied with executive function, has been studied in children with dyscalculia using the WCST (Bull et al., 1999). The central executive, which is responsible for coordinating the actions of the phonological loop and visual-spatial sketchpad, was significantly weaker in children with dyscalculia. The phonological loop, which is involved in processing of verbal material, is also indicated in counting and holding information during more complex calculations; the visual-spatial sketchpad, which is involved in the processing of visual or spatial information, has been linked to multidigit problems where alignment of numbers into columns is required (McLean & Hitch, 1999).

As noted earlier, it has been suggested that ability and disability in relation to math problem solving is associated with the phonological system and the phonological loop (Fürst & Hitch, 2000; S. E. Gathercole & Pickering, 2000; S. E. Gathercole, Pickering, Ambridge, & Wearing, 2004). This premise has not been supported consistently in that studies have not consistently yielded deficits in verbal memory among those with dyscalculia (Bull & Johnston, 1997). Alternatively, results support an association between visual-spatial skills and visual working memory with counting skills (Kyttälä, Aunio, Lehto, Van Luit, & Hautamäki, 2003) and overall math ability through adolescence (Jarvis & Gathercole, 2003). In early grades, nonverbal ability, short-term memory, and working memory predict math skills; however, longitudinally, working memory emerges as the better predictor (Passolunghi & Cornoldi, 2008). Over time, visual short-term memory (e.g., spatial span tasks) and visual working memory have been found to predict math achievement (Bull, Espy, & Wiebe, 2008; McLean & Hitch, 1999). These findings suggest involvement of the visual-spatial sketchpad in math disabilities (McKenzie, Bull, & Gray, 2003).

Passolungui and Siegel (2004), in their study of working memory, examined the role of the central executive in dyscalculia. Similarly, scores on the visual-spatial sketchpad are more strongly related to 8-year-old children's mathematical performance than to 10-year-old students' performance (J. Holmes & Adams, 2006). In contrast, measures of working memory and shifting abilities did not explain unique variance in the preschool sample; however, scores on working memory measures have predicted unique variance in the mathematical performance in school-age children (Bull & Scerif, 2001; Xuan et al., 2007). Factor modeling revealed that the central executive as well as visual-spatial sketchpad components of working memory accounted for unique variance in scores on different mathematical skills (J. Holmes & Adams, 2006). Unique variance in 7-year-old children's scores on a group mathematics test was explained by measures of working memory, inhibition, and flexibility scales when intelligence quotient scores and reading ability were controlled (Bull & Scerif, 2001a).

While most have focused on evaluating the impact of working memory on mathematics skills (Bull et al., 1999; J. Holmes & Adams, 2006; Jenks et al., 2007), research specific to short-term memory is equivocal (McLean & Hitch, 1999; Passolunghi & Cornoldi, 2008; Silver, Ring, Pennett, & Black, 2007; J. L. White, Moffitt, & Silva, 1992). Many researchers believe that long-term memory plays a role in dyscalculia, but exactly what that role is seems uncertain (Bull & Johnston, 1997). One theory links number-sense difficulties to difficulty with retrieval from long-term memory; because their understanding of numbers is weaker, children with dyscalculia do not find number facts to be meaningful enough to be stored in long-term memory (Robinson et al., 2002).

Processing Speed

Other tasks revealed that children with dyscalculia had a significantly slower processing speed than their peers (Bull & Johnston, 1997). In fact, processing speed was the best predictor of math abilities. There are concerns, however, about implicating processing speed in dyscalculia, because the deficit may be at least partially environmental. It is unclear whether processing speed deficits stand alone or are due to a lack of automaticity with facts that could be remediated or even a lack of familiarity with the material (Hitch & McAuley, 1991).

Visual-Perceptual Ability

Others have examined the profiles of children with math learning disabilities in relation to visual-spatial skills (Proctor et al., 2005). Although no general cognitive differences emerged, visual-spatial thinking emerged as a relative weakness for the sample with math disabilities. The association between visual-spatial skills and math reasoning has been identified in previous research as well (Geary, 1994; Rourke, 1993; Strawser & Miller, 2001).

Assessment Considerations

The current emphasis in Individuals with Disabilities Education Improvement Act (IDEIA) for math learning disability is less focused on fluency and more focused on calculation skills and math reasoning. The Cross-Battery Assessment (Flanagan et al., 2007) includes a domain for math that incorporates conceptual and calculation subtests

Table 3.2 Evidence-Based Interventions for Math

Interventions	Target	Status/Reference
Mathematics Recovery (Wright, Stewart, Stafford, & Cain, 1998)	Early math skills	Promising practice (Griffin, 2007)
Number Worlds Program	Number concepts and meaning	Promising practice (Griffin, 2007)
Round the Rug Math (Casey, 2004)	Early childhood: Spatial sense	Promising practice (Griffin, 2007)
Building Blocks (Sarama & Clements, 2004)	Early childhood: Spatial sense and geometry	Promising practice (Griffin, 2007)
Sequential Direct Instruction	Computation/Algorithms	Promising practice (S. Baker et al., 2002; Kroesbergen & Van Luit, 2003; Kroesbergen, Van Luit, & Maas, 2004)
Use of Manipulatives	Computation	Promising practice (F. M. Butler, Miller, Crehan, Babbitt, & Pierce, 2003; Cass, Cates, Smith, & Jackson, 2003)
Mnemonic Strategies	Computation/Algorithms	Promising practice (Maccini & Hughes, 2000)
Self-Monitoring and Performance Feedback	Computation	Promising practice (S. Baker et al., 2002; K. Bennett & Cavanaugh, 1998; Shimabukuro, Prater, Jenkins, & Edelen-Smith, 1999)
FAST-DRAW (Strategy Instruction)	Computation/Algorithms	Promising practice (The Learning Toolbox, n.d.)
Reciprocal Peer Tutoring	Computation/Algorithms	Positive practice (S. Baker et al., 2002; Fantuzzo, King, & Heller, 1992; Rathvon, 2008)
Cognitive Tutor® Algebra I	Middle school math/Algebra	Promising practice (Institute of Educational Sciences, 2007)
Copy-Cover-Compare	Automaticity (math facts)	Promising practice (Institute of Educational Sciences, 2007)
Connected Mathematics Project©	Middle school math	Inconclusive (Institute of Educational Sciences, 2007)
I CAN Learn® Pre-Algebra and Algebra	Middle school math/Algebra	Positive practice (Institute of Educational Sciences, 2007)
Metacognitive Strategies	Math problem solving	Promising practice (Montague, 2008)
Saxon Middle School Math©	Middle school math/Algebra	Positive practice (Institute of Educational Sciences, 2007)
The Expert Mathematician™ (TEM)	Middle school math	Promising practice (Institute of Educational Sciences, 2007)
Transition Mathematics	Middle school math	Inconclusive (Institute of Educational Sciences, 2007)
University of Chicago School Mathematics Project (UCSMP) Algebra	Middle school math/Algebra	Positive practice (Institute of Educational Sciences, 2007)

from standard achievement tests including the WJ III, the Kaufman Test of Educational Achievement, Second Edition, and the Wechsler Individual Achievement Test, Second Edition. Alternatively, benchmarking as part of response to intervention program (RtI) or curriculum-based measurement is more likely to take a fluency or automaticity of math facts approach; this is also possible to do using the Math Fluency subtest of the WJ III. These measures provide an indication of the child's mathematical abilities in two or three specific areas but do not address or identify any causal factors to the difficulties. Consistently, weaknesses in visual-spatial skills are associated with math learning disabilities, and with so many instructional approaches to mathematics relying on visual-spatial methods, identification of a weakness in this area should translate into a change in instructional methods. Given the research evidence that both working memory and other aspects of executive function are implicated in math disabilities, it is imperative that these domains of function also be assessed. Specific measures that can be used to assess visual-spatial memory, working memory, and executive function domains are identified in Chapter 1.

EVIDENCE-BASED INTERVENTIONS

Key factors in the prognosis for individuals with math learning disability include the effectiveness of classroom instruction and interventions. Because the component of math difficulty may vary across individuals, interventions need to vary depending on the type(s) of problems encountered. Many times the studies that are available related to math interventions do not meet methodological criteria, often not specifying how low math achievement was defined or conceptualized (S. Baker, Gersten, & Lee, 2002); variation in how math disability is defined further complicates review of math interventions. Table 3.2 provides a listing of interventions; however, many of the studies reviewed and referenced may be specific to children with low math achievement as opposed to a math disability.

From a neuropsychological perspective, the metacognitive skills and use of strategies (e.g., executive function processes) also may be the target of interventions. There is some support for the use of mnemonics, explicit goal setting, and self-monitoring, for example, to address deficits in executive processes, including attention and working memory, that affect math performance (Hayden & McLaughlin, 2004; Hayter, Scott, McLaughlin, & Weber, 2007; Schraw, 1998; Seabaugh & Schumaker, 1994). Teaching of metacognitive strategies has been found to result in improved math performance for children with math learning disability (Montague, 2008; Montague, Applegate, & Marquard, 1993).

CASE STUDY: CARL—DYSCALCULIA

The next report is from a hospital-based clinic. Identifying information, such as child and family name, teacher or physician name, and school information, has been altered or fictionalized to protect confidentiality.

Reason for Referral

Carl is a 13-year-old male referred for evaluation by his mother due to concerns with academic progress, particularly in math.

Assessment Procedures

Behavioral observations
Clinical interview
Differential Abilities Scale, Second Edition (DAS-II)
Wechsler Individual Achievement Test, Second Edition (WIAT-II)
Delis-Kaplan Executive Function System (D-KEFS)
Clinical Evaluation of Language Fundamentals (CELF-IV)
Wechsler Intelligence Scale for Children, Fourth Edition (WISC-IV) Integrated (selected subtests)
Neuropsychological Assessment, Second Edition (NEPSY-2)
Behavior Assessment System for Children, Second Edition (BASC-2)

Background Information

Home

A 13-year-old teenager from a working-class suburb in a major metropolitan area in the Northeast, Carl was described as somewhat of a loner, and had few friends in school, but he did enjoy playing fantasy computer games online with others. Carl lived at home with his mother, an employed worker in a retirement home, and had little contact with his frequently unemployed father, who had legal and housing problems. Carl was described as a "sweet" but "lonely" youth, who frequently spent time in his room watching television or using the computer. Although his mother reported a positive relationship with Carl, she said they were not close, in part because her work required evening and weekend hours.

Medical

The birth and developmental histories were reportedly unremarkable, other than Carl being slow to interact with others. He had no history of major illness, but he did have a fall resulting in a laceration above his right eye from falling on a coffee table at age 5. The mother reported that he was evaluated for a concussion and received four sutures, but no further treatment was undertaken. Carl reportedly had adequate vision and hearing and was in good health at the time of the evaluation. He seemed to have difficulty going to sleep at night and getting up in the morning, according to his mother and self-report. Despite his slim appearance, Carl reported that he "ate like a horse" and this had not changed in recent times.

Educational

School was never a priority for Carl, according to his mother. He seemed to enjoy reading fantasy or science fiction books, but often balked at other academic subjects and had few aspirations aside from completing high school. Although the teacher reported he was quite good at reading, Carl was described as a "quiet" youth who had considerable difficulty with math computation and problem solving. He also had poor planning, organization, and self-management skills, and his locker was a "chaotic mess." He had difficulty with work completion, and his homework was seldom done or turned in to the teacher.

Behavioral Observations

Classroom Observations

Carl was observed during language arts and mathematics classes. Little change in behavior was observed during the observation periods. Carl was not disruptive or overtly noncompliant but instead was quiet, reserved, and withdrawn. He looked frequently at others and out the window but rarely interacted with his teachers or peers. Although these inattentive behaviors resulted in frequent off-task behaviors, Carl was on task more in language arts (78%) than in mathematics (52%) class yet did not complete the assignment or turn in homework in either class. When the math teacher asked Carl about his work, he said "I forgot"; when pressed, he complained it was "too hard."

Assessment Observations

Carl presented as a 13-year, 6-month-old slim youth with dark hair and eyes. Dressed casually in jeans and a sweatshirt, Carl appeared to have adequate hygiene, but his hair was disheveled and he had dark circles under his eyes. During the initial conversation with the examiner, Carl was reluctant to respond and did not make eye contact; however, he became more engaged when asked to discuss the computer games he enjoyed. During testing, Carl was fairly focused and persistent, but his response style was reflective, measured, and slow. He stared blankly during oral instructions and asked for repetition at times but did not have difficulty with oral directions, suggesting he was temporarily distracted. Oral expression was accurate but limited in output, and occasionally his grammar was awkward, as words were spoken out of sequence. Sequencing problems also were noted on rote and more complex cognitive and neuropsychological tasks. Carl's affect was generally flat, with little change in oral or facial expression regardless of the task or his success rate.

Assessment Results

Cognitive and Neuropsychological Functioning

On the DAS-II, Carl obtained a General Conceptual Ability (GCA) Scaled Score (SS; mean = 100, standard deviation = 15; higher scores = better performance) of 87, placing him in the upper end of the low average range compared to his same age peers. There was considerable variability among factor scores, ranging from average Verbal Ability (SS = 103), to impaired Processing Speed (SS = 68). As a result of this within and between factor variability, the GCA does not appear to be a reliable and valid indicator of Carl's global intellectual functioning (see Table 3.3). Instead, an idiographic approach to interpretation was undertaken.

Although Carl had some qualitative difficulty with expressive output, his Verbal Ability scores were solidly in the average range. He had little difficulty with defining vocabulary terms or identifying similarities among words, suggesting he has adequate crystallized ability, lexical-semantic knowledge, receptive and expressive language, and concordant-convergent thought. Consistent with this impression, Carl had no difficulty with encoding and retrieval of meaningful information presented both verbally and visually, suggesting adequate long-term memory. In addition to some of the grammatical/word order problems noted during oral expression, sequencing problems also were observed when Carl was asked to use sensory attention and working memory skills for immediate recall of

Table 3.3 Psychometric Summary for Carl

	T-Score	Standard Score
Differential Ability Scales-II		
Verbal Ability		103
Word Definitions	48	
Verbal Similarities	56	
Nonverbal Ability		82
Matrices	44	
Sequential/Quantitative Reasoning	34	
Spatial Ability		84
Recall of Designs	44	
Pattern Construction	37	
Working Memory		85
Recall of Digits Forward	40	
Recall of Digits Backward	46	
Recall of Sequential Order	35	
Processing Speed		68
Speed of Info Process	30	
Rapid Naming	35	
Object Memory		
Recall of Objects-Immediate	52	
Recall of Objects-Delayed	44	
Delis-Kaplan Executive Function System (D-KEFS)	**Scaled Score**	
Verbal Fluency Test		
Letter Fluency	7	
Category Fluency	12	
Category Switching Total	8	
Trail Making Test		
Letter Sequencing	7	
Number Sequencing	5	
Letter-Number Switching	6	
Visual Search	11	
Motor Speed	9	
Color Word Interference Test	**Scaled Score**	
Inhibition	4	
Inhibition/Switching	5	
Color Naming	9	
Word Reading	8	
Auditory Attention	6	
Clinical Evaluation of Language Fundamentals, Fourth Edition (CELF-IV)	**Scaled Score**	
Recalling Sentences	8	
Concepts	7	
Following Directions	7	

(continued)

Table 3.3 *(Continued)*

	Scaled Score	Standard Score
Wechsler Intelligence Scale for Children, Fourth Edition (WISC-IV) and WISC-IV Integrated		
Digit Span Forward	6	
Visual Digit Span Forward	7	
Digit Span Backward	9	
Spatial Span Forward	9	
Spatial Span Backward	11	
Block Design	7	
Block Design Multiple Choice	11	
Neuropsychological Assessment, Second Edition (NEPSY-2)	**Scaled Score**	
Speeded Naming	6	
Auditory Attention and Response Set	8	
Animal Sorting	4	
Visuomotor Precision	5	
Woodcock Johnson Tests of Cognitive Ability, Third Edition (WJ-III Cognitive)		
Decision Speed		81
Wechsler Individual Achievement Test, Second Edition (WIAT-II)		
Reading Composite		93
Word Reading		100
Pseudoword Reading		96
Reading Comprehension		91
Math Composite		66
Numerical Operations		76
Mathematical Reasoning		64
Written Language Composite		93
Spelling		97
Written Expression		92
Oral Language		
Listening Comprehension		104

orally presented meaningful and numeric stimuli. At the same time, he was inconsistent on working memory tasks, with scores in the average to low-average range.

Carl appeared to have fairly adequate novel problem solving, hypothesis testing, and fluid inductive reasoning skills with visual-spatial stimuli, but there were qualitative differences between his performance on the Matrices subtest and the Sequential and Quantitative Reasoning subtest, with the latter possibly reflecting difficulty with part-whole inductive reasoning or sequential processing of numeric information. This pattern also could account for the finding that constructional praxis or visual-spatial-motor integration skills were adequate, yet he struggled on some items and displayed a slow response style on a task that required analysis and synthesis of block patterns, again demonstrating difficulty with integrating part/detail and whole/global perceptual relationships (see Table 3.3).

Carl had the greatest difficulty with quick efficient responding when asked to identify similar numbers among a group of distracters and rapid confrontation naming. Although

Carl was accurate, he responded to few items on both tasks, suggesting difficulty with processing or psychomotor speed. Graphomotor concerns were not observed during testing; and Carl's handwriting was reportedly good, and an examination of written products revealed very neat, careful letter formation and word/letter spacing, yet this was entertained as a possible cause for poor processing speed during subsequent hypothesis testing.

Cognitive Hypothesis Testing

On the basis of history, prior data collection, and intellectual/cognitive screening, several hypotheses were developed and subsequently evaluated. First, despite adequate skills in many domains, Carl appeared to struggle with sequential processing, understanding of part-whole relationships, and processing speed, which secondarily appeared to negatively affect oral expression, working memory, and other executive functions. As a result, a number of additional measures were administered to test these hypothesized deficit areas.

Although language was not a significant concern, results and observations suggest Carl could have had difficulty with language formulation and sequential processing, both of which can affect oral expression. The Delis-Kaplan Executive Function System (D-KEFS; $M = 10$, SD = 3) Verbal Fluency Letter (SS = 7), Category (SS = 12), and Category Switching (SS = 8) subtests were in the average to low-average range, suggesting lexical/semantic and categorical information facilitates verbal retrieval. His Clinical Evaluation of Language Fundamentals (CELF-4) Recalling Sentences (SS = 8) and Concepts and Following Directions (SS = 7) subtest scores were fairly adequate, but sequencing problems were noted on both tasks, as he would occasionally reproduce the right stimuli, but in the wrong order.

Consistent with these findings, Carl struggled somewhat with sequencing information, but not digit recall, on the auditory WISC-IV/WISC-IV Integrated Auditory Digit Span Forward (SS = 6) and Visual Digit Span Forward (SS = 7) tasks. In addition, his Digit Span Backward (SS = 9) score was adequate, similar to the DAS-II findings, and he did not have similar problems on the Spatial Span tasks (Forward SS = 9, Backward SS = 11), suggesting the addition of spatial information for working memory demands facilitated Carl's performance. As might be expected given his DAS-II performance, Carl's NEPSY-2 Speeded Naming (SS = 6) subtest score was well below average. These findings suggest Carl has some difficulty with quick, efficient verbal retrieval from long-term memory, especially during confrontation naming situations and/or when required to order or sequence information, which could be due to executive deficits. Although not significant deficits, these findings could explain some difficulty with expressive language output, accuracy, or efficiency.

Further evaluation of executive functioning revealed Carl indeed had considerable difficulty with quick efficient performance, decision speed, sequencing, and online monitoring of performance. Although accurate, Carl's performance on the WJ III Decision Speed subtest was in the low-average range (SS = 81), suggesting difficulty with quick, efficient decision making. His D-KEFS Trail Making Test Letter Sequencing (SS = 7), Number Sequencing (SS = 5), and Letter-Number Switching (SS = 6) were quite low given his adequate Visual Search (SS = 11) and Motor Speed (SS = 9) subtest scores. He also had considerable difficulty with Color-Word Interference Test Inhibition and Inhibition/Switching subtests (SS = 4 and SS = 5 respectively), but not the Color Naming (SS = 9) or Word Reading (SS = 8) ones. He had some difficulty with initial sustained auditory attention (SS = 6) but did better when flexibility and inhibition were required on the response set task (SS = 8) on the NEPSY-2 Auditory Attention and Response Set subtest. Although his Animal Sorting (SS = 4) score was quite low, Carl focused on card arrangements rather than details within the cards, thereby apparently invalidating the results.

Although processing speed problems appeared to be due to executive deficits, it was important to determine if problems could be related to visual, motor, or integration problems. Carl's NEPSY-2 Visuomotor Precision score was adequate for accuracy (26–50th percentile), but slow (SS = 5). Finger tapping was adequate for both hands (26–50th percentile), yet he had some difficulty with sequencing finger movements (6–10th percentile right hand, 11–25th percentile left hand). His performance on the WISC-IV Block Design subtest was in the low average range (SS = 7), yet his WISC-IV Integrated Block Design Multiple Choice performance was average (SS = 11), suggesting he could correctly identify spatial relationships among component parts. Although visual-spatial explanations for Carl's processing speed issues could be ruled out on the basis of hypothesis testing results, the findings suggested some minor difficulty with motor coordination and control (praxis), which could secondarily affect visual-motor coordination and processing speed. Ordering and sequencing information, performing tasks quickly and efficiently, easily accessing stored lexical/semantic information, and simultaneous integration of multiple psychological processes, especially in unstructured situations, appears to be difficult for Carl.

Academic Functioning

The achievement testing completed by an educational diagnostician resulted in average scores in reading, writing, and language functioning but considerable difficulty with math skills. Problems with math concepts, computation/algorithm adherence, and math fact automaticity were noted.

Social-Emotional and Behavioral Functioning

In addition to these cognitive and neuropsychological findings, the Behavior Assessment System for Children, Second Edition (BASC-2) teacher report indicated few externalizing problems, but considerable problems with lethargy, anhedonia, negative affect, withdrawal, inattention, and learning problems.

Summary and Diagnostic Impressions

Carl was a quiet, reserved, and withdrawn 13-year-old youth with considerable math difficulty and psychosocial concerns. Although his difficulty could be explained in part by his poor motivation and work completion, his pattern of performance suggests considerable problems with integration of multiple psychological processes, sequencing of information, decision making, and processing speed. He also evidenced subtle difficulties with oral expression and praxis. Taken together, these results are consistent with executive dysfunction that affects not only Carl's mathematics performance but also his psychosocial functioning. The interaction between his cognitive, academic, and psychosocial functioning provide a framework from which to develop multiple interventions designed to meet Carl's unique needs.

Recommendations

Educational Implications

For the math problems, Carl was given direct metacognitive instruction designed to help him use self-talk strategies to work through math problems. He was given direct instruction and a step-by-step algorithm sheet that showed him how to break down math tasks into subcomponent parts, change sentences into equations, and then complete each step in the calculation. After these steps, Carl checked his work against the algorithm sheet, thereby allowing him to monitor his progress, completion, and successful response to math problems (i.e., a modification to cover-copy-compare). He also was given math fact fluency instruction, as automaticity in math fact retrieval would free working memory to address the sequential problem solving issues. Additional interventions were designed to foster verbal retrieval and fluency as well as grammar (for the word choice/sequencing issues), use of a timer to self-chart time to homework completion, and a home-school report card with privileges as reinforcers to foster work completion in the class and home. Although graphomotor skills appeared to be adequate, the team thought they would monitor Carl for difficulty with praxis.

Psychological Implications

For psychosocial functioning, Carl was encouraged to join the computer club at school, a place where he could share his interest with others. Finally, Carl was provided with cognitive-behavior therapy and a psychiatric consult to consider possible difficultics with lethargy, anhedonia, withdrawal, and depression. Although attention concerns were reported, Carl did not have problems with hyperactivity, and the team felt that the psychiatric consult could further address whether his attention problems were secondary to sleep disturbance and/or depressive symptoms with appropriate medical interventions.

Accommodations and Modifications

Strategy instruction and positive reinforcement for strategy use combined with self-monitoring are the major components of classroom accommodations. Carl may need additional scaffolding and positive prompts in order for interventions to be successful in effecting change.

Further Discussion of Case Study

The case conceptualization here used the Cognitive Hypothesis Testing (CHT) model (Hale & Fiorello, 2004; Hale et al., 2003). CHT is intended to provide a framework for integrating cognitive assessment into the problem-solving model that assists in hypothesis testing initially based on individualized single-subject interventions and progress monitoring. Taken together, the case study information (child response to intervention and progress or lack thereof) with theoretical knowledge of neuropsychology links assessment to empirically supported interventions (Hale & Fiorello, 2004). CHT is further intended to improve the reliability of the more traditional attempts at profile analysis through the continued incorporation of case study data as interventions are implemented, monitored, evaluated, and recycled. This is a unique component of the CHT approach: The conclusion is a hypothesis that includes not only a problem identification but a potential solution; the approach is a continuing process that uses individual responsiveness to add further to problem clarification. It is based theoretically in cognitive and neuropsychological theory and has a growing base of support (Hale & Fiorello, 2004). CHT assigns specific subtypes—fluid/quantitative reasoning subtype, executive/working memory subtype, numeric-quantitative knowledge, right-hemisphere nonverbal learning disability, and dyscalculia-Gerstmann syndrome—based on the pattern of strengths and weaknesses across specific ability areas (Hale et al., 2008). As noted earlier in the chapter, there is a clear association of executive function with some mathematical skills; the CHT framework as employed here identified executive function as the underlying psychological process that was contributing to Carl's learning disability in mathematics. Consistent with this premise, the interventions suggested address deficits in executive function as well as math skills.

An alternate model of conceptualizing math achievement and disability relies more directly on the hierarchical model of intelligence derived from Cattell-Horn-Carroll (Floyd, Keith, Taub, & McGrew, 2007; Hale, Fiorello, Kavanaugh, Hoepner, & Gaither, 2001). Using a large sample and examining the general and broad cognitive abilities, it was found that regardless of age, fluid reasoning, crystallized intelligence, and processing speed demonstrated statistically significant direct effects on achievement (Taub, Floyd, Keith, & McGrew, 2008). Of these, the Fluid Reasoning component comes closest to measuring executive function. Taub et al. further found that, regardless of age, the general intelligence score had only indirect effects on math achievement.

CONCLUDING COMMENTS

The incidence of math learning disability, or dyscalculia, is comparable to that of other disorders; moreover, math disability co-occurs with many other disorders (Shalev et al., 2000). Unfortunately, the same level of extensive research has not been done in this area; only recently has math disability become an area of research. Although multiple perspectives can be used in identification and conceptualization of math disabilities (CHT, CHC, nonverbal learning disabilities), on an individual basis, it is important to identify those neuropsychological domains that are or are not intact in order to inform intervention planning. Of the neuropsychological domains, those abilities most related to working memory and executive function seem to be implicated most often in conjunction with difficulties in mathematics (dyscalculia). Which mathematical tasks (i.e., arithmetic, algorithmic calculation, word problems) are best predicted by which measures of executive function has not been studied extensively, particularly among adolescents and adults. The extent to which math difficulties can be habilitated, the means to intervene effectively, and the longitudinal outcomes associated with math difficulties all require more research.

Chapter 4

SPECIFIC LANGUAGE IMPAIRMENT/ DYSPHASIA

DEFINITION

Specific language impairment (SLI) is a developmental disorder defined by unexplained delayed language learning in children with normal global intellectual functioning, hearing acuity, and exposure (Stark & Tallal, 1981; Tomblin, Smith, & Zhang, 1997). Children with SLI typically exhibit limited vocabulary knowledge, underdeveloped or unusual syntax, and impaired grammatical morphology (Bishop, 1992; Bishop & McArthur, 2005). Language impairment may be primary and occur in the context of otherwise normal development, or the impairment may be secondary to mental retardation, autism, or other disorder (Schuele, Spencer, Barako-Arndt, & Guillot, 2007). In research, children with SLI are those children who exhibit a deficit in expressive and/or receptive language despite normal nonverbal ability (Bartlett et al., 2002; Newbury, Bishop, & Monaco, 2005; D. Williams, Stott, Goodyear, & Sahakian, 2000); those children with nonverbal ability below 85 may be identified with nonspecific language impairment (H. Catts, Fey, Tomblin, & Zhang, 2002). The *Diagnostic and Statistical Manual of Mental Disorders*, Fourth Edition Text Revision (*DSM-IV*-TR) (American Psychiatric Association [APA], 2000) identifies three types of specific language disorders: expressive language disorder, mixed receptive-expressive language disorder, and phonological disorder.

Expressive language disorder is the most prevalent language disorder among young children (B. A. Lewis, Freebairn, & Taylor, 2000) and is characterized by a child's limited ability to learn new vocabulary, restricted speech production, and difficulty in the acquisition of grammatical aspects of language (L. B. Leonard, 1998). Children with mixed receptive-expressive language disorder not only exhibit limited vocabulary but also demonstrate comprehension difficulties. Receptive deficits have been linked with verbal short-term memory deficits as well as phonological processing problems in adulthood (Clegg, Hollis, Mawhood, & Rutter, 2005). Phonological disorder is characterized by the child's inability to make age-appropriate speech sounds. These language deficits hinder a child's ability to acquire new vocabulary, contributing to deficits in global language learning and academic difficulties (Tallal, 2003, 2004).

In neurological or neuropsychological contexts, disorders of language usually are identified as acquired (aphasia) or developmental (dysphasia); regardless of whether acquired or developmental, there are multiple levels and types of language disorders (Schuele et al., 2007). For children, although some of these disorders may in fact be acquired, the effects are delays in language development. *Dysphasia* is then a disorder of language produced by deviation or early injury to brain areas specialized for these functions; dysphasia (or specific language impairment) can be broken down into various types, depending on function(s) impacted (see Table 4.1). In most cases, regardless of the type of language disorder, children may be eligible for special educational services under the category of speech impaired.

Auditory Processing Disorders

Related to language disorders are a range of auditory processing disorders. Auditory processing disorder (APD) encompasses auditory perceptual deficits in the individual's ability to localize, discriminate, recognize patterns, store, filter, sort, or attach meaning to auditory signals despite normal hearing (American Speech-Language-Hearing Association, 1996). With APD, there is little disruption of sensitivity to changes in sound

Table 4.1 Types of Language Disorders

Term	Definition
Dysarthria	Disorder in coordination of musculature of mouth
Paraphasia	Production of unintended syllables, words, or phrases during the effort to speak; sounds articulated correctly, but they are the wrong sounds (e.g., saying "pike" instead of "pipe")
Fluent aphasias	Speech is fluent but difficulties either in auditory verbal comprehension or in the repetition of words, phrases, or sentences spoken by others
Nonfluent aphasias or Broca's aphasia	Difficulty in articulating but relatively good auditory verbal comprehension
Wernicke's aphasia	Inability to comprehend words or arrange sounds into coherent speech
Transcortical aphasia (isolation syndrome)	Individuals can repeat and understand words and name objects but cannot speak spontaneously or cannot comprehend words/sentences even though they can repeat them (echolalia)
Conduction aphasia	Individual can speak easily, name objects, and understand speech but cannot repeat words; some debate as to whether this is aphasia or a memory problem
Anomic aphasia	Comprehension, production of meaningful speech, and repetition intact; individual has difficulty remembering the actual names of objects; frequently talks around the name of the object, thus indicating knowledge of the object (circumlocution). In fluent speech, individual may use the object name at other times, demonstrating that it is not that he or she just doesn't "know" the word; described as partial amnesia for words
Agnosia	Inability to name an object although individual recognizes object
Aprosodia	Disorder (expressive or receptive) of prosody: rhythm, intonation, emotional expression in speech
Auditory processing disorder	Deficits in individual's ability to localize, discriminate, and/or recognize patterns, and/or store, filter, sort, or attach meaning to auditory signals despite normal hearing
Ataxic dysarthria	Slower production of syllables, unusual prosodic patterns, loss of distinct phonological contrasts: /da/ versus /ta/

frequency or intensity; however, the individual may have difficulty with discriminating sounds at specific rates or in judging simultaneity of sounds, or impairment in judging the order in which the sounds were heard. With unilateral temporal lobe damage, processing is impaired such that the individual may complain that others are talking too quickly due to his or her inability to discriminate between sounds rapidly. The impact is more severe if there is damage to the left temporal lobe as opposed to the right temporal lobe; the left temporal lobe is seen as particularly important in discrimination of speech sounds and related to Wernicke's aphasia (J. Katz & Smith, 1991). Auditory processing is believed to be neuromaturational in nature (Bishop & McArthur, 2005), with delays or deviations in the developmental process resulting in similar symptoms as cortical deafness or unilateral damage to temporal lobes. In general, there is a high co-occurrence of auditory processing deficits within the group of individuals with language impairment as well as those with reading disability (Bishop & McArthur, 2005; McArthur, Ellis, Atkinson, & Coltheart, 2008).

In addition to language and auditory disorders, there are multiple speech-related disorders. These include the mechanical disorders of speech (e.g., dysarthria, speech apraxia) that are due to incoordination or motor impairment of musculature of mouth or vocal apparatus. It is not unusual for children or adults with fine motor problems also to have articulation problems, and vice versa. When all possible facets of SLI are considered, the importance of considering individual differences, rather than group characteristics, is evident (Bishop & McArthur, 2005).

Differential Diagnosis

One of the more difficult tasks facing clinicians is that of differential diagnosis of SLI as opposed to hearing impairment, global intellectual disability, and pervasive developmental disorder/autistic spectrum disorder. This is particularly true of autism, where the chief complaint of parents is frequently that of language disorder or communicative deficits (see Chapter 5). Early diagnosis of SLI often is hampered because the child may appear to be intellectually disabled (D. J. Cohen, Caparulo, & Shaywitz, 1976); language delays are also frequent among children with Down syndrome (see Chapter 15). Adaptive behavior is one means that is frequently used to distinguish between children with global impairments of cognition and children with more narrowly defined disorders (Grossman, 1983). It has been found that, in particular, children with SLI who did not obtain equivalent scores across all adaptive domains were more likely to evidence a relative weakness in the area of communication than in any other adaptive behavior domain (T. W. Powell & Germani, 1993).

Incidence and Prevalence

Because language impairment can occur in conjunction with other disorders, it is estimated that up to 20% of children have some form of language learning impairment (Beitchman, Brownlie, & Wilson, 1996; S. E. Shaywitz, Shaywitz, Fletcher, & Escobar, 1990). That said, depending on how it is defined, SLI occurs in approximately 3% to 15% of children ranging in age from 3 to 21 years (APA, 2000; L. B. Leonard, 1998; Riccio & Hynd, 1993; Tomblin et al., 2005). An estimated 5% to 10% of these children evidence difficulties of sufficient severity to warrant referral and subsequent intervention (Aram & Hall, 1989; Bliss, Allen, & Walker, 1978; H. Catts et al., 2002). In one large epidemiological study, 7.4% of kindergarten children were identified as delayed in language areas

(Tomblin et al., 2005). Thus, disorders of language are among the most common disorders of higher cerebral function in children.

ETIOLOGY

Genetic Influences

A number of family studies have been completed and indicate a genetic contribution to SLI (Barry, Yasin, & Bishop, 2007; Bishop, Laws, Adams, & Norbury, 2006; Conti-Ramsden, Falcaro, Simkin, & Pickles, 2007; M. L. Rice, 2007; Spitz, Tallal, Flax, & Benasich, 1997; Tallal et al., 2001). For example, in one study, SLI occurred in 13.0% of children when neither parent was affected, 40% of children with one parent affected, and 71.4% of children in families when both parents were language impaired (Tallal et al., 2001). In another study (Conti-Ramsden et al.), there was a strong relationship between proband severity and the increased occurrence of SLI in first-degree relatives. Further, there is some indication that deficits in nonword repetition serve as a marker for familial SLI (Barry et al., 2007; M. L. Rice, 2007). Some of the difficulties in determining the heritability of SLI are related to variance in how SLI is defined, whether children are identified through universal screening, speech problems, or limited to more severe cases (Bishop & Hayiou-Thomas, 2008).

Genetic components of SLI are not well defined, but there are indications that genetic contributions to SLI may be most similar to the genetic contributions to the language problems associated with autism as opposed to reading disability/dyslexia (S. D. Smith, 2007). There has been some indication of the involvement of 16q and 19q in SLI; when considering these two regions and two aspects of language—phonological short-term memory and tense or verb grammar morphology, respectively—results indicated a strong familial association on the phonological task (Falcaro et al., 2008). Family aggregation was evident only on the morphology (tense) task when results were considered dichotomously (i.e., normal, not normal) as opposed to continuously.

Of the components of SLI, speech sound disorder has been associated with linkage to 15q14–21 (Stein et al., 2006). Chromosome 15 also has been associated with oral-motor function, articulation, and phonological memory. Linkages have also been identified on chromosome 13q21 with additional loci on chromosome 2 and 7 (Bartlett et al., 2004; Bartlett et al., 2002). The language deficits associated with speech sound disorder are evident across disorders including SLI, autism (see Chapter 5), and reading disability (see Chapter 2) as well as Prader Willi syndrome and Angelman's syndrome (see Chapter 15).

Environmental Factors

A number of prenatal, perinatal, and postnatal factors may play a role in the disruption or delay of normal language development. Prenatal or perinatal factors that may predispose the child to language disorders include anoxia, congenital or perinatal infections (including rubella, herpes, and cytomegalovirus), jaundice, low birth weight, and the mother's use of cigarettes, drugs, and/or alcohol; data continue to be correlative, and results of studies examining these factors are equivocal (Aram, Hack, Hawkins, Weissman, & Borawski-Clark, 1991; M. Lahey, 1988).

Otitis Media with Effusion

Research suggests that the occurrence of multiple ear infections (otitis media with effusion [OME]) in the first postnatal year is highly correlated with auditory perception problems and delayed language development (Nittrouer & Burton, 2005; Tallal & Benasich, 2002). Animal studies demonstrated that blocking off of the ear (lack of stimulation) will result in lack of development of the auditory cortex. Further, there is evidence that three to five or more ear infections in first year of life decreases auditory stimulation and therefore impacts later learning. Previously it was believed that the auditory cortex would be affected only at the discrete interval or point in time when "infection" occurred. It is now believed that there is a period, before and after the pain associated with recognition of infection, when the auditory signal is degraded or affected somehow (Nittrouer & Burton, 2005). The time before and after the occurrence of pain therefore may affect the differentiation of the auditory cortex. Moreover, ear infections are treated with antibiotics that are themselves ototoxic (impact on the auditory system and in particular the cochlea, including hair loss); antibiotics as a result can impact on the signal:noise ratio (auditory figure ground). As a result, prolonged or frequent otitis media may lead to problems in hearing, attending to, or comprehending auditory communication (J. E. Roberts & Schuele, 1990).

Although there is some consensus that phonological deficits may be genetically determined, auditory processing deficits are explained more often by environmental factors not related to medical issues (Bishop, 2002). In fact, it is widely accepted not only that genetics contribute to SLI but that environmental factors are involved (Conti-Ramsden et al., 2007). For example, it has been proposed that environmental factors play a role in the development of language asymmetry. The notion has been that during the first year, the auditory cortex needs to receive "k" amount of stimulation (auditory) to help with the differentiation of the auditory cortex and develop auditory perception skills. For example, study of individuals who are illiterate or deaf demonstrates that experience with language somehow influences cerebral asymmetry. Three hypotheses are:

1. Disuse of the left hemisphere results in degeneration.
2. In the absence of auditory stimulation, the left hemisphere is inhibited somehow by the right hemisphere.
3. The left hemisphere takes on some other function when it is not stimulated auditorally (Conti-Ramsden et al., 2007).

Home Environment

The hypotheses just described not only attempt to explain why frequent loss of hearing due to otitis media may affect language even after the infection has passed but also implicate the level of stimulation in the home as contributing to language development. For example, studies with individuals who are exposed to two languages from birth suggest that early exposure to more than one language can affect the cognitive development of children (Bialystok, 2001). Alternatively, low socioeconomic status and presumed low language exposure is associated with language delays comparable to that associated with otitis media (Nittrouer & Burton, 2005). This is consistent with findings from studies related to early literacy and the literacy environment of the home (V. J. Molfese, DiLalla, & Lovelace, 1996).

Neurological Correlates

Most children with SLI do not have obvious signs of focal deficit on neurological examination, do not demonstrate electroencephalographic abnormality, and do not exhibit identifiable lesions on standard computed tomography or magnetic resonance imaging (MRI) of the brain. There is some indication of greater likelihood of diffuse polymicrogyria in the area of the sylvian fissure on neuropathological investigation (M. J. Cohen, Campbell, & Yaghmai, 1989) and MRI (Guerreiro et al., 2002). These are shown in Figures 4.1 and 4.2. Results of functional MRI (fMRI) studies indicate that individuals with SLI evidence abnormal activation of both the temporal and frontal areas as compared to controls, with weaker bilateral activation (Hugdahl et al., 2004). Assuming that the majority of these children are left-hemisphere dominant for propositional language, these findings would indicate that these children are experiencing dysfunction involving the left (language-dominant) cerebral hemisphere contrasted by relatively spared functioning of the right cerebral hemisphere. This interpretation is consistent with the findings reported in neuropathological (M. J. Cohen et al., 1989) and neuroimaging studies (E. Plante, Swisher, & Vance, 1989; E. Plante, Swisher, Vance, & Rapcsak, 1991) of children with SLI that indicate that significant pathology or variation exists in the morphological development of language-related cortex and associated subcortical systems.

For the majority of individuals with SLI, there is no major neurological anomaly (Im, Park, Kim, Song, & Lee, 2007), but there may be some indication of neurological abnormalities when structural differences in morphometry are considered (Trauner, Wulfeck, Tallal, & Hesselink, 2000). For example, there are indications of reduced overall cortical and subcortical volume in children with SLI (Jernigan et al., 2002) as well as reduced volume of areas associated with language (e.g., pars triangularis in Broca's area) in some individuals with SLI (Gauger, Lombardino, & Leonard, 1997). It has been suggested

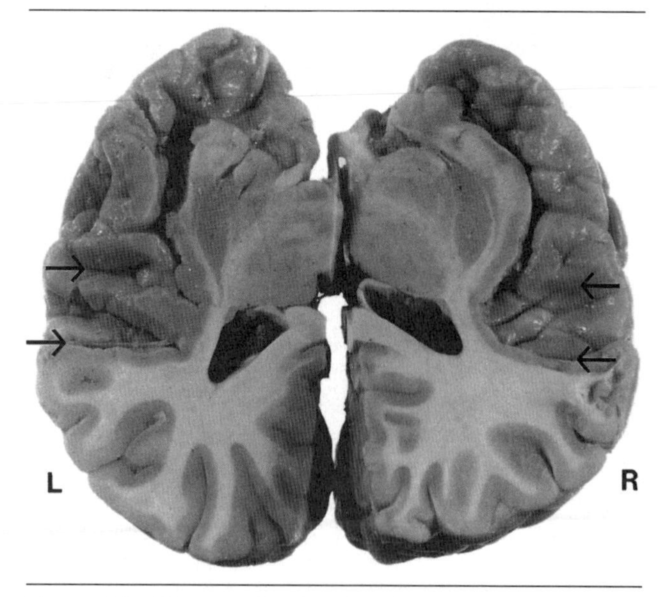

Figure 4.1 Photograph of brain showing symmetry of the plana temporale as measured from the sulcus of Heschl (top arrow) to the posterior margin of the planum temporale (bottom arrow) on the left (L) and right (R).

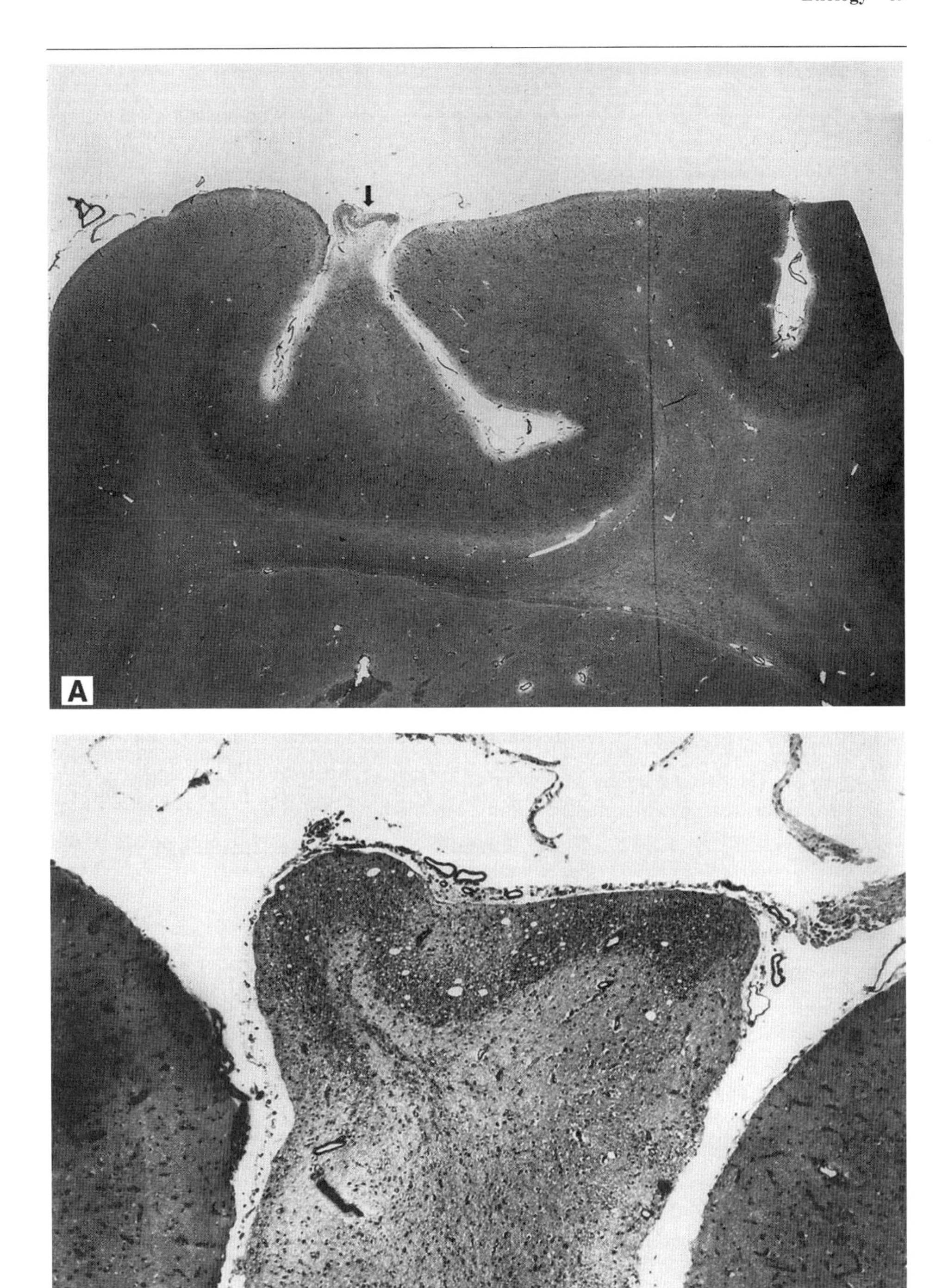

Figure 4.2 (A) Section of the left insular cortex showing a single dysplastic microgyrus (arrow) adjacent to normal gyri. (B) Detail of the dysplastic gyrus showing an abnormal presence of a subpial band of myelinated fibers in the usual location of the molecular layer. Underneath this sparse zone is a population of large, medium, and small neurons. Thus, the normal laminar arrangement of cortical neurons is absent.

that relatively smaller symmetrical brain structures are associated with the level of difficulties in comprehension evidenced with SLI; this is a different pattern than is associated with reading disability (C. M. Leonard et al., 2006). Glucose metabolism, as measured with positron emission tomography and indicates decreased metabolism in bilateral frontal and temporal as well as right parietal regions (Im et al., 2007). Consistent with these findings, fMRI studies indicated that children with SLI exhibit significant hypoactivation in those areas with both attention and memory as well as language processing with reliance on a less functional network than controls (Weismer, Plante, Jones, & Tomblin, 2005). Functional MRI also indicated abnormal activation of the temporal and frontal lobes during language encoding and recognition tasks (Hugdahl et al., 2004). Further, children with SLI evidenced increased metabolism bilaterally in the occipital lobes (Im et al., 2007). Notably, frontal and cingulate areas were activated by individuals with SLI on a task-switching paradigm but were not activated by controls (Dibbets, Bakker, & Jolles, 2006).

The interaction and extent of integration of functional systems in speech and language is evident from multiple studies, and includes not only specific structures and nuclei but also underlying white matter. For example, with developmental stuttering, it was found that there was reduced integrity of the white matter underlying the regions of the ventral premotor cortex (Giraud et al., 2008; Packman, Code, & Onslow, 2006); the white matter then connects to the posterior superior temporal and inferior parietal cortex. It is this latter connection that allows for the articulatory planning and sensory feedback necessary for fluent speech and that, in turn, connects to the motor cortex. These same structures and others are intricately involved in aspects of speech and language (Giraud et al., 2008). The cerebral cortex and caudate have been found to be relatively smaller in individuals with SLI, but given that whole brain white matter was larger than controls, differences were not significant (Herbert, Ziegler, Makris et al., 2003). Another study with children with SLI indicated decreased white matter volumes in the left hemisphere and the motor cortex, the dorsal premotor cortex, the ventral premotor cortex, and the planum polare of the superior temporal gyrus (Jäncke, Siegenthaler, Preis, & Steinmetz, 2007).

Laterality of Language Function

In the majority of individuals, language dominance is associated with the left hemisphere. Lateralization of language is believed to occur early in development and increase with age (Hiscock, 1988; Ressel, Wilke, Lidzba, Lutzenberger, & Krägeloh-Mann, 2008). Using dichotic listening tasks as a measure of language lateralization as well as temporal lobe integrity, as a group, children with SLI demonstrated left, rather than right, ear advantage (M. J. Cohen, Riccio, & Hynd, 1999); however, this is not consistent across studies. In fact, when individual rather than group results are considered, there appear to be subgroups of those with deficient right ear performance, those with deficient left ear performance, and those with deficient performance bilaterally. These differences may reflect lateralization of language and present qualitative differences in terms of prognosis and developmental trajectory of language skills (M. J. Cohen et al., 1999).

Asymmetry

Whole-brain study suggested right-asymmetrical cortex in both individuals with SLI and those with autism; asymmetry differences were greatest in higher order association areas (Herbert et al., 2005). Rightward asymmetry of the inferior frontal region (Broca's area) as well as the posterior superior temporal cortex have also emerged in conjunction with SLI and autism (De Fosse et al., 2004). These similarities are not unexpected given the extent to which communication deficits are a part of autism spectrum disorders (see Chapter 5).

Additional studies also indicate reversed or absent expected asymmetry. For example, individuals with SLI have been shown to lack the normal left greater than right asymmetry of the planum temporale (Cowell, Jernigan, Denenberg, & Tallal, 1995; C. M. Leonard et al., 1993; A. E. Morgan & Hynd, 1998; Tallal et al., 1990); the planum temporale is believed to have a role in speech comprehension and phonological processing with nonleftward asymmetry associated with linguistic deficits (Chiarello, Kacinik, Manowitz, Otto, & Leonard, 2004; Hiemenz & Hynd, 2000; A. E. Morgan & Hynd, 1998). Comparison of children with SLI and children with dyslexia yielded significant differences in plana asymmetry as well as the size of a single left Heschl's gyrus (Lester et al., 2002). Notably, at least one study did not find any evidence of nonleftward asymmetry of the planum temporale or the planum parietale (Preis, Jäncke, Schittler, Huang, & Steinmetz, 1998); this may reflect differences in age of participants, methodology, or sampling. Atypical asymmetry of the frontal lobes also has been found for individuals with SLI (Jernigan, Hesselink, Sowell, & Tallal, 1991; J. P. Larsen, Hoien, Lundberg, & Odegaard, 1990). Finally, atypical asymmetrical findings have emerged for the parietal region (Cowell et al., 1995; Jernigan et al., 1991). The combined differences in patterns of asymmetry are believed to be reflected in decreased activation of frontal and posterior temporal regions (Hagman et al., 1992; Rumsey et al., 1992).

Cytoarchitectonic Findings

It is hypothesized that brain abnormalities associated with SLI include ectopias and polymicrogyria (Guerreiro et al., 2002). Polymicrogyria evident across the sylvian fissure on MRI were associated with both phonological and syntactic deficits; more parietal locations of the polymicrogyria were associated with predominantly phonological deficits (Guerreiro et al., 2002). Across children with SLI, it was found that those with posterior cortical involvement tended to have milder forms of SLI than those with profuse polymicrogyria in the perisylvian cortex, who presented with more severe SLI (de Vasconcelos Hage, Cendes, Montenegro, Abramides, Guimarães, & Guerreiro, 2006). The presence of polymicrogyria also has been associated not only with SLI in children but with reading disorder in parents, supporting a familial link (Oliveira et al., 2008).

Frontal Lobes

The frontal lobe is believed to be involved in paralinguistic deficits, including deficits in speech output, associated with medial frontal regions. This often is tested by asking individuals to generate words beginning with a target letter (usually F, A, or S) or specific category; these types of frontal tasks generally are believed to reflect left frontal function (Perret, 1974). Frontal damage may be evidenced in lexical retrieval of words for which there are multiple associations (e.g., verb associates to "cat") but not when there are limited associations possible, such as to "scissors." On these types of tasks, the activation is in the left inferior frontal region in typically developing individuals and is related to the need to "select" which associations to generate (Justus & Ivry, 2001). An fMRI study indicated significant differences in brain activation in the inferior frontal and temporal regions in response to auditory stimuli for families with SLI as compared to controls (Hugdahl et al., 2004). Morphology of the inferior frontal gyrus was examined in parents of children with SLI and controls (M. M. Clark & Plante, 1998). The two groups could be discriminated based on the presence of morphometric anomaly (e.g., extra sulcus) of the inferior frontal gyrus. The association of SLI with Attention-Deficit/Hyperactivity

Disorder (ADHD; see Chapter 6) also has been considered to support frontostriatal dysfunction in SLI (D. Williams et al., 2000).

Cerebellar Deficits

Cerebellar deficits are widely reported in individuals with SLI. Cerebellar damage has been associated with ataxic dysarthria (e.g., slower production of syllables, unusual prosodic patterns, loss of distinct phonological contrasts:/da/ versus /ta/). Further, the temporal differences (voice onset time, stress) may be evident not only in production but in perception with cerebellar dysfunction (Ackermann, Gräber, Hertrich, & Daum, 1999; Ackermann, Mathiak, & Ivry, 2004; Murdoch & Whelan, 2007). Based on several studies, right cerebellar lesions are associated with atypical responses on word generation tasks that involve categories (lexical retrieval) as opposed to phonemic retrieval (Fabbro et al., 2000; Ravizza et al., 2006). Cerebellar damage also is associated with verbal fluency for both phonemic and semantic tasks (Ghosh, Tourville, & Guenther, 2008). Problems in retrieval and fluency do not appear to be directly associated with speech production problems that may be associated with cerebellar damage; the problems may reflect the need to engage articulatory representations for linguistic processing (Justus & Ivry, 2001).

COURSE AND PROGNOSIS

The prognosis for children with SLI, based on retrospective data, is relatively guarded with a direct relationship between prognosis and the severity of the language impairment (Aram, Ekelman, & Nation, 1984; M. Lahey, 1988; Schuele et al., 2007). In about 25% of cases, children identified at age 5 will not demonstrate continued difficulty with intervention; in about 75% of cases, the SLI will continue to be present through age 12 and into adulthood (Beitchman et al., 1994). Research consistently suggests that speech and language impairments have a negative impact on the acquisition of reading and writing skills (Puranek, Petscher, Al Otaiba, Catts, & Lonigan, 2008; Schuele et al., 2007). Children who evidence language delays prior to age 3 are at risk for other neuropsychiatric disorders, including autism (see Chapter 5) and ADHD (see Chapter 6) by age 7 (Miniscalco, Nygren, Hagberg, Kadesjö, & Gillberg, 2006); in effect, the language impairment may be secondary to some other disorder; or other disorders, such as ADHD, may be secondary to the SLI. Of those children with SLI, regardless of the etiology, children with severe receptive language disorder are more likely to have less positive outcomes and more long-term problems (A. Clark et al., 2007).

The extent to which SLI is associated with reading problems is such that it has been argued that language impairment and learning disabilities often are distinguished only by the age of the child at the time of diagnosis (H. Catts et al., 2002). Where the SLI is less severe, language problems may not be recognized until school entry. Language disorders often can be quite subtle and may manifest as a learning disorder rather than language impairment because these language problems surface in the child's difficulty learning to read, keeping up with peers, attending to group lessons, and getting organized (Paul, 1992; Wallach, 1984). Over time, those children with speech problems or whose language problems are resolved early have a better prognosis than those who continue to evidence SLI in elementary grades (C. J. Johnson et al., 1999; Young et al., 2002). By young adulthood, individuals with an early history of language impairment are at risk of being behind controls in all areas of academic achievement, not just reading and written expression.

Rates of learning disabilities are also higher for those individuals with SLI than base rates in the community (Young et al., 2002).

Neuropsychological Correlates

Cognitive Ability

One study examined the cognitive ability and achievement profiles of 21 children with developmental language disorders as compared to 26 children with learning disabilities (Rose, Lincoln, & Allen, 1992). Both groups of children demonstrated similar degrees of reading, spelling, and arithmetic disability; however, they differed markedly on verbal subtests of cognitive measures. Specifically, the children with SLI were significantly more impaired than children with learning disabilities on verbal subtests. Further, while the subtests comprising the verbal comprehension cluster (Information, Similarities, Vocabulary, Comprehension) were significantly intercorrelated for the children with learning disabilities, these subtests did not intercorrelate significantly for the children with SLI. Rose and colleagues suggested that these findings would be indicative of less integrated verbal capacities in some children with SLI (Rose et al., 1992). Similar qualitative differences on verbal and nonverbal tasks also have been demonstrated in other studies (see Table 4.2).

For example, another study (Riccio, Cash, & Cohen, 2007) indicated that for children with SLI, nonverbal intelligence was generally in the low-average to average range with the children tending to exhibit a significant language/visual-spatial discrepancy in favor of their nonverbal/perceptual abilities. This discrepancy was found to be significantly greater for those children with more global impairments (Receptive/Expressive subtype). In fact, across areas of cognition, academic achievement, and behavior problems, the children in the Receptive/Expressive subtype demonstrated a pattern of greater impairment as compared to the Expressive-only subtype. Comparison of the Receptive/Expressive and Expressive subtypes revealed not only significant differences for receptive vocabulary, as would be expected, but also for Verbal IQ and Full Scale IQ. The borderline nonverbal ability by the Receptive/Expressive subtype was believed to be highly related to difficulty in comprehending the complex verbal directions and/or the extent to which verbal mediation may facilitate performance on the nonverbal tasks presented (Riccio et al., 2007) and supports previous findings of differential performance of children with SLI on nonverbal tasks (Kamhi, Minor, & Mauer, 1990; Swisher & Plante, 1993).

Phonological Awareness and Skills

In particular, children with SLI are initially at risk for phonological difficulties; alternatively, they may master phonological decoding without difficulty but have significant difficulties with comprehension. The latter manifests as hyperlexia (see Chapter 2). Characteristics of hyperlexia include advanced word recognition skills in the absence of comprehension (Glosser et al., 1996, 1997; Huttenlocher & Huttenlocher, 1973; C. M. Temple, 1990). The combination of strengths and weaknesses suggests that visual pattern recognition is a key component to the presentation of hyperlexia in children with specific language impairment (M. J. Cohen et al., 1997). As noted in Chapter 2, *hyperlexia* is the term used to describe children who read words at levels beyond that expected (Silberberg & Silberberg, 1967). The high frequency with which this occurs in conjunction with SLI suggests that this is a disorder of language rather than one of reading. Characteristics of hyperlexia include advanced word recognition skills in combination with reading comprehension that is more consistent with impaired language

Table 4.2 Neuropsychological Domains and Effects of Specific Language Impairment

Domains	Specific Deficits
Cognition	Verbal abilities less integrated; nonverbal abilities tend to be in average to low-average range
Auditory-linguistic/ Language function	Prosody Pragmatics Right ear deficiency on dichotic listening tasks Difficulty with verbal fluency
Visual perception/ Constructional praxis	Difficulty with mental rotation tasks
Learning and Memory	Updating of working memory found to be impaired Deficits in verbal memory Deficits in verbal working memory Deficits in visual-spatial memory
Processing speed	Some indication of slower processing of verbal information but results equivocal
Executive function	Difficulty in metacognition, planning, problem solving, self-regulation Ability to shift mental set may be spared Difficulty with inhibition of prepotent response No difficulty noted on task-switching
Attention/Concentration	Difficulty with attentional capacity Subgroup may evidence attentional control difficulties
Motor function	Mild delays in acquisition of gross motor skills; some difficulties with fine motor dexterity
Achievement/Academic skills	Hyperlexia Learning disability In young adults, individuals with SLI from early childhood tend to lag significantly behind in all areas of academic achievement
Emotional/Behavioral functioning	At-risk for anxiety and social phobia by late adolescence SLI correlated with attention deficits, conduct disorder, internalizing disorders, aggression

(M. J. Cohen et al., 1987; Glosser et al., 1996, 1997; Huttenlocher & Huttenlocher, 1973; C. M. Temple, 1990). Despite the fact that 96% of the children with learning disabilities demonstrated significant deficits consistent with SLI, only 2% were receiving services to address these linguistic deficits (Gibbs & Cooper, 1989). When these data are taken into account, it is very likely that the current prevalence of SLI is significantly underestimated.

Memory

One theoretical perspective on SLI is that the language deficits manifest as a result of problems or deficits in phonological short-term memory. Specifically, it has been asserted that short-term auditory memory, as represented by the phonological loop, has an important role in language acquisition and vocabulary development (Baddeley, Gathercole, & Papagno, 1998). Within this context, short-term auditory memory can be defined as the retention of small amounts of information over brief periods of time (Baddeley, 2000). Working memory provides a system for holding (via rehearsal) and manipulating incoming information during the performance of a complex cognitive task (Baddeley, 2000); thus, working memory requires one to attend to, concentrate on, and manipulate auditory information. In addition, early research demonstrated that children with SLI experienced difficulty repeating sentences of increasing length (Menyuk & Looney, 1972) and performed more poorly on the Token Test as the length of the command increased (Tallal, 1975). Further, it has been demonstrated that children with SLI experienced deficient immediate auditory working memory as the linguistic/semantic demands of the tasks increased; in contrast, immediate visual working memory was spared (M. J. Cohen et al., 1999).

In one of the first studies designed to examine learning and immediate recall of pictured objects, children with SLI had decreased verbal short-term storage "capacity," presumably due to diminished ability to process, organize, and maintain information in working memory (Sininger, Klatzky, & Kirchner, 1989). Studies employing different list learning procedures, such as the California Verbal Learning Test—Children's Version (CVLT-C) (Shear, Tallal, & Delis, 1992) and the Rey Auditory Verbal Learning Test (Records, Tomblin, & Buckwalter, 1995) as well as a study that used a digit-span backward test (D. Williams et al., 2000) provide further support for the "diminished verbal capacity" theory.

While research to date appears to support the contention that children with SLI exhibit poorer performance on auditory short-term memory tasks and auditory working memory tasks, little available research has looked at auditory long-term retention and visual/nonverbal learning and memory in this population. In one study, the children with SLI were not significantly impaired on the delayed free recall component (20-minute delay) of the CVLT-C (Shear et al., 1992). This finding would appear to indicate that although the children with SLI were less efficient in learning the word list, their delayed recall of the list was not significantly below that of the normal children. It is not clear whether these children have a dysfunctional immediate auditory/verbal working memory system or merely give the appearance of having dysfunctional auditory/verbal memory as a secondary manifestation of the SLI (M. J. Cohen et al., 1997).

Research has found that children with auditory short-term memory deficits have impaired expressive language ability (N. J. Cohen et al., 2000), lagged behind their counterparts on standardized measures of language by 18 to 24 months (S. Gathercole & Baddeley, 1989, 1990), have difficulty learning the phonological form of new words (Baddeley, Papagno, & Vallar, 1988; Newbury et al., 2005; Trojano & Grossi, 1995), and exhibit deficits in retaining sequentially ordered information (Montgomery, 1996). Furthermore, phonological working memory and vocabulary growth were highly correlated (S. Gathercole, Willis, Emslie, & Baddeley, 1992) while working memory skills were shown to predict performance on phonemic awareness tasks in 7- and 8-year-old students (Oakhill & Kyle, 2000). Supporting the connection between auditory working memory ability, language development, and achievement, children with poor attainment on reading comprehension and vocabulary subtests on standard achievement tests at age 7 demonstrated significantly impaired performance on working memory assessment (S. Gathercole & Pickering, 2001).

Attention/Concentration

Based on studies with behavior rating scale data obtained from the parents and teachers of children with SLI, there is an increased (higher than base rate) incidence of children with behavioral features of ADHD. When comparing visual attention in children with normal hearing, children with hearing aids, and children with cochlear implants using a visual continuous performance test and visual cancellation task, groups did not differ on either of the visual attention tasks (Tharpe, Ashmead, & Rothpletz, 2002). In a follow-up study of preschoolers with unresolved language delay, there was higher than typically expected incidence of attention problems in adolescence (Snowling, Bishop, Stothard, Chipchase, & Kaplan, 2006). While the finding of a comorbid relationship between SLI and ADHD is generally consistent with previous research (L. Baker & Cantwell, 1990; Cantwell & Baker, 1991; Riccio & Hynd, 1995; Riccio, Hynd, Cohen, Hall, & Molt, 1994), the increased frequency raises the intriguing question of whether these children possess two independent disorders or if the behavioral features of inattention are a secondary manifestation of SLI.

Executive Function

It has been suggested that there is significant interaction between language processes and executive function (i.e., metacognition) as well as self-regulation (Denckla, 1996; Hayes, Gifford, & Ruckstuhl, 1996; B. D. Singer & Bashir, 1999). Hayes et al. (1996) asserted that executive functions are "all about the connection between . . . verbal abilities and actual behavior regulation" (p. 300). On typical card-sorting and tower tasks of problem solving, children with SLI demonstrated increased perseverative errors as well as rule violations as compared to controls (Marton, 2008). In contrast, shifting of mental set was not found to be impaired in children with SLI relative to a control group (Im-Bolter et al., 2006).

Processing Speed

There is research to suggest that children with SLI may process information at a slower rate than their peers (L. B. Leonard et al., 2007). Correlations between processing speed and language level have not been shown to be significant, suggesting that some factor other than language accounts for the slowed processing (M. Lahey et al., 2001). Results of other studies suggest that verbal working memory may be the underlying cause of the apparent sluggish cognitive tempo. Nonverbal working memory also may account for some of the variance in processing speed (L. M. D. Archibald & Gathercole, 2007; L. B. Leonard et al., 2007).

Academic Achievement

Deficits in auditory short-term memory and working memory not only hinder the language development of children with SLI, but they also have been shown to place them at risk for inadequate academic achievement and identification as learning disabled (A. Adams & Gathercole, 2000; Tomblin et al., 2000). Differences in auditory short-term memory have been found to be related to, and predictive of, vocabulary skills, depending on the age of the subjects (Jarrold, Baddeley, Hewes, Leeke, & Phillips, 2004). In effect, the connection is greater for younger children and decreases after age 8. At the same time, however, some research suggests that even if the language impairment resolves during elementary school, the children continue to be at risk for learning disabilities in reading and written expression (Snowling, Bishop, & Stothard, 2000; Stothard, Snowling, Bishop, Chipchase, & Kaplan, 1998).

Other studies have indicated that those children with speech impairments may be at even greater risk for difficulties in reading (Carroll & Snowling, 2004; Sutherland & Gillon, 2007). A recent study that used oral reading fluency for benchmarking found that a large proportion of students with speech or language impairment were not able to meet grade-level benchmarks in first to third grades, with lowest scores among those students with speech/language impairment who had been identified with specific learning disability (Puranek et al., 2008).

Emotional/Behavioral Problems

Individuals with SLI are at increased risk of psychiatric disorder across the life span (Brownlie et al., 2004; Clegg et al., 2005; Tomblin et al., 2000), with some indication that emotional and behavioral problems are mediated by reading disability (Tomblin et al., 2000). Studies consistently indicate a higher rate of anxiety and depression in adolescents with a history of SLI, particularly among girls (Benasich, Curtiss, & Tallal, 1993; Conti-Ramsden & Botting, 2008; Riccio & Hynd, 1993; Snowling et al., 2006). Most recently, it has been determined that SLI increases the likelihood of social phobia in particular (Voci et al., 2006). Alternatively, rates of aggression, delinquency, and conduct disorder tend to be more frequent among boys with SLI (Brownlie et al., 2004). Prognosis is particularly poor for those children with receptive language problems (Beitchman, Brownlie, Inglis et al., 1996) and for those whose language deficits are not resolved by age 6 (Snowling et al., 2006). At 15-year follow-up, for those with unresolved language delays, by adolescence there was an increased incidence of social problems, particularly in those with both expressive and receptive difficulties (Snowling et al., 2006). Further, it has been found that preschool children with SLI frequently demonstrate behavior problems (e.g., hyperactivity, inattention, social withdrawal, immaturity, dependency). It has been suggested that these behavioral problems may be secondary to the SLI (N. J. Cohen et al., 2000). Studies have indicated a frequent codiagnosis of ADHD, in particular, for children with SLI (L. Baker & Cantwell, 1990; Beitchman, Hood, & Inglis, 1990; Cantwell & Baker, 1991; Riccio & Hynd, 1995).

Assessment Considerations

Comprehensive evaluation of language function, usually requiring the collaboration of a speech language pathologist, is critical in developing an appropriate intervention plan for children and adolescents with SLI. Additional evaluation should be undertaken with measures selected that are able to parse out the language problems from the domain being assessed. For example, in selecting a measure of cognitive ability, it is imperative that the language loading of the measure (even if nonverbal in response requirements) be considered. At the same time, psychometric properties need to be considered. The Leiter International Performance Scale—Revised (Leiter-R), Universal Nonverbal Intelligence Test (UNIT), Wechsler Nonverbal Scale, and Naglieri Nonverbal Ability Test are examples of some nonverbal measures with adequate psychometric abilities. Memory is also important to consider, both in assessment and in designing appropriate instructional programs. Additionally, it is important not to ignore the potential confounding behavioral and emotional problems. Interventions that focus only on the language component may not be as effective as when combined with other interventions to address co-occurring problems. Identification of appropriate target behaviors for intervention requires comprehensive evaluation of domains other than language.

EVIDENCE-BASED INTERVENTIONS

The most obvious targets of intervention are in language areas (see Table 4.3). Children with SLI frequently are referred and receive speech/language services either individually

Table 4.3 Evidence-Based Status of Interventions for Specific Language Impairment

Interventions	Target	Status
Explicit instruction in phonological processing	Phonological awareness	Promising practice (Schuele et al., 2007; Troia, 1999)
Parent-child shared reading	Phonological awareness	Emerging (Justice, Kaderavek, Bowles, & Grimm, 2005)
Computer-assisted phonological awareness training	Phonological awareness	Emerging (Segers & Verhoeven, 2004)
Fast ForWord®	Language	Promising practice (W. Cohen et al., 2005; Gillam et al., 2008; Merzenich et al., 1999; Tallal, 2000)
Phonemic awareness or phonological processing training	Reading	Emerging (Blischak, Shah, Lombardino, & Chiarella, 2004)
Parent training/Shared reading	Reading	Emerging (Justice et al., 2005; Skibbe, Justice, Zucker, & McGinty, 2008)
Hybrid language intervention	Reading	Emerging (Munro, Lee, & Baker, 2008)
Mental imagery training	Reading comprehension	Emerging (Joffe, Cain, & Maric, 2007)

or in small groups; few studies have examined differing methods of providing language therapy. One such study (Boyle, McCartney, Forbes, & O'Hare, 2007) explored five different approaches and found no significant differences between direct and indirect modes of therapy, on one hand, or between individual and group modes, on the other, across language outcome measures. They did, however, find that direct therapy with a speech language therapist delivered three times a week for 30 to 40 minutes over a 15-week period yielded significant improvements in age-corrected standardized scores for expressive language, although not for receptive language, relative to those receiving community-based services. Overall, those children with expressive language delay were more likely to show improvement than those with mixed receptive-expressive difficulties (Boyle et al., 2007).

In addition to language, children with SLI potentially present with myriad difficulties; for that reason, a multidisciplinary collaboration is needed to ensure that a comprehensive intervention program is designed that addresses not only the linguistic deficits but the associated neurocognitive deficits and behavioral difficulties as well (Riccio & Hynd, 1995; Riccio, Hynd et al., 1994). For example, given the high rate of attentional problems associated with SLI (L. Baker & Cantwell, 1990; Cantwell & Baker, 1991; Riccio & Hynd, 1995; Riccio, Hynd et al., 1994), it would seem appropriate to identify and address attentional issues as well as linguistic ones. Doing this would best utilize an interdisciplinary approach to intervention planning; however, the majority of research with regard to children with SLI comes from the field of speech language pathology. Given the potential impact of home environment, early intervention that addresses the home language and literacy environment is seen as one approach to improving outcomes (Justice et al., 2005; Skibbe et al., 2008).

Reading

It has been argued that early intervention in the area of phonological awareness for children with SLI is beneficial. The difference in instruction may be removal of corresponding requirements to map speech sounds to print for those children with SLI (Justice, Chows, Capellini, Flanigan, & Colton, 2003; O'Connor, Jenkins, Leicester, & Slocum, 1993; van Kleeck, 1990). Specific interventions that target rhyming, blending, and segmenting of sounds have been found to be generally effective (Justice et al., 2005; S. Laing & Espeland, 2003; O'Connor et al., 1993; van Kleeck, Gillam, & McFadden, 1998), with some variability. Indications are that for children with SLI, instruction may need to be in small groups rather than classroom based. Further, children with SLI may have difficulty with generalization, thus necessitating explicit instruction (S. Laing & Espeland, 2003). Explicit instruction also may be required to affect the mapping of speech sounds to print; this is not likely to be as intuitive for children with SLI as it is with typically developing children. Because of their deficits in comprehension, children with SLI rely more on the graphophonemic strategies for decoding than language; they are not able to use context cues to identify unfamiliar words in text (Kouri, Selle, & Riley, 2006).

CASE STUDY: NAYA—DYSPHASIA/SLI

The next report is from a hospital-based clinic. Identifying information, such as child and family name, teacher or physician name, and school information, has been altered or fictionalized to protect confidentiality.

Reason for Referral

Naya is a 10-year-old fifth grader who is being initially evaluated by the pediatric neuropsychology service at the request of her pediatrician, who is following Naya for a history of language and learning/memory difficulties. As a result, neuropsychological evaluation was undertaken in order to assess higher cortical functioning and make appropriate recommendations regarding school placement and the need for supportive therapies.

Assessment Procedures

- Clinical interview (parent)
- Behavioral observations
- Wechsler Intelligence Scale for Children, Fourth Edition (WISC-IV)
- Neuropsychological Assessment (NEPSY)/Neuropsychological Assessment, Second Edition (NEPSY-2; selected subtests)
- Peabody Picture Vocabulary Test, Fourth Edition (PPVT-IV)
- Boston Naming Test (BNT)
- Clinical Evaluation of Language Fundamentals, Fourth Edition (CELF-IV; selected subtests)
- Kaufman Assessment Battery for Children, Second Edition (KABC-2; selected subtests)
- Dichotic Listening Test

Finger Oscillation Test
Delis-Kaplan Executive Function Scale (D-KEFS; selected subtests)
Developmental Test of Visual Motor Integration, Fifth Edition (DTVMI-V)
Children's Memory Scale (CMS)
Gray Oral Reading Test, Fourth Edition (GORT-4)
Wechsler Individual Achievement Test, Second Edition (WIAT-II)
Behavior Assessment System for Children, Second Edition (BASC-2; Parent and Teacher Rating Scales)
DSM-IV ADHD Checklist (Parent)

Background Information

Home

Naya resides with her mother. Naya's parents were never married. Naya's father is 36 years of age. He completed high school and is currently employed as a manager of a Wal-Mart. He has since married and has a 6-year-old daughter who is doing well in the first grade and is in good health. Naya's mother is 34 years of age, has a college degree in education, and works as a kindergarten teacher. Both parents are reported to be in good health. The paternal family medical history is significant for a great-uncle with depression and a second great-uncle with intellectual disability of unknown etiology. The maternal family medical history is negative for neurological and psychiatric disorder.

Developmental and Medical History

Review of developmental and medical history with Naya's mother indicates that Naya is the product of a normal full-term pregnancy and vaginal delivery requiring the use of forceps. Naya weighed 6 pounds 2 ounces at birth, did well as a newborn, and went home with her mother on day 3. Developmental motor milestones were obtained within normal limits, with sitting up occurring at 6 months of age and walking at 10 months of age. Developmental language milestones were delayed in that Naya was only babbling at 2 years of age. As a result, she underwent speech/language evaluation and began receiving therapy. At 3 years of age, the therapy was provided at Naya's daycare as part of her preschool special education services. Toilet training was fully accomplished at 3 years of age. Aside from the usual childhood illnesses, Naya's past medical history is unremarkable. There is no reported history of seizures or head injury, and Naya has a normal appetite and sleep pattern.

Educational History

Review of educational history indicates that Naya began receiving significantly developmentally delayed (SDD) special education preschool services at her daycare when she turned 3. At 4, Naya attended a preschool classroom at her daycare, where her mother reported that Naya continued to receive SDD preschool special education services along with speech/language therapy. Naya began attending elementary school for kindergarten. According to her mother, speech/language therapy and preschool special education services were discontinued. In first grade, Naya began having difficulty grasping spoken language and with reading comprehension although her reading skills were good. Even though Naya was beginning to experience difficulty, she passed all of the state Criterion Referenced Competency Testing (CRCT) at the end of the year. According to Naya's mother, second grade was a "difficult year" in that her teacher reported that Naya was having problems focusing and her grades began to fall. As a result, a student support team referral was implemented. When the team met, difficulty with reading comprehension, math problem solving, memory, short attention span, auditory perceptual problems, and speech/language problems were noted. According to Naya's mother, suggestions for intervention were made, but the team never reconvened. Further, Naya did not pass CRCT testing in reading and English in the spring of that year.

During the summer, the family moved to a neighboring county and Naya began attending third grade. Naya did well that year without services. Fourth grade "was a disaster" in that Naya struggled throughout the year to earn passing grades. As a result, her mother requested a response to intervention (RtI) program for reading comprehension and mathematics, which began the following September or October. No written record of this was provided by the mother or the school system. Review of a school report form completed by Naya's teacher indicated that she was very concerned about

> Naya's ability to listen and comprehend spoken language. When she does give an answer, it doesn't always match the question. Often she will just stare and give no response at all and will appear anxious as though she wants to answer. She will nervously try to take some action like erase things on her paper even without having an eraser.

At present, Naya is attending the fifth grade, where she has four different teachers. Her mother stated that she is also attending Early Intervention Program (EIP) classes for reading and mathematics. Naya's pediatrician requested an audiological and a neuropsychological evaluation. In the spring of fifth grade, Naya was evaluated by an audiologist in private practice. Audiometric testing revealed normal pure tone responses across all frequencies in both ears. Further, assessment of auditory processing was undertaken with the Test for Auditory Processing Disorders in Children—Revised (SCAN-C). Naya performed poorly on Filtered Words, Auditory Figure-Ground, Competing Words, and Competing Sentences. Based upon these results, it was felt that Naya had normal peripheral hearing in conjunction with significant auditory processing problems.

Behavioral Observations

Naya presented herself for testing as a pleasant, somewhat reserved, and neatly groomed young lady who was casually dressed in a gray top and jeans. She separated appropriately from her mother and accompanied the examiners to the testing room without difficulty. Naya was oriented and demonstrated good eye contact, although she did not readily interact with the examiners, speaking only when she was spoken to or when she was required to answer an examination question. In response to direct questions, Naya's language usage was fluent although at times she was observed to speak rapidly with mild word-finding difficulty evident. In general, her verbal comprehension was poor. As a result, directions were repeated when permissible to ensure adequate understanding of task demands. Throughout the evaluation, which consisted of two sessions separated by a lunch break, Naya's attention span, activity level, and impulsivity within the context of this one-to-one assessment were felt to be age appropriate. When confronted with more challenging tasks, Naya exhibited a slow response style with good task persistence. In general, Naya appeared eager to please and responded well to praise and encouragement from the examiners. Lateral dominance is firmly established in the right hand for paper-and-pencil manipulation. Vision with corrective lenses for nearsightedness was felt to be adequate for the purposes of this evaluation. Hearing was formally assessed and reported to be within normal limits bilaterally.

Assessment Results

Cognitive and Neuropsychological Functioning

The results of neuropsychological evaluation indicate that Naya currently is functioning within the average range of nonverbal intellectual ability as measured by the Perceptual Reasoning Index of the Wechsler Intelligence Scale for Children, Fourth Edition (WISC-IV). Due to the significant verbal-performance discrepancy noted between the Verbal Comprehension and Perceptual Reasoning Index scores, and Naya's history of language delay and auditory processing disorder, it is felt that the Perceptual Reasoning Index score represents Naya's best estimate of intellectual potential (see Table 4.4). Additional assessment indicates that Naya demonstrated significant difficulty on the Tower subtest of Neuropsychological Assessment (NEPSY), which is a measure of sequential reasoning/problem-solving capability.

Language Functioning

Naya's expressive and receptive language skills are generally in the borderline to low-average range, consistent with her history of language delay. Further, Naya's depressed right ear score on a Dichotic Listening Test for consonant vowel syllables in the face of normal left ear performance and a normal hearing evaluation would support the interpretation of dysfunction involving the left geniculotemporal pathway and central auditory processing difficulty.

Visual-Spatial and Motor Functioning

Visual-spatial perception and visual-motor integration/construction were found to be solidly average and consistent with her performance on the WISC-IV. Fine motor tapping speed was found to be relatively depressed in the right (dominant) hand as measured by the Finger Oscillation Test.

Memory and Learning

Analysis of Naya's performance on the Children's Memory Scale indicates that, at the present time, she is exhibiting average to above-average ability to hold material in immediate/working memory. When asked to learn and remember (30 minutes later) newly presented material, Naya demonstrated above-average ability to learn and immediately recall rote verbal material, such as a list of 14 word pairs presented over three learning trials, contrasted by low-average immediate recall of stories that were read to her. Thus, Naya appeared to experience difficulty processing large amounts of verbal information. Delayed recall for the same verbal information was low average to average. It should be noted that Naya's recall of the word pairs was aided by the use of a cued recall paradigm that would be indicative of organization and retrieval difficulty. This pattern of performance on verbal memory assessment is commonly seen in individuals who have difficulty processing and storing lengthy verbal material due to auditory processing and/or a language disorder. Naya's ability to learn and recall visual information is generally average with superior delayed recall of spatial location (where).

Academic Achievement

Academically, Naya demonstrated above-average oral reading fluency and spelling and average word recognition, reading comprehension, and written expression. Naya's numerical reasoning and calculation skills were low average to average.

Table 4.4 Psychometric Summary for Naya

	Scaled Score	Standard Score
Wechsler Intelligence Scale for Children, Fourth Edition (WISC-IV)		
Full Scale IQ		87
General Ability Index		94
Verbal Comprehension Index		83
Similarities	10	
Vocabulary	7	
Comprehension	4	
Perceptual Reasoning Index		106
Block Design	11	
Picture Concepts	8	
Matrix Reasoning	14	
Working Memory Index		94
Digit Span	10	
Letter-Number Sequencing	8	
Processing Speed Index		73
Coding	9	
Symbol Search	1	
Delis-Kaplan Executive Function System (D-KEFS)		
Verbal Fluency Test (Letter Fluency)		85
Neuropsychological Assessment (NEPSY) Tower		65
Neuropsychological Assessment—Second Edition (NEPSY-2)		
Phonological Processing		80
Comprehension of Instructions		70
Arrows		100
Peabody Picture Vocabulary Test, Fourth Edition (PPVT-IV)		89
Boston Naming Test (BNT)		77
Clinical Evaluation of Language Function, Fourth Edition (CELF-IV)		
Sentence Repetition		75
Formulated Sentences		85
Kaufman Assessment Battery for Children, Second Edition		
Gestalt Closure		105
Clock Face Drawing Test		
Form		110
Time (10:20)		109
Developmental Test of Visual Motor Integration–Fifth Edition (DTVMI-V)		103
Children's Memory Scale (CMS)		
General Memory Index		103
Attention/Concentration Index		122
Numbers	11	
Sequencing	16	

(continued)

Table 4.4 *(Continued)*

	Scaled Score	Standard Score
Picture Location (supplemental)	12	
Verbal Immediate Index		106
Stories	8	
Word Pairs	14	
Visual Immediate Index		109
Dot Locations	11	
Faces	12	
Verbal Delayed Index		91
Stories	9	
Word Pairs	8	
Visual Delayed Index		110
Dot Locations	14 (Max)	
Faces	10	
Delayed Recognition Index		103
Stories	8	
Word Pairs	13	
Learning Index		112
Word Pairs	15	
Dot Locations	9	
Gray Oral Reading Test, Fourth Edition (GORT-4)		
Fluency		110
Comprehension		100
Wechsler Individual Achievement Test, Second Edition (WIAT-II)		
Word Reading		108
Pseudoword Decoding		108
Written Expression		109
Spelling		111
Mathematical Reasoning		93
Numerical Operations		93

Behavior Assessment System for Children, Second Edition (BASC-2)

	T-Scores	
	Parent	Teacher
Clinical Scales		
Hyperactivity	45	44
Aggression	46	46
Conduct Problems	51	45
Anxiety	70*	42
Depression	72*	48
Somatization	39	43
Atypicality	62	45
Withdrawal	62	74*
Attention Problems	61	73*
Learning Problems	NA	64

(continued)

Table 4.4 *(Continued)*

	T-Scores	
	Parent	Teacher
Adaptive Scales		
Adaptability	44	52
Social Skills	37	29*
Leadership	34	35
Study Skills	NA	40
Activities of Daily Living	39	NA
Functional Communication	38	21*
DSM-IV ADHD Checklist	**Raw Score**	
Inattention	14/27	22/27*
Hyperactivity/Impulsivity	4/27	3/27

Notes. NA = Not applicable. Asterisk (*) denotes a significant score.

Social/Emotional and Behavioral

Behaviorally, analysis of rating scales completed by Naya's mother and teacher indicates that, at the present time Naya appears anxious and depressed in the home. Although not clinically significant, parent report also endorses a high level of inattentive behavior. Naya's teacher endorsed significant concern related to short attention span, withdrawal, social skills deficits, and poor functional communication skills.

Summary and Diagnostic Impressions

Taken together, this pattern of neuropsychological test performance is consistent with a picture of dysfunction involving the left cerebral hemisphere and a diagnosis of central auditory processing disorder and specific language impairment, mixed type. The inattention and poor social skills that Naya appears to be exhibiting at school are felt to be secondary manifestations of her language disorder. Further, even though this evaluation was carried out in a quiet, distraction-free setting, it is still remarkable that a child with Naya's history of auditory processing and language disorder was able to perform as well as she did on individually administered achievement testing, given that she does not appear to be performing at this level on a daily basis in the classroom.

Recommendations

It is recommended that Naya continue to receive EIP classroom placement along with the RtI program at her school. Naya's mother is strongly encouraged to stay involved in this process. When meeting with the RtI team members, she should feel comfortable that adequate steps are being taken to ensure that:

1. Chosen interventions involve the use of research-based methodologies.
2. Appropriate assessment tools are being used to monitor Naya's progress over the two 8- to 12-week intervention time periods.
3. The instructor is properly trained in the implementation of the interventions.

If the interventions prove to be ineffective, a referral for special education learning disability services should be initiated. In addition, Naya should be referred for a formal language evaluation and language therapy through the special education program. Thirteen additional recommendations are:

1. Given Naya's pattern of strengths and weaknesses, it is recommended that academic instruction in reading/written expression emphasize visual and multisensory approaches.
2. In light of her auditory processing disorder, teachers, therapists, and parents should keep in mind several general "rules" while interacting with Naya.
   - Eye contact should be ensured.
   - A prompt to look at the speaker before directions are presented will be helpful.
   - Instructions and directions should be kept short, simple, and concrete, and should be presented several times.
3. In order to enhance Naya's learning/retention, new material should be presented in an organized format that is meaningful to her. The material to be learned should be pretaught, broken down into smaller components/steps, and presented in a highly structured format with frequent repetition to facilitate new learning.
4. Instruction should be supplemented with visual aids, demonstrations, and experiential/procedural learning.
5. Naya would benefit from being taught how to use mnemonic strategies when learning new material and studying for tests. These include but are not limited to:
   - Rehearsal—showing Naya how to repeat information verbally, to write it, and look at it a finite number of times.
   - Transformation—instructing her in how to convert difficult information into simpler components that can be remembered more easily.
   - Elaboration—showing Naya how to identify key elements of new information and to create relationships or associations with previously learned material.
   - Chunking—instructing Naya in how to group or pair down long strings of digits or different items into more manageable units and thereby facilitating encoding and retention.
   - Imagery—showing Naya how to visualize and make a "mental picture" of information to be learned.
6. When studying for tests or doing multiple homework assignments on the same day, similar subject material should be separated in order to lessen interference. Additionally, Naya should be provided with periodic review of previously learned material in order to enhance long-term retention.
7. Accommodations will be necessary to enhance Naya's ability to succeed in the classroom, including preferential seating and additional time to complete assignments and tests.
8. Given her auditory processing disorder, consideration should be given for a trial with an auditory trainer within the classroom.
9. Given Naya's difficulty with verbal information retrieval, testing should be carried out using multiple choice/matching/true-false testing paradigms.
10. Study skills training also will be warranted emphasizing such techniques as the appropriate outlining of lecture notes and how to study for tests.

11. Naya also will benefit from being taught how to take notes on text material and plan written reports using an outlining method. In a related vein, training in word processing is strongly encouraged.
12. Given the social skills deficits reported by Naya's previous and current teachers, Naya would benefit from participation in a social skills training group.
13. Finally, if Naya continues to demonstrate significant anxiety/depressed mood at home, consideration should be given for individual therapy. Specifically, therapy should focus on reducing Naya's anxiety/depression along with enhancing her self-esteem and coping skills.

Further Discussion of Case Study

This case study illustrates research findings from various studies (Cowan, 1996; Daneman & Merikel, 1996; S. Gathercole, Hitch, Service, & Martin, 1997; Menyuk & Looney, 1972; Records et al., 1995; M. L. Rice, 2007; D. Williams et al., 2000) that children with SLI perform significantly below normal control children on measures of short-term memory for lengthy auditory/verbal material. Naya's profile is consistent with Kirchner and Klatzky's (1985) contention that children with SLI have a "diminished verbal capacity" to process, organize, and maintain auditory information in working memory. Further, children with SLI tend to do better on verbal immediate as compared to verbal delayed recall. Also of note is the finding that, although it is expected that the meaningful context of stories would support recall, children with SLI, including Naya, do more poorly on immediate story recall than on immediate recall of a list of rote word pairs or a list of words. This finding suggests that the episodic buffer proposed by Baddeley (2000) is not sufficiently intact or does not provide sufficient contextual support for children with SLI for semantically based recall. This case study demonstrates that children with SLI may possess normal or even exceptional ability to process, maintain, and manipulate visual/nonverbal information; working memory for visual/nonverbal material does not evidence the same level of impairment. Thus, the working memory system associated with the storage and retrieval of visual/nonverbal material (e.g., the visual-spatial sketchpad of Baddeley's model) appears to be intact in Naya, as is often the case for children with SLI (Riccio et al., 2007). Regardless, these findings would appear to indicate that intervention planning and programs that link verbal short-term memory with visual/nonverbal information may be useful with children with SLI. Naya has received continuous support and her academics are surprisingly within expectancy; however, the "cost" may be apparent in her anxiety and withdrawal/social skills deficits. She clearly will need continued support, given her attentional problems and deficits in functional communication.

CONCLUDING COMMENTS

For whatever reason, universal screening of language development is not conducted routinely; only those children who exhibit significant articulation or expressive language difficulties are likely to be identified at an early age (Tallal & Benasich, 2002). Others with more subtle deficits will not be identified until they enter school and encounter academic, behavioral, or social problems. In light of the risk for reading difficulties and below-average academic achievement for children with SLI (B. A. Lewis et al., 2000; H. J. Swanson, 2000), identification of possible memory deficits in young children with phonological awareness difficulties may serve to expedite the development and implementation of appropriate remediation programs and possibly divert later academic difficulty or failure (Riccio et al., 2007). At the same time, language is the basis of emotional and behavioral self-regulation. Research suggests a high co-occurrence of other disorders, particularly ADHD and autism spectrum disorders. As such, screening for behavioral and attention problems that may co-occur also is seen as critical in averting additional problems.

Chapter 5

AUTISM SPECTRUM DISORDERS

DEFINITION

The terms *autism spectrum disorders* (ASDs) and *pervasive developmental disorders* (PDDs) encompass autistic disorder, Rett's disorder, childhood disintegrative disorder, Asperger's disorder, and pervasive developmental disorder not otherwise specified (PDD-NOS) (American Psychiatric Association [APA], 2000). Due to overlapping symptoms and few absolute distinctions between autism and the other disorders on the spectrum, classical autism often serves as the prototype for ASD or PDD (Lord & Risi, 2000; Minshew, 1997; Ozonoff & Rogers, 2003). These disorders occur on a continuum of severity and represent a spectrum of disorders (Best, Moffat, Power, Owens, & Johnstone, 2008; Newschaffer et al., 2007; Strock, 2004; Whitman, 2004). Based on this conceptualization of the relation among these five disorders, the term *autism spectrum disorder* (ASD) often is used in place of the term *PDD* in an effort to underscore the presence of a continuum or spectrum. ASDs comprise a group of complex neurobiological disorders that typically lasts throughout a person's lifetime (Billstedt, Gillberg, & Gillberg, 2005; Newschaffer et al., 2007). Although the same psychological processes may occur in all individuals to some extent, the ASDs comprise a behavioral syndrome defined by deficient social interaction, language and communication difficulties, and bizarre restricted or repetitive behavior (motor) patterns (APA, 2000; Klinger & Dawson, 1996; Remschmidt & Kamp-Becker, 2006). These three characteristic domains are sometimes referred to as the autism triad (Parikh, Kolevzon, & Hollander, 2008). Symptoms exhibited by individuals on the spectrum tend to vary in severity and pattern, with some individuals having severe impairment while others having only minor impairment; extent of impairment also may vary across the behavioral triad.

Prevalence and Incidence

ASD cases in the 1960s had an estimated prevalence rate of 4 to 5 per every 10,000 live births; with changes in the diagnostic criteria and increased awareness of ASD over the years, the current incidence rate for the broad spectrum is estimated at 4 to 6 per 1,000 births (Hertz-Picciotto et al., 2006). The prevalence of autistic disorder is estimated at between 10 and 16 per 10,000 (Fombonne, 2005; Tidmarsh & Volkmar, 2003; Volkmar, Lord, Bailey, Schultz, & Klin, 2004). Because of these differences in rates, there is a perception that the incidence of ASDs is on the rise. Others argue that increases in prevalence rates do not necessarily reflect increases in incidence rates of ASDs but most likely are the result of confounding variables, such as increases in the awareness of ASDs, improvements in early detection and identification of ASDs, increases in service availability for persons with ASDs, and flaws in methodology of some epidemiological studies (Fombonne, 2005). Some methodological problems in these studies consist of population sampling errors and inconsistent diagnostic criteria used for identification.

Prevalence and incidence varies by type of ASD as well. Although it is considered a low-incidence disability (Bryson, 1996; Bryson & Smith, 1998; Ford, Riggs, Nissenbaum, & LaRaia, 1994), autistic disorder historically has been the most prevalent of the ASDs (Klinger & Dawson, 1996), with prevalence rates cited as ranging from 5 to 10 per 10,000 children (APA, 2000; Fombonne, 2003; G. Gillberg, 1993). It has been suggested that the prevalence of Asperger's disorder is much higher than that of autistic disorder, at 36 per 10,000 live births (Ehlers & Gillberg, 1993). Both autistic disorder and Asperger's disorder are three to four times more likely to occur in males than females (APA, 2000; Fombonne, 2003; G. Gillberg, 1993; Hertz-Picciotto et al., 2006; Muhle, Trentacoste, & Rapin, 2004). Data regarding the prevalence of Rett's disorder and childhood disintegrative disorder are lacking, with research often limited to case studies. Rett syndrome occurs predominantly in females, while there is some indication that childhood disintegrative disorder is more common among males (APA, 2000). The prevalence of PDD-NOS diagnoses is unknown as well; however, PDD-NOS is considered to be the most common of the ASD diagnoses in recent years (Constantino & Todd, 2003; Fombonne, Simmons, Ford, Meltzer, & Goodman, 2001), in many cases reflecting the milder end of the spectrum. With a tendency to generalize all the ASDs, including PDD-NOS, under the general term *autism*, particularly in educational settings where the legal, educational label of autism refers to the entire spectrum, accurate determination of the prevalence of the individual ASD may be compromised.

Theoretical Perspectives

Three major theoretical models are proposed to account for ASD. The most discussed over the years has been meta-representational theory or theory of mind (Baron-Cohen, 1988, 1995; Baron-Cohen, Leslie, & Frith, 1985). This perspective conceptualizes ASD as a central disorder of empathy such that individuals on the spectrum are unable to understand mental states of self or others. This disorder is related to their inability to represent (or mentalize) the states or perspectives of others such that they cannot predict behaviors of others (or presuppose how/what others will feel/think); subsequently, pragmatic communication skills are impaired. Theory of mind is believed to consist of more than emotion recognition but also an understanding that other persons may not share the same belief system. Neurological substrates implicated for perspective taking include the temporoparietal junction, superior temporal sulcus, and medial prefrontal cortex (M. F. Mason & Macrae, 2008). It has been suggested that the deficits observed across the spectrum extend beyond what can be explained by theory of mind (Tager-Flusberg, 2007). Debate continues regarding the extent to which theory of mind and the primary deficits in social reasoning are dependent on executive function and language (Apperly, Samson, & Humphreys, 2005; Perner & Lang, 2000).

A second theoretical model, weak central coherence theory (Happé, 1993, 2005), suggests that individuals with ASDs engage in sporadic processing of information (Joseph, 1999), particularly in the establishment of meaningful connections between stimuli

(Joliffe & Baron-Cohen, 1999). The main idea is that individuals with ASD have difficulty switching from details to general concepts (Happé, 2005; Happé, Briskman, & Frith, 2001); this model is based in part on some evidence that individuals with ASDs perform better on specific tasks than on complex, metacognitive or global tasks (Ehlers et al., 1997; Frith, 1989; Frith & Happé, 1994). This finding is also related to why they can retain words in a passage in the absence of understanding (Happé et al., 2001); it may be related to the frequent occurrence of hyperlexia (see Chapter 4) in children with ASDs as well. No particular neurological association is made with this theory other than that the deficit is familial (Happé et al., 2001) and may be related to executive dysfunction (South, Ozonoff, & McMahon, 2007; M. A. Turner, 1997). It has been suggested that this weak central coherence affects social processing and related social-cognitive skills (Burnette et al., 2005; Pellicano, Maybery, & Durkin, 2005). At the same time, others have argued that central coherence can occur on two levels, conceptual and perceptual, and that different individuals with ASDs may have weak central coherence in one, the other, or both (López, Leekam, & Arts, 2008).

ASDs also have been explained from the perspective of executive dysfunction (Ozonoff, Pennington, & Rogers, 1991; Russo et al., 2007). In effect, learning in ASD is characterized by perseveration, poor self-regulation, difficulties adapting to change, reduced forward planning, poor problem solving, and ineffective use of feedback; all of these behaviors are consistent with deficits in executive function. Several studies have provided support for the notion that individuals with ASDs evidence problems with planning, mental flexibility, inhibition, generativity (fluency), and self-monitoring (C. Hughes, 1996, 1998). Further, there is considerable evidence that individuals with ASD have difficulty with cognitive shifts (Minshew, Meyer, & Goldstein, 2002; Ozonoff, 1995). Although it has been hypothesized that there would be an association between the ASD and performance on measures of executive function, such a connection has been only partially supported (Pellicano, 2007; South et al., 2007; Thede & Coolidge, 2007; M. A. Turner, 1997; Yerya, Hepburn, Pennington, & Rogers, 2007). One of the issues in understanding the components of executive function that may be implicated in ASDs is the need for a developmental perspective in the selection of measures and comparison groups as well as in the interpretation of research results (Russo et al., 2007).

ETIOLOGY

With the exception of Rett syndrome, which is directly associated with mutations of the methyl-CpG-binding protein 2 (MeCP2) gene, the etiology of ASDs still remains unknown (Muhle et al., 2004). When autism was first described, attributions were made to a familial/parenting style as a causative factor (Kanner, 1943); at the same time, it was implied that there was a biological basis to autism. Unfortunately, the psychogenic basis of autism gained more attention until others endorsed a more biological-based etiology, changing the focus of research on autism (Rimland, 1964). Several decades past Kanner, much more is known about the etiology. It is now recognized, for example, that there is significant heterogeneity across individuals with autism; severity varies as well. These differences support the notion of disorders on a spectrum. Most recently, it has been suggested that there needs to be consideration of genetic, epigenetic, and environmental influences (Persico & Bourgeron, 2006).

Environmental Influences

It is believed that, in some cases, autism is due to a disruption (e.g., prenatal viral infection, mid-trimester bleeding) of normal brain development. For example, during the 1964 rubella outbreak, 8% to 13% of children born developed autism along with other problems associated with congenital rubella syndrome (Hertz-Picciotto et al., 2006; Muhle et al., 2004). Additional nongenetic causes may include exposure to teratogens (e.g., fetal alcohol syndrome, fetal valproate syndrome; see Chapter 14). Some questions have been raised in relation to thimerosal in vaccines as well as exposure to pollutants and heavy metals (see Chapter 13); the relation between vaccination and autism has not been supported by research (K. Madsen et al., 2002). In general, children with nongenetic forms of ASDs tend to have experienced complications prenatally or perinatally and show a high rate of "soft" neurological signs (Lannetti, Mastrangelo, & Di Netta, 2005). Further, in many instances, ASD co-occurs with mental retardation, epilepsy (Ciaranello & Ciaranello, 1995), chromosomal abnormalities, neurocutaneous disorders, or metabolic disorders (A. Bailey, Phillips, & Rutter, 1996; M. Barton & Volkmar, 1998). In these cases, the same factor that results in the co-occurring disorder may be the cause of the ASD.

Genetic and Epigenetic Influences

Alternatively, various studies (A. Bailey et al., 1995; Pisula, 2003; Rutter, 2005) have highlighted research conducted among families and identical twins that provides confirmation that genetics appear to play an important role in the etiology of ASDs. Estimates are that among monozygotic twins, there is an 82% to 92% concordance rate; among siblings, there is an estimated 2% to 3% risk; heritability estimates are as high as 90% (Folstein & Rosen-Sheidley, 2001; Veenstra-VanderWeele & Cooke, 2004). No single biological or clinical marker for autism has yet been discovered, nor has a single gene been found to be responsible for its expression (Pickett & London, 2005). When etiology is genetic, it is believed that ASD is due to mutations in genes that control brain development. ASD is believed to be polygenetic, with as many as 5 to 20 genes implicated (Folstein & Rosen-Sheidley, 2001; Liu et al., 2001; Muhle et al., 2004); the polygenetic basis of ASD may explain the variations across the ASD. In addition, others have identified gene mutations that form "nonsyndromic" or "syndromic" variants. Finally, some genes have been identified as "vulnerability" genes with potential increased risk, but they are not associated directly with ASD itself (Persico & Bourgeron, 2006). A person has a 10- to 20-fold increase compared to the general population of developing autism if he or she has a sibling with autism, and a number of studies have demonstrated a family history of social and language deficits in persons with autism. In all, a number of proteins involved in neurodevelopment and synaptic function have been identified; to some extent, these have been linked with one of the genetic pathways or gene-environment interactions. In particular, there are X-linked disorders (Rett, fragile X syndrome) where ASD is a secondary manifestation of the primary disorder; while Rett disorder is classified among the ASDs, 20% to 40% of individuals with fragile X also meet criteria for ASD.

The variations in genes and associated proteins further contributes to the heterogeneity of individuals with ASDs (Persico & Bourgeron, 2006). In some cases, it is not solely the genetic makeup that affects the manifestation of ASDs. Further, the phenotypic expression of the disorder varies widely, even within monozygotic twins, suggesting a combination of genetic and environmental factors (Amaral, Schumann, & Nordahl, 2008). Autistic diathesis theory proposes that genetic predisposition makes the individual vulnerable; it is the interaction of the individual vulnerability with specific psychosocial and environmental stressors that produces the disorder (Persico & Bourgeron, 2006).

Neurological Correlates

Regardless of the theoretical model or etiology, the majority of behaviors associated with ASDs are believed to be a manifestation of physiological dysfunction. Notably, on neurological assessment, gross abnormality in the brain (e.g., tumors) is not generally evident. More recently, with functional magnetic resonance imaging (fMRI), it was found that among higher-functioning individuals with ASDs, there were no differences in the functional organization and activation of brain regions for attention and goal-directed cognitive tasks; however, significant difference in the activation of brain regions was found for social and emotional processing, suggesting that altered organization of a specific neurological network underlies behavioral components in ASDs (D. Kennedy & Courchesne, 2007). In contrast, however, approximately 30% to 47% of children with ASDs exhibit abnormalities on electroencephalography (EEG) (Akshoomoff, Farid, Courchesne, & Haas, 2007; Delacato, Szegda, & Parisi, 1994; L. Y. Tsai, Tsai, & August, 1985). EEG tends to be abnormal in about half the individuals with ASDs with excessive slow-wave activity and decreased alpha activity; absence of abnormality on EEG in conjunction with autism is associated with higher cognitive ability (Coben, Clarke, Hudspeth, & Barry, 2008). Across individuals with ASDs, there is evidence of subclinical epileptiform activity, particularly in the perisylvian regions and the right hemisphere (Muñoz-Yunta et al., 2008). Event-related potentials tend to be abnormal for auditory stimuli to a greater extent than visual stimuli, with abnormal P3b (associated with attention and alertness to environmental stimuli) associated with autism (Courchesne, 1987; Courchesne, Courchesne, Hicks, & Lincoln, 1985). Lateralization of language function is also indicated as notable among children with autism (Kleinhans, Müller, Cohen, & Courchesne, 2008). For example, on letter fluency, the group with autism had significantly greater activation in the right frontal and right superior temporal lobes as compared to controls, suggesting significantly reduced lateralization of activation patterns; the same pattern did not emerge for category fluency. These findings were interpreted to indicate reduced hemispheric differentiation for certain verbal fluency tasks in ASDs (Kleinhans et al., 2008).

Mechanisms believed to be involved include reduced programmed cell death and/or increased cell proliferation, altered cell migration with subsequent abnormalities at the cytoarchitectonic level, abnormal cell differentiation, and altered synaptic function (Bauman & Kemper, 2005; Pickett & London, 2005). At the cortical level, this is evident in increased cell density, smaller cortical columns, and neuronal disorganization (A. Bailey et al., 1998; Casanova, Buxhoeveden, Switala, & Roy, 2002). Across studies and methods, at the structural level, a number of researchers have conducted studies using magnetic resonance imaging (MRI) to advance knowledge of what is known about ASDs (Belmonte et al., 2008; Bloss & Courchesne, 2007; Courchesne, Townsend, & Saitoh, 1994; Hashimoto et al., 1995; Luna et al., 2002; Piven, Bailey, Ranson, & Arndt, 1997; Piven et al., 1992). Relative to brain volume, there are indications of increased brain size and ventricles; this was most evident in males with ASDs (Bigler et al., 2003). More recent research suggests, however, that these differences are not significant when head size is taken into consideration (Bigler et al., 2003; Neeley et al., 2007). Enlarged ventricles are evident in 81% of cases, particularly for the right ventricle (Delacato et al., 1994). There is also some indication that the splenium of the corpus callosum is significantly smaller in individuals with autism (Hazlett, Poe, Gerig, Smith, & Piven, 2006).

Other areas and structures of the brain have been implicated as well. In particular, the structures of the brain stem that involve gating of sensory input based on the sensorimotor components are believed to be impacted in ASDs (Delacato et al., 1994; Ornitz, Atwell, Kaplan, & Westlake, 1985). In support of this finding, both the midbrain and medulla oblongata are smaller in children with autism (Hashimoto et al., 1993). In other brain regions, the proportion of thalamus to total brain volume is not comparable in individuals with autism (Harden et al., 2007). Still others have suggested involvement of the parietal lobe, with most of the behavioral manifestations a result of spatial neglect (Wainwright & Bryson, 1996). In exploring similarities and differences among children with Attention-Deficit/Hyperactivity Disorder (ADHD) or ASD, it was found that children in both groups demonstrated reduced gray matter volume in the left medial temporal lobe as well as increased gray matter in the left inferior parietal lobe (Brieber et al., 2007). The similarity was proposed to explain the similarity in attention problems exhibited by children in these groups. In contrast, only the ASD group evidenced increased gray matter in the right supramarginal gyrus at the temporoparietal junction. This difference was proposed to be associated with their difficulties in theory of mind and empathy (Brieber et al., 2007). In addition to specific structures, migration anomalies (focal pachygyri) have been found (Bauman & Kemper, 2007; F. Keller & Persico, 2003).

Although there is supporting evidence for involvement of multiple systems, there is no conclusive evidence for any one system; this lack of evidence may support the notion of a developmental disruption with diffuse synergistic effects. Initial overgrowth of white matter in the first 2 years of life, as well as subsequent differences in myelination, has been posited as being significant in explaining the neurobiology of ASDs (Courchesne et al., 2007; J. R. Hughes, 2007). Related to this assertion, it was found that increased white matter volume of the motor cortex for both the right and left hemispheres predicted poorer motor skill (Mostofsky, Burgess, & Larson, 2007). This predictive association was not found for children with other disorders. It was suggested that the implications of the increased white matter in motor areas likely was only one aspect of a global pattern of atypical brain development that related not only to motor dysfunction but also to communication and social functioning in ASDs due to reduced intracortical connectivity (Just, Cherkassky, Keller, Kana, & Minshew, 2007) and associated with the size of the anterior portion of the corpus callosum (R. A. Mason, Williams, Kans, Minshew, & Just, 2008). The lack of seizure behavior in the presence of epileptiform discharges shows that autistic children may have a deficiency of corticocortical fibers that typically spread the discharges through the brain to cause seizure behavior (J. R. Hughes & Melyn, 2005). Other research has examined other areas of brain development in ASDs. Specific areas of the brain implicated include the hippocampus, amygdala, other limbic nuclei, the frontal-striatal system, and the cerebellum (Bachevalier, 1994; Bachevalier & Loveland, 2006; Hazlett et al., 2006; Loveland, Bachevalier, Pearson, & Lane, 2008; Piven, Arndt, Bailey, & Andreasen, 1996; Piven et al., 1992). Additional findings related to specific brain structures and systems are detailed next.

Temporal Lobe and Limbic System

The limbic system hypothesis (Joseph, 1999) attributes social and communication deficits observed in children with autism to medial temporal and limbic structures of the brain. The temporal lobe, particularly language areas, is implicated due to the communication deficits of individuals with autism. In a single case study of a child with autism, there was partial absence of the left temporal lobe (C. P. White & Rosenbloom, 1992). Similarly, with a case with Asperger's disorder, computed tomography exposed damage to the left temporal lobe (P. B. Jones & Kerwin, 1990). Children with autism had reduced amplitude in temporal areas, particularly the left temporal lobe on EEG (Dawson, Klinger, Panagiotides, Lewy, & Castelloe, 1995). Similarly, single photon emission computed tomography (SPECT) and positron emission tomography (PET) studies indicated reduced cerebral blood flow in the temporal lobes (I. C. Gillberg, Bjure, Uvebrant, Vestergren, & Gillberg, 1993; Zilbovicius et al., 2000). With auditory information, children with autism demonstrated increased slow wave and prolonged N1 peak latency for speech stimuli in the left temporal lobe as compared to children with mental retardation and typically developing children (Narita & Koga, 1987). Taken together, studies consistently indicate some abnormality or difference in temporal lobe functioning.

Within the temporal lobe, the medial temporal lobe (limbic system) and particularly the hippocampus and amygdala are implicated due to similarities between autism and Klüver-Bucy syndrome (DeLong, 1992; Hetzler & Griffin, 1981) as well as the role of the hippocampus in language, construction of meaning, and integration of motivation, experience, memory, and learning. Differences in hippocampal volume and cell number (E. H. Aylward et al., 1999; Courchesne, 1997; Herbert, Ziegler, Deutsch et al., 2003; B. F. Sparks et al., 2002) are believed to be associated with the memory disturbances specific to working memory and more complex tasks, while rote memory and echolalia are intact (Coldren & Halloran, 2003; Luna et al., 2002). In a single case study of a child with autism who had a left temporal tumor involving the hippocampus and the amygdala, some autistic behaviors were found to improve after tumor resection; however, other behaviors persisted (Hoon & Reiss, 1992). Further, hippocampal involvement is indicated in increased cell density, reduced neuronal size, and decreased dendritic branching in CA4 and the subiculum (Minshew & Goldstein, 1993). These differences often are associated with long-term memory deficits; however, not all research indicates long-term memory deficits with autism (Minshew, 1997). Although the hippocampus has been studied extensively in a range of persons with autism disorder, the contribution of the hippocampus to the disorder is yet to be fully understood; however, there are indications of a potential genetic basis for hippocampal abnormalities in autism (D. C. Rojas et al., 2004).

Social behavior is also dependent on the amygdala, orbital frontal cortex, and temporal lobe (Abell et al., 1999; Amaral et al., 2008). Amygdala enlargement is associated with anxiety and difficulties with social and communication skills, the latter of which are diagnostic features of autism (Schumann et al., 2004). The amygdala in boys with autism appears to undergo an abnormal developmental course with a period of enlargement early in life that does not persist through late childhood. The amygdala appears initially to be larger in children with autism but does not undergo the same preadolescent age-related increase in volume that takes place in typically developing boys (Schumann et al., 2004). Qualitative observations in six postmortem cases of autism ages 9 to 29 years indicated that neurons in certain nuclei of the amygdala of autism cases appeared unusually small and more densely packed than in age-matched controls (Kemper & Bauman, 1993). In a comparison of 9 boys with autism and 10 typically developing age-matched male controls, the autism group had significantly fewer neurons in the total amygdala and in the lateral nucleus than the controls (Schumann & Amaral, 2006). These researchers did not find the increased neuronal density or decreased size of neurons as Kemper and Bauman (1993) had reported. Others have investigated the biochemical abnormalities in the amygdale as potentially contributing to social impairment in autism (Kleinhans et al., 2009).

Both the communication and the social deficits in autism may be related to impaired functioning of the superior temporal sulcus (Amaral et al., 2008; Redcay, 2008; Zilbovicius et al., 2006). As with the hippocampus, there is increased cell density and reduced neuronal size in the amygdale (Bauman, 1991). Further, there is evidence of increased gray matter in the frontal and temporal lobes in young children with ASDs (Carper, Moses, Tigue, & Courchesne, 2002) with associated shifting of the superior temporal sulcus (Levitt et al., 2003). Histological study (autopsy) of six brains of individuals with autism revealed abnormalities in the limbic forebrain (Kemper & Bauman, 1993); histological study also has revealed abnormalities in the hippocampus, entorhinal (olfactory) cortex, septal nuclei, mamillary body, and amygdale (Bauman & Kemper, 1985). Finally, reversed asymmetry of frontal and temporal lobes, as in learning disability, has been found in individuals with ASDs (Hier, LeMay, & Rosenberger, 1979). Related to the communication deficits associated with ASD, there are also indications of malformation and decreased activation of the temporal lobe (Pierce, Muller, Allen, & Courchesne, 2001; Sweeten, Posey, Shekhar, & McDougle, 2002).

Fronto-Striatal Model

Frontal lobe and basal ganglia are also believed to be related to ASDs (Amaral et al., 2008; Hollander et al., 2005; Rinehart, Bradshaw, Brereton, & Tonge, 2002; Rinehart et al., 2006). Rinehart et al. (2002) presented tasks of increasing cognitive complexity to individuals with autism, Asperger's disorder, and normal controls. Across tasks, the Asperger group performed comparably to the controls; however, as the task complexity increased, the autistic group displayed deficits in inhibition. Additional support has been provided by PET studies. For example, individuals with autism evidenced atypical activation of the left anterior cingulate gyrus during language tasks (R.-A. Müller et al., 1999). Another PET study used a continuous performance test (CPT) and found that individuals with autism lacked the normal (i.e., right greater than left) cortical hemispheric asymmetry for attentional tasks (Buchsbaum et al., 1992). Buchsbaum et al. also found decreased relative metabolic rate in the right posterior thalamus and the right putamen. Also using PET, high metabolic rate in the left inferior frontal cortex and an inverse correlation between activation of the medial superior frontal gyral area with performance on CPT was found, as was decreased metabolic rate in the left posterior putamen (B. V. Siegel et al., 1992). Finally, it has been found that children with autism had reduced amplitude in frontal areas, particularly the left frontal area, on EEG (Dawson et al., 1995). Developmental differences emerged such that at 3 to 4 years of age, children with autism evidenced hypoperfusion (decreased blood flow) to the frontal area; however, by age 7, blood flow to the frontal area was normal (Zilbovicius et al., 1995). In addition to the frontal-striatal model, other models have posited dysfunction of the mesolimbic cortex of the temporal and frontal lobes, neostriatum (basal ganglia) and anterior and medial groups of the thalamus (Maurer, 1986). Still another systemic model involves the hippocampus and amygdala as well as the interrelated neurochemical systems (oxytocin and vasopressin, serotonin, and endogenous opiate) and the temporal and parietal association areas; these structures and circuitry interact to produce the deficits associated with autism (Waterhouse et al., 1996).

Notably, individuals with autism exhibited lower glucose metabolic activity in limbic areas as compared to controls (Haznedar et al., 2000). In contrast to normal controls, on a theory of mind task, individuals with Asperger's disorder activated a completely different area located in the left medial frontal lobe, suggesting that areas of physiological dysfunction determine type and manifestation of ASD (Happé et al., 1996). Neuropsychologically, the anterior cingulate cortex (ACC) is linked to awareness of mental states in self and others (Abell et al., 1999), so associated differences in the ACC would be expected. Finally, related to the motor perseveration, the basal ganglia has been the focus of study, with indications of structural changes (Kates et al., 1998; Sears et al., 1999) and functional impairments (R. A. Müller, Pierce, Ambrose, Allen, & Courchesne, 2001).

Minicolumn Hypothesis

The basic anatomical and physiological unit of the neocortex is the minicolumn; information is transmitted through the core of the minicolumn and is prevented from activating neighboring minicolumns by surrounding inhibitory fibers (Casanova et al., 2006). The minicolumns in the brains of individuals with autism tend to be smaller in size, although there are the same total number of cells per column and more columns; these differences would affect information processing, potentially enhancing the ability to process stimuli that require discrimination, but at the expense of generalizing the relevance of a particular stimulus. This finding could be related to the tendency of individuals with autism to focus on smaller parts of objects rather than the object as a whole and could be a potential explanation for difficulties experienced filtering sensory information (Casanova et al., 2006).

Cerebellum

The cerebellum is implicated functionally in ASDs due to the deficits in integration of attention, movement, and thought processes (Courchesne, 1997; Piven et al., 1992). On autopsy, abnormalities have been found of cerebellar circuits (Kemper & Bauman, 1993), neocerebellar cortex, the roof nuclei of the cerebellum, and inferior olivary nucleus (Bauman & Kemper, 1985). At the cell level, there are findings of decreased Purkinje cells and a modest decrease in granule cells (Bauman, 1991; Courchesne, 1997); there is further indication of an association of specific autistic-like behaviors in association with changes in cerebellar cell level and volume (Pierce & Corchesne, 2001). For example, the cerebellum, particularly the vermis, has been shown to modulate sensory input at the level of the brain stem, thalamus, and cerebral cortex (Amaral et al., 2008). Stimulation of the vermis can cause hypersensitivity to touch and sound. Persons with autism sometimes respond in peculiar ways to sensory stimuli and can be hypersensitive to stimuli (Amaral et al., 2008). The right cerebellum has been shown to work with the left frontal and anterior cingulate areas in word generation tasks (Fiez et al., 1996). The cerebellum is also involved in language function. Lesions of the right cerebellum result in problems in word selection and production. Lesions of the vermis can result in dysarthria and abnormal speech rhythm (Fiez et al., 1996). Finally, these same areas are involved in the shifting of attention; individuals with autism can have difficulty with shifting of attention, and can become fixated with certain stimuli; they may stare into space, avoid eye contact, or look at objects from unusual angles (Amaral, et al., 2008; Fiez et al., 1996).

Studies of individuals with autism suggest that for a majority of cases, there was hypoplasia of vermal areas of cerebellum (Courchesne, 1997); others had hyperplasia of the vermal area (Redcay & Courchesne, 2005). The pons/cerebellum vermian lobules seemed to have developed more rapidly in the group with autism while the posterior fossa was smaller in children with autism, suggesting early maldevelopment and hypoplasia (Hashimoto et al., 1995). Others have not found any differences in the cerebellar vermal area, pons, or fourth ventricle (Garber & Ritvo, 1992; Holttum, Minshew, Sanders, & Phillips, 1992; Rumsey et al., 1988). The cerebellum has been the target of study in postmortem studies of autism with findings of decreased density of Purkinje cells and 40% less expression of GAD67 mRNA in the cerebellar Purkinje cells of individuals with autism (Yip, Soghomonian, & Blatt, 2007). The postmortem finding of fewer Purkinje cells appears to differ from MRI findings of an enlarged cerebellum in autism; this difference was likely due to the heterogeneous groups and presence of co-occurring disorders across studies (Kern, 2003).

Mirror Neuron System

At the cellular level, mirror neurons have been implicated, particularly with individual response to perceptual events, imitation, empathy, and language learning (Gallese, 2003; Iacoboni & Mazziotta, 2007; Iacoboni et al., 1999; Leslie, Johnson-Frey, & Grafton, 2004; Uddin, Iacoboni, Lange, & Keenan, 2007). Mirror neurons are a group of premotor neurons that provide a simple means for understanding the actions of others (Triesch, Jasso, & Deák, 2007). Although initially identified in studies with monkeys (Rizzolatti, Fadiga, Gallese, & Fogassi, 1996), comparable studies have implicated mirror neurons for the same functions in humans (Decety, Chaminade, Grezes, & Meltzoff, 2002; Decety & Grezes, 1999; Fadiga, Craighero, & Oliver, 2005). Mirror neurons are activated in response to specific actions performed by the individual as well as by similar actions that are observed in others (J. H. G. Williams, Whiten, Suddendorf, & Perrett, 2001a, 2001b); it is the mirror neuron system that allows people to connect an observed action with a corresponding motor representation in their brains (Buccino & Amore, 2008; Iacoboni, 2007). As such, this system would be most consistent with the conceptualization of ASD and deficits related to theory of mind and the inability to presuppose the feelings and actions of others. It would further be consistent with perspectives that social relating and understanding is dependent on the individual's capacity not only to perceive others as similar to self (Meltzoff & Moore, 1995) but also to simulate the behaviors of others in the individual's mental representation of his or her own emotions, cognitions, and movements. There is evidence of the role of mirror neurons and simulation in typically developing individuals; it is believed that this internal simulation and representation overlaps or mediates the imitation of behavior as well as the perception of the behavior (Oberman & Ramachandran, 2007) and understanding of others' intentions (Iacoboni, 2007). It should be noted that support for mirror neurons as explaining intention and attribution is not without controversy (Borg, 2007).

The exact nature and function of the mirror neuron system has not been determined. It has been suggested that damage or developmental failure of these mirror neurons, located in the frontal lobes, may underlie the deficits in empathy and theory of mind in ASDs (Buccino & Amore, 2008; Iacoboni, 2007; Oberman et al., 2005; Oberman & Ramachandran, 2007; Schulte-Rüther, Markowitsch, Fink, & Piefke, 2007; J. H. G. Williams et al., 2001b). In effect, the lack of activation of the mirror neuron system on observing similar movements of others may be related to perspective taking and social cognition (Pfeifer, Iacoboni, Mazziotta, & Dapretto, 2008). Anatomical differences, specifically decreased gray matter in the areas of mirror neuron system, has been found in a group of individuals with high-functioning autism; cortical thinning of the gray matter in this region was associated with symptom severity (Hadjikhani, Joseph, Snyder, & Tager-Flusberg, 2006). Brain activity associated with emotional and facial stimuli in nondiagnosed adults has been identified using fMRI (Schulte-Rüther et al., 2007). Also with fMRI, group comparisons indicated that children with ASDs showed an absence of mirror neuron activity in the inferior frontal gyrus (pars operculis) despite comparable performance on the task (Dapretto et al., 2006). Further, Dapretto and colleagues found that the level of activity at the inferior frontal gyrus was inversely related to symptom severity such that decreased levels of activity were associated with increased severity. Based on PET scans and fMRI, the frontal operculum and the anterior parietal cortex have also been implicated (Decety et al., 1997; Iacoboni et al., 1999), with somatotropic distribution in the premotor and parietal areas similar to that found for monkeys (Buccino et al., 2001). Additionally, the superior temporal sulcus appears to have somatotropic distribution (Pelphrey, Morris, & McCarthy, 2005). Of brain waves, the *mu* wave is associated with execution, imagination, and observation of human action and is believed to be associated with mirror neuron activity. Using EEG and measuring *mu* frequency to self and observed movements, Oberman and colleagues (2001) found that individuals with high-functioning autism did not evidence *mu* suppression to observed hand movements but did evidence the *mu* suppression on self movements, supporting the hypothesis of a dysfunctional mirror neuron system in ASDs. In the insula and anterior cingulate cortex, activation of mirror neurons associated with empathy (i.e., observing facial expressions of disgust or pain) has been observed with fMRI (I. Morrison, Lloyd, DiPellegrino, & Roberts, 2004; T. Singer et al., 2004; Wicker et al., 2003). Mirror neurons are believed to be related not only to empathy and social competence but also to the language difficulties associated with ASDs, particularly the frequency of echolalia, neologisms, and pronoun reversal (Oberman & Ramachandran, 2007).

Neurotransmitters

In addition to specific structures, neurotransmitters implicated include serotonin (B. Devlin et al., 2005), monoamines (Martineau, Barthélémy, Jouve, & Müh, 1992), and opiatergic transmitters (due to high levels of opiate activity in the CSF; C. Gillberg, 1995). Serotonin is considered pivotal to brain development and associated with many of the behavioral characteristics of ASDs (Chugani, 2002); decreased serotonin synthesis has been found in individuals with ASDs, particularly in the left frontal cortex, basal ganglia, and thalamus as well as in the dentate nuclei of the cerebellum (Chugani et al., 1997). Research has yielded some indications of elevated levels of serotonin among individuals with autism (E. H. Cook & Leventhal, 1995; B. Devlin et al., 2005; McBride et al., 1989); levels of serotonin were associated with clinical state, particularly whole-blood 5-hydroxytryptamine (5-HT) levels (Hérault et al., 1996). In an attempt to alter serotonin levels, and presumably address the level of clinical symptoms, use of levodopa (L-dopa) has been studied (Ritvo et al., 1971). Although the L-dopa had the intended effect on the serotonin levels, there were no associated changes in clinical symptoms. In contrast, the use of selective serotonin reuptake inhibitors has been helpful in determining the role of serotonin in autism. For example, positive results have been found with fluoxetine and fluvoxamine (DeLong, 1992; DeLong, Teague, & Kamran, 1998; Ghaziuddin, Tsai, & Ghaziuddin, 1991; McDougle, Price, & Goodman, 1990). DeLong proposed that the serotonergic dysfunction was specific to the left hemisphere in high-functioning autism with bilateral dysfunction in low-functioning autism; Asperger's disorder is hypothesized to reflect serotonergic dysfunction of the right hemisphere only.

Behaviors of self-stimulation and nonresponsiveness to conditioning are indicative of dopamine dysfunction within the mesocortex. Children with autism have been found to have high levels of D2 receptor binding in the caudate and putamen (Fernell et al., 1997); other studies have indicated differences in D2, D3, and D5 (Martineau, Hérault, & Petit, 1994). In addition, levels of homovanillic acid—a metabolite in the breakdown of dopamine—in the cerebrospinal fluid of children with autism has been found to be much higher than levels in normal children (C. Gillberg & Svennerholm, 1987). Dopamine antagonists (e.g., haloperidol) can be effective in decreasing autistic behaviors in about 50% of cases, further supporting dopaminergic influences.

The neurotransmitter oxytocin is related to social attraction, behavioral response, and memory; as such, oxytocin may be involved in ASDs. Oxytocin is a 9–amino acid peptide that is synthesized in the hypothalamic neurons and transported down axons of the posterior pituitary. Oxytocin levels are important both in the birthing process and in breastfeeding, with oxytocin transmitted from the mother to the infant during feeding. Notably, research suggests that there are low blood plasma levels of oxytocin in individuals with ASDs (Modahl et al., 1998). In addition to serotonin, dopamine, and oxytocin, glutamate receptors also have been implicated in ASDs (Hussman, 2001; Purcell, Jeon, Zimmerman, Blue, & Pevsner, 2001; Serajee, Zhong, Nabi, & Huq, 2003).

COURSE AND PROGNOSIS

Course and prognosis vary based on the type of ASD but consistently revolve around the autistic triad: communication, social interaction, and repetitive/restrictive behavior (Parikh et al., 2008).The various behavioral manifestations that may result in a diagnosis of ASD include cognitive impairment, poor or limited social relationships, underdeveloped or impaired communication skills (verbal and/or nonverbal), and repetitive behaviors, interests, and/or activities (APA, 2000; National Institute of Mental Health, 1999). Each of the disorders in the spectrum includes some combination of these manifestations, with subtle or more obvious differences. From a theoretical perspective, cognitive processes related to dealing with ambiguity, theory of mind, and central coherence continue to be predictive of behaviors associated with ASDs through adolescence and adulthood (Best et al., 2008).

Communicative Impairment

Communication and the ability of the individual to acquire language are key features of ASDs. At the same time, a distinguishing feature between autistic disorder and Asperger's disorder is that individuals with Asperger's disorder exhibit "no clinically significant delays or deviance in language acquisition" (APA, 2000, p. 80); they do, however, often demonstrate difficulty with understanding the emotional content of communication, exhibit problems with pragmatic responses, and evidence difficulty integrating affective and cognitive aspects of a situation or conversation (Blacher, Kraemer, & Schalow, 2003). In fact, several language phenotypes have been identified within the spectrum (Kjelgaard & Tager-Flusberg, 2001), with language abilities in children with autism showing profiles of unevenness such that abilities range from muteness to verbal speech with some residual language deficits (Minshew, 1997). Impairments exist in language comprehension and in receptive and expressive verbal as well as nonverbal communication, especially in the areas of gestures, facial expressions, rhythm and pitch of speech, and eye contact (Minshew, 1997; Whitman, 2004). Pragmatic language deficits are most evident across all disorders on the spectrum (Bishop & Norbury, 2002) and are most likely to persist across the life span (Rutter, 2001).

Approximately 25% to 50% of the children with autism never develop receptive and expressive language, nor do they compensate through the use of nonverbal communication (Minshew, 1997; Osterling, Dawson, & Munson, 2002). At the same time, however, for children with autism, language development tends to follow a distinctive and abnormal pattern. The verbal language of children with autism may develop in the sequence of

> simple immediate echolalia, complex delayed echolalia, the functional use of echolalia to communicate needs resulting in pronoun reversals (e.g., I for you), original or nonechoed language with grammatical errors or grammatically correct language that is stereotyped, grammatically correct simple sentences, and complex sentences (Minshew, 1997, p. 820)

that is more protracted and not likely to include the same level of abstraction. Similar to children with speech language impairment (SLI), children with ASDs may perform poorly on nonword repetition (Kjelgaard & Tager-Flusberg, 2001). Communication deficits with ASDs differ from those of children with SLI (see Chapter 4) in that both verbal and nonverbal communication is affected (Whitehouse, Barry, & Bishop, 2007). SLI or level of language at age 6 to 8 years was found to account for the greatest variation in outcome in adolescents on the spectrum, with decreased language at age 6 or 8 predictive of outcome in adolescence (T. Bennett et al., 2008). This highlights the importance of language/communication not only during childhood but as individuals on the spectrum enter adulthood.

Out of those children with autism who develop language, 25% of these children maintain a rudimentary stage of verbal and nonverbal language (Minshew, 1997). When communicating with others, children with autism may interrupt others frequently, have difficulty holding an extensive conversation with spontaneous dialogue, and have difficulty understanding satire, jokes, or nonliteral language (Happé, 1993; Whitman, 2004). Pragmatic communication is similarly impaired (Loth, Gómez, & Happé, 2008). Nonverbal communication oftentimes follows a similar sequence as language with (a) initially no eye contact; (b) distant glancing that is constant; (c) the use of the glancing eye in social situations; (d) eye contact that is prolonged in social situations; and (e) engaging in eye contact in social situations that is normal in quantity (Minshew, 1997). Another component to nonverbal communication is facial expression. Facial expressions in children with autism typically are expressionless or consist of a smile that is unvarying (Minshew, 1997).

Social Interaction

Related to their pragmatic communication deficits, individuals with autism may have difficulty with social relations and in making friends; a basic deficit is the lack of orientation toward a social stimulus and associated nonverbal and verbal behaviors (M. J. Weiss & Harris, 2001). When engaging in an activity, individuals with autism do not make attempts to bring others into their activity and do not appear to be aware of the existence of other individuals aside from themselves or one other (Ozonoff & Rogers, 2003). In addition, children with autism have difficulty generalizing their experiences from one situation to the next. While they may know what is expected of them and behave accordingly in one situation, they have difficulty adapting that information to new similar, situations (Aarons & Gittens, 1999). Components of social cognition that are affected in ASDs include:

- Perspective taking (LeBlanc et al., 2003; Warreyn, Roeyers, Oelbrandt, & De Groote, 2005)
- Sense of agency (David et al., 2008)
- Meaningful imitation (Meltzoff, 2002; Meltzoff & Moore, 1995)
- Joint attention (Baron-Cohen, Baldwin, & Crowson, 1997; Naber et al., 2007; Roos, McDuffie, & Gernsbacher, 2008; Warreyn et al., 2005)
- Mentalizing (Baron-Cohen et al., 1997; David et al., 2008; Sigman, Dijamco, Gratier, & Rozga, 2004)

Across studies, there are indications of deficits in joint attention and imitation (Baron-Cohen et al., 1997; Meltzoff, 2002) as well as face recognition/discrimination despite intact object recognition/discrimination (Klin et al., 1999; B. R. López et al., 2008; Wilson, Pascalis, & Blades, 2007). Even among individuals with average cognitive abilities, or at least average verbal abilities, there are continued deficits in social interactions (Klin et al., 2007). Social deficits are most evident in social situations that are unstructured or ambiguous, where structured routines and patterns do not provide prompts (Loth et al., 2008). It is in these unstructured settings that deficits in theory of mind and the inability to presuppose what is likely to happen and what is expected in terms of behavior become more evident. Similarly, individuals on the spectrum have difficulty predicting the behaviors or motivations of others (Loth et al., 2008).

Early on, the deficits in social behavior are noted in difficulty with early social behaviors, including joint attention, gaze following, pretend play, and imitation (Baron-Cohen, 1995; Charman et al., 1997; Meltzoff, 2002; Rogers, 1999). Facial recognition and emotion recognition strategies are atypical (Baron-Cohen, Wheelwright, Hill, Raste, & Plumb, 2001; Schultz, 2005). Research suggests that individuals with ASDs pay less attention to social cues and are less able to derive social meaning from varying contexts (Klin, Jones, Schultz, Volkmar, & Cohen, 2001a, 2001b). Children with ASDs evidence difficulty with comprehending even the most common of social events (Loveland & Tunali-Kotoski, 2005; Volden & Johnston, 1999). Taken together, it has been suggested that the deficits in theory of mind in conjunction with the social-perceptual style affect the acquisition of common event schemas (Loth et al., 2008). Notably, the social deficits and associated pragmatic skills continue to be evident in adults with high-functioning autism or ASDs, with some indications that the social impairments give rise to pragmatic communication deficits (Colle, Baron-Cohen, Wheelwright, & van der Lely, 2008). Individuals with ASDs continue to demonstrate difficulty in social areas throughout adulthood; the social difficulties may significantly impair not only social functioning but employability (Venter, Lord, & Schopler, 1992).

Restricted or Stereotyped Behaviors

The restriction of ideas and interests that characterizes autism also impedes social relationships. Often, in conversations, children with ASDs will converse in great detail about their topics of interest and may not recognize that they are violating social norms by dominating the conversation with these single topics. Children with ASDs are known to be extremely knowledgeable about specific topics, such as airplanes or cars, and will develop a memory for extensive minute details or facts regarding these restricted topics (Mesibov, Adams, & Klinger, 1997). Related to the restricted interests, individuals with autism may exhibit splinter skills or circumscribed abilities. These may include the ability to recall entire scripts of films or rapidly decode words in the absence of comprehension (hyperlexia) (Newman et al., 2007). Alternatively, children with ASDs often will become fixated on parts of objects. For example, a child with ASD may only spin the wheels on a car and ignore the real purpose of the car.

The restriction or repetitiveness is not limited to topics of conversation or specific objects. Children with autism tend to engage in behaviors that are atypical, stereotyped, and ritualistic. For example, children with ASDs may engage in a high frequency of self-stimulatory behaviors, such as twirling or rocking their body or objects, or engage in self-injurious behaviors, such as head banging; often these behaviors become evident between 3 and 5 years of age (Rutter, 2001). In addition, they may engage in ritualistic behaviors, such as lining up objects or adhering strictly to a specific and inflexible routine. Interrupting their ritualistic behavior or routine or changing something in their environment can result in emotions of extreme irritation, anxiety, or anger (Loth et al., 2008; Whitman, 2004). Underlying reasons for this behavior are not known; however, dual cognitive deficits—high level of awareness for detail combined with impairments in abilities of abstract reasoning—have been suggested (Minshew, 1997). In regard to what causes stereotyped behaviors, it has been postulated that children with ASD engage in stereotyped behaviors as a way to reduce anxiety or tension or as a means to find stimulation when they are experiencing a low internal state of arousal (Whitman, 2004).

Neuropsychological Profiles

There is continued controversy among those doing research and clinical practice in the PDD area; neuropsychological research suggests differing cognitive profiles for individuals with Asperger's disorder versus autism (Minshew, 1997). It has been argued that Asperger's disorder is most closely associated with the profile of nonverbal learning disability as discussed in Chapter 3; strengths exist in auditory perception, attention and memory, simple motor production, and rote learning while deficits exist in nonverbal areas including problem solving, visual perception and memory, pragmatics, and prosody. Although in preschool, children with autism may show deficits in understanding object permanence and spatial relations (Dawson & Adams, 1984), there is evidence that by adolescence, these children evidence strengths in visual perceptual and visual-spatial areas in conjunction with deficits on tasks requiring verbal skills, simultaneous performance of multiple operations, and complex language and memory skills (Frith & Happé, 1994). Both groups demonstrate deficits in executive functioning; however, the problem exhibited by the group of children with autism was in the inability to shift set (perseveration), indicating limited cognitive flexibility. In constructing potential profiles, it is important to note that only the group of children with autism demonstrates deficits on some theory of mind tasks (Ziatas, Durkin, & Pratt, 2003). In a recent study, it was found that individuals identified with high-functioning autism did not differ from those identified as having Asperger's disorder on more global scales of verbal and nonverbal functioning (Spek, Scholte, & van Berckelaer-Onnes, 2008). The two groups differed, however, on patterns of functioning across subtests such that the high-functioning autism group performed more poorly on the Coding and Processing Speed tasks but better on the Information and Matrix Reasoning tasks (Spek et al., 2008). In a second study with children with high-functioning autism, indications were that they did better on perceptual reasoning and particularly motor-free tasks as well as verbal comprehension tasks as compared to working memory and processing speed (Mayes & Calhoon, 2008). Taken together with results from other studies, Mayes and Calhoon concluded that the profile on traditional measures of cognition reflected attention, graphomotor, and processing speed weaknesses of children with high-functioning autism while allowing their verbal and nonverbal reasoning to be demonstrated. General deficits associated with ASDs are presented in Table 5.1.

There is some consensus that children with ASDs demonstrate difficulty on various tasks of executive function (B. R. López, Lincoln, Ozonoff, & Lai, 2005; South et al., 2007; Yerys, Hepburn, Pennington, & Rogers, 2007). Examples include increased perseverative errors on the Wisconsin Card Sorting Test as well as decreased efficiency on the Tower of Hanoi (Bennetto, Pennington, & Rogers, 1996; Ozonoff, Pennington, & Rogers, 1991). Similarly, adolescents and adults with ASDs tend to have difficulty with organization and effective strategy use (Minshew & Goldstein, 1993). In a study with adults with ASDs, deficits continued to be evident in areas of working memory and planning (L. Bernard, Muldoon, Hasan, O'Brien, & Steward, 2008). Others evaluated executive function in preschoolers ($n = 18$) with autism in comparison to a control group ($n = 18$); no significant

Table 5.1 Neuropsychological Domains and Specific Deficits with Autism Spectrum Disorders

Domains	Specific Deficits
Cognition	Global decreased functioning with 40% to 60% below the average range
Auditory-linguistic/ Language function	Comprehension (verbal and nonverbal) Expressive (verbal and nonverbal) Prosody Pragmatics
Visual perception/ Constructional praxis	Difficulty when motor components, speed of processing, or memory involved (motor-free visual perception often spared)
Perceptual sensory functioning	Increased sensitivity
Learning and memory	Rote memory usually intact; deficits most evident in working memory
Processing speed	Slow to respond and complete tasks
Executive function	Disinhibition Impaired cognitive flexibility Perseveration
Attention/Concentration	May be hypervigilant and unable to shift attention
Motor function	Perseverative or repetitive behaviors or patterns of behaviors Evidence graphomotor difficulties
Achievement/Academic skills	Hyperlexia
Emotional/Behavioral functioning	Joint attention Imitation Face recognition/memory/discrimination Empathy, mentalizing, perspective taking
Other: Stereotypy	Restricted interests Self-stimulating behavior Self-injurious behaviors

difference in executive function performance was found; however, the children in the autism group exhibited less social interaction (Griffith, Pennington, Wehner, & Rogers, 1999). In a follow-up study of 13 children in the autism group, similar findings were revealed. These results are counter to the executive dysfunction hypothesis of autism based on research with adults. It has been proposed that the executive deficits in autism originate, at least partially, from the inability of individuals with autism to use internal speech to self-regulate behavior and emotions (J. Russell, 1997).This same internal language would be responsible for the deficits in working memory (Joseph, McGrath, & Tager-Flusberg, 2005; J. Russell, 1997).There are some indications of an association between theory of mind and executive function deficits, but research has been equivocal (Bach, Happé, Fleminger, & Powell, 2005; C. Fine, Lumsden, & Blair, 2001; C. Hughes & Graham, 2002). Finally, one study investigated brain activation during a mental rotation task and concluded that there was insufficient activation of the prefrontal cortex in the boys with autism as compared to those in the control group but that parietal activation was similar in the two groups; these findings were seen as supporting a dysfunction in the frontro-striatal networks (Silk et al., 2006).

Prognosis and Associated Features

The level of cognitive functioning of individuals with autism spans a broad range, from profound mental retardation to superior intellect (Pickett & London, 2005). Although individuals with ASD evidence a range of ability levels, a large percentage of those identified with ASD exhibit impaired cognition (E. H. Cook & Leventhal, 1995; DiCicco-Bloom et al., 2006). Additionally, there is a high rate of co-occurrence with epilepsy (see Chapter 10) and attentional disorders, including ADHD (see Chapter 6), as well as other externalizing disorders (E. H. Cook & Leventhal, 1995).

Overlap and similarities in behavioral manifestations also have been noted with Tourette syndrome (see Chapter 7), particularly in relation to echolalia, perseverations, and stereotypic movements (Canitano & Vivanti, 2007; Geurts et al., 2008). Additional associated features include hypersensitivity to sounds, tactile stimulation, or odors. Across studies, there are some indications of difficulty with imitation of motor movements. Motor and movement abnormalities have been identified as early as infancy from home videos in some cases, but this is most noticeable in those children who have developmental delays in addition to autism (Ozonoff et al., 2008). Some of the motor difficulties relate to gait, knee flexion, and posturing (Damasio & Maurer, 1978; Jansiewicz et al., 2006; Minshew, Sung, Jones, & Furman, 2004; Vilensky, Damasio, & Maurer, 1981).

Little research has examined the outcomes of individuals with ASDs, but what research has been done has not been overly optimistic. Some of the early research found that 60% to 75% of those with autism had poor outcomes, as defined by living in institutions and/or not receiving appropriate residential or vocational services (Lotter, 1978). A recent study found that outcome was related to severity of autism (as measured by a rating scale) and cognitive ability at age 11 (Eaves & Ho, 2008). Eaves and Ho found that at age 24, the most common emotional or psychiatric problem was that of "emotional difficulty" (p. 742); additional co-occurring disorders included bipolar disorder, depression, conduct disorder, Tourette syndrome, and anxiety disorder. Of children with ASDs in a population-based cohort, 70% had at least one comorbid diagnosis; 41% had two or more diagnoses in addition to the ASD (Simonoff et al., 2008). The majority continued to live at home, received government disability, and had a case worker. Families noted unmet needs particularly in the social arena (Eaves & Ho, 2008). Research generally suggests continued difficulties with special obsessions, naiveté, self-centeredness, a tendency to talk incessantly about a topic of interest to them, and low empathy; these difficulties at times contribute to the likelihood of their involvement with the legal system (D. Allen et al., 2008). Furthermore, it is hypothesized that these behaviors make negotiating the legal system more difficult for individuals with Asperger's disorder than for others, thus increasing the likelihood of negative outcome for even a minor offense. In the Allen et al. study, the mean age of first offense was 25.8 years but occurred as early as age 10 or as late as age 61. Self-reported factors that precipitated the offense in at least 50% of cases included social rejection, bullying, sexual rejection, or family conflict. The types of offenses ranged from physical or verbal aggression to other types of offenses (e.g., drugs, traffic offenses).

Assessment Considerations

Assessment of children and adolescents on the autism spectrum requires planning and preparation. Practice parameters for the assessment of ASDs have been offered (Filipek et al., 2000; Klin, Saulnier, Tsatsanis, & Volkmar, 2005; Volkmar et al., 1999). Taken together, the parameters include obtaining sufficient background information related to symptom presentation, history, intensity, and frequency; information from multiple informants related to current (and past) symptom presentation; and direct observation of symptom presentation related to the autism triad (Kanne, Randolph, & Farmer, 2008). Specific measures suggested for these components and specific to ASDs include the Autism Diagnostic Interview—Revised (ADI-R), the Social Communication Questionnaire (SCQ), the Social Responsiveness Scale (SRS), and the Autism Diagnostic Observation System (ADOS) as well as various other rating scales (e.g., Childhood Autism Rating Scale, Gilliam Autism Rating Scale). In addition to assessing the specific symptoms and severity of the ASD, it is also important to obtain information related to cognitive ability, language skills, and adaptive functioning. The choice of the measure to use for determination of cognitive functioning must be based on the language abilities and cooperation level of the individual child; considerations would be similar to those discussed in Chapter 4. In language areas, and particularly with higher functioning or Asperger's disorder, language assessment will need to include measures of pragmatics; the Test of Pragmatic Language may be appropriate in this regard (Kanne et al., 2008). Most important, continuing assessment (progress monitoring) of all domains will be needed over time.

EVIDENCE-BASED INTERVENTIONS

A number of different approaches have been used in the past, and continue to be used, in the treatment of ASDs; the extent to which there is an evidence/research base to support some of these interventions is provided in Table 5.2. Interventions for children with ASDs may focus on specific behaviors or be more comprehensive in scope (J. M. Campbell, Herzinger, & James, 2008). The comprehensive approaches include the use of applied behavior analysis (ABA; Lovaas, 1987), the Treatment and Education of Autistic and Related Communication Handicapped Children (TEACCH) program of structured teaching (Schopler, 1997), and Learning Experiences . . . an Alternative Program (LEAP) (Kohler, Strain, & Goldstein, 2005). Based on multiple reviews and meta-analyses

Table 5.2 Evidence-Based Status of Interventions for Autism Spectrum Disorders

Interventions	Target Behavior	Status
Treatment and Education of Autistic and Related Communication Handicapped Children (TEACCH) program	Comprehensive	Promising practice (J. M. Campbell et al., 2008)
Learning Experiences ... an Alternative Program (LEAP)	Comprehensive	Promising practice (J. M. Campbell et al., 2008)
University of Colorado Health Science Center (UCHSC) program	Comprehensive	Promising practice (Rogers & DiLalla, 1991; Rogers & Lewis, 1989)
Discrete trial training	Communication and other behaviors	Promising practice (J. M. Campbell et al., 2008; H. Goldstein, 2002)
Adult-directed teaching	Communication	Promising practice (Odom et al., 2003)
Incidental teaching	Communication	Promising practice (H. Goldstein, 2002)
Functional communication training	Communication	Promising practice (H. Goldstein, 2002)
Pivotal response treatment	Range of behaviors	Promising practice (Koegel et al., 2001; Rogers & Vismara, 2008; Shearer & Schreibman, 2005)
Differential reinforcement	Communication; stereotypic behavior	Promising practice (J. M. Campbell, 2003; Odom et al., 2003)
Visual systems and supports (e.g., Picture Exchange Communication System; PECS)	Communication	Emerging to promising practice (Odom et al., 2003)
Facilitated communication	Communication	Ineffective (American Academy of Pediatrics Committee on Children with Disabilities, 1998; Simpson, 2005a; Zimmer & Molloy, 2007)
Social skills training (generic)	Social interaction	Inconclusive (Rao et al., 2008)
Social stories	Social interaction	Promising practice (Ali & Frederickson, 2006; Bellini & Peters, 2008)
Video modeling/Video self-modeling	Social communication skills	Promising practice (Bellini & Akullian, 2007)
Peer-mediated training	Socialization, communication	Promising practice (H. Goldstein et al., 1992; McConnell, 2002; Odom et al., 2003)
Self-monitoring	Social interaction	Emerging (Odom et al., 2003)

(continued)

Table 5.2 ***(Continued)***

Interventions	Target Behavior	Status
Positive behavior support	Problem behaviors; functional communication	Promising practice (Odom et al., 2003)
Differential reinforcement	Self-injurious behaviors	Inconclusive (Odom et al., 2003)
Verbal and auditory cues, pictorial cues, activity schedules, video priming	Transition between activities	Promising practice (Sterling-Turner & Jordan, 2007)
Inclusive education	Socialization, communication	Inconclusive (Rogers & Vismara, 2008)
Punishment/overcorrection	Self-injurious behaviors	Inconclusive but may be effective when positive approaches are not successful (Matson & LoVullo, 2008)
Secretin	General ASD behaviors	Ineffective with negative effects (Zimmer & Molloy, 2007)
Glutein-free/casein-free diet	General ASD behaviors	Minimal to ineffective with possible adverse effects (Levy & Hyman, 2008)
Small carbohydrate diet	General ASD behaviors	Minimal to ineffective with possible adverse effects (Levy & Hyman, 2008)
DMG, other nutritional supplements	General ASD behaviors	Minimal to ineffective with possible adverse effects (Bolman & Richmond, 1999; Kern et al., 2001)
Auditory integration training	Sensitivity to sound	Inconclusive (American Academy of Pediatrics Committee on Children with Disabilities, 1998)
Sensory integration training, massage therapy	Sensitivity to stimuli	Inconclusive (Zimmer & Molloy, 2007)
Risperdal (Risperidone)	Aggression, irritability, hyperactivity, stereotypy	Positive practice (Chavez et al., 2006; Gleason et al., 2007; McDougall et al., 2005; Parikh et al., 2008)
Revia (Naltrexone)	Aggression and self-injurious behavior	Inconclusive (Parikh et al., 2008)
Haldol (Haloperidol), Anafranil (clomipramine hydrochloride), Depakote (sodium valproate), Lamictal (lamotrigine)	Aggression and self-injurious behavior	Adverse effects (Parikh et al., 2008)
Other medications: Prozac (fluoxetine), Ritalin, Concerta (methylphenidate), Strattera (atomoxetine)	Repetitive behavior, hyperactivity	Inconclusive (Gleason et al., 2007; Posey et al., 2005)

(J. M. Campbell, 2003; J. M. Campbell et al., 2008; Iovannone, Dunlap, Huber, & Kincaid, 2003; Odom et al., 2003; Rao, Beidel, & Murray, 2008; Rogers & Vismara, 2008), a growing body of research provides information on the extent to which there is evidence to support various practices. At the same time, generally there is a lack of sufficient evidence for any of the treatments to meet criteria for "probably efficacious" or "exemplary" based on criteria for empirically supported treatments (J. M. Campbell et al., 2008). A number of approaches and programs, however, have sufficient studies to be considered "promising practices" or "possibly efficacious" (Rogers & Vismara, 2008). Most often, the criterion not met is that of random assignment to condition as typically accomplished with randomized clinical trials. In many cases, the research evidence is further limited by treatment integrity, differences in treatments across studies, child characteristics, generalizability, and follow-up assessment (J. M. Campbell, 2003; Rao et al., 2008). For example, while many studies have been done with ABA or Lovaas-type interventions, there are often variations across studies.

Of the comprehensive interventions with the most support, many programs or approaches draw from ABA. For example, differential reinforcement of appropriate and desired behaviors (Charlop-Christy, Carpenter, Le, LeBlanc, & Keller, 2002; Drasgow, Halle, & Phillips, 2001; Nuzzolo-Gomez, Leonard, Ortiz, Rivera, & Greer, 2002) and positive behavioral supports have been used to increase communication skills, increase social interactions, and decrease problem behaviors (Keen, Sigafoos, & Woodyatt, 2001). The approach may make use of discrete trial learning based on principles of operant conditioning (Lovaas, 1987), incidental teaching, and functional communication training (H. Goldstein, 2002). Across behavioral approaches, whether positive or aversive, or combination, the behavioral approach has been found to be more effective when the treatment is designed following functional assessment (J. M. Campbell, 2003). Age, treatment intensity, treatment duration, and cognitive level also have been identified as predictors in determining success (Luiselli, Cannon, Ellis, & Sisson, 2000; Rogers, 1998). Across the comprehensive programs, all of which have promising support, common elements incorporate these components. While presenting a problem in comparison and replication across studies, particularly with single-subject design, another common component is that of tailoring the intervention to the specific needs of the individual (J. M. Campbell et al., 2008).

Additional interventions are available with varying levels of support. Various modeling procedures have been used to increase communication and social interaction among children with ASDs, including adult-directed teaching strategies, with the adult providing verbal modeling or prompts (G. Williams, Donley, & Keller, 2000), peer-mediated strategies with peers modeling and providing the prompts (H. Goldstein, Kaczmarck, Pennington, & Shafer, 1992), and the use of video models (Schreibman, Whalen, & Stahmer, 2000). With some children, there is some indication that self-monitoring may be as effective as adult-directed training (Shearer, Kohler, Buchan, & McCullough, 1996). Involvement of various family members in the intervention has been found to increase effectiveness (M. J. Baker, 2000; Dunlap & Fox, 1999; Steibel, 1999). Finally, some studies have attempted to use the child's interests and preferred activities (Koegel, Koegel, & McNerney, 2001), as well as choices, to improve communication and social interaction (C. M. Carter, 2001; Ducharme, Lucas, & Pontes, 1994). Specific accommodations may include providing class notes or outlines, modifying tests to reduce the graphomotor component, allowing additional time for written work, and decreasing written work requirements (Mayes & Calhoon, 2008); the extent to which these accommodations would meet criteria for "evidence based" is unknown. Inclusion often is advocated as an alternative to self-contained programming, but there is little empirical evidence in this regard, and some argue that the intensity of programming needed for individuals with ASDs is not possible within an inclusive setting (Rogers & Vismara, 2008).

In addition to the traditional or conventional approaches to treatment of ASDs, there are a number of unconventional or alternative treatments (Levy & Hyman, 2003, 2005; Zimmer & Molloy, 2007). Biologic treatments (e.g., secretin, diets) tend to address the belief that gastrointestinal problems are responsible for ASDs. Related to dietary interventions, some have recommended the use of digestive enzymes and probiotics for children with ASDs (Levy & Hyman, 2005). Other supplements, including dimethylglycine (DMG), tryptophan, and tyrosine may be recommended but have minimal to no scientific evidence to support their use and in some cases may have negative side effects (Bolman & Richmond, 1999; Kern et al., 2001; Zimmer & Molloy, 2007). Nonbiologic alternative treatments include auditory integration training, sensory integration training, and massage therapy. Supporters claim that benefits of auditory integration training (AIT) include improved attention, improved auditory processing, decreased irritability, reduced lethargy, improved expressive language, and improved auditory comprehension; however, conclusions were that there was insufficient evidence to support AIT in the treatment of ASDs (American Academy of Pediatrics Committee on Children with Disabilities, 1998). There are few well-designed clinical trials examining sensory integration therapy, massage therapy, movement therapy, or cranio-sacral manipulation for treatment of ASDs (Zimmer & Molloy, 2007). A new approach uses neurofeedback to modulate *mu* rhythms to address the dysfunctional mirror neuron system (Oberman, Ramachandran, & Pineda, 2008); studies are under way to see if this is effective. It should be noted that some of these "therapies" may be dangerous or at least very costly to implement and have no proven or potentially harmful effects (see Table 5.2).

Finally, psychopharmacological interventions have been tried with children and adults on the spectrum. Published studies with young children on the spectrum have focused on risperidone with two randomized clinical trials (Luby et al., 2006; Nagaraj, Singhi, & Malhi, 2006) as well as one open trial (Masi, Cosenza, Mucci, & Brovedani, 2003). Consistently, across studies, there are indications of decreased behaviors, particularly those related to irritability, aggression, and stereotypy (McDougall et al., 2005); at the same time, there is little evidence of effect on other core autistic behaviors (Chavez, Chavez-Brown, & Rey, 2006; Gleason et al., 2007).

CASE STUDY: JOHN—ASPERGER'S DISORDER

The next report is from a hospital-based clinic. Identifying information, such as child and family name, teacher or physician name, and school information, has been altered or fictionalized to protect confidentiality.

Reason for Referral

John is a 12-year-old Caucasian male who was referred for a neuropsychological assessment to determine his current neurocognitive functioning. John's parents reported declines across various areas of functioning including speech/language skills, vision, academic functioning, and social-emotional functioning (i.e., withdrawn, social rejection). Past medical history is significant for a diagnosis of Asperger's disorder; this diagnosis was based on behavioral criteria in areas of pragmatic communication, social relationships, and stereotypy/restricted behavior by a licensed professional specializing in ASDs; diagnosis was not the purpose of this evaluation. John's parents are searching for the most appropriate and optimal school placement and programming; they have requested this neuropsychological to assist in the intervention planning.

Assessment Procedures

John's parents provided information via questionnaire and interview format. Available medical records and a previous evaluation were reviewed. These assessment measures were utilized during the evaluation:

Wechsler Intelligence Scale for Children, Fourth Edition (WISC-IV)
Woodcock-Johnson Tests of Achievement, Third Edition—Form A (WJ III Achievement)
Developmental Test of Visual Motor-Integration, Fifth Edition (DTVMI-V)
Motor-Free Visual Perception Test, Third Edition (MVPT-3)
Grooved Pegboard Test
Rey Complex Figure Test (RCFT)
Wide Range Assessment of Memory and Learning, Second Edition (WRAML-2)
Wisconsin Card Sort-64 (WCST-64)
Behavior Rating Inventory of Executive Function (BRIEF; Parent Form)
Achenbach Child Behavior Checklist (CBCL; Parent & Teacher Forms)

Background Information

Home

John is an only child and resides with his parents. No recent psychosocial stressors within the home were reported.

Medical

John was born following a full-term pregnancy that was complicated by his mother having the flu during the second trimester. He was delivered vaginally via a lengthy labor (27.5 hours) and weighed 7 pounds 12 ounces at birth. John remained in the hospital for 2 days due to dehydration. John has been a relatively healthy child, with no hospitalizations, surgeries, or long-term medications. Medical history is significant for Asperger's disorder, vision problems (accommodative spasm, very nearsighted), allergies, occasional headaches, and one febrile seizure at 5 years of age. With regard to early development, John's speech, motor, and self-help milestones reportedly were achieved within normal limits. Per parents, family history is significant for bipolar disorder (cousin) and alcohol/substance abuse (aunt, grandparents).

John's parents reported that approximately 10 months ago, he began experiencing declines across various areas of functioning. John reported vision problems, eye pain, headaches, decline in academic functioning, fatigue, and increased social withdrawal. John's parents also reported hair loss on the top/back portion of his head that was suspected to be alopecia or trichotillomania. He is currently prescribed a topical steroid. Magnetic resonance imaging and all blood work performed by the hospital was reportedly within normal limits. He has a scheduled appointment at the Genetics Clinic next week.

John was diagnosed with Asperger's disorder. He reportedly has difficulties with distinguishing between real and fiction, understanding nonverbal cues, social/peer interactions, some sensory stimuli, unusual types of interests, focused/intense interests, atypical use of objects, and withdrawal when overstimulated. Specific social-emotional concerns included difficulty expressing emotion, naiveté, poor eye contact, preference for solitary play, anxiety, and limited social interaction. John has a long history of language/pragmatics therapy from a local university-based clinic twice a week; despite the interventions, language/pragmatics are reported to be atypical.

Educational

John is currently enrolled in the seventh grade at a local junior high school; no previous grade retentions were reported. Per teacher report, John receives Section 504 accommodations, including preferential seating and study guides. He currently maintains a C–F average across subjects, which is a significant decline compared to his grades in the sixth grade. John's parents reported that he also receives tutoring at school and privately, particularly for math. He is noted to "work better verbally than visually." John's teachers reported that he is a "pleasant young man and respectful," but he has problems with following directions, inconsistent work performance, loses interest easily, appears withdrawn, isolates himself, avoids eye contact, and twirls/pulls out his hair. One teacher also noted John's significant difficulties with sequential math and basic math skills.

Behavioral Observations

John was a quiet boy who presented with an awkward shyness but transitioned well to the testing session. He demonstrated poor eye contact, no spontaneous conversation, and flat affect. Verbal output was characterized by "yes/no" or short answers to questions, and his speech was somewhat muffled. John was appropriate in height and weight compared to same-age peers and was dressed appropriately for weather and setting. He did not wear glasses during the evaluation, and no hearing difficulties were reported or observed. John appeared able to see the test materials presented at a normal distance, and he was able to hear verbal instructions spoken at a normal conversational tone. John appeared to give his best effort on all tasks but was slowed in his mental processing and psychomotor speed. He maintained good attention to tasks; however, he displayed anxiety symptoms including picking at eyebrows and nails. Poor gross motor skills were observed including awkward gait, poor balance, and clumsy walking movements. In terms of upper extremities, he was right-hand dominant, with an immature pencil grip (thumb over two fingers). No tremors or associated movements were observed on motor output tasks. Results from this evaluation should be considered a valid indication of John's current neurocognitive functioning.

Assessment

Intellectual Functions

John's intellectual functioning was assessed using the WISC-IV and was found to be in the low-average to borderline impaired range. Scores were: Full Scale IQ = 79, Verbal Comprehension Index = 87, Perceptual Reasoning Index = 86, Working Memory Index = 91, and Processing Speed Index = 70. John appeared to have great difficulty with tasks involving mental processing speed, visual scanning, visual-perceptual discrimination, and psychomotor speed; however, his short-term sequential memory and working memory skills were intact (see Table 5.3).

Academic Functioning

John's academic functioning was assessed using selected subtests from the Woodcock-Johnson Tests of Achievement, Third Edition (WJ III): Form A. All scores were in the average to very superior range. Scores were: Letter-Word Identification = 126, Passage Comprehension = 107, Calculation = 105, Applied Problems = 100, Spelling = 138, and Writing Samples = 103. John appeared to have greater ease with more basic tasks and tasks requiring rote memory, such as spelling and reading increasingly difficult words.

Table 5.3 Psychometric Summary for John

	Scaled Score	Standard Score
Wechsler Intelligence Scale for Children, Fourth Edition (WISC-IV)		
Full Scale IQ		79
Verbal Comprehension Index		87
Perceptual Reasoning Index		86
Working Memory Index		91
Processing Speed Index		70
Developmental Test of Visual Motor Integration, Fifth Edition (DTVMI-V)		76
Motor-Free Visual Perception Test, Third Edition (MVPT-3)		81
Grooved Pegboard Test		57
Wide Range Assessment of Memory and Learning, Second Edition (WRAML-2)		
General Memory Index Score		76
Verbal Memory Index		97
Visual Memory Index		76
Attention/Concentration Index		73
Story Memory	11	
Design Memory	5	
Verbal Learning	8	
Picture Memory	7	
Finger Windows	1	
Number/Letter	10	
Story Memory Recall	11	
Verbal Learning Recall	7	
Design Recognition	9	
Behavior Rating Inventory of Executive (BRIEF), Parent Form		
Clinical Scales	T- Scores	
Inhibit	45	
Shift	59	
Emotional Control	42	
Initiate	59	

(continued)

Table 5.3 *(Continued)*

	T-Scores	Standard Score
Working Memory	62	
Plan/Organize	61	
Organization of Materials	52	
Monitor	60	
Indices		
Behavioral Regulation Index	48	
Metacognition Index	61	
General Executive Composite	57	
Woodcock-Johnson Tests of Achievement, Third Edition (WJ III)		
Letter-Word Identification		126
Calculation		105
Spelling		138
Passage Comprehension		107
Applied Problems		100
Writing Samples		103

Visual-Perceptual and Visual-Motor Functions

Visual-motor integration and visual-motor output skills were assessed using the Developmental Test of Visual-Motor Integration (VMI). John demonstrated a right-handed immature pencil grip (thumb over two fingers) and completed only 20 out of 30 simple figure designs. He obtained a Standard Score of 76 (5th percentile), suggesting borderline impaired visual-constructional abilities. Figures were distorted for age, but no directional confusion was noted.

With regard to visual-perceptual skills, John was administered the Motor-Free Visual Perception Test, Third Edition (MVPT-3). On this task, he obtained a Standard Score of 81 (10th percentile), which fell within the low-average range. In examining his profile, he had particular difficulty with items involving visual discrimination, spatial orientation, visual closure, and embedded figure/figure ground tasks. In combination, these scores indicated significant problems in the areas of visual-perceptual and visual-constructional skills. These problems are negatively affecting his academic functioning, particularly in math and written output.

John demonstrated significant difficulty on the copy performance portion of the Rey Complex Figure Test. He scored in the $\leqslant$ 1st percentile (raw score = 28) compared to others his same age. He was unorganized in his copy approach, and the design was significantly distorted. Problems with this task are likely related to poor visual-perceptual and visual-constructional skills as well as poor motor planning and organization.

Psychomotor speed and fine motor coordination were measured using the Grooved Pegboard Test. John demonstrated significant psychomotor slowing across hands bilaterally, with an appropriate dominant hand advantage. He had particular difficulty with his left hand (Scaled Score = 57; 2 dropped pegs), including motor slowing and poor fine motor coordination.

Memory Functions

John was administered the Wide Range Assessment of Memory and Learning, Second Edition (WRAML-2) as a measure of general memory processing skills. John's General Memory Index Score was in the borderline impaired range of functioning; however, there was a significant difference between his verbal and visual memory scores as well as within verbal memory areas. John did much better on recall of verbal information that is meaningful and semantically related (i.e., story recall); he had more difficulty on recall of unconnected words (i.e., list learning). In visual areas, John had particular difficulty with encoding, transfer, and retrieval of visual information, which is consistent with his measured difficulties with visual-perceptual stimuli, as noted. John also demonstrated difficulty with short-term sequential visual memory tasks, which lowered his overall Attention/Concentration Index score. These memory problems are adversely impacting academic performance and support the idea that he tends to learn better verbally. John's verbal memory strength should be used in teaching him; however, he would benefit from multiple modes of input, including verbal, visual, and tactile, in his learning. He also will benefit from repetition in his learning and cues/prompting to aid in memory retrieval processes.

Executive Functions

The results of the Behavior Rating Inventory of Executive Function (BRIEF)—Parent Form are presented in Table 5.3. This form was completed by John's mother to assess current executive skills functioning. Overall, John's profile fell within the average range, with no significant areas of weakness.

John also was administered the Wisconsin Card Sort-64 (WCST-64) as an objective measure of executive functioning. His problem-solving and mental flexibility skills fell in the low-average to impaired range. John had 31 total errors, 28 perseverative responses, 2 completed categories, and 0 failures to maintain set. John was able to perform basic problem solving when given verbal feedback on his performance; however, he began to guess when categorization of set became more difficult. He had specific difficulties with mental set shifting and perseveration.

Social-Emotional and Behavioral Functioning

Behavior and social-emotional functioning was measured using the Achenbach Child Behavior Checklist (CBCL)—Parent & Teacher Forms. John's mother reported problems with depression, somatic complaints, social interactions, and attention problems. On the same scale, John's teacher reported the same areas of problems as well as behaviors consistent with anxiety and thought problems.

Summary

- John has a previous diagnosis of Asperger's disorder with reported general decline across areas of functioning beginning 10 months ago. He is currently enrolled in the seventh grade and receives Section 504 modifications and tutoring for math.
- Intellectual skills were found to be in the low-average to borderline impaired range, with particular difficulty with tasks involving mental processing speed, visual scanning, visual-perceptual discrimination, and psychomotor speed.

- Academic abilities were in the average to superior range. No learning disabilities were indicated. He performed better on basic and rote memory tasks.
- Significant difficulties were noted with visual-perceptual and visual-constructional skills as well as motor planning and organization.
- John exhibited slowed mental processing speed, especially with visual-perceptual tasks. Psychomotor speed was slowed across hands, with greater difficulty with his left hand (nondominant).
- Significant problems with visual memory processes, retrieval functions, and higher level memory organization were identified. In addition, John evidenced difficulties with problem-solving skills and mental flexibility (perseveration and set shifting).
- Per parent and teacher report, John has continued difficulties with poor motivation and limited social interaction as well as problems with attention and anxiety. Behavior observations were consistent with flat affect, poor eye contact, limited conversation, and limited social interaction.

Diagnostic Impressions

- Results from the current neuropsychological evaluation indicated significant difficulties with visual-perceptual and visual-constructional skills as well as visual memory functions (encoding and retrieval). These problems are consistent with his reported areas of academic underachievement, especially involving math and written output. John also demonstrated significant slowing with mental processing speed and psychomotor output, more with his left hand. This pattern of problems suggests difficulties with right temporal and right frontal lobe functioning.
- Difficulties with inattention, problem solving, set shifting, and mental flexibility also indicate problems with prefrontal lobe functioning. This pattern of problems likely will adversely impact his math abilities, written output, inconsistencies in classroom performance, ability to complete multistep directions, and planning and organizational skills.
- John's profile is consistent with a diagnosis of Asperger's disorder. He also demonstrates a pattern of symptoms similar to that of a person with nonverbal learning disorder (NVLD). It should be noted that NVLD and Asperger's disorder have similar patterns of symptoms and are often difficult to differentiate.

Recommendations

- John's parents were provided with a detailed packet on Asperger's disorder at today's evaluation.
- John's parents are encouraged to share this report with his school and consider the need for placement as a child with a disability under the Individuals with Disabilities Education Improvement Act (Autism Spectrum Disorder or Part B; Other Health Impaired; e.g., special education and related services). John's diagnosis of Asperger's disorder should qualify him for these services; however, determination of an educational disability is made by the student's educational committee. If these services are not available, John should continue to receive services under Section 504 of the Rehabilitation Act of 1973 (e.g., modification plan designed, implemented, and evaluated in the regular classroom). In any case, John requires

additional classroom modifications and possible resource classes for math if he is to achieve at his potential.

These are suggested recommendations for the home and school:

- John's difficulties with constructional tasks and motor planning skills likely will affect his efficacy on writing tasks. He should be allowed extra time to complete writing tasks and to utilize printing if this is a more effective means for written communication. Alternatives to conventional writing also may need to be considered, such as a laptop computer, word processor, and/or tape recorder. A tape recorder will be particularly effective since it will allow John to dictate initial drafts of writing assignments, eliminating any significant motor output requirements. For essay-type tests, he may benefit from the option of dictating his response or from oral testing.
- It is suggested that his school provide John with all of his textbooks as audio recordings. This will give him the opportunity to gain access to information without relying strictly on his reading abilities. It also will allow him to utilize his strengths with verbal memory.
- Due to John's significant difficulty with visual-perceptual and visual-constructional tasks, these modifications should be considered:
  - Relaxed grading for handwriting.
  - Relax time limits for written material.
  - Pair visual material with an auditory presentation of material.
- John should not be required to complete lengthy copying tasks. He would benefit from copies of the lecture notes, slide presentation, and so on prior to the lecture.
- John may benefit from the option of dictating his response or from oral testing.
- Allow the use of computers or typewriters for written assignments.
- These classroom modifications should be considered to help with attention and concentration problems:
  - John should be given preferential seating in his school classes. He should be seated close to the teacher in order to minimize distractions, and away from windows, doors, and pencil sharpeners in order to minimize distractibility.
  - The teacher should provide necessary prompts and cues (preferably unnoticeable to other children).
  - Larger tasks should be broken into smaller, more manageable tasks, such as presenting John with only one worksheet at a time. Also, parts of an assigned worksheet page can be covered up (hidden) to reduce distraction or stress.
  - Teachers should try to keep instructions and directions concise and simple as possible.
  - John should be allowed to take breaks when possible.
  - Multiple modalities should be used when presenting directions, explanations, and instructional content (e.g., auditory, visual, tactile, etc.), especially visual aids (e.g., schedule of events, written instructions on board).
  - Teachers should provide John with ample time (preferably one week) and specific/detailed study guides to help with exam/project preparation.
  - Due to John's visual-perceptual processing and slowed mental processing speed, he would benefit from modified assignments (e.g., reduced length or number of

problems) and increased time limits on tests and assignments. Another option would be a modified grading system in which John is graded based on completed work if an appropriate amount of work is attempted. This will also help to reduce John's test and performance anxiety.

- John appears to benefit from cuing and structure in order to facilitate retrieval of information. Given this finding, it is suggested that teachers give him multiple-choice or matching format tests whenever possible. Word banks also would be beneficial in cuing recall of information.
- John would benefit from a structured environment and as much one-on-one teaching as possible. He also would benefit from a visual schedule attached to his desk to help with changes in schedule and self-monitoring. A male "buddy" also may help John with increasing social skills and transitioning between classes.
- John is quite perseverative in his response style; this interferes with his skills at shifting effectively and efficiently within or between tasks. Teachers need to monitor his performance on in-class worksheets as he will require extra time and direct cues to facilitate subtle shift (e.g., changing from addition to subtraction on a math worksheet). John also will require a brief break or extra warm-up time when expected to change from one task to another.
- Due to John's problems with visual-perceptual processing, it will be extremely difficult for him to complete "bubble answers" on most standardized test forms. He should be allowed to write his answers, dictate into a voice recorder, or dictate the answers to someone who can complete the form.
- John is encouraged to engage in activities involving visual-perceptual skills (e.g., putting puzzles together or models).
- It is suggested that John use a daily assignment/homework notebook. He will need direct teacher assistance as he adjusts to using this organizational/memory tool. Teachers will need to provide him with cues as to what needs to be logged into the notebook. A lead teacher then will need to review the notebook at the end of each school day and provide direct cues as to what materials are needed for that evening's homework. John's mother should maintain close contact and monitoring with the school, including signing off on the notebook each night, to ensure success with this tool.

These recommendations are to be considered for working memory problems:

- John should be taught strategies to help him better retain basic concepts, including making meaningful/applied connections of instructional material as well as the use of mnemonic devices or associative cues to assist with his memory.
- Repeated drill and practice of basic skills presented through multiple formats will increase the likelihood of retention. Software programs may provide this drill in a more gamelike format.
- John should create environmental cues to aid with memory, such as a schedule of daily events on his desk, to-do lists, and the like.

John's current social skills should continue to be fostered at home, through therapy, and at school through the use of modeling emotions and social stories portraying appropriate pictures and labels of emotions. The next social stories books and authors are suggested:

- *Comic Strip Conversations: Colorful Illustrated Interactions with Students with Autism and Related Disorders* by Carol Gray
- *The Original Social Story Book* and *The New Social Story Book* by Carol Gray
- Encourage John's participation in activities in and outside of school to maximize his opportunities for socialization with his same-age peers.
- John should have a follow-up neuropsychological evaluation in two years to continue to map his neurocognitive development.

Further Discussion of Case Study

John's history and progress are consistent with the pattern often evident with youth with Asperger's disorder. He demonstrates the decreased nonverbal/visual spatial abilities as well as impaired executive function. Notably, John had difficulty with the embedded figures task; this is often an area of strength for youth with Asperger's disorder, but not in this case. As often occurs with ASDs, individual differences preclude the assumption of a specific pattern of strengths and weaknesses. The extensive list of recommendations addresses all aspects of impairment noted; multiple suggestions are offered to allow flexibility by the service providers in choosing interventions and prioritizing target behaviors. Because John's behaviors did not emerge as being particularly problematic, there is less reliance on Applied Behavior Analysis (ABA) methods, but a structured setting with consistent expectations continues to be recommended.

CONCLUDING COMMENTS

In the popular press as well as in the professional community, there is increased concern for the numbers of children being identified with ASDs as well as potentially negative or limited outcomes for these children as they grow into adulthood. It has been suggested that ASDs are the most severely debilitating of the neurocognitive disorders (Pelios & Lund, 2005); only mental retardation is considered to occur at the same frequency (Newschaffer et al., 2007). A number of theories have been proposed and with advances in neuroscience, more is known about ASDs now than previously. At the same time, much still is unknown about the highly heterogeneous group of individuals who fall somewhere on the spectrum; no specific genotype or endophenotype has been identified (Newschaffer et al., 2007).

One of the major points of consensus is the need for early identification and early intervention if potential success and positive outcomes are to be maximized. The broad range of deficits that can be associated with ASDs and the variations in manifestation across the behavioral triad of communication, social interaction, and stereotypy/restricted range make it virtually impossible to develop a phenotype for the ASDs. Assessment and subsequent intervention need to be determined on an individual basis (Myles, Grossman, Aspy, Henry, & Coffin, 2007). As with all neurocognitive disabilities, there is a need for further research relative to scientifically based and effective practices (Simpson, 2005a,b). At the same time that there is increased concern with the evidentiary base to choosing interventions, attention also is being given to social validation and the extent to which various stakeholders support the use of various interventions (Callahan, Henson, & Cowan, 2008).

Chapter 6

ATTENTION-DEFICIT/HYPERACTIVITY DISORDER

DEFINITION

Attention-Deficit/Hyperactivity Disorder (ADHD) is defined as "a persistent pattern of inattention and/or hyperactivity-impulsivity that is more frequently displayed and more severe than is typically observed in individuals at a comparable level of development" (American Psychiatric Association [APA], 2000, p. 85). The *Diagnostic and Statistical Manual of Mental Disorders* (*DSM*) classifies these symptoms into three subtypes of ADHD: predominantly inattentive type (persistent symptoms of inattention), predominantly hyperactive-impulsive type (persistent symptoms of hyperactivity and/or impulsivity), and combined type (persistent symptoms of inattention in combination with persistent symptoms of hyperactivity-impulsivity). The combined type is thought to be the most common subtype among children and adolescents. In order to warrant a diagnosis of ADHD, some of the symptoms must have been seen before the child reached 7 years of age. This does not mean that ADHD must be diagnosed in early childhood but points to the importance of a thorough developmental history when diagnosing older children and adolescents. Further, the symptoms must be seen in more than one setting (e.g., academic, social, occupational) and must cause significant interference in everyday functioning (APA, 2000).

Prevalence/Incidence

Research suggests that ADHD may look somewhat different in girls as compared to boys, with girls being more likely to demonstrate inattentive symptoms than hyperactive-impulsive symptoms (Staller & Faraone, 2006). ADHD appears to be diagnosed among boys more often than among girls, and boys are referred for ADHD evaluations at a higher rate, perhaps due to higher levels of oppositional and externalizing behaviors that are disruptive and therefore lead to referral (Stefanatos & Baron, 2007). The estimated prevalence of ADHD is 5% to 10% among children and adolescents and 4% among adults (Biederman, 2005); prevalence among preschoolers (children from 2 to 5 years of age) has been estimated at 2% to 8% (Egger, Kondo, & Angold, 2006).

The hyperactive-impulsive subtype appears to be the rarest and tends to occur mostly in young children, while the combined subtype appears to be the most common subtype (Pelham, Fabiano, & Massetti, 2005). Interestingly, those young children who are initially diagnosed as hyperactive-impulsive may be reclassified as the combined subtype later in school, when the attentional demands of tasks increase and attention deficits become more pronounced (Egger et al., 2006; B. B. Lahey, Pelham, Loney, & Willcutt, 2005). Further, the gender difference in prevalence (i.e., males diagnosed more than females) appears to be less drastic with the predominantly inattentive type (APA, 2000).

Diagnostic Process

Various measures commonly used in assessing the different domains and symptoms of ADHD were identified in Chapter 1. Assessment of ADHD in childhood and adolescence typically involves gathering information from multiple sources, including parent interviews and behavioral rating scales, teacher interviews and behavioral rating scales, detailed developmental history, classroom observations across several different tasks and subject areas, review of educational records (e.g., grades, pattern of discipline referrals), and clinical information from the child or adolescent (e.g., interview, tests of academic achievement and cognitive functioning) (American Academy of Pediatrics, 2000). All of these pieces of information are essential in determining whether the child meets *DSM* criteria (e.g., symptoms present before 7 years of age, impairment in more than one setting) and also to account for possible comorbidity or alternative explanations for symptoms, as many behaviors associated with ADHD may be explained by other conditions or problems (e.g., vision or hearing problems, learning disabilities, cognitive deficits, situational factors). A comprehensive assessment battery was used as part of the Multimodal Treatment Study of Children with ADHD, which provides an example of what a multicomponent assessment approach might look like (Hinshaw et al., 1997).

Omnibus behavioral rating scales often are used to examine the potential for comorbidity, such as depression and anxiety. These scales typically have parent-, teacher-, and self-report components, thereby allowing the clinician to examine differences in symptom manifestation based on factors such as rater and setting. Examples of frequently used rating scales with children and adolescents include the Behavior Assessment System for Children, Second Edition (BASC-2) (Reynolds & Kamphaus, 2004) and the Conners' Rating Scales Revised (C. K. Conners, 1997, 2008). One of the interesting issues encountered by clinicians when using these rating scales is the potential for low cross-informant consistency in behavioral ratings. Low to moderate correlations across parent and teacher ratings were observed based on the normative data for the BASC-2 and Conners' scales (C. K. Conners, 2008; Reynolds & Kamphaus, 2004), suggesting variability across informants. Similarly, a recent study (Sullivan & Riccio, 2007) examining the Conners' Rating Scales Revised—Short Form (Conners, 1997) and Behavior Rating Inventory of Executive Function (BRIEF) (Gioia, Isquith, Guy, & Kenworthy, 2000) rating scales indicated that correlations between parent and teacher ratings on parallel scales were statistically significant but moderate in magnitude; cross-informant coefficients for the BRIEF ranged from .31 to .59 (median $r = .48$) and coefficients for the Conners' scale ranged from .51 to .58 (median $r = .54$). In a way, the moderate magnitude of these correlations seems desirable in light of the purpose of ADHD assessment using multiple informants: If consistency between raters is too low, the behavioral symptoms of ADHD may be related primarily to a specific setting or context; if consistency between raters is extremely high, we gain only limited additive information by gathering ratings from multiple sources. Moderately correlated ratings suggest a degree of behavioral stability across settings and contexts while also allowing for both some differences in perspective among raters and the possibility that the child's behaviors may be more conspicuous or disruptive in some situations than in others (e.g., based on the unique characteristics of a particular classroom, social situation, or academic subject). Another study compared the results of the BRIEF and the BASC (Jarratt, Riccio, & Siekierski, 2005), with results indicating that the BASC and BRIEF scales appear to be measuring similar, but still distinct, constructs pertaining to behaviors associated with ADHD. The findings suggested that use of both the BASC and BRIEF in ADHD assessment provided additional, rather than redundant, information and may be useful in designing a comprehensive treatment plan.

Results of the Sullivan and Riccio (2007) study also suggested that while the BRIEF and Conners' scales were able to distinguish children with ADHD or other clinical diagnoses from children without any diagnosis, the scales were less successful at discriminating children with ADHD from those with other clinical diagnoses. This pattern of results also suggests that, to some extent, the characteristics of ADHD and executive dysfunction measured by the BRIEF and the widely used Conners' scales may not be specific to children and adolescents with ADHD. This is consistent with research suggesting that executive dysfunction may be involved in psychiatric disorders other than just ADHD (Gioia et al., 2002; P. K. Shear, DelBello, Rosenberg, & Strakowski, 2002), thereby contributing to the difficulty in accurately differentiating ADHD from other conditions or disorders. When conducting ADHD evaluations (or psychological assessments of any type, for that matter), behavioral rating scales provide critical pieces of information, but these data must be corroborated by other sources in order to make the most accurate diagnostic decisions.

The extent to which patterns in intelligence test scores can distinguish children with ADHD from children without ADHD has been subject to debate, with one consistent pattern showing that children with ADHD score lowest on the Working Memory and Processing Speed indexes on the Wechsler scales (Mayes & Calhoun, 2006). Tests of intelligence and academic achievement often are used in the assessment process in order to assess the possibility of learning disabilities or cognitive deficits as better (or additional) explanations for the student's difficulties.

Nigg (2005) conducted a review of the psychological assessment literature related to ADHD, in order to identify those assessment methods best able to distinguish children with ADHD from those without. Some of these tasks (and their associated effect sizes) include Spatial Working Memory (0.75 to 1.14), Response Suppression Tasks (0.61 to 0.94), Continuous Performance Tests (0.72), Stroop Naming Speed (0.69), Full Scale IQ (0.61), Trails B Time (0.55 to 0.75), Tower Tasks (0.51 to 0.69), Mazes (0.58), Verbal Working Memory (0.41 to 0.51), Decision Speed Tasks (0.49), Wisconsin Card Sort Test Perseverative Errors (0.35 to 0.53), Fluency (0.27), and Stroop Interference (0.25) (Nigg, 2005). The ability of many neuropsychological tests to detect or distinguish ADHD has been questioned, as some individuals with ADHD do not demonstrate deficits in executive function or other relevant neuropsychological constructs. That is, some tests demonstrate satisfactory sensitivity to ADHD but inadequate specificity (Seidman, 2006); however, this may be less an indictment of our tests and more an indication that ADHD is multidetermined and may have different etiological pathways (and therefore varying neuropsychological deficits or profiles) for different people.

Pelham et al. (2005) reviewed methods of assessing ADHD in children and adolescents and, based on psychometric properties and clinical utility, concluded that evidence-based methods include behavioral rating scales designed to identify ADHD, omnibus rating scales, structured interviews based on the *DSM* system, and behavioral observations. The review also supports the collection of data (i.e., from rating scales) from both parents and teachers, in order to provide a comprehensive perspective. Notably, tasks such as continuous performance tests and tower tasks were not identified as evidence-based assessment methods for diagnosing ADHD; nor were imaging procedures such as magnetic resonance imaging (MRI) or positron emission tomography (PET) scans (Pelham et al., 2005). This makes sense given the current behavioral (as opposed to biological or neurological) definition of the disorder. Functional behavior assessment also may be informative in order to identify targets for intervention based on what factors might be triggering and maintaining the problematic behaviors (i.e., antecedents and consequences).

ETIOLOGY

Genetic Contributions

Recent research suggests a strong genetic contribution to the etiology of ADHD. For example, in a comprehensive review, high heritability indexes were found in numerous twin studies (Waldman & Gizer, 2006). Similarly, based on a review of 18 twin studies, the mean heritability index was found to be .77 (Biederman, 2005). Further, other studies have focused on the potential contribution of specific genes and neurotransmitter systems (e.g., dopamine transporter gene, dopamine receptor D4, serotonin transporter gene, serotonin receptor genes) to the manifestation of ADHD characteristics. The role or observed contribution of these various genes and neurotransmitters to ADHD has been somewhat inconsistent across studies (J. M. Swanson et al., 2007); see Swanson et al. (2007) and Waldman and Gizer (2006) for a complete description of the current status of knowledge in this area.

Neurological Correlates

Regardless of whether the behavioral constellation of ADHD is the result of genetics or other causes, several neuropsychological constructs have been implicated as playing roles in the development and manifestation of ADHD. Some of these constructs with empirical support include sustained attention, behavioral inhibition, working memory, and planning ability; these abilities often are included within the multifaceted construct called executive function (Barkley, 1997; Stefanatos & Baron, 2007). It follows that specific areas and structures of the brain that may be involved in ADHD include the frontal lobe, mesocortical pathway from the substantia nigra to the prefrontal cortex, mesolimbic pathway, nigrostiatal pathway, basal ganglia, limbic system, thalamus, corpus callosum, and cerebellum (Krain & Castellanos, 2006; Nigg, 2005). Broadly speaking, evidence suggests that ADHD is related to frontal lobe dysfunction and abnormal connections between the frontal lobe and subcortical areas of the brain (Biederman, 2005). See Figure 6.1 for an illustration of some of the more well-documented neurological correlates and pathways contributing to ADHD.

Swanson et al. (2007) provided a review of the literature supporting the dopamine deficit hypothesis, which postulates that dysfunction of the neurotransmitter dopamine is a causal factor in the development of ADHD. The authors explain that dopamine is involved in carrying out some of the behaviors affected by ADHD, such as planning and self-regulation. In addition, the authors review the literature on other dopamine-related biological factors contributing to ADHD, citing findings such as: Compared to control participants, individuals with ADHD have smaller brain structures such as the caudate nucleus and globus pallidus. In addition, children with ADHD show reduced blood flow and metabolism in the frontal lobes; and stimulant medications, such as methylphenidate, reduce ADHD symptoms by increasing dopamine levels. The pattern of findings

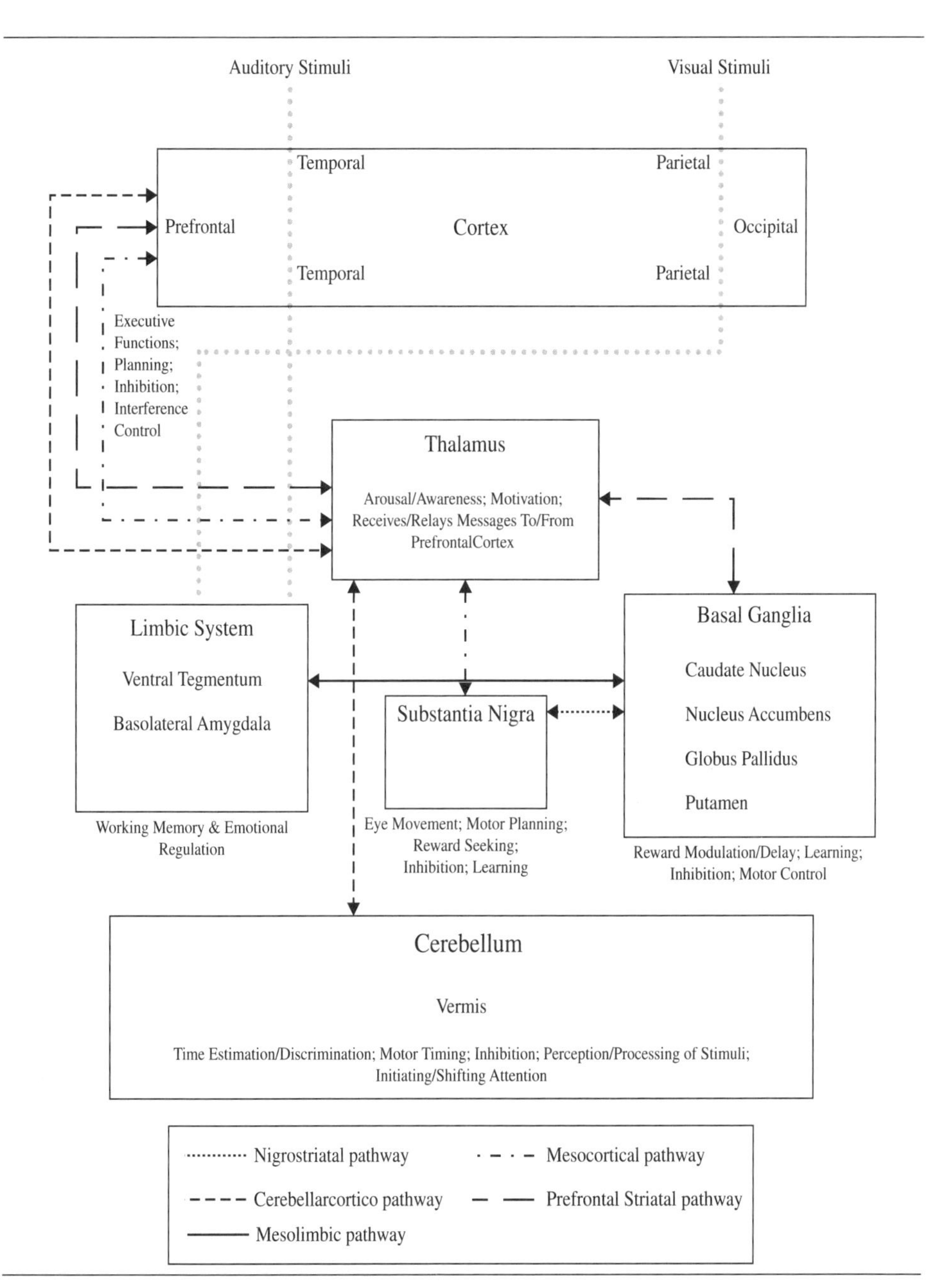

Figure 6.1 Pathways involved in ADHD.

presented in the Swanson et al. review supports the hypothesis that dopamine deficiencies play a role in the development and manifestation of ADHD.

Several imaging studies conducted by Castellanos and colleagues (2001, 2003) support anatomic differences between children with and without ADHD. For example, using MRI scans on nine pairs of monozygotic twins (with one twin in each pair having ADHD and the other twin not having ADHD), twins with ADHD had significantly smaller total caudate volume with no significant differences in other areas (e.g., frontal lobes, temporal lobes, cerebellum), suggesting a link between prefrontal-striatal circuitry and ADHD (Castellanos et al., 2003). Similarly, these authors have found that both boys and girls with ADHD had smaller total brain volume compared to those without ADHD, in addition to significantly smaller volumes in the posterior-inferior cerebellar vermis (Castellanos et al., 2001). A similar study also reported decreased volume of the superior cerebellar vermis among children with ADHD, thereby supporting the involvement of the cerebellum identified by Castellanos's team (Mackie et al., 2007). Interestingly, the Castellanos et al. (2001) study described findings in which brain variables (e.g., total cerebral volume, posterior-inferior vermal volume) were significantly correlated with Full Scale IQ and scores on parent rating scales such as attention problems and anxiety-depression. With all of these correlations, smaller cortical volumes were associated with greater levels of pathology. Thus, these anatomic brain variables may be able to predict important intellectual and behavioral variables, but much more research is needed in order to identify the relationships between interconnected systems and cognitive-behavioral outcomes.

Two recent reviews summarized MRI studies examining neuroanatomical differences between children with and without ADHD. Krain and Castellanos (2006) noted that most MRI research on ADHD has examined total cerebral volume, prefrontal regions, basal ganglia, corpus callosum, and cerebellum. The most consistent finding across MRI studies identified by Krain and Castellanos is related to overall brain size: Children and adolescents with ADHD tend to have significantly smaller brains than control children. Numerous studies also have found significantly smaller prefrontal cortex and cerebellum (especially the posterior-inferior cerebellar vermis) in children with ADHD. With regard to the basal ganglia (including the caudate and putamen) and corpus callosum, studies have been less consistent: Some report smaller structures among children with ADHD while several studies report no significant difference. Differences in the caudate may be age dependent, as the differences tend to get smaller with adolescence. A comprehensive review of imaging studies reached similar conclusions and provides further confirmation of involvement of the frontal-striatal circuit in ADHD (Willis & Weiler, 2005), which also supports theoretical models of ADHD that conceptualize the disorder as a behavioral manifestation of deficits in executive function and behavioral inhibition (Barkley, 1997).

Most MRI studies have small sample sizes due to the expense of MRI scans; these small sizes, in conjunction with other methodological issues (e.g., whether comorbidity is accounted for, whether IQ is used as a covariate, whether females are included in addition to males, whether ADHD subtypes are differentiated, whether participants are medication naive) likely contribute to inconsistencies across studies (Krain & Castellanos, 2006; Willis & Weiler, 2005). As the methodological rigor of these imaging studies increases, it is likely that consistency of results across studies will increase as well. Imaging methods have not been recommended as part of the diagnostic process for ADHD but are recognized as valuable procedures for research on the etiology of ADHD.

Environmental Factors

Correlational data suggest a relationship between several environmental factors and the development of ADHD characteristics; these factors include prenatal exposure to nicotine, exposure to low levels of lead during early childhood, and complications surrounding pregnancy (J. M. Swanson et al., 2007). These relationships have been observed across multiple studies. Another environmental factor identified in the development and manifestation of ADHD is chaotic or inconsistent parenting, although this may represent an interactive relationship in which inconsistent or negative parenting develops in response to the child's disruptive behaviors associated with ADHD, thereby exacerbating these very behaviors (Daley, 2006).

Overall, research supports neurological, genetic, and environmental factors as causal agents of ADHD, but the specific contributions of these factors, and their interactions with one another, are not yet completely understood. Mounting evidence suggests that ADHD is not caused by a single area of the brain or developmental pathway. Further, most research on etiology has examined individuals with ADHD—combined type, and different etiological factors or neuropsychological deficits may be observed in those with the other ADHD subtypes (Nigg, 2005).

COURSE AND PROGNOSIS

ADHD often is diagnosed in elementary school, as the academic and behavioral expectations of the school environment become more demanding (APA, 2000). Symptoms often persist into adolescence, although the severity of hyperactive symptoms tends to decline while academic difficulties and problems with peers become more pronounced (Wolraich et al., 2005). Similarly, inattentive symptoms tend to persist into adolescence and adulthood, manifesting as disorganization and poor time management (Hervey, Epstein, & Curry, 2004; J. S. Wadsworth & Harper, 2007). For example, with 182 adolescents ages 13 to 17 years (43 predominantly inattentive, 42 combined, 97 control), those with ADHD were impaired compared to controls; differences from controls were in a composite executive function factor related to inattention rather than hyperactive-impulsive symptoms, and no subtype differences emerged (Martel, Nikolas, & Nigg, 2007). Thus, it appears that, by adolescence, predominant problems relate to executive function (inattention/organization) as opposed to hyperactivity-impulsivity.

Findings from two recently published meta-analytic reviews (Hervey et al., 2004; Schoechlin & Engel, 2005) suggested that, among adults, the most consistent neuropsychological deficits associated with ADHD include deficits in attention, behavioral inhibition, working memory, and verbal memory. According to the *Diagnostic and Statistical Manual of Mental Disorders*, Fourth Edition Text Revision (APA, 2000), some of the associated features of ADHD include poor achievement in school, being perceived by others as lazy or irresponsible, oppositional-defiant behaviors, and rejection by peers. The potential for comorbidity is also high, especially with regard to learning disabilities, oppositional defiant disorder, conduct disorder, mood disorders, substance use, and anxiety disorders (S. Clarke, Heussler, & Kohn, 2005; Wolraich et al., 2005); children with ADHD also are at elevated risk for engaging in antisocial behaviors and illegal activities as adolescents and young adults (Barkley, Fischer, Smallish, & Fletcher, 2004). Social and disruptive behavior problems continue to be more frequently associated with combined type as compared to the inattentive type. Research suggests that children with the hyperactive-impulsive or combined types are more likely to have a comorbid conduct disorder or oppositional defiant disorder (Baumgartel, Wolraich, & Dietrich, 1995; Eiraldi, Power, & Nezu, 1997; Faraone, Biederman, Weber, & Russell, 1998; Gaub & Carlson, 1997; Manning & Miller, 2001; A. E. Morgan, Hynd, Riccio, & Hall, 1996) than those with the inattentive type. Further, children with combined type also have been found to have greater impairment as evidenced by lower global assessment of functioning (APA, 2000) relative to inattentive or hyperactive-impulsive subtypes (Faraone, Biederman, & Friedman, 2000). Alternatively, research suggests that children with inattentive type are more likely to have internalizing disorders and learning disabilities (Baumgartel et al.,

1995; Faraone et al., 1998; Gaub & Carlson, 1997; Manning & Miller, 2001; M. Weiss, Worling, & Wasdell, 2003). For example, in a recent study (Bauermeister et al., 2005), Latino/Hispanic children in the inattentive group were less social but had fewer reported externalizing problems and higher adaptive functioning than children in the combined-type group. Similarly, it was found that children with inattentive type were rated as less socially adept by teachers but not evidencing significant behavior problems relative to other ADHD subtypes (Gadow et al., 2000). Others found that both combined and inattentive groups were less socially preferred but that inattentive was associated with decreased social interactions and combined was associated with aggression (Hodgens, Cole, & Boldizar, 2000). In contrast, Gadow et al. (2004) found that boys with combined type were more socially impaired than those with inattentive type. These associated features and comorbid conditions likely contribute to the potential difficulties that may accompany ADHD into adolescence and adulthood (Gadow et al., 2004). Some of the factors associated with persistence of symptoms into adulthood include family history of ADHD, the presence of comorbid disorders, and psychosocial stressors (e.g., poverty, marital discord, parental psychopathology) (Biederman, 2005). Gender differences in symptom presentation may contribute to differences found in comorbidity as well (Breen, 2006; Carlson, Tamm, & Gaub, 1997; Gaub & Carlson, 1997).

Outcome and manifestation in cognitive and academic areas may differ somewhat by subtype as well. Multiple studies examined the differences in subtypes as specified in the *Diagnostic and Statistical Manual of Mental Disorders*, Third Edition (*DSM-III*) (Barkley, 1998; Goodyear & Hynd, 1992; B. B. Lahey, Schaughency, Hynd, Carlson, & Nieves, 1987; Marshall, Hynd, Handwerk, & Hall, 1997; Marshall, Schafer, O'Donnell, Elliott, & Handwerk, 1999). Using the *DSM-III* criteria, children diagnosed with Attention-Deficit Disorder (ADD) without hyperactivity were more likely to experience cognitive processing problems and learning disabilities as well as to have a higher likelihood of internalizing disorders. In academic areas, for example, Marshall et al. (1997) and Marshall et al. (1999) found that math achievement was significantly lower for children diagnosed with ADD without hyperactivity. These findings replicated findings of others suggesting impaired math achievement for ADD without hyperactivity (Ackerman, Anhalt, Holcomb, & Dykman, 1986; Carlson, Lahey, & Neeper, 1986; Hynd et al., 1991). These differences have continued to be found with the respecification of criteria for ADHD subtypes; a number of studies support the notion that academic problems are linked to attention problems (Rabiner, Murray, Schmid, & Malone, 2004). Further, it has been suggested that inattention is related to poor reading comprehension among children with predominantly inattentive type (P. Aaron, Joshi, & Phipps, 2004). In a study of children with ADHD, the predominantly inattentive group evidenced lower performance on calculation and written expression tasks; however, these differences dissipated when IQ was included as a covariate (Riccio, Homack, Jarratt, & Wolfe, 2006). For executive function domains, differences emerged for interference, but only when girls were excluded from the analysis and no control for IQ was made. For parent ratings of executive function using the BRIEF, expected differences were found on the Inhibit scale with the combined group evidencing greater problems in this area; this difference remained even when girls were excluded and IQ was controlled (Riccio et al., 2006).

With regard to real-life functioning, research suggests that compared to adolescents with no diagnosis of ADHD, adolescents with ADHD are at much greater risk for failing classes, getting lower grades, repeating grades, scoring low on standardized achievement tests, dropping out of high school, being involved in a teenage pregnancy, contracting a sexually transmitted disease, abusing substances, having at-fault car accidents, being arrested and incarcerated, and getting fired from a job (Mannuzza & Klein, 1999; Steele, Jensen, & Quinn, 2006). Thus, symptoms and manifestations of ADHD can persist into adolescence and young adulthood, and functional impairment can be more far-reaching than the classroom or school setting.

ADHD symptoms may continue to cause academic difficulty for college students who have been diagnosed with the disorder, as they are still attempting to function in a demanding academic environment (Weyandt & DuPaul, 2006). In a study that examined the learning and study strategies employed by college students with ADHD, compared to students either with learning disabilities or with no diagnosis of ADHD or learning disabilities (Reaser, Prevatt, Petscher, & Proctor, 2007), based on responses to the Learning and Study Strategies Inventory, Second Edition (Weinstein & Palmer, 2002), results indicate that compared to students in the no-diagnosis group, students with ADHD scored more negatively on most scales, including Anxiety, Motivation, Concentration, Information Processing, Self-Testing, Selecting Main Ideas, Test Strategies, and Time Management. Students in the ADHD group also scored more negatively than students in the learning disability group on Concentration, Selecting Main Ideas, Study Aids, Test Strategies, and Time Management. Further analyses suggest that for students in the ADHD group, ipsative weaknesses included the areas of Concentration, Selecting Main Ideas, and Test Strategies (Reaser et al., 2007). These findings support the notion that symptoms related to inattention, poor self-regulation, and academic difficulties can persist into adult educational settings. These results are supported in part by another study of college students with ADHD, students with other clinical disorders, and a no-diagnosis comparison group (Riccio et al., 2005). Compared to both comparison groups, the adults with ADHD evidenced problems with follow-through, forgetting, organization, and losing things. Related to sense of time, adults with ADHD endorsed problems with meeting deadlines, not completing tasks, not planning ahead, and having a poorer sense of time significantly more frequently than adults in either comparison group. Table 6.1 summarizes the clinical manifestations of ADHD from young childhood to adolescence.

EVIDENCE-BASED INTERVENTIONS

This section describes several recent meta-analyses and review papers that have summarized the literature on ADHD treatments and outcome. It also reviews some of the most important findings from the Multimodal Treatment Study of Children with ADHD. Table 6.2 summarizes the evidence-based status of ADHD interventions.

Reviews and Meta-Analytic Findings

Several reviews have evaluated the evidence-based status of psychosocial interventions for ADHD. Psychosocial treatment approaches often involve working with other people in the child's system; parents and teachers are trained to implement strategies based on social learning theory and operant conditioning in order to reduce problem behaviors and increase adaptive behaviors. Pelham and Fabiano (2008) noted that while stimulant medications have been shown to produce short-term improvements in ADHD symptoms, they have not demonstrated long-term changes, thereby pointing to the importance of psychosocial interventions. Behavioral parent training programs, behavioral classroom management interventions such as teacher consultation based on behavioral

Table 6.1 Clinical Manifestations of ADHD by Age

Age Level	Clinical Manifestations
Preschool	Impulsivity Hyperactivity Limited emotional self-regulation Noncompliance Inattention Difficulty with interpersonal relationships (adults and peers)
Childhood	Deficits in executive function Difficulty with sustained attention Distractibility High reactivity Hyperactivity High impulsivity Poor emotional regulation Difficulty with peer relations Academic underachievement Noncompliance
Adolescence/Adulthood	Deficits in executive function Disorganization Planning deficits Limited future orientation Academic underachievement Difficulty with peer relations Difficulty with sustained attention Emotional immaturity Irritability Negative self-perceptions Aggression Sensation-seeking behaviors Increased risk for substance abuse Increased risk for antisocial behaviors

principles (e.g., consultation on the use of point systems and time-out procedures), and behavioral peer-focused interventions (e.g., summer programs) have been identified as evidence-based treatments (Chronis, Jones, & Raggi, 2006; Daly, Creed, Xanthopoulos, & Brown, 2007; Pelham & Fabiano, 2008). Parent training involves teaching parents how to use behavior modification principles to reduce ADHD symptoms and associated behaviors (e.g., aggressive or acting-out behaviors), often using manualized approaches. Chronis et al. reported an average effect size of 0.87 (ranging from –0.09 to 2.25) based on studies examining the effect of parent training on behaviors associated with ADHD. School-based behavioral interventions include a range of strategies designed to impact behavioral and academic variables. For example, classroom behavior management interventions involve the psychologist consulting with the classroom teacher, conducting functional behavior assessments to identify what environmental factors may be maintaining the problem behaviors, designing specific strategies to reduce the behaviors, instructing the teacher in behavior modification principles and in the implementation of specific strategies, and conducting follow-ups to assess reduction in problem behaviors. Chronis et al. reported strong effects for these consultative behavior modification interventions,

Table 6.2 Evidence-Based Status of Interventions for ADHD

Interventions	Target	Status
Stimulant medications (e.g., methylphenidate [Ritalin, Concerta], dextroamphetamine [Adderall])	Attention Impulsivity Hyperactivity On-task behavior Compliance	Positive practice (Pelham & Fabiano, 2008; Pliszka, 2007)
Nonstimulant medications (i.e., atomoxetine [Strattera])	Attention Impulsivity Hyperactivity	Positive practice (Cheng et al., 2007)
Behavioral parent training	Impulse control On-task behaviors Oppositional behaviors Parent-child interactions	Positive practice (Chronis et al., 2006; Daly et al., 2007; Pelham & Fabiano, 2008)
Combined treatment (medication plus behavioral)	Comprehensive	Positive practice (Daly et al., 2007; Majewicz-Hefley & Carlson, 2007)
Behavioral classroom management/ Classroom modifications (e.g., point systems, daily report card)	Impulse control On-task behaviors Work completion Social skills	Positive practice (Chronis et al., 2006; Daly et al., 2007; Pelham & Fabiano, 2008)
Electroencephalogram biofeedback	Attention	Emerging (Riccio & French, 2004; Rojas & Chan, 2005)
Traditional counseling approaches (e.g., individual counseling, play therapy, cognitive therapy)	Comprehensive	Ineffective (Pelham & Fabiano, 2008)
Behavioral-focused summer treatment program (which includes a social skills training component)	Social skills Compliance Conduct problems	Positive practice (Pelham & Fabiano, 2008; Pelham et al., 2000)
Office-based social skills training groups	Social skills	Emerging (Chronis et al., 2006; Pelham & Fabiano, 2008)
Academic interventions (e.g., peer tutoring, instructional modifications, computer assisted instruction)	Academic achievement	Emerging (Chronis et al., 2006; Daly et al., 2007)
Dietary modifications (e.g., elimination of refined sugar, Feingold diet)	Attention Hyperactivity	Ineffective (Rojas & Chan, 2005)

as they often result in improvements in students' classroom behaviors. Finally, the summer treatment programs evaluated by Pelham and Fabiano (2008) are intensive and seek to produce generalizable social and behavioral skills, given the context in which they are implemented (team-based sports activities), and are implemented within larger contingency management systems.

Categories of psychosocial treatments identified as needing further research and replication in order to establish stronger evidence for efficacy include academic interventions and social skills training (Chronis et al., 2006; Daly et al., 2007). These treatment approaches appear promising based on initial research efforts, but additional studies are needed in order to more fully understand their efficacy. Further, traditional counseling approaches such as office-based, weekly social skills groups do not have consistent empirical support (Pelham & Fabiano, 2008). There also is a need for additional research on psychosocial treatments with adolescents, as most research has focused on children with ADHD (Chronis et al., 2006).

A specific behavioral strategy reviewed by DuPaul (2007) attempts to reduce ADHD symptoms and related behaviors by enhancing communication between home and school. Often referred to as a "daily report card," this strategy involves teachers, parents, and students working together to develop behavioral goals for the classroom and establish rewards that can be consistently delivered at home when classroom goals are met. This approach requires constant communication between school and home and therefore may help the student feel accountable and closely supervised from one setting to the next. The research summarized suggests the daily report card is useful in improving students' classroom behaviors (DuPaul, 2007).

Clearly, psychosocial interventions represent an important modality in the treatment of ADHD; other interventions include pharmacological and combined approaches. Daly et al. (2007) noted that the combined treatment approach is often considered the "gold standard" in ADHD treatment. Within this context, "combined" treatments refer to those treatments that combine psychosocial and pharmacological approaches to provide a comprehensive intervention. Thus, combined approaches address both the biological contributors to ADHD and some of the associated features that can render medication-only approaches insufficient (e.g., parent-child conflict, oppositional behaviors, academic difficulties, comorbidity). Majewicz-Hefley and Carlson (2007) conducted a meta-analysis (based on eight studies) examining combined treatments for children with ADHD. After looking at relevant variables across the eight studies, the authors calculated these mean effect sizes for the ADHD-relevant variables (with standard errors in parentheses): inattention = 1.27 (.23), hyperactivity = 1.27 (.24), impulsivity = 0.91 (.17), social skills = 0.90 (.20), and academics = 0.19 (.09). Thus, across the eight studies included in the analysis, the combined treatment approach had a significant influence on reported ADHD and associated symptoms, with the weakest impact on academic difficulties (Majewicz-Hefley & Carlson, 2007).

The authors also cited and reviewed two important meta-analyses that examined the effects of stimulant medications alone on ADHD symptoms, in order to provide comparisons between effect sizes obtained for combined treatment (i.e., those obtained in the Majewicz-Hefley and Carlson study) and those obtained for pharmacological treatment. The first stimulant meta-analysis (Crenshaw, Kavale, Forness, & Reeve, 1999) reported an effect size of 0.72 for the "core" features of ADHD, including impulsivity, hyperactivity, and inattention, and effect sizes ranging from 0.41 to 0.61 for associated features such as aggressive and noncompliant behaviors, academic performance, and prosocial behaviors. The second stimulant meta-analysis (Faraone & Biederman, 2002) examined the effects of dextroamphetamine (Adderall) on the combined "core" ADHD symptoms, as compared to placebo conditions. The authors found effect sizes (across six studies) of varying strengths depending on the source of behavioral ratings: clinicians = 1.41, teachers = 0.94, and parents = 0.83; effect size differences also were observed for the type of measure used: measures of ADHD symptoms = 0.91, measures of aggressive symptoms = 1.10, and global ratings = 1.66. The pooled effect size across the six studies was 1.00. Overall, the results of these meta-analyses support the use of combined treatment approaches in addressing ADHD, as effect sizes for combined approaches compare favorably to those obtained for medication-only approaches; Majewicz-Hefley and

Carlson (2007) concluded that combined approaches may be especially effective at treating the associated or "peripheral" features of ADHD, such as social skill deficits, although additional work is needed in this area.

Similar conclusions about combined treatments were reached by others (R. T. Brown et al., 2005); researchers summarized reports from several large lines of inquiry on ADHD and found that:

1. Different stimulant medications (including methylphenidate [Ritalin, Concerta], dextroamphetamine [Adderall], and pemoline [Cylert]) did not have significantly different effects; all performed similarly in reducing ADHD symptoms.
2. Using combined approaches led to increased acceptance by parents and teachers.
3. Using combined approaches reduced the amount of medication required to realize the same level of behavioral change as accomplished through medication alone.

Thus, reviews suggest that combined treatment approaches may make important contributions to comprehensive ADHD treatment that go above and beyond stimulant treatment alone.

In a recent review of medication treatments for ADHD, the more recently developed long-acting (e.g., extended release, transdermal) stimulants demonstrate similar response rates to those demonstrated by the traditional stimulants, when compared to placebo conditions (Pliszka, 2007). Atomoxetine (Strattera) has recently been identified as an effective nonstimulant medication for treating ADHD (Cheng, Chen, Ko, & Ng, 2007; Michelson et al., 2002), although effect sizes are somewhat smaller than those for stimulant medications (Newcorn et al., 2008). Research suggests that atomoxetine may be especially useful in treating children with ADHD who have comorbid depression, anxiety, oppositional defiant disorder, or Tourette syndrome (Bangs et al., 2007; Cheng et al., 2007; Spencer et al., 2008), and in treating ADHD among children who do not respond to stimulant medications (Newcorn et al., 2008).

A recent study examined the effectiveness of a methylphenidate transdermal system (MTS) on ADHD symptoms among 6- to 12-year-old children with ADHD (McGough et al., 2006). The MTS is a patch worn on the child's skin, delivering a consistent dose of methylphenidate throughout the day. Behavioral ratings of children using the MTS were compared with ratings of children using a placebo (ratings were made by observers who were blind to medication versus placebo status), and results suggest that the MTS intervention significantly reduced behaviors associated with ADHD when participants were observed in a laboratory classroom setting. Data supporting the efficacy of stimulant medication among preschool-age children with ADHD is sparse, as most efficacy studies have focused on school-age children and adolescents (Kollins & Greenhill, 2006). Further, most of the preschool studies include relatively small sample sizes, thereby preventing firm conclusions regarding the effectiveness of stimulants with children in this age group.

Multimodal Treatment Study of Children with ADHD

One of the most important and large-scale lines of research on ADHD treatment is the Multimodal Treatment Study of Children with ADHD (MTA study), which was coordinated by the National Institute of Mental Health (MTA Cooperative Group, 1999a, 1999b). In this multisite study, 579 children with ADHD combined type (from 7.0 to

9.9 years of age, many with a range of comorbidities) were followed over 14 months after being randomly assigned to one of four treatment conditions:

1. Medication management (typically including stimulant medication three times a day, monitoring, monthly follow-up visits, and providing parents with materials to read, all of which occurred after a titration process to determine ideal dose for each child)
2. Behavioral treatment (including 35 sessions of group or individual parent training in behavioral management techniques in addition to regular teacher consultation sessions and an 8-week summer program focusing on social and academic skills)
3. Combined treatment (including all features of the medication management and behavioral treatment conditions, with the added feature of regular communication between school professionals and pharmacotherapists)
4. Routine community care (this was the comparison group; families were referred to community resources and received a variety of services—most often stimulant medication—of less intensity than those received by the experimental groups).

Children in the MTA study were assessed at four timepoints: baseline, 3 months, 9 months, and 14 months.

This study produced numerous findings reported in multiple peer-reviewed journal articles. P. S. Jensen et al. (2001) summarized some of the most important results, including:

- Children in all four conditions exhibited reduced ADHD symptoms over time.
- The medication and combined approaches were most effective at reducing ADHD symptoms, with no significant differences between these two conditions when only ADHD symptoms were considered.
- Combined treatment generally was most effective with associated features of ADHD (e.g., academic difficulties, problems with peer relations, oppositional behaviors, affective symptoms) when significant differences were detected.
- The medication and combined treatments generally were statistically superior to the community care condition considering ADHD symptoms only, while behavioral treatment was not consistently superior to community care.
- Combined treatment resulted in the greatest rate of "normalization," or percentage of children who exhibited very few symptoms at the end of the study.
- Parent satisfaction ratings were significantly higher for the combined and behavioral conditions as compared to the medication management condition.
- Moderators included comorbid anxiety and familial receipt of public assistance, as these participants benefited most from combined and behavioral treatments.
- Mediators included acceptance/attendance, meaning these factors were significantly related to children's outcomes, especially for those participants in the medication management condition.

This pattern of results suggests that medication management should include more than simply prescribing medication: This approach should include regular (e.g., monthly) monitoring and follow-up in order to facilitate communication among parents and professionals. As pointed out by Greene and Ablon (2001), the behavioral treatment condition may have resulted in greater effects if the treatment had been individualized. That is, all children and parents received the same number of sessions addressing the same behavioral and academic skills regardless of individual needs, which was very different from the medication management condition, in which ideal doses for each participant were determined through a rigorous titration procedure (Greene & Ablon, 2001). This finding raises the question of whether the behavioral treatment would have a greater effect if the treatment were based on a functional behavior assessment or similar individualized process, so that the components of the intervention were matched with the child's individual needs.

An additional investigation based on the summer treatment program component of the MTA study (Pelham et al., 2000), which was provided as part of the behavioral treatment condition, compared two groups of children: those who were on medication during the summer program (combined treatment group) and those who were not on medication during the summer treatment program (behavioral treatment group). The summer treatment was an intensive 8-week program that included behavioral approaches such as time out, a response-cost point system, social reinforcement, daily report card, modeling, and group social skills training that included instruction, practice, and feedback. This program also included a weekly parent training component. All children attended the program on weekdays from 8:00 a.m. to 5:00 p.m. and spent each day in small cohorts attending classroom sessions and participating in recreational group activities (e.g., playing soccer or softball). The only difference between the two treatment groups was whether medication was used in conjunction with the summer program; the behavioral treatment component was identical for both groups. Results indicated that at the end of the intervention, children in the combined treatment group (i.e., those receiving medication during the summer treatment program) scored significantly better on several dependent measures as compared to children in the behavioral treatment group: following activity rules, following classroom rules, sportsmanship, number of negative peer nominations, and teacher ratings of inattention/hyperactivity. Normalization rates indicated that many children in both groups were functioning within the normal range by the end of the study across most behavioral domains. Normalization rates were significantly higher for children in the combined treatment group for following activity rules, rule violations, conduct problems, negative verbalizations, following classroom rules, and teacher ratings of oppositional-defiant behaviors. At the same time, there were no significant group differences on most dependent measures in the study, suggesting that medication had an additive effect on some behaviors but not others. The authors suggested that if a behavioral treatment program is intensive enough (such as the intensity of the summer program), concurrent medication treatment may not add much to the outcome of the intervention because the behavioral treatment is sufficient (Pelham et al., 2000).

A study of changes in parenting behaviors based on MTA treatment groups found that the combined treatment (which included a parent training component) was associated with more constructive and positive parenting behaviors at the end of the MTA study as compared to the medication treatment and control groups (Wells et al., 2006). Thus, the combination of behavioral intervention, parent training, and medication management resulted in the best parenting behavioral outcomes, suggesting that a combined approach may be the ideal treatment for changing these parenting variables. Importantly, these findings are based on observational results during a laboratory task rather than on a parent or teacher report, and thus are not subject to the same type of rater bias. Further, observers were blind to children's treatment condition when making their behavioral ratings of parent-child interactions and used a formal system for coding behaviors. These experimental conditions and measurement procedures are different from those used in the prior MTA studies, which relied on parent report of parenting variables.

Several follow-up studies with the MTA sample suggest longer-term intervention effects. For example, follow-up assessment 10 months after the end of the MTA intervention phase indicated that the medication management and combined treatments continued to show greater effects on ADHD and oppositional-defiant symptoms as compared to the other treatments (MTA Cooperative Group, 2004). No significant differences were found between the medication and combined groups, or between the behavioral and control groups. Further, no significant long-term treatment effects were observed for academic achievement, social skills, or negative/ineffective discipline (by parents) dependent variables. The superiority of medication (i.e., both groups that included a medication component: the medication management and combined treatment groups) over the other treatments was somewhat diminished over time based on comparison of follow-up effect sizes with effect sizes obtained in the prior MTA studies. Further diminishment of effect was observed at 2-year follow-up, as children in all four treatment groups performed similarly on all outcome measures; no significant differences were observed in ADHD symptoms, oppositional-defiant symptoms, social skills, or reading scores based on treatment group (P. S. Jensen et al., 2007). At the same time, children in all four groups showed improvement at the 2-year follow-up compared to their functioning at baseline assessment, with treatment effect sizes ranging from 0.1 (for reading) to 1.7 (for ADHD symptoms). Finally, some of the changes in effects from the initial MTA findings, to the 10-month follow-up, to the 2-year follow-up may be attributed to a wide degree of variability and change in terms of the percentage of children in each group who were using medication at the time of the follow-up assessments; increases or decreases in the use of medication may have diluted some of the group differences in outcome variables. In any event, the superior effects of the medication and combined treatments wore off over time, thereby pointing to the importance of long-term treatment approaches in which adherence is closely monitored.

In sum, findings from the MTA study have made major contributions to our understanding of empirically supported interventions for ADHD. Perhaps the main advantage of this study is the rigor of the methodology and procedures (e.g., diagnostic and treatment procedures, long-term follow-up), which enhance the reliability of the results. The study certainly has shaped practice in terms of providing a basis for using medication and behavioral treatments for children with ADHD and also has facilitated the identification of additional research questions that need to be answered.

Alternative Treatments

In contrast to the well-studied interventions discussed thus far, several interventions are considered "alternative" treatments for ADHD; these treatments include biofeedback and dietary modifications. Numerous studies have examined electroencephalogram biofeedback and attentional functioning among children with ADHD. However, most of these have been case studies or suffer from a host of methodological limitations, such as small sample sizes, lack of a control group, lack of long-term follow-up, lack of relevant dependent measures, and heterogeneous groups of participants (Riccio & French, 2004; N. L. Rojas & Chan, 2005), thereby preventing definitive conclusions regarding the treatment effects of biofeedback.

Related to diet, N. L. Rojas and Chan (2005) reviewed extant studies on the effects of eliminating refined sugar and food additives (e.g., artificial colors and flavors, preservatives) from children's diet (the additive-free diet is also called the Feingold diet), targeting only those studies employing placebo-controlled, double-blind, randomized clinical trials that included either a crossover design or comparison group. The authors report an interesting trend with regard to the Feingold/additive-free diet: The older studies conducted in the 1970s and early 1980s generally found little support for the diet, usually using hyperactivity as the outcome variable (Kavale & Forness, 1983; Mattes, 1983), but several more recent studies suggest an association between hyperactivity and food additives. At the same time, many children in these more recent studies did not meet diagnostic criteria for ADHD, suggesting that food additives may have behavioral effects on some children but not necessarily children with an ADHD diagnosis; this clearly calls into question the use of dietary modifications as a treatment for ADHD. Rojas and Chan reached similar conclusions with regard to the elimination of refined sugar from children's diet: The methodologically sound studies to date do not support the use of sugar elimination as a treatment for ADHD based on limited effects on behavioral or cognitive variables (Wolraich, Wilson, & White, 1995). Some of these diet studies have shown effects on parent ratings of the child's behavior but not on other measures, such as teacher ratings, classroom observations, and achievement tests (Schnoll, Burshteyn, & Cea-Aravena, 2003). One of the reasons why studies on dietary modifications sometimes show behavioral improvement based on parent ratings might be the parents' expectations and strong desire to observe changes in their children's behavior (Eigenmann & Haenggeli, 2004). Of course, some of these dietary modifications may have some effects for some children (e.g., those with certain food allergies or sensitivities) and therefore may be beneficial for some children, but behavioral effects with children with ADHD have not been consistent enough to support their use in treating ADHD (N. L. Rojas & Chan, 2005). In sum, there is a reason why these treatments still are considered "alternative" rather than first-line options in the treatment of ADHD symptoms. More systematic and rigorous research will be necessary before their routine use in the treatment of ADHD can be recommended.

Interacting Factors

Finally, factors identified in the literature as potentially complicating the treatment of ADHD (and which therefore should be considered in designing treatment approaches) include parental stress and psychopathology, comorbidity, parental attributions of ADHD symptoms as internal and stable characteristics of the child, age of the child or adolescent, and poverty with its resulting lack of resources (Chronis et al., 2006; Daly et al., 2007). Treatment approaches must consider these factors in order to make interventions individualized rather than generic.

CASE STUDY: EDDIE—ATTENTION-DEFICIT/HYPERACTIVITY DISORDER, COMBINED TYPE

The next report is from a hospital-based clinic. Identifying information, such as child and family name, teacher or physician name, and school information, has been altered or fictionalized to protect confidentiality.

Reason for Referral

Eddie is a 6-year 6-month-old African American male kindergarten student who is being initially evaluated at the request of his pediatrician and his parents due to a history of short attention span, difficulty following multipart directions and classroom routines, poor handwriting, and difficulty with fine motor skills. Neuropsychological evaluation was undertaken in order to assess higher cortical functioning and make appropriate recommendations regarding school placement and the need for supportive services.

Assessment Procedures

Eddie's parents (Mr. and Mrs. Jones) provided information via questionnaire and interview format. Available medical records and a previous evaluation were reviewed. These assessment measures were utilized during the evaluation:

Wechsler Intelligence Scale for Children, Fourth Edition (WISC-IV)
Wechsler Individual Achievement Test, Second Edition (WIAT-II)
Neuropsychological Assessment (NEPSY)/ Neuropsychological Assessment, Second Edition (NEPSY-2)
Peabody Picture Vocabulary Test, Fourth Edition (PPVT-IV)
Clinical Evaluation of Language Fundamentals, Fourth Edition (CELF-IV)
Boston Naming Test (BNT)
Dichotic Listening Test
Finger Oscillation Test
Kaufman Assessment Battery for Children, Second Edition (KABC-2)
Developmental Test of Visual-Motor Integration, Fifth Edition (DTVMI-V)
Clock Face Drawing Test
Children's Memory Scale (CMS)
Behavior Assessment System for Children, Second Edition (BASC-2)
DSM-IV ADHD Checklist

Background Information

Home

Eddie resides in Paradise with his parents, James and Rebecca, and his two siblings, Lisa and Anna. Lisa is 15 years old, an A/B student in the ninth grade, and in good health. Anna is 2 years old, developing normally, and in good health as well. Mr. Jones is 34 years old, a college graduate with a degree in computer science, who is employed as an information technology executive. According to Mrs. Jones, her husband had febrile seizures as a child and struggled somewhat in elementary school. Eddie's mother is 34 years of age, has earned a bachelor's degree in nursing, and is currently a full-time homemaker. She reports having articulation therapy in kindergarten and first grades. Both parents are in good general health. Aside from Parkinson's disease in the maternal grandfather, the family history is negative for neurological disorders, including mental retardation.

Medical

Review of developmental and medical history with Mrs. Jones indicates that Eddie is the product of a normal 36-week gestation pregnancy and vaginal delivery, weighing 7 pounds 6 ounces at birth. Eddie did well as a newborn and went home from the hospital with his mother the next day. During the first 6 months, Eddie experienced feeding difficulty and reflux, which eventually resolved with Zantac. Developmental motor milestones were obtained within normal limits with sitting up occurring at 4 to 5 months of age and walking at 12 months of age. Developmental language milestones also were attained within normal limits with first words at 5 months of age and short phrases at 2 years of age. Toilet training was fully accomplished at 3 years of age. Aside from the usual childhood illnesses, Eddie's past medical history is significant for frequent ear infections from 4 months to 2 years of age and allergies to peanuts, walnuts, grasses, and pollen. There is no history of seizures or head injury.

Educational

Mrs. Jones reports that she and Eddie's prekindergarten teacher first became concerned about his attention span when he was 4 years of age. The teacher was also concerned about his fine motor skill development and "out-of-seat" behavior. As a result, the parents elected to have Eddie repeat prekindergarten the next year. Eddie continued to exhibit difficulty with short attention span, wandering away from group activities, and poor fine motor skills, and he was "always on the go." At present, Eddie is attending kindergarten at Land Elementary School within the Paradise School System. He continues to have a short attention span, has difficulty following multipart directions, and his fine motor skills continue to be of concern. As a result, Eddie underwent an occupational therapy evaluation. Results of the evaluation indicated that Eddie was exhibiting mild delays in visual-motor integration, upper limb coordination, functional handwriting, and short attention span. Based on these results, Eddie began outpatient therapy once each week, which has continued to the present. Earlier this year, Eddie underwent a speech/language evaluation. Based on the results of that evaluation, it was felt that Eddie demonstrated average auditory processing and language skills; however, his attention span was short and "his hands and arms" moved constantly. Speech/language therapy was not recommended at that time.

Finally, review of a school report form completed by Eddie's teacher, Ms. Bell, indicates that she characterizes Eddie as a healthy 6-year-old boy. She provided this description:

> He is happy and seems to like school. He likes to tell weird stories about adventures. Eddie has a difficult time following a daily routine of walking and stopping at specific spots, going to lunch and coming back. He doesn't respond when his name is called. It takes at least three times for Eddie to respond when his name is called. Eddie sometimes appears to be zoned out in his own world, not aware of what is going on around him.

She reported that areas in need of improvement include listening, following directions, and handwriting.

Behavioral Observations

Eddie presented himself for testing as a happy, neatly groomed youngster who was casually dressed in a Power Rangers shirt, warm-up pants, and sneakers. He separated appropriately from his mother and accompanied the examiners to the testing room without difficulty. Eddie was oriented and related appropriately toward the examiners with good social eye contact and a broad range of affect noted. In response to direct questions as well as when conversation was spontaneous, Eddie's use of language was fluent and prosodic with mild linguistic planning difficulty noted. Throughout the evaluation, which consisted of two sessions separated by a lunch break, Eddie's attention span and impulse control within the context of this one-to-one assessment setting were felt to be significantly below age level expectancy. For example, Eddie often would drift off task during his conversation. He periodically required repetition of directions when permissible to ensure appropriate comprehension. Eddie was impulsive with manipulatives and did not always scan choices properly. As a result, Eddie required periodic breaks, frequent prompting, and verbal redirection from the examiners. Lateral dominance appears to be established in the right hand for paper-and-pencil manipulation. However, it should be noted that initially Eddie used his left hand for drawing but quickly switched to the right. Eddie uses his left hand and foot for gross motor activities, such as throwing and kicking a ball. Vision and hearing were screened by the school system, and Mrs. Jones reported that they were normal. Given the adequacy of the testing conditions and Eddie's general cooperation toward the tasks, results of this evaluation should be considered a valid reflection of Eddie's current neuropsychological functioning (with the exception of one of the Children's Memory Scale subtests, as explained later).

Assessment Results and Interpretation

Cognitive and Neuropsychological Functioning

Individual subtest and composite scores for all measures are presented in the Psychometric Summary (see Table 6.3). The results of neuropsychological evaluation indicate that Eddie currently is functioning within the average range of intellectual ability as measured by the WISC-IV. Additional assessment indicates that Eddie's sequential reasoning/problem-solving capability is in the low-average range. Eddie's expressive and receptive language skills are generally in the low-average to average range with relative strengths noted in his receptive and expressive vocabulary development and confrontational picture naming ability. In contrast, a relative weakness was noted on tasks sensitive to linguistic planning. Further, it should be noted that Eddie's performance on receptive language assessment also was impacted by his short attention span.

Language appears to be lateralized in the left cerebral hemisphere as evidenced by a right ear advantage in Eddie's ability to report Consonant Vowel syllables presented simultaneously to each ear on a Dichotic Listening Test (Left Ear = 7/30 Correct, Right Ear = 15/30 Correct). Eddie's performance on measures of visual-spatial perception was also highly variable as a result of difficulty sustaining attention to task. Specifically, Eddie performed in the average to high-average range on a measure of visual closure contrasted by deficient performance when asked to judge spatial orientation; however, he often responded impulsively on this task without adequately scanning all possible choices before answering. Visual-motor integration/construction was found to be well within the average range when Eddie was asked to construct geometric designs with blocks. In contrast, his constructional ability declined significantly when the fine motor and motor planning requirements of the task were increased with the use of paper and pencil. Fine motor tapping speed is found to be relatively depressed in the right (dominant) hand as measured by the Finger Oscillation Test; right (dominant) hand = 23.3 taps per 10 seconds, left (nondominant) hand = 25.3 taps per 10 seconds.

Analysis of Eddie's performance on the CMS indicates that, at the present time, he is exhibiting average ability to hold material in immediate auditory working memory contrasted by borderline visual working memory. When asked to learn and remember (30 minutes later) newly presented material, Eddie demonstrated average to above-average ability to learn and recall verbal information, such as stories that were read to him and a list of 10 word pairs presented over three structured learning trials. In contrast, Eddie exhibited low-average ability to learn and recall the spatial location of dots on a page presented over three learning trials. Further, it should be noted that Eddie's

Table 6.3 Psychometric Summary for Eddie

	Standard Score
Wechsler Intelligence Scale for Children, Fourth Edition (WISC-IV)	
Full Scale IQ	94
General Ability Index	99
Verbal Comprehension Index	96
Similarities	105
Vocabulary	100
Comprehension	85
Perceptual Reasoning Index	102
Block Design	105
Picture Concepts	95
Matrix Reasoning	105
Working Memory Index	94
Digit Span	100
Letter-Number Sequencing	90
Processing Speed Index	88
Coding	85
Symbol Search	95
Neuropsychological Assessment, Second Edition (NEPSY-2)	
Tower (from NEPSY)	85
Phonological Processing	90
Sentence Repetition	85
Comprehension of Instructions	90
Word Generation	95
Arrows	65
Peabody Picture Vocabulary Test, Fourth Edition (PPVT-IV)	101
Boston Naming Test (BNT)	117
Clinical Evaluation of Language Fundamentals, Fourth Edition (CELF-IV)	
Formulated Sentences	80
Kaufman Assessment Battery for Children, Second Edition (KABC-2)	
Gestalt Closure	110
Developmental Test of Visual Motor Integration, Fifth Edition (DTVMI-V)	96
Clock Face Drawing Test	
Form	74
Time	80
Finger Oscillation Test	
Right (dominant) Hand	90
Left (nondominant) Hand	110
Children's Memory Scale (CMS)	
General Memory Index	93
Attention/Concentration Index	97
Numbers	95
Sequences	100
Picture Locations	75
Verbal Immediate Index	125

(continued)

Table 6.3 *(Continued)*

		Standard Score
Stories		110
Word Pairs		130
Visual Immediate Index		72
Dot Locations		80
Faces		75 (NV)
Verbal Delayed Index		106
Stories		100
Word Pairs		110
Visual Delayed Index		75
Dot Locations		90
Faces		70 (NV)
Delayed Recognition Index		97
Stories		80
Word Pairs		115
Learning Index		106
Word Pairs		135
Dot Locations		75
Wechsler Individual Achievement Test-II (WIAT-II)		
Word Reading		95
Pseudoword Decoding		89
Written Expression		79
Spelling		88
Mathematical Reasoning		89
Numerical Operations		95
Behavior Assessment System for Children, Second Edition (BASC-2)		
	T-Scores	
	Parent	Teacher
Clinical Scales		
Hyperactivity	51	52
Aggression	48	48
Conduct Problems	40	49
Anxiety	34	50
Depression	61	56
Somatization	50	42
Atypicality	46	72
Withdrawal	58	66
Attention Problems	67	71
Learning Problems	NA	60
Adaptive Scales		
Adaptability	32	45
Social Skills	30	39
Leadership	36	38
Study Skills	NA	40
Activities of Daily Living	34	NA
Functional Communication	39	41
DSM-IV ADHD Checklist	**Raw Score**	
Inattention	15/27	26/27
Hyperactivity/Impulsivity	9/27	12/27

Notes. NA = Not applicable; NV = Not valid.

performance on the Faces subtest of the CMS was deemed invalid due to poor comprehension of the task demands. This would cause the Visual Index scores to be depressed as well.

Academic Functioning

The WIAT-II was administered as a measure of academic achievement. Eddie appears to be gaining basic readiness skills at a level that is generally commensurate with intellectual expectancy with the exception of his writing ability.

Social-Emotional and Behavioral Functioning

Behaviorally, analysis of rating scales completed by Eddie's mother and kindergarten teacher indicates that, at the present time, they both have significant concerns regarding Eddie's ability to focus and sustain his attention to task. At the same time, behaviors indicative of hyperactivity, impulsivity, aggression, and conduct problems were not rated as significant, indicating typical functioning in these areas. Mrs. Jones rated Eddie as exhibiting significant difficulty adapting to changes in routine along with poor social skills. Eddie's teacher noted concerns related to social-emotional immaturity and social withdrawal in the classroom, and his mother reported somewhat elevated levels of depressed mood.

Summary and Diagnostic Impressions

Taken together, this pattern of test performance in conjunction with behavioral observations and Eddie's developmental history are consistent with a diagnosis of ADHD, combined type in conjunction with executive functioning deficits (poor sequential reasoning/problem solving, attention regulation, linguistic and motor planning) and developmental coordination disorder, which are significantly impacting Eddie's ability to successfully perform at school. Although Eddie's mother and teacher did not report elevated hyperactivity or impulsivity via norm-referenced behavior ratings, qualitative reports and behavioral observations suggest difficulty in these areas as well, thereby leading to the diagnosis of the combined type of ADHD. In addition, these deficits are beginning to affect his social-emotional development, and place Eddie at risk for developing a learning disability in the area of written expression in the future.

Recommendations

- It is recommended that Eddie be referred to the response to intervention or student support team at his school so that a response to intervention program can be developed as soon as possible in order to improve his attention regulation, listening skills, classroom behavior, and socialization skills. Eddie's parents are strongly encouraged to become involved in this process. They should feel comfortable that adequate steps are being taken to ensure that:
  - The interventions involve the use of research-based methodologies.
  - Appropriate assessment tools are being used to monitor Eddie's progress over the 8- to 12-week intervention time period.
  - Instructors are properly trained in the implementation of the interventions.

If the interventions prove to be ineffective in significantly improving Eddie's classroom behavior, an immediate referral for special education resource/inclusion services under the eligibility category of "Other Health Impaired" should be initiated.

- As part of the response to intervention behavioral plan, rules and expectations should be simply, clearly, and consistently presented and reviewed frequently. The plan should place a large emphasis on consistently rewarding Eddie's "good" behavior, such as positive social interactions, working on classwork, and following directions, rather than having a punitive system that primarily calls attention to his mistakes. In other words, he should have a high ratio of positive reinforcement (gaining points, tokens, etc.) to punishment (losing points, etc.; ratio = 5:1). Consequences for both appropriate and inappropriate behavior should be enforced on a consistent basis through "positive reinforcement" and "response cost." This could be managed in the form of a token economy, given Eddie's age. The behavioral plan should be coordinated with the parents to ensure consistency between home and school, including target behaviors, reinforcers, and punishments.
- Given Eddie's pattern of strengths and weaknesses, it is recommended that academic instruction in reading/writing emphasize phonetic and multisensory approaches. In order to enhance Eddie's learning/retention, new material should be presented in an organized format that is meaningful to him. The material to be learned should be pretaught, broken down into smaller components/steps, and presented in a highly structured format with frequent repetition to facilitate new learning. Instruction should be supplemented with visual aids, demonstrations, and experiential/procedural learning whenever possible. Eddie should be provided with periodic review of previously learned material in order to enhance long-term retention.
- In light of his inattention and impulsivity, teachers, therapists, and parents should keep in mind several general rules when interacting with Eddie.
  - Eye contact should be ensured.
  - A prompt to look at the speaker before directions are presented will be helpful.
  - Instructions and directions should be kept short, simple, and concrete.
  - Requests should be limited to single commands.
  - Instructions should be presented several times as necessary.
- Accommodations will be necessary to enhance Eddie's ability to succeed in the classroom, including preferential seating away from bulletin boards, doorways, windows, or other students, if necessary, where excessive stimuli might prove distracting. Instruction should be provided in small-group settings, and efforts should be made to redirect his attention. Given his ADHD, a reduction in the amount, but not the difficulty level, of assignments may assist Eddie in completing classroom tasks and homework in a timely manner. Moreover, whenever possible, he should be given additional time to complete assignments. Tests should be in multiple choice/matching/short answer formats instead of an essay format and should be administered individually/orally, with additional time provided when necessary. Eddie also will benefit from the use of graph paper or different color highlighter pens to help maintain place value when he begins doing written calculation. Finally, Eddie may require copies of classroom lecture notes and the use of a computer with word processing capability as he progresses through school. Most word processing

programs are equipped with spell checks and cut and paste and can be adapted for voice dictation if necessary.

- As Eddie approaches middle school, study skills training will be warranted, emphasizing such techniques as the appropriate outlining of lecture notes and how to study for tests. He also will benefit from being taught how to take notes on text material and plan written reports using an outlining method. In a related vein, training in word processing is strongly encouraged. Eddie also may require instruction on how to organize and plan his approach to his studies as executive functioning is an area of weakness for him. In addition, direct instruction in basic organizational strategies will assist Eddie in knowing what to do, when to do it, and how to do it. Specifically, he should be guided in the use of checklists and other organizational aids such as a daily planner. With help from teachers and parents, ideally he will plan each day of the week, including time after school.
- Eddie should continue to receive occupational therapy to improve his fine motor functioning as it relates to his school performance.
- Speech/language reevaluation should be considered in order to determine if Eddie's linguistic planning difficulties warrant direct intervention.
- Eddie would benefit from participation in a social skills training group, and his parents are encouraged to enroll in a parent effectiveness training group in order to develop their parenting skills.
- If these interventions, classroom accommodations, and a behavioral plan prove ineffective at managing Eddie's symptoms of inattention, overactivity, and impulsivity, consultation with his pediatrician regarding a trial of medication management should be considered.

Further Discussion of Case Study

Eddie's case illustrates the point that many children who are referred for an ADHD evaluation also have other significant issues (in this case coordination difficulties, executive function deficits, and emotional symptoms) that interfere with academic and behavioral functioning. An important aspect of the assessment process involves consideration of comorbidity and identification of deficits that may contribute to or result from the primary ADHD diagnosis. These additional diagnoses or deficits should then lead to individualized intervention approaches based on the unique needs of the student, in addition to addressing the ADHD symptoms.

CONCLUDING COMMENTS

ADHD continues to be a frequent reason for referral for school- and clinic-based evaluations (DuPaul & Stoner, 2003). Given the commonality of these concerns, there has been a commensurate research effort aimed at identifying the underlying causes and mechanisms of dysfunction, examining different assessment modalities (e.g., rating scales, continuous performance tests), and evaluating the effectiveness of interventions. As a result of this research effort, our understanding of the neurological basis of ADHD has improved dramatically over the last decade, and continuing research promises even greater advances in the near future.

While our knowledge of how to assess and treat ADHD symptoms improves with advances in the research literature, practitioners have at their disposal a collection of well-established interventions, such as behavioral parent training programs, behavioral classroom management, classroom modifications, and stimulant medications. Future research may focus on refining these identified intervention approaches in order to maximize their effectiveness and improve implementation. Additional research also is needed on the effectiveness of interventions designed to improve academic outcomes (as opposed to behavioral and social outcomes) among children and adolescents with ADHD.

Chapter 7

TOURETTE SYNDROME

DEFINITION

Tourette syndrome (TS; also referred to in the literature as Gilles de la Tourette's syndrome and Tourette's disorder) is classified as a tic disorder in the *Diagnostic and Statistical Manual of Mental Disorders*, Fourth Edition Text Revision (*DSM-IV-TR*; American Psychiatric Association [APA], 2000). The *DSM-IV-TR* defines a tic as "a sudden, rapid, recurrent, nonrhythmic, stereotyped motor movement or vocalization" (p. 108). Thus, tics include both motor and vocal behaviors. (Note that vocal tics are sometimes referred to as phonic tics.) Tics often are classified as simple or complex (APA, 2000). For example, simple motor tics include eye blinking, nose twitching, and neck jerking; complex motor tics include touching, smelling, head shaking, jumping, grooming behaviors, copropraxia (i.e., making obscene gestures), and echopraxia (i.e., imitating gestures used by others). Similarly, simple vocal tics include grunting, barking, sniffing, and throat clearing; complex vocal tics include echolalia (i.e., repeating sounds or words used by others), coprolalia (i.e., uttering obscene words), and repeating words without appropriate context (APA, 2000; Jankovic, 2001). Although coprolalia tics receive much attention in the popular media, these symptoms are relatively rare, occurring in less than 10% of people diagnosed with TS (APA, 2000). A factor analysis of tic symptoms suggested that in addition to purely motor and vocal tics, tic symptoms in TS also may be categorized into aggressive behaviors such as argumentativeness and temper fits, compulsive behaviors such as touching objects or other people, and tapping in the absence of grunting (Alsobrook & Pauls, 2002). Tics are often thought of as completely involuntary, but many tics appear to be at least partially controllable by the child. Some of the interventions described later in this chapter rely on the child's ability to suppress the urge to tic or on restructuring the child's environment to minimize antecedent variables that lead to the urge to tic (Swain, Scahill, Lombroso, King, & Leckman, 2007).

Also included under tic disorders are chronic motor or vocal tic disorder, transient tic disorder, and tic disorder not otherwise specified. Professionals must differentiate TS from these other tic disorders when reaching a diagnosis; and differential diagnosis is based on the type of tics, chronicity of symptoms, and age at onset. TS includes four diagnostic criteria:

1. The presence of both multiple motor tics and at least one vocal tic.
2. Occurrence of tics on a frequent and consistent basis for more than one year.
3. Onset before 18 years of age.

4. Tics are not accounted for by substance use or a general medical condition such as Huntington's disease or multiple sclerosis (APA, 2000).

Although the *DSM-IV-TR* requires the occurrence of tics on a frequent and consistent basis, it also is recognized that tics often vary in frequency and severity over time (Swain et al., 2007).

In the special education setting, children with TS are likely to receive services under the Other Health Impaired category of the Individuals with Disabilities Education Improvement Act (IDEIA), although they may be classified under the Emotional Disturbance, Learning Disability, or other categories depending on the nature of their symptom presentation; comorbidity; and specific emotional, behavioral, and academic difficulties. Common academic consequences of tics include interference with reading and handwriting due to motor tics and avoidance of reading aloud and asking questions in class due to interfering vocal tics and related embarrassment (Packer, 2005).

Prevalence/Incidence

The prevalence of TS is estimated at approximately 5 to 30 children per 10,000, which appears to decrease to 1 to 2 adults per 10,000 (APA, 2000), although other estimates are closer to 1% of children and adolescents (A. S. Davis & Phelps, 2008; Robertson, 2003) and epidemiologic studies have presented wide ranges of prevalence estimates (Scahill, Tanner, & Dure, 2001). Further, tic behaviors alone are much more common among children than the TS diagnosis, but tics in the absence of TS are typically mild and brief (Snider et al., 2002). TS is diagnosed between three and five times more frequently in males than in females in clinical settings, but only about two times more frequently in males in some community samples (APA, 2000). Research suggests that TS has been found across all countries, cultures, and ethnic groups (Robertson, 2000).

ETIOLOGY

Genetic Contributions

Tourette syndrome is considered a genetic neurodevelopmental disorder due to strong evidence for genetic influences in its etiology (APA, 2000; A. S. Davis & Phelps, 2008; Pauls, 2003). Researchers have observed high concordance rates in twin studies, especially among monozygotic twins (A. S. Davis & Phelps, 2008; Hoekstra et al., 2004; Verkerk et al., 2006), and one prospective study found that children had a much higher probability of developing TS (in addition to obsessive-compulsive disorder [OCD] and Attention-Deficit/Hyperactivity Disorder [ADHD]) if one parent had been diagnosed with TS and even higher probability if *both* parents were diagnosed with TS (McMahon, Fredine, & Pauls, 2003). The specific genes that contribute to TS are under investigation, and numerous models for inheritance (e.g., mixed model with genetic and environmental variables, polygenic inheritance, bilineality, genetic heterogeneity) have been proposed, but the genetics of TS are not yet fully understood (Robertson, 2000; Swain et al., 2007). Possible genetic markers have been identified on chromosomes 3q, 4q, 8p, 5, 9q, 10, 11q23, and 13q, in addition to errors on chromosomes 6, 9, 7q, 8q, and 19q21.1–q22.2 (C. L. Barr et al., 1999; Phelps, 2008; Verkerk et al., 1991). The fact that so many sites have been studied and implicated suggests that TS is caused by multiple genes rather than by a single predictable gene (Leckman, 2002). Further, while genetics provide a level of vulnerability, it is likely that genetic makeup interacts with nongenetic factors to determine who will develop symptoms of TS (APA, 2000).

Neurological Correlates

Recently, much research on TS has examined the neurological correlates of the disorder, largely using brain imaging methods to identify neuroanatomical differences or abnormalities among individuals with TS. Generally speaking, TS is believed to be related to abnormal neurotransmitter activity causing disinhibition of cortico-striatal-thalamic-cortical circuitry, or circuits that link regions of the frontal lobes with subcortical structures (Jankovic, 2001; H. S. Singer & Minzer, 2003; Ziemann, Paulus, & Rothenberger, 1997). More specifically, decreased motor inhibition due to impaired modulation of neuronal activity in the basal ganglia and thalamus has been implicated, which likely involves the circuit from the prefrontal cortex to the caudate, then to the globus pallidus and substantia nigra, then to the thalamus, and finally back to the cortex (B. S. Peterson et al., 1998). Research suggests a shorter cortical silent period in adults with TS as compared to controls, reflecting impaired motor inhibition in the motor cortex (Ziemann et al., 1997).

Research has most consistently implicated the basal ganglia in TS and in tics more generally (Amat et al., 2006; Mink, 2001; Phelps, 2008; Segawa, 2003), as imaging studies show reduced basal ganglia volume and lack of the typical asymmetry in the basal ganglia among children with TS (Robertson & Baron-Cohen, 1996). Specifically, the basal ganglia may activate the motor cortex, premotor area, and cingulate motor area to cause motor tics (Mink, 2001), since the basal ganglia interact with other areas (e.g., brain stem, motor thalamus, motor cortex) to determine motor functioning and produce movement (Joseph, 1996). The basal ganglia also could be involved in the symptoms of ADHD and OCD, which may explain the high rates of comorbidity with TS and these disorders via a common etiologic pathway through the basal ganglia (Amat et al., 2006; Mink, 2001; Phelps, 2008).

Further, B. S. Peterson et al. (2003) found significant reduction in caudate volume among a large sample of children and adults with TS compared to controls; adults with TS also showed a trend toward reductions in the putamen and globus pallidus volumes. Regional volumes were not associated with severity of TS symptoms in childhood. A prospective study, however, found that caudate volumes in children with TS predicted severity of TS and OCD symptoms in early adulthood, with smaller volumes associated with more severe symptoms (Bloch, Leckman, Zhu, & Peterson, 2005). These findings are consistent with earlier studies implicating the limbic system in TS, which suggested that TS results from disinhibition of functions that are regulated by the limbic system, which in turn is regulated at the cortical level by the prefrontal cortex (B. G. Comings & D. E. Comings, 1987). In another study, boys with TS showed a larger proportion of white matter in the right frontal lobe, which supports the involvement of frontal-striatal circuitry in TS and may serve as a possible reason for abnormalities of the basal ganglia (Fredericksen et al., 2002). Frontal abnormalities also have been identified with single photon emission computed tomography (SPECT) studies (Robertson & Baron-Cohen, 1996).

Other findings support the involvement of diffuse cortical systems in the etiology of TS. For example, a relatively large sample of children and adults with TS had larger volumes in the dorsal prefrontal region and parieto-occipital region, and smaller volumes in the inferior occipital region, as compared to controls (B. S. Peterson et al., 2001).

Considering children separately, those with TS showed larger dorsal prefrontal volumes in boys and girls, smaller premotor volumes in boys, larger parieto-occipital volumes in boys and girls, smaller orbitofrontal and subgenual volumes in boys, and larger inferior occipital volumes in boys and girls. Further, tic severity was associated with cerebral volumes of the orbitofrontal, midtemporal, and parieto-occipital regions. B. S. Peterson et al. (2007) also found significantly larger overall volumes of the hippocampus (resulting primarily from enlarged head and medial surface) and amygdala (resulting primarily from enlarged dorsal and ventral surfaces) among children with TS, suggesting involvement of these areas of the limbic cortico-striatal-thalamic-cortical circuit. Interestingly, volumes of these areas declined with age (cross-sectionally) for TS subjects, with volumes for TS subjects becoming smaller than those for controls by adulthood (B. S. Peterson et al., 2007). This pattern may be explained by the fact that the TS adults in this study were highly symptomatic even as adults; thus, these results do not conflict with research suggesting a typical reduction in tics with age (discussed later).

Widespread abnormalities (i.e., immaturity) in the neural functional connectivity were observed among adolescents with TS, especially in the fronto-parietal network, resulting in unwanted behaviors and reduced control (Church et al., 2009). Plessen et al. (2004) also found evidence of involvement of the corpus callosum in the pathophysiology of TS, as children with TS showed a smaller corpus callosum area as compared to controls and adults with TS showed a larger corpus callosum area as compared to controls. Size of the corpus callosum also was positively correlated with severity of motor tics but not severity of vocal tics (Plessen et al., 2004). Thus, TS symptoms may be partially explained by limited interhemispheric connectivity and reduced input to inhibitory neurons in the prefrontal cortical regions. As with the B. S. Peterson et al. (2007) study, the TS adults in this study were still highly symptomatic even as adults; thus, the pattern suggesting increased corpus callosum size with age suggests the possibility of a developed compensatory mechanism in response to persistent tic symptoms, in which the corpus callosum helps regulate tic severity.

A functional magnetic resonance imaging (fMRI) study of adults with TS showed that tic suppression involved activation of the basal ganglia, thalamus, and prefrontal cortical areas, suggesting that tics are related to neuronal modulation deficits in subcortical circuits resulting in difficulty inhibiting behavioral impulses (B. S. Peterson et al., 1998). Similarly, an fMRI study with children showed that subjects with more severe tics demonstrated increased activation of the substantia nigra and ventral tegmental area (which regulate diffuse areas of the brain), premotor cortex, superior frontal gyrus, inferior frontal gyrus pars triangularis, middle frontal gyrus, thalamus, putamen, and right nucleus accumbens when completing a cognitive control task. These results suggest that children with more severe tics activated multiple regions of the cortico-striatal-thalamic-cortical circuit when completing the task; this may serve as an adaptive compensatory mechanism for these children (i.e., they rely more heavily on these areas to help them complete the challenging task) (Baym, Corbett, Wright, & Bunge, 2008).

Specific neurotransmitter systems identified as potential causal factors in TS include dopamine, serotonin, acetylcholine (ACh), gamma-aminobutyric acid (GABA), and others (Jimenez-Jimenez & Garcia-Ruiz, 2001; Robertson, 2000). Dopamine receptor genes, dopamine transporter genes, adrenergic genes, and serotonin transporter genes also have been implicated (Phelps, 2008; H. S. Singer, 2005). It is hypothesized that abnormalities in multiple areas produce a cumulative effect rather than these individual areas acting independently to determine TS (Swain et al., 2007). TS may be related to dysfunction in the regulation of dopamine release and uptake (Jankovic, 2001; Nomura & Segawa, 2003), but research has been inconsistent on the role of dopamine in the development of TS (Phelps, 2008). Evidence for the involvement of dopamine is found in pharmacological research in which medications that block dopamine receptors also reduced the number of tics, whereas medications that increase dopamine transmission increased number of tics (H. S. Singer, 2005). SPECT studies also have shown increased dopaminergic innervation of the striatum of individuals with TS (Swain et al., 2007). Also, dopamine has been shown to have a role in the inhibition of behavior, with reductions in dopamine in the prefrontal cortex associated with greater hyperactivity and disinhibition, while dopamine neurons projecting to the nucleus accumbens are responsible for stimulating motor activity (Comings, 1987). An important area for future investigation will be to follow up on preliminary evidence of abnormalities in the tangential migration of GABAergic cells in the basal ganglia among individuals with TS, which may contribute to increased levels of cortical excitability and motor system activity (Swain et al., 2007).

In sum, a number of different areas, structures, and neurotransmitters have been implicated in the pathophysiology of TS. Longitudinal studies are needed to better understand how abnormalities in these different areas cause, or are caused by, TS. It is also important to keep in mind that neuroanatomical differences observed among children and adults with TS may not represent causal factors in the disorder; these differences may instead represent consequences or even compensatory changes in the brain in response to TS symptoms (Gerard & Peterson, 2003).

Environmental Factors

Environmental influences have been related to TS and tic severity including prenatal and perinatal insults such as maternal stress during pregnancy, maternal use of stimulant medications and smoking during pregnancy, low birth weight, and birth complications, but a lack of controlled studies prevents definitive conclusions about these variables (Leckman, 2002; Mathews & MacDorman, 2006; Robertson, 2000). The finding that experiencing more psychosocial stress leads to increased future tic severity supports the notion that stress can influence the manifestation of TS (Leckman et al., 1997; Swain et al., 2007). Several case study investigations have raised hypotheses about associations between TS and herpes simplex 1, Lyme disease, and pneumonia (Robertson, 2000; Swain et al., 2007), but these should be considered only hypotheses or clinical observations at this time.

Recently, TS (along with OCD and tic disorder) has been investigated as a pediatric autoimmune neuropsychiatric disorder associated with streptococcal infections (PANDAS) due to the hypothesis that TS is related to autoimmune mechanisms. *PANDAS* refers to conditions that are thought to be brought on or exacerbated by streptococcal infections (H. S. Singer & Loiselle, 2003). For example, a case control study found that children diagnosed with TS were more likely than control children to have experienced a streptococcal infection several months before onset of their disorder. Further, this risk was even higher among children who had experienced multiple streptococcal infections (especially group A beta-hemolytic streptococcal infections) in the year before being diagnosed (Mell, Davis, & Owens, 2005). It has been speculated that these infections affect areas of the brain that are also affected by TS, such as the basal ganglia (Leckman, 2002). Alternatively, it may be that antibodies directed toward group A beta-hemolytic streptococcal infections attack brain cells such as those of the caudate nucleus, thereby resulting in the onset or exacerbation of TS symptoms (Hoekstra, Kallenberg, Korf, & Minderaa, 2002; H. S. Singer & Loiselle, 2003; Swain et al., 2007). At the same time, however, prospective studies have at this point found no significant association between group A beta-hemolytic streptococcal infections and (a) symptom exacerbations among children with TS (Luo et al., 2004) or (b) onset of tic symptoms among children without TS (Perrin et al., 2004). Thus, investigations of the PANDAS explanation for TS have produced somewhat inconsistent results, and many children experience streptococcal infections without developing TS symptoms (H. S. Singer & Loiselle, 2003). The best summary statement may be that there appears to be an association based on retrospective studies, but there is no evidence for a causal relationship based on prospective data.

It is thought that environmental factors may interact with genetic and neurobiological factors to determine whether children with the genetic predisposition for TS actually will develop the disorder, and may determine the severity of the disorder (Leckman et al., 1997; Robertson, 2000). For example, streptococcal infections may interact with genetic and other environmental and biological variables to determine onset of TS (Mell et al., 2005). The study of environmental risk factors represents an important area for future inquiry, especially with regard to the interaction among environmental, genetic, and neurological factors in determining onset and severity of TS.

COURSE AND PROGNOSIS

The mean age at onset of TS is between 6 and 9 years (APA, 2000; A. S. Davis & Phelps, 2008), although some studies suggest that age at onset is often younger (Jankovic, 2001; Leckman et al., 1998). Development of motor tics often precedes the onset of vocal tics by several years (Leckman, 2002). Diagnosis of TS usually occurs by early adolescence (R. D. Freeman et al., 2000). Severity of tics can range from very mild, causing little or no distress, to very severe, causing extreme distress due to the intrusiveness and social stigmatization of the tics (APA, 2000). The course of TS is quite variable (Coffey et al., 2000), but tics typically are the worst between 8 and 12 years of age, and this worst-ever period usually is followed by a gradual decline in tic severity into young adulthood (Leckman et al., 1998; Swain et al., 2007). Thus, some symptoms may last into adulthood, but short- and long-term periods of remission may occur, and the severity and frequency of symptoms usually decrease in adolescence and adulthood (APA, 2000; Leckman, 2002; Robertson, 2000), with some adults reporting minimal or no tics (Burd et al., 2001). In fact, it is estimated that only about 20% of children with TS experience at least a moderate level of impairment by young adulthood, but those who continue to experience TS symptoms as adults are more likely to experience the most severe symptoms, such as self-injurious tics and coprolalia (Leckman, 2003; Swain et al., 2007). These typical developmental decreases in TS symptoms over time seem to explain the lower prevalence in adulthood compared to childhood.

In addition to decreases in tic severity and frequency, longitudinal data suggest decreases in comorbidity by adulthood and improvement in global psychological functioning for many adults with TS (Burd et al., 2001). At this time, little is known about predictors of TS remission or persistence into adulthood; limited evidence suggests that better outcomes are associated with female sex, less severe tics, fewer comorbid symptoms, higher socioeconomic status, and longer duration of treatment (Coffey et al., 2000).

Frequency and types of tics may vary over time and may get worse when under stress (e.g., stressful events such as death of a parent, separation of parents, beginning school, experiencing an illness, stressful social events) or during times of excitement or fatigue, overstimulation, waiting, multitasking, socializing, watching television, being observed by others, engaging in academic tasks, talking about tics, and being alone (Conelea & Woods, 2008b; A. S. Davis & Phelps, 2008; Jankovic, 2001; Robertson, 2000). Tics may become less severe or frequent when children are expending their energy concentrating on physical or mental tasks, such as playing a musical instrument, relaxing, studying, reading, playing sports, habitual activities, and socializing with familiar people (Conelea & Woods, 2008b; Jankovic, 2001; Swain et al., 2007). Although it seems to be a common belief that tics become significantly more frequent or severe after a period of voluntary tic suppression (i.e., a rebound effect due to a buildup of tension), research generally does not support this phenomenon (Meidinger et al., 2005; Verdellen, Hoogduin, & Keijsers, 2007). For some children, tics occur during sleep and may cause sleep disturbance (Swain et al., 2007), which may lead to fatigue during the day. Children with TS also may experience sleep disturbances such as difficulty falling asleep, more wakefulness after sleep onset, reduced sleep efficiency, increased arousal, and sleepwalking (Kostanecka-Endress et al., 2003).

Physical sensations, discomfort, or feelings of anxiety or tension often occur before tics, and these feelings are then relieved after the child engages in the tic; these feelings have been termed *premonitory urges* (Jankovic, 2001; Leckman, 2003). Premonitory urges appear to occur most commonly as physical sensations in the shoulders, upper back, stomach, and hands but can occur throughout the body (Leckman et al., 1997). In this way, tics seem to be similar to compulsions, as the premonitory urges may be relieved only when the tics are performed in a certain way or a certain number of times, and tics may be accompanied by feelings of anxiety if they are not performed (Jankovic, 2001). Indeed, it is sometimes difficult to distinguish between complex motor tics and compulsions (Mansueto & Keuler, 2005), especially in light of the fact that TS is often comorbid with OCD (see the next discussion on comorbidity).

Comorbidity

Comorbidity is an especially important issue in the course and prognosis of TS, as children diagnosed with TS often demonstrate additional behavioral symptoms such as obsessions, compulsions, inattention, hyperactivity, and impulsivity, and many may experience embarrassment, depression, and peer rejection due to their tics (APA, 2000). Common comorbid diagnoses include ADHD, OCD, and learning disabilities (LD) (APA, 2000; A. S. Davis & Phelps, 2008), in addition to anxiety disorders, mood disorders, sleep disturbances, self-injurious behaviors, difficulty controlling temper, and oppositional-defiant disorder (Gaze, Kepley, & Walkup, 2006; Jankovic, 2001; Robertson, 2000; Robertson & Baron-Cohen, 1996). Recent data suggest that tic disorders also are frequently observed among children with autism spectrum disorders (Canitano & Vivanti, 2007). A multisite, international database of 3500 individuals diagnosed with TS found that, on average, only about 12% of all participants reported TS without some comorbid condition (the range across all sites was 2% to 35% of participants with TS alone; R. D. Freeman et al., 2000). Thus, comorbidity appears to be a typical characteristic of TS.

Prevalence rates for comorbid diagnoses vary somewhat depending on whether clinical or community samples are considered (Swain et al., 2007). ADHD co-occurs in greater than 50% of children with TS in many clinical and epidemiological studies (APA, 2000; Robertson, 2006a), OCD co-occurs in about 35% to 50% of children with TS (APA, 2000), and LD co-occurs in about 10% to 25% of children with TS (Burd, Freeman, Klug, & Kerbeshian, 2005; Lewandowski, 2005). At the same time, most children who are diagnosed with ADHD, OCD, or LD do not meet criteria for TS.

The combination of TS and ADHD is associated with more aggressive and noncompliant behaviors than TS alone, in addition to family conflict, academic difficulties, and rejection by peers (Swain et al., 2007). Children with comorbid TS and ADHD may have greater difficulty with tic suppression due to ADHD interfering with the child's ability to engage in activities requiring focus and concentration, activities that have been shown to facilitate tic suppression (Gaze et al., 2006). There is some evidence that children with comorbid TS and ADHD often develop ADHD first, then develop motor and vocal tics several years later (D. E. Comings & B. G. Comings, 1987a). Research also suggests that children with TS plus ADHD are likely to have greater deficits in overall psychosocial functioning, are more likely to receive special education services, and are more likely to have additional comorbid conditions (e.g., mood and disruptive disorders) than children with either diagnosis alone (Spencer et al., 1998).

Specific OCD symptoms commonly seen among individuals with TS include counting rituals, checking and arranging behaviors, and obsessions related to symmetry and to aggressive and sexual themes (Robertson & Baron-Cohen, 1996; Shavitt, Hounie, Campos, & Miguel, 2006); this collection of symptoms is distinct from the obsessions with contamination and compulsions to clean often seen in pure OCD (Robertson, 2000). In fact, a specific subtype of OCD has been proposed in which TS diagnostic criteria are combined with OCD symptoms that include more aggressive behaviors, earlier age at onset, higher frequency among males, and less response to selective serotonin reuptake inhibitors (SSRIs; APA, 2000; Mansueto & Keuler, 2005). Indeed, measuring event-related brain potentials (ERPs) among small samples of adults with TS, OCD, or no diagnosis demonstrated that as compared to controls, those subjects with TS and those subjects with OCD exhibited altered electrophysiological activity in the frontal cortex (indicative of altered frontal inhibition) while engaging in a Stroop task. Subjects with TS and subjects with OCD were very similar on several measures of ERPs, providing support for neurological similarities of the two disorders (Johannes et al., 2003).

The combination of TS and LD is associated with male sex, greater likelihood of perinatal problems, younger age when first seen by a professional, younger age at diagnosis, more severe tics, and greater likelihood of comorbid ADHD, social skills deficits, anger problems, and other psychiatric disturbance (Burd et al., 2005).

Comorbid diagnoses may cause more academic, social, and emotional impairment than symptoms of TS alone (Jankovic, 2001; Robertson, 2000), as children with TS and comorbid ADHD, OCD, or LD often perform more poorly on neuropsychological tests than those diagnosed with TS only. Thus, it is likely that these comorbid conditions interact to influence performance on neuropsychological tests (Lewandowski, 2005; Robertson & Baron-Cohen, 1996). This hypothesis has been borne out in several studies in which children with TS-only performed better than comorbid groups on a range of neuropsychological tasks and emotional/behavioral ratings (E. L. Harris et al., 1995; Ozonoff, Strayer, McMahon, & Filloux, 1998; Schuerholz, Singer, & Denckla, 1998; Shin, Chung, & Hong, 2001). Comorbidity also seems to contribute significantly to stress among parents of children with TS, as comorbid symptoms are reported as more stressful than TS symptoms alone (Wilkinson, Marshall, & Curtwright, 2008). Thus, the neuropsychological, emotional-behavioral, and family functioning profile may be quite different when TS is combined with other diagnoses, which will have implications for treatment. This high association between comorbid conditions and neuropsychological performance complicates the study of neuropsychological deficits associated with pure TS, as TS-only children appear to be the exception. High comorbidity rates also suggest the possibility that TS, ADHD, and OCD are partially caused by common neurological pathways and neuroanatomical factors (e.g., the neuropathology of all three disorders likely involves the basal ganglia and related circuits) and also may share some degree of genetic vulnerability (Sheppard, Bradshaw, Purcell, & Pantelis, 1999; Swain et al., 2007). Additional research is needed to sort out these neurological and genetic mechanisms.

Neuropsychological Deficits

At this time, more is known about genetic and neurological factors that contribute to TS than is known about neuropsychological functioning among children with TS (Robertson & Baron-Cohen, 1996). Thus, this discussion (and the content of Table 7.1) is tentative as our understanding of the neuropsychology of TS will continue to evolve. Further, many of the studies on which we base our understanding of neuropsychological functioning used heterogeneous samples of children diagnosed with TS plus other conditions, making it difficult to reach firm conclusions about the neuropsychological performance of children with TS alone.

TS has been associated with deficits in multiple areas of neuropsychological functioning, including intelligence, language, perceptual-motor skills, memory, academic achievement, executive function, and psychosocial functioning (Robertson &

Table 7.1 Neuropsychological Deficits Associated with TS

Global Domain	Specific Deficits
Cognition	Verbal IQ greater than Performance IQ, although overall intellectual function often in the average range
Auditory-linguistic/Language function	Verbal fluency impaired, expressive language (organizing and monitoring linguistic output) impaired, problems with making inferences, difficulty in discourse processing, difficulty understanding abstract language, and speech dysfluency (e.g., stuttering)
Learning and memory	Areas of memory affected include strategic memory, working memory, short-term nonverbal memory, long-term nonverbal memory, procedural memory, retention of information, probabilistic classification learning, rate of learning
Visual perception/Constructional praxis	Impairments in visual-spatial function, visual scanning, visual discrimination, fine motor skills, nonconstructional abilities and constructional abilities, visual-motor integration, motor coordination, motor inhibition, handwriting
Executive function	Problems with attention, sustained attention, vigilance, inhibition, self-monitoring, reaction time, interference control, impulse control, working memory
Academic achievement	Problems in arithmetic, writing, reading; frequent learning disabilities; frequent placement in special education settings
Emotional/Behavioral functioning	Anxiety, obsessions, compulsions, schizotypal behaviors, depression, problems with peer relationships/socialization, peer victimization, impulsivity, hyperactivity, conduct problems, aggression, withdrawal, somatic complaints, self-injurious behaviors, anger control

Note. These deficits often are strongly related to comorbid diagnoses in addition to TS.

Baron-Cohen, 1996). Comings and Comings (B. G. Comings & D. E. Comings, 1987; D. E. Comings & B. G. Comings, 1987a–e) published a series of studies examining neuropsychological and behavioral functioning among 246 children and adults (mostly children and young adults) with TS, comparing these children to controls. Some of the central findings include:

- Significant reading difficulties (e.g., slow reading, letter, number, or word reversal)
- Stuttering
- Poor retention of information
- Test anxiety
- Attention deficits
- Hyperactivity
- Impulsivity
- Conduct problems (e.g., lying, stealing, vandalism, violence, drug and alcohol abuse)
- Phobias
- Panic attacks
- Obsessions
- Compulsions
- Schizoid and paranoid symptoms
- Depressive symptoms (including suicidal ideation and attempts)
- Mania
- Sleep problems (e.g., sleepwalking, night terrors)
- Developmental delays in bowel and bladder control
- Greater likelihood of special education services, such as placement in adaptive behavior classrooms

While most of these difficulties certainly did not characterize all or even most of the subjects with TS, the deficits generally were *much* more frequent and severe for TS subjects than for controls. Many problems, such as conduct problems and manic symptoms, were strongly related to having comorbid ADHD, as subjects with TS and ADHD were much more likely to report these problems than subjects with TS only. This finding supports the notion that some of the problems experienced by individuals with TS are associated with comorbid conditions. The studies by Comings and Comings greatly contributed to our initial understanding of the neuropsychological deficits associated with TS. Results of more recent investigations are summarized next.

Cognition

Children with TS often score in the average range on IQ tests but sometimes exhibit a significant Verbal IQ (VIQ) > Performance IQ (PIQ) pattern (Bornstein, 1990; Robertson & Baron-Cohen, 1996) and sometimes score lower than the control group (A. S. Carter et al., 2000; Mahone, Koth, Cutting, Singer, & Denckla, 2001; Spencer et al., 1998). Lower PIQ scores may be largely attributable to comorbid ADHD, as a group of children with TS alone scored higher on PIQ than VIQ and also scored higher on all Performance subtests than a group of children with comorbid TS and

ADHD (E. Dykens et al., 1990). Similar results were reported by Brand et al. (2002), Rizzo et al. (2007), and Shin et al. (2001), in which children with comorbid TS and ADHD scored lower on VIQ and PIQ as compared to children with TS alone. Those children with TS alone scored above 100 on both domains (Brand et al., 2002; Rizzo et al., 2007; Shin et al., 2001). Comorbid OCD also may contribute to lower IQ scores, as one study found differences of over 10 points between children with TS only and children with TS plus OCD symptoms on Full Scale, Verbal, and Performance IQ, with the TS-only group scoring over 100 on all three measures (de Groot, Yeates, Baker, & Bornstein, 1997). Thus, children with pure TS are probably similar to healthy controls on most measures of intellectual functioning.

Language

With regard to verbal fluency, in one study children with comorbid TS and ADHD scored lower than children with TS only (Brand et al., 2002), but children with TS only have shown deficits in verbal fluency when compared to controls; this is especially true for girls with TS (Schuerholz et al., 1998). In a small sample of adolescents with TS, several subjects showed weaknesses in organizing and monitoring linguistic output, making inferences, discourse processing, and understanding abstract language. At the same time, there was much variability in language skills across subjects, with several subjects showing average language skills (Legg, Penn, Temlett, & Sonnenberg, 2005). Additional limited evidence suggests language problems related to speech dysfluency, such as stuttering, cluttering, interjections, and phrase repetitions (Burd, Leech, Kerbeshian, & Gascon, 1994; Jankovic, 2001; Van Borsel & Tetnowski, 2007; Van Borsel & Vanryckeghem, 2000). Due to small sample sizes and much variability among children with TS on measures of language functioning, it is difficult to reach firm conclusions or descriptions that characterize most children with TS in terms of language skills.

Memory and Learning

Most research suggests no significant deficits on measures of memory and learning, including measures of immediate and delayed story recall, immediate and delayed visual reproduction, verbal learning, recognition, working memory, visual working memory, and short-term memory (S. W. Chang, McCracken, & Piacentini, 2007; Channon, Pratt, & Robertson, 2003; S. Crawford, Channon, & Robertson, 2005; Ozonoff & Strayer, 2001; Verte, Geurts, Roeyers, Oosterlaan, & Sergeant, 2005). At the same time, not much research in this area has been conducted with children with TS, and there is some evidence for selective memory impairment (specifically, impairment on measures of strategic, working, short-term nonverbal, long-term nonverbal, and procedural memory, and no impairment of measures of immediate, semantic, verbal, and declarative memory) among adults with TS (Lavoie, Thibault, Stip, & O'Connor, 2007; Stebbins et al., 1995).

Several studies found that children and adults with TS were impaired on a probabilistic classification learning task (i.e., weather prediction task) and showed slower improvement over multiple trials when compared to controls, with slower rate of learning correlated with greater tic severity (Keri, Szlobodnyik, Benedek, Janka, & Gadoros, 2002; Marsh, Alexander, Packard, Zhu, & Peterson, 2005; Marsh et al., 2004). At the same time, children and adults with TS were not impaired on tasks of perceptual-motor skill learning (Marsh et al., 2005). Thus, learning deficits may be specific to probabilistic classification tasks, and these difficulties with learning would be consistent with the abnormalities of the basal ganglia described earlier in the chapter.

Visual Perception/Constructional Praxis

Bornstein (1990) found normal performance on most neuropsychological tasks but norm-referenced impairment on sensory-perception and psychomotor measures, which would be consistent with abnormalities of the basal ganglia. Sensory abilities such as vision and hearing are typically normal, but there is some evidence for deficits in visual scanning and visual discrimination skills (Robertson & Baron-Cohen, 1996). Some of the more consistent perceptual-motor findings include deficits in visual-motor integration, fine motor skills, handwriting, and motor coordination, based on performance on measures such as the Bender-Gestalt Test, Rey-Osterreith Complex Figure, Beery Visual-Motor Integration Test, and Purdue Pegboard (Bloch, Sukhodolsky, Leckman, & Schultz, 2006; Schultz et al., 1998). For example, Schultz et al. (1998) found that both groups of children with TS in their study (TS without ADHD and TS plus ADHD) showed deficits in visual-motor integration, visual-perceptual skills, and motor inhibition (errors of commission) as compared to the control group. In contrast, they did not differ from each other, suggesting that on these constructs, children with TS with and without ADHD are relatively similar. Deficits on fine motor tasks in childhood also have been found to predict greater tic severity in late adolescence (Bloch et al., 2006).

At the same time, results presented by Shin et al. (2001) suggest that comorbid ADHD greatly contributed to deficits in fine motor skills, as children with tic disorders alone performed similarly to the control group. S. W. Chang et al. (2007) and Verte et al. (2005) also found normal visual-motor integration and constructional skills among their samples of TS children, and other studies found intact motor dexterity and finger-tapping speed among adults with tic disorders (Lavoie et al., 2007; S. V. Muller et al., 2003).

Some research suggests deficits on Wechsler subtests such as Coding and Block Design, in addition to deficits on copying tasks, which would indicate deficits in both constructional and nonconstructional visual-spatial abilities (Robertson & Baron-Cohen, 1996). At the same time, results in this area have been inconsistent, with some research suggesting no impairment on these tasks among children with pure TS (e.g., Rizzo et al., 2007; Shin et al., 2001). Finally, Schuerholz, Cutting, Mazzocco, Singer, and Denckla (1997) found that motor movements were not significantly slowed among children with TS alone, but motor slowing was observed among children with TS and comorbid ADHD, especially for more complex sequences of motor movements.

Executive Function

While earlier research suggested that children with TS demonstrated significant impairment on measures of executive function, more recent research with better-defined groups of children with TS only and TS with comorbidity suggests that many deficits are accounted for by comorbid ADHD among children with TS. For example, TS has been characterized as a disorder of inhibitory control, and deficits in inhibition are often reported among children with TS (Stern, Blair, & Peterson, 2008), which would be consistent with disruption of the cortico-striatal-thalamic-cortical circuitry and basal ganglia function described previously (S. V. Muller et al., 2003). In contrast, Ozonoff et al. (1998) found that deficits in inhibition were largely dependent on comorbidity, as children with TS alone performed similarly to controls but children with TS plus ADHD and/or OCD showed deficits compared to the control group. Interestingly, inhibition deficits also were related to number and severity of TS symptoms. In another study, children with TS alone and children with ADHD alone showed more intrusions (i.e., inhibition errors) than controls on one verbal list learning task, but the children with TS performed in the average range overall on other measures of disinhibition and response organization (Mahone et al., 2001). Similarly, a sample of adults with TS plus OCD showed deficits on measures of response inhibition and performance monitoring as compared to controls but did not show deficits in measures of memory or attention and still scored within the average range on most tasks (S. V. Muller et al., 2003).

Channon et al. (2003) found impairment on a measure of inhibition among a group of adolescents with TS alone, but impairment on a measure of multitasking was observed only for adolescents with TS plus ADHD; no groups showed significant impairment in rule following or set shifting. Similarly, in one study, it was found that among children with comorbid tic disorders and ADHD, deficits in executive function (i.e., cognitive flexibility, sustained attention, interference control, impulse control) were explained by ADHD rather than by the presence of tic symptoms (Roessner, Becker, Banaschewski, & Rothenberger, 2007). In another sample, children with tic disorders alone performed similarly to the control group on measures of vigilance, signal detection, reaction time, and information processing while children with tic disorders plus ADHD showed deficits on these measures (Shin et al., 2001). Using the Behavior Rating Inventory of Executive Function (BRIEF) Parent Form, children with comorbid TS and ADHD were rated as more impaired than children with TS only and controls on indices of working memory, inhibition, metacognition, behavior regulation, and global executive function. Notably, children with TS only and controls were rated similarly on all of these scales except for working memory, where children with TS alone showed mild impairment relative to controls (Mahone et al., 2002).

Attention deficits have been hypothesized since TS may interfere with the child's ability to maintain attention due to the effort and concentration required to suppress tics (Jankovic, 2001; Lewandowski, 2005). This notion is supported by data indicating that children with TS had greater difficulty maintaining attention on a continuous performance test when trying to suppress their tics (Conelea & Woods, 2008a). This difficulty also may manifest as attention problems in the classroom when children are attempting to suppress their tics during academic tasks.

Children with TS showed no deficits in planning as measured by the Tower of Hanoi, cognitive flexibility as measured by the Wisconsin Card Sorting Test, or inhibition as measured by the Stroop task; this pattern was observed for TS children with no comorbidity and for TS children with comorbid ADHD and/or OCD (Ozonoff & Jensen, 1999a). In another study, children with TS did not differ significantly from control children on measures of inhibition, visual working memory, planning, cognitive flexibility, and verbal fluency, thereby suggesting normal functioning on these tasks (Verte et al., 2005). Similar findings have been reported for adults with tic disorders, as adults with TS performed similarly to controls on the Tower of London, Trail Making Test, Stroop task, and Wisconsin Card Sorting Test (Lavoie et al., 2007). Thus, in these studies, individuals with TS performed similarly to controls across executive function measures. Impaired reaction time has been observed among children with TS compared to controls (E. L. Harris et al., 1995; Shucard, Benedict, Tekok-Kilic, & Lichter, 1997).

In sum, research on executive function has produced inconsistent findings. Many studies suggest that severe executive function deficits are not part of the typical profile for children with TS alone but may be observed among children with TS plus comorbid diagnoses (especially ADHD) and may be present on narrow aspects of executive function, such as inhibition and monitoring. It also has been suggested that these inconsistent findings are related to overall intellectual functioning, with TS children with higher cognitive ability being less likely to show deficits in executive function and TS children with lower cognitive ability more likely to show these deficits (Mahone et al., 2001). Thus, executive function deficits observed in children with TS likely will vary based on comorbid conditions, severity of symptoms, and overall intellectual functioning, thereby pointing to the importance of considering these factors when interpreting neuropsychological assessment data and making predictions.

Academic Achievement

Academic achievement has not been the focus of many studies; sometimes it is used as a descriptive or demographic variable (or covariate) rather than a variable of interest to the study. Thus, our understanding of the impact of TS on academic functioning is quite limited. In one sample of children with TS, 51% met criteria for a learning disability in at least one academic area (i.e., reading, reading comprehension, math, spelling) based on a significant IQ–achievement discrepancy; frequencies of learning disabilities in spelling and math were especially high (Burd, Kauffman, & Kerbeshian, 1992).

Many difficulties with academic achievement among children with TS seem to be related to comorbid conditions. For example, one study revealed weakness in mental and written arithmetic among children with comorbid TS and ADHD but average functioning among children with TS alone (E. Dykens et al., 1990). Similarly, another study found that learning disabilities in reading, math, and written language were much more prevalent among children with TS plus ADHD than children with TS only (Schuerholz et al., 1998), and Mahone et al. (2002) reported average scores in reading and math achievement for children with TS only. In yet another study, children with TS performed more poorly than controls on a measure of arithmetic achievement, but this poorer performance on the arithmetic task was related largely to deficits in attention among the children with TS, as those children without attention problems did not show arithmetic deficits (Huckeba, Chapieski, Hiscock, & Glaze, 2008). Finally, children with TS plus ADHD and OCD symptoms scored significantly lower on reading, spelling, and arithmetic achievement than children with TS only, and children with TS only scored over 100 on all three measures (de Groot et al., 1997).

Emotional/Behavioral Functioning

Based on sociometric ratings, children with TS showed increased risk for peer relationship problems, such as aggression and withdrawal (this was especially true for children with TS plus ADHD), but not for self-rated social skills deficits or low self-esteem (Bawden, Stokes, Camfield, Camfield, & Salisbury, 1998). Children with tic disorders also are more likely to be teased and bullied than other children, and this peer victimization has been associated with greater tic severity, loneliness, and anxiety (Storch et al., 2007). A study using the Vineland Adaptive Behavior Scales also found significant weakness in socialization skills (e.g., interpersonal relationships) among children with TS (E. Dykens et al., 1990).

As with other constructs, comorbidity contributes to problems with behavioral and emotional adjustment, as children with TS plus a comorbid diagnosis tend to show poorer adjustment than children with TS alone. For example, in one study, children with comorbid TS and ADHD demonstrated significantly more problems than control children and children with TS alone across multiple parent-rated externalizing behaviors, internalizing problems, and social problems, while children with TS alone showed more internalizing problems (i.e., anxious/depressed, somatic complaints), school problems, and attention problems than controls (A. S. Carter et al., 2000). Similar results, in which children with TS alone are rated as having more difficulty with broad behavioral domains than control children, although not to the same extent as those with comorbid conditions, have been reported in several additional studies (Rizzo et al., 2007; Robertson, 2006a; Roessner et al., 2007; Shin et al., 2001). Further, the likelihood of experiencing anger problems, sleep problems, self-injurious behaviors, and coprolalia seems to increase with the number of comorbid conditions (R. D. Freeman et al., 2000).

Findings related to increased internalizing symptoms are consistent with research indicating greater risk for mood disorders and depressive symptoms as compared to controls. These internalizing symptoms may be related partly to TS medication side effects, comorbid OCD and ADHD, tic severity, external locus of control, and the social consequences of TS (E. Cohen, Sade, Benarroch, Pollak, & Gross-Tsur, 2008; Lin et al., 2007; Robertson, 2006b; Robertson, Williamson, & Eapen, 2006). Greater levels of stress and comorbid anxiety also have been observed among children with TS, which may be explained partly by comorbid depression and ADHD and external locus of control (E. Cohen et al., 2008), and which may contribute to tic severity given the association between psychosocial stress and exacerbation of tics (Gaze et al., 2006; Lin et al., 2007). In one study, tic severity among adolescents with TS was positively correlated with somatization, obsessive-compulsive symptoms, interpersonal sensitivity, depression, anxiety, and global distress (H. Chang, Tu, & Wang, 2004); however, the study did not examine the influence of comorbidity on self-reported psychopathology; these symptoms may have been related to comorbid conditions such as OCD or ADHD rather than tic severity alone.

In addition to depression and anxiety, adults with TS appear to be at greater risk for schizotypal personality traits and schizotypal personality disorder (Cavanna, Robertson, & Critchley, 2007). Finally, episodic rage and problems with anger control sometimes are observed in children with TS, but these behaviors often are related to comorbid conditions, such as ADHD or oppositional defiant disorder (Budman, Rockmore, Stokes, & Sossin, 2003).

Summary

Numerous studies suggest that the neuropsychological deficits among children with TS are accounted for largely by comorbid conditions, as significant impairment across a range of neuropsychological constructs is much less likely for children with TS alone (Osmon & Smerz, 2005). Further, many children with TS score in the average range on neuropsychological measures or demonstrate only mild impairment. Below-average performance on neuropsychological measures has been associated with later age at onset and greater complex tic severity (Bornstein, 1990); greater severity of tics also has been associated with poorer psychosocial functioning (Brand et al., 2002). Thus, it appears that the likelihood of significant neuropsychological impairment increases as does the number of comorbid conditions or symptoms, and other variables such as tic severity may be predictive of neuropsychological and psychosocial problems. Future studies, in which children with TS alone are examined separately from children with ADHD, OCD, and other comorbid conditions, will shed light on which areas of neuropsychological deficit are related to TS and which are better accounted for by comorbid diagnoses.

Assessment Process

Assessment of TS seems straightforward, given the *DSM* criteria necessary for diagnosis. However, assessment is complicated by comorbidity and the need to differentiate TS from other psychiatric, neuropsychological, and medical disorders that feature motor or vocal tic behaviors (Jankovic, 2001; Phelps, 2008). The assessment process should focus on identifying comorbid conditions, strengths and weaknesses, and functional implications of TS in the school setting in order to inform intervention development, as interventions will vary based on comorbidity and unique neuropsychological profile (A. S. Davis & Phelps, 2008; Osmon & Smerz, 2005). For example, comorbid ADHD and/or OCD (or other disorders) certainly will have implications for psychosocial and pharmacological interventions (Mansueto & Keuler, 2005; Robertson, 2006a). Thus, in addition to gathering specific information (e.g., type, frequency, environmental antecedents) about the tics themselves, the assessment should consider a range of comorbid symptoms (e.g., hyperactivity, impulsivity, inattention, obsessions), neuropsychological constructs (e.g., executive function, visual-motor skills), learning difficulties, and possible social and emotional sequelae related to the tics (Burd et al., 2005; Lewandowski, 2005; Osmon & Smerz, 2005; Phelps, 2008). The assessment process also should consider how the child's tics impact functioning across educational, social, and home settings, including the potential for embarrassment and teasing or peer rejection due to tics (Gilbert, 2006; Leckman, 2002). Taking all of these pieces of data into account will help the clinician identify multiple potential areas of deficit and therefore targets for intervention programs.

In addition to omnibus rating scales used to assess multiple emotional and behavioral symptoms (e.g., Behavior Assessment System for Children—Second Edition, Child Behavior Checklist), Phelps (2008) described several measures specifically designed to provide information about tics. These scales include the Yale Global Tic Severity Scale (Leckman et al., 1989; Storch et al., 2005), Shapiro Tourette's Syndrome Severity Scale (Shapiro & Shapiro, 1984), and Tourette's Syndrome Global Scale (Harcherik, Leckman, Detlor, & Cohen, 1984). A more recently developed TS scale is the Tourette Syndrome Diagnostic Confidence Index (Robertson et al., 1999), which assesses lifetime likelihood of ever having TS. These scales may help the clinician organize information about the type, history, intensity, frequency, and antecedents of tics. It also has been recommended that clinicians monitor the tics over several months in order to determine fluctuations in frequency and severity and to assess the impact of the tics on the child's and family's adjustment (Swain et al., 2007). Functional behavior assessment also can play an important role in identifying the environmental (e.g., classroom) antecedents and consequences of tic behaviors, which may identify potential targets for classroom interventions (Watson, Dufrene, Weaver, Butler, & Meeks, 2005).

School-based practitioners play an important role in assessing the child's progress after pharmacological and/or psychosocial interventions have been implemented, as these practitioners have access to data regarding the child's functioning in the school setting. Thus, for school-based practitioners, the assessment process may include gathering baseline data on tics and other symptoms of concern in order to facilitate these pre-post comparisons (Walter & Carter, 1997).

EVIDENCE-BASED INTERVENTIONS

Evidence-based interventions for TS may be categorized into pharmacological and psychosocial approaches. Currently there is greater empirical support for pharmacological approaches, as these appear to be the most commonly used interventions for TS (Carr & Chong, 2005; C. R. Cook & Blacher, 2007), although evidence is starting to accumulate for psychosocial interventions, such as habit reversal training and response prevention. The current status of evidence-based interventions is summarized in Table 7.2. Whether

Table 7.2 Evidence-Based Status of Interventions for TS

Interventions	Target	Status
Typical antipsychotic medications (e.g., haloperidol [Haldol], pimozide [Orap])	Motor and vocal tics	Positive practice (Robertson, 2000; Swain et al., 2007)
Risperidone (Risperdal; atypical antipsychotic medication)	Motor and vocal tics	Positive practice (Robertson, 2000; Swain et al., 2007)
Ziprasidone (Geodon; atypical antipsychotic medication)	Motor and vocal tics	Promising practice (Robertson, 2000; Swain et al., 2007)
Alpha-adrenergic agents (e.g., clonidine [Catapres] and guanfacine [Tenex])	Motor and vocal tics, impulsivity, hyperactivity, comorbid ADHD	Promising practice (Gaffney et al., 2002; Robertson, 2000; Scahill et al., 2001; Swain et al., 2007; Tourette's Syndrome Study Group, 2002)
Metoclopramide [Reglan]	Motor and vocal tics	Emerging practice (R. Nicolson, Craven-Thuss, Smith, McKinlay, & Castellanos, 2005)
Selective serotonin reuptake inhibitors (e.g., fluoxetine [Prozac], sertraline [Zoloft], paroxetine [Paxil])	Compulsive behaviors (TS with comorbid OCD and/or depression symptoms)	Promising practice (Pediatric OCD Treatment Study Team, 2004; Robertson, 2000)
Tricyclic antidepressants (e.g., desipramine [Norpramine], imipramine [Tofranil])	Symptoms of depression, ADHD, and OCD among children with TS	Emerging practice (Robertson, 2000)
Habit reversal training	Motor and vocal tics	Promising practice (Carr & Chong, 2005; Himle et al., 2006; Swain et al., 2007)
Response prevention	Motor and vocal tics	Emerging practice (C. R. Cook & Blacher, 2007; Verdellen et al., 2004)

pharmacological or psychosocial interventions (or a combination of treatments) are used, the treatment approach should:

- Be carefully designed to address specific areas of functional impairment for the individual child.
- Address comorbid symptoms identified during the assessment process.
- Build capacity for coping skills and social support that may serve as protective factors and reduce the impact of tics on the child's overall functioning (B. S. Peterson & Cohen, 1998).

The assessment process should inform intervention planning, as children with TS represent a heterogeneous group who require individualized approaches based on severity of TS, comorbid diagnoses, and impact on academic and social functioning.

Pharmacological Interventions

Many different medications have been investigated in the treatment of TS (Jimenez-Jimenez & Garcia-Ruiz, 2001), and investigations of different pharmacological agents are ongoing. Antipsychotic medications have been studied extensively with TS and appear to be effective by blocking dopamine receptors to decrease dopaminergic transmission from the substantia nigra to the basal ganglia (Phelps, 2008; Swain et al., 2007). For example, haloperidol (Haldol) is one of the most commonly used medications in the treatment of TS. While it is recognized as an established treatment, it also produces adverse side effects that may compromise treatment compliance (Robertson, 2000). Other typical antipsychotics that have demonstrated efficacy in the treatment of TS include pimozide (Orap), substituted benzamides, and sulpiride (Robertson, 2000). Atypical antipsychotic medications such as risperidone (Risperdal) and ziprasidone (Geodon) also have been investigated; an advantage of these medications is that they produce fewer extrapyramidal side effects, such as muscular rigidity and tremor, than the typical antipsychotics while showing similar levels of efficacy (Bruggeman et al., 2001; Gilbert, Batterson, Sethuraman, & Sallee, 2004; Phelps, 2008; Sallee et al., 2000). The atypical antipsychotics act on serotonin and dopamine receptors; involvement of serotonin may serve to prevent the adverse side effects of the typical antipsychotics (Swain et al., 2007). Much less is known about the medication metoclopramide (Reglan), but initial evidence suggests it was effective at reducing tics (R. Nicolson, Craven-Thuss, Smith, McKinlay, & Castellanos, 2005).

Several researchers have noted that when the child has comorbid conditions such as ADHD, OCD, or depression, often the initial target for treatment of TS should be the comorbid conditions, as these coexisting conditions likely contribute more to psychological and social impairment than TS, and often treatment of these conditions reduces the severity of tics (Gilbert, 2006; Roessner et al., 2007; Swain et al., 2007). The most effective pharmacological treatment for comorbid TS and OCD or depression may be a SSRI combined with a dopamine antagonist such as haloperidol or pimozide (Bystritsky et al., 2004; Denys, de Geus, van Megen, & Westenberg, 2004; Eapen & Robertson, 2000; Robertson, 2000). Clonidine (Catapres) and guanfacine (Tenex) may be especially useful in the treatment of comorbid TS and ADHD due to their effect on symptoms of both disorders (Eapen & Robertson, 2000; Gaffney et al., 2002; Scahill, Chappell et al., 2001). Clonidine or guanfacine combined with methylphenidate (Ritalin, Concerta) may be indicated for children with comorbid TS and ADHD, as clonidine and guanfacine appear to be effective at reducing both tics and impulsive behaviors and methylphenidate seems to be most helpful for inattentive symptoms (Gaffney et al., 2002; Scahill, Chappell et al., 2001; Tourette's Syndrome Study Group, 2002). Stimulant medications such as methylphenidate, dextroamphetamine (Adderall, Dexedrine), and pemoline (Cylert) have been found to improve attention and hyperactivity problems among children with TS and comorbid ADHD, but stimulant medications may exacerbate tics among some children with TS (Robertson, 2000). Many children can tolerate these stimulant medications in low doses without long-term increases in tics (Jankovic, 2001; Jimenez-Jimenez & Garcia-Ruiz, 2001; Poncin, Sukhodolsky, McGuire, & Scahill, 2007; Robertson, 2006a), but children undergoing stimulant treatment should be closely monitored for worsening tics. Using atomoxetine (Strattera) for ADHD symptoms among children with comorbid TS and ADHD may be a preferable treatment approach because atomoxetine is a nonstimulant medication and therefore is less likely to exacerbate tics (Poncin et al., 2007; Spencer et al., 2008).

Some children with mild TS, in which symptoms do not significantly interfere with daily functioning, may not require pharmacological intervention (Gilbert, 2006; Poncin et al., 2007). For all children, severity of symptoms and likely benefit of medication should be weighed against the potential adverse effects of medication (Sandor, 2003). When evaluating the effectiveness of medications for tics, clinicians must keep in mind that tics often show natural variation in severity and frequency, and these natural patterns should be considered before concluding that a medication is effective or ineffective for a particular child (Leckman, 2003; Swain et al., 2007).

Psychosocial Interventions

As noted, tics often are preceded by physical sensations or feelings of anxiety, making it possible for the child to sense on oncoming tic (Jankovic, 2001). Habit reversal has been studied as a behavioral intervention to reduce tics and appears to be the most studied psychosocial intervention method for children with TS (Himle, Woods, Piacentini, & Walkup, 2006; Piacentini & Chang, 2005). This compensatory approach involves learning to detect oncoming tics (including physiological and environmental cues) and stopping them before they occur by performing a physically competing response (Phelps, 2008). Identifying environmental antecedents during the assessment process is important, as this information can be used to help the child understand what types of environmental stressors or settings may increase the likelihood of tics. Thus, habit reversal training involves five steps:

1. The child describes or defines the exact tic behaviors.
2. He or she increases awareness of environmental antecedents (e.g., learns to detect premonitory urges or situations that exacerbate tics).
3. He or she learns to detect the initial movements of the tics.
4. The child learns the process of relaxation training.
5. He or she also practices a competing physical behavior (e.g., contracting muscles) to use when an oncoming tic is detected, so that this behavior is completed instead of the tic until the urge has passed (Himle et al., 2006; Phelps, 2008; Piacentini & Chang, 2005).

Once the child has learned these steps, he or she practices the process in real-world settings and receives social support in the form of prompts and reinforcement for using the competing response, thereby facilitating generalizability of the learned skills

(Himle et al., 2006). Habit reversal training has been identified as a promising practice through numerous multiple-baseline single-subject studies, open clinical trials, and randomized controlled trials (Carr & Chong, 2005; Himle et al., 2006). The most recent comprehensive review concluded that habit reversal is a "well established" treatment for TS (C. R. Cook & Blacher, 2007). Additional controlled studies, however, are needed to firmly establish this practice with children (Swain et al., 2007). Further, most studies using habit reversal training were designed to treat motor tics as the outcome variable, so effectiveness with vocal tics is less established (Carr & Chong, 2005). Habit reversal training is thought to be effective through the self-monitoring component involved in increasing awareness of tics and by teaching a physically competing response that may serve the same function (i.e., satisfying the premonitory urge) as the tic behaviors (Himle et al., 2006).

As an example of one of the multiple-baseline studies on habit reversal training, M. A. Clarke, Bray, Kehle, and Truscott (2001) described the use of a habit reversal and self-modeling intervention with four children with TS. The habit reversal component involved sessions with the school psychologist in which each child operationally defined and identified his or her tics, identified environmental variables surrounding the tics, and practiced competing responses that were incompatible with the tics (e.g., tensing neck muscles instead of head jerking, pressing arms tightly against the body instead of shoulder jerking, deep breathing through the mouth instead of sniffing or vocal tics). The self-monitoring component involved the subjects observing themselves exhibiting tic-free behaviors in the classroom on videotape, in order to promote observational learning and self-efficacy. At 5- to 10-week follow-up, three children showed significant decreases in tics while the fourth demonstrated moderate decreases (M. A. Clarke et al., 2001). This study is particularly notable because it demonstrates the implementation of habit reversal training in the school setting, thereby supporting the use of this intervention beyond the clinic setting.

Response prevention is an emerging practice that involves prolonged exposure to the conditions that typically precede tics (including premonitory urges or sensations) while physically suppressing the tics, thereby preventing the behavioral response due to habituation to the premonitory urges (Phelps, 2008; Verdellen, Keijsers, Cath, & Hoogduin, 2004). The response prevention process is facilitated by clinicians who help the child monitor tics and provide encouragement for them to suppress tics. Cook and Blacher (2007) identified response prevention as a promising practice; initial research suggests it was as effective as habit reversal in reducing tics among children and adults with TS, and this intervention has been effective for children with OCD (Pediatric OCD Treatment Study Team, 2004; Verdellen et al., 2004). However, more research is necessary to establish the effectiveness of this method with children and adolescents with TS, as very few studies have been conducted at this time.

Cook and Blacher (2007) also reviewed the evidence base for self-monitoring, contingency management, massed negative practice (i.e., over-rehearsal), and cognitive-behavioral interventions for reducing tics and concluded that these interventions do not meet evidence-based criteria primarily due to a lack of research and methodological limitations of the few existing studies. Thus, additional research may either support or not support the inclusion of these approaches in the collection of evidence-based or promising treatments for TS.

Numerous educational and classroom accommodations have been advocated in the treatment of TS, such as preferential seating, individual testing, extra time for tests, reduced work, provision of visual cues, breaking large tasks into smaller steps, and modified assignments (Lewandowski, 2005). Survey data suggest that frequently employed accommodations for children with TS in the school setting include allowing the student to leave the room, providing extended time for assignments and tests, preferential seating in the classroom, individual testing, providing a word processor, and reducing homework (note that many of these accommodations are related to difficulties with handwriting and inattention; Packer, 2005). Psychoeducational approaches (i.e., educating the family, teachers, and child about TS) and supportive psychotherapy to address issues such as coping skills, self-esteem, and social stress that may accompany TS also have been advocated in the literature (Jankovic, 2001; Leckman, 2002; B. S. Peterson & Cohen, 1998; Swain et al., 2007); however, classroom modifications, psychoeducational approaches, and psychotherapy have not been studied systematically among child TS populations. There is some evidence that simple behavioral methods such as positive reinforcement for tic-free periods of time, have been effective and that publicly commenting on the child's tics or drawing additional attention to the child may increase anxiety, which in turn may increase tics (Conelea & Woods, 2008b). In all, the field is in need of additional research on evidence-based behavioral interventions for TS (Phelps, 2008).

CASE STUDY: MOSES—TOURETTE SYNDROME

The next report is from a hospital-based clinic. Identifying information, such as child and family name, teacher or physician name, and school information, has been altered or fictionalized to protect confidentiality.

Reason for Referral

Moses is an adolescent aged 15 years 11 months who is being initially evaluated by the pediatric neuropsychology service at the request of his pediatric neurologist (Dr. Elliott), who has been following Moses for a history of Tourette syndrome and academic difficulty. At present, Moses is taking clonidine .05 mg three times per day (t.i.d.) in order to help in the management of his vocal and motor tics. Due to increasing academic difficulty during the current tenth-grade school year, Dr. Elliott requested neuropsychological evaluation in order to assess higher cortical functioning and make appropriate recommendations regarding school placement and the need for supportive therapies.

Assessment Procedures

Wechsler Intelligence Scale for Children, Fourth Edition (WISC-IV)
Wisconsin Card Sorting Test (WCST)
Peabody Picture Vocabulary Test, Fourth Edition (PPVT-IV)
Clinical Evaluation of Language Function, Fourth Edition (CELF-IV)
Boston Naming Test (BNT)
Delis-Kaplan Executive Function System (D-KEFS)
Judgment of Line Orientation Test (JLO)
Developmental Test of Visual-Motor Integration, Fifth Edition (DTVMI-V)
Rey Complex Figure Copying Task (RCF)
Clock Face Drawing Test

Finger Oscillation Test
Test of Variables of Attention (TOVA)
Children's Memory Scale (CMS)
Wechsler Individual Achievement Test, Second Edition (WIAT-II)
Gray Oral Reading Test, Fourth Edition (GORT-4)
Test of Written Language, Third Edition (TOWL-3)
Behavior Assessment System for Children, Second Edition (BASC-2)
DSM-IV ADHD Checklist

Background Information

Home

Moses resides with his parents and his 12-year-old brother who is an A/B student in the seventh grade and in good health. Moses's father is 46 years of age, a college graduate, currently employed as a manager for an insurance company. He is in good physical health; however, he does report experiencing panic attacks. The paternal family history is negative for neurological disorder including mental retardation. Moses's mother is 40 years of age, a high school graduate with two years of college coursework who is currently employed as a data processing clerk. She too is in good physical health. The maternal family history is also negative for neurologic disorder including mental retardation.

Medical

Review of developmental and medical history indicates that Moses is the product of a normal 36-week gestation pregnancy and vaginal delivery weighing 9 pounds 14 ounces at birth. He did well as a newborn and went home with his mother from the hospital on schedule. Moses attained his developmental motor milestones within normal limits with sitting up occurring at 5 months of age and walking at 10 months of age. Language development also was felt to be normal, with first words coming at 12 months of age, two-word phrases at 15 months of age, and short sentences at 18 months of age. Toilet training was accomplished at 30 months without difficulty. Aside from the usual childhood illnesses, Moses's past medical history is essentially unremarkable with the exception of the Tourette syndrome. Moses's parents report that he always has been immature and poorly organized with poor penmanship skills. Attention span has not been a major problem until this school year.

Educational

Throughout Moses's elementary school years, which were divided between public and private schools, Moses was generally an A/B student. Moses first began exhibiting motor and vocal tics during the autumn of seventh grade (12 years of age). At that time he was attending private school, where he was generally characterized as a C student. During the beginning of the school year, Moses's parents noticed eye blinking and unusual head movements and some soft swallowing or coughing noises. Moses was referred by his pediatrician to Dr. Elliott, a neurologist, who felt that Moses might have mild Tourette syndrome. Since the symptoms were not causing any major problems, medication was not prescribed; however, the tics gradually worsened over time, and Dr. Elliott prescribed clonidine, which appeared to be helpful in controlling the tics. Unfortunately, Moses reported that the medicine made him tired; as a result, it was discontinued towards the end of the seventh-grade year. Moses continued to attend private school for the eighth grade, making Cs and Bs without medication. In August, Dr. Elliott wrote a letter advising the school system of Moses's condition and that the tics could be aggravated by anxiety or stress. He requested that this be taken into consideration during the school year. During the ninth grade, which Moses also spent in private school, his parents reported that he did take clonidine "off and on" during the school year, making Cs and Bs.

During the summer after ninth grade, Moses was invited to participate on a traveling baseball team and encouraged by the public high school baseball coach to attend the high school for tenth grade so that he could play on the baseball team and receive more exposure. Moses elected to make the switch and began attending tenth grade at the local high school. With the increasing stress of playing competitive baseball during the summer in conjunction with the school change, Moses's vocal tics became more frequent and he began to exhibit facial twitching. According to his parents, Moses made As and Bs during the first four weeks of school; however, by the nine-week grading period, his grades began to drop primarily in math (Algebra I), science, and his forestry elective. As a result, Moses's parents initiated tutoring in math three evenings a week at home. Even with the tutoring, Moses earned a failing semester grade in Algebra I and the forestry elective. Due to the increased frequency of the vocal tics, which was causing problems for some of his classroom teachers, Moses was reevaluated by Dr. Elliott. At that time, Dr. Elliott increased the clonidine to .05 mg in the morning and .1 mg at night. In addition, he wrote another letter to the school requesting that Moses be placed within the "Other Health Impaired" special education program so that he could receive modifications in instruction and testing. With the increased dosage of clonidine, Moses began falling asleep at school. As a result, the medication dosing was changed to .05 mg. t.i.d. During the Christmas break, Moses's parents reported that he began to experience evidence of coprolalia (uncontrolled use of obscene language as part of a vocal tic).

Prior to the beginning of the second semester of ninth grade, Moses's father met with the principal and requested that Moses be considered for a 504 plan so that he could begin receiving classroom modifications. In addition, he alerted the principal to the coprolalia that Moses was exhibiting. With the beginning of the second semester, Moses was allowed to retake his forestry elective examination, which he passed. Further, he was dropped from Algebra I; however, he continued to meet with his tutor so that he could retake the first-semester examination and receive credit for that half of the course. In January, a student support team meeting was convened and several accommodations were put into place, including:

- Providing an alternate testing environment when Moses requests this (media center)
- The use of an assignment sheet or notebook initialed by his teachers
- Preferential seating
- Additional time for tests as needed
- Modified semester exams (reduce overall test items by one-quarter to one-half)

In March, Moses's father reported in a phone conversation that Moses's grades continued to be poor, particularly in classes in which his parents were not informed of his assignments in the event that Moses forgets. Additionally, at this time, Moses's tics were worsening, often consisting of coprolalia. Moses's level of school-related frustration had increased as well. As a result, Moses saw Dr. Elliott in order to try to better control his vocal and motor tics. Dr. Elliott switched his medication from clonidine to haloperidol (Haldol). A phone conversation with Moses's father in April revealed that after the medication change, Moses's tics dramatically decreased.

Behavioral Observations

Moses presented himself for testing as a pleasant, neatly groomed teen who was in no apparent physical distress aside from his frequent tics. The tics were evident throughout the day, but they were worse when beginning testing in the morning, as his anxiety was likely the highest at this time. His tics consisted of loud vocal outbursts, facial grimaces, hand jerks, echolalia, coprolalia (once), lip smacking, and light coughing. Moses separated appropriately from his parents and accompanied the examiner to the testing room without difficulty. He was oriented and related appropriately toward this examiner throughout the evaluation, which consisted of two sessions separated by a lunch break. In response to direct questions, as well as when conversation was spontaneous, Moses's use of language was fluent and prosodic. Moses's attention span, activity level, and impulsivity within the context of this one-to-one assessment were mostly age appropriate. It was noted that Moses was very drowsy at times during testing, likely due to medication side effects. On more challenging tasks, Moses responded to frustration with good sustained effort. Lateral dominance is firmly established in the right hand and foot. Moses's fine motor skills, including handwriting and drawing, were poor. Vision was not formally screened; however, his parents reported that this has been evaluated in the past and reported as requiring correction for nearsightedness. It should be noted that Moses did not wear his corrective lenses during this assessment. Hearing was not formally assessed but appeared to be adequate for this evaluation. Due to his frequent tics throughout testing, the results may be an underestimate of his potential, but the testing appears to be reflective of his current level of functioning.

Assessment Results and Interpretation

Intellectual functioning as measured by the Wechsler Intelligence Scale for Children, Fourth Edition (WISC-IV) is found to be in the low-average range. Specifically, Moses obtained a Full Scale IQ of 83 (Average Score = 100 + 15; 95% confidence interval = 79–88). Analysis of Index scores indicates that Moses's understanding of verbal material is in the low-average to average range and his visual-perceptual skills are lower, in the borderline to low-average range (Verbal Comprehension Index = 87, Perceptual Reasoning Index = 84). His processing speed is in the borderline to low-average range as well, and Moses's working memory/focused attention is higher, in the low-average to average range (Processing Speed Index = 83, Working Memory Index = 94). Additionally, Moses's Verbal Comprehension Index may be a slight underestimate of his true verbal ability, due to his frequent tics in the beginning of testing, which may have lowered his scores on the first few subtests. Individual subtest scores are presented in the Psychometric Summary in Table 7.3.

In order to assess higher-order executive functions, Moses was administered the Wisconsin Card Sorting Test. This instrument required him to sort cards according to rules he had to determine based on examiner feedback as to the correctness of the response. This test provides information about problem-solving skills and mental flexibility. On this measure, Moses was able to obtain 6 out of a possible 6 categories. This level

Table 7.3 Psychometric Summary for Moses

	Scaled Score	Standard Score
Wechsler Intelligence Scale for Children, Fourth Edition (WISC-IV)		
Full Scale IQ		83
Verbal Comprehension Index		87
Similarities	5	
Vocabulary	9	
Comprehension	9	
Perceptual Reasoning Index		84
Block Design	8	
Picture Concepts	6	
Matrix Reasoning	8	
Working Memory Index		94
Digit Span	10	
Letter-Number Sequencing	8	
Processing Speed Index		83
Coding	4	
Symbol Search	10	
Wisconsin Card Sorting Test (WCST)		
Categories Achieved		106
Perseverative Errors		112
Failures to Maintain Set		108
Peabody Picture Vocabulary Test, Fourth Edition (PPVT-IV)		87
Clinical Evaluation of Language Function, Fourth Edition (CELF-IV)		
Sentence Imitation		105
Concepts and Directions		75
Formulated Sentences		85
Boston Naming Test (BNT)		73
Delis-Kaplan Executive Function System (D-KEFS)		
Verbal Fluency Test		75
Judgment of Line Orientation Test (JLO)		87
Developmental Test of Visual-Motor Integration—Fifth Edition (DTVMI-V)		77
Rey Complex Figure Copying Task		97
Clock Face Drawing Test		
Form		75
Time		106
Finger Oscillation Test		
Right (dominant) Hand		120
Left (nondominant) Hand		121
Test of Variables of Attention (TOVA)		
Omission Errors		98
Commission Errors		108
Response Time		96
Variability		88
Children's Memory Scale (CMS)		
General Memory Index		67

(continued)

Table 7.3 *(Continued)*

	Scaled Score	Standard Score
Attention/Concentration Index		91
Numbers		100
Sequences		85
Picture Locations		90
Verbal Immediate Index		69
Stories		95
Word Pairs		55
Visual Immediate Index		82
Dot Locations		75
Faces		95
Verbal Delayed Index		72
Stories		95
Word Pairs		60
Visual Delayed Index		85
Dot Locations		75
Faces		100
Delayed Recognition Index		60
Stories		80
Word Pairs		55
Learning Index		63
Word Pairs		55
Dot Locations		85
Wechsler Individual Achievement Test, Second Edition (WIAT-II)		
Word Reading		104
Pseudoword Decoding		105
Spelling		105
Mathematical Reasoning		77
Numerical Operations		100
Gray Oral Reading Test, Fourth Edition (GORT-4)		
Fluency		85
Rate		85
Accuracy		100
Comprehension		80
Test of Written Language, Third Edition (TOWL-3)		
Written Language Quotient		87
Contextual Conventions		90
Contextual Language		80
Story Construction		100
Behavior Assessment System for Children, Second Edition (BASC-II)		
	T-Scores	
	Parent	Teacher
Clinical Scales		
Hyperactivity	37	52
Aggression	42	41
Conduct Problems	43	43
Anxiety	42	43

Table 7.3 *(Continued)*

	T-Scores	
	Parent	Teacher
Depression	42	49
Somatization	42	49
Atypicality	39	48
Withdrawal	37	39
Attention Problems	68	64
Learning Problems	NA	53
Adaptive Scales		
Adaptability	49	54
Social Skills	52	44
Leadership	46	46
Study Skills	NA	42
Activities of Daily Living	58	NA
Functional Communication	49	42
DSM-IV ADHD Checklist	**Raw Score**	
Inattention	21/27	21/27
Hyperactivity/Impulsivity	8/27	16/27

Note. NA = Not applicable.

of performance is significantly higher than what one would expect based on the current estimate of Moses's intellectual potential. Further, no significant evidence of perseveration (repeated incorrect responding) or failure to maintain mental set (off-task behavior) was noted. Moses scored in the average/high-average range on this task, indicating well-developed problem-solving skills.

Assessment of linguistic functioning was conducted in order to evaluate receptive and expressive language development. Analysis of his performance indicates that Moses's receptive language is variable. Specifically, his understanding of vocabulary words is low average and his repetition of sentences is average; however, Moses struggled on a task requiring understanding of complex multipart directions, scoring in the borderline range. Analysis of Moses's expressive language development indicates that these skills are also variable. In particular, his skills at defining words are average, and his linguistic planning (formulating sentences) is low average. However, he exhibited a word finding/retrieval deficit, as he scored in the borderline range on measures of picture naming and verbal fluency (quickly naming words beginning with a certain letter) tasks. In sum, Moses's language skills range from borderline to average, with poor word retrieval and complex comprehension skills, but these abilities are generally consistent with his verbal intellectual ability.

In order to assess visual spatial perception/discrimination ability without a motor component, Moses was administered the Judgment of Line Orientation Test (JLO). Analysis of his performance indicates that his visual perceptual functioning is in the low-average range. Constructional praxis, as measured by the Developmental Test of Visual-Motor Integration (DTVMI-V), the Rey Complex Figure (RCF) copying task, and a Clock Face Drawing with the requested time of 10:20 is found to be variable, ranging from borderline to average. Notably, Moses's drawings were marked by motor planning difficulties, which lowered his scores on several tasks. These results, taken together with Moses's low-average to average performance on the Block Design subtest of the WISC-IV, indicate that his visual spatial/constructional functioning is adequate but marked by poor motor planning and fine motor difficulties when constructing with paper and pencil. Fine motor finger oscillation as measured by a manual finger tapper is found to be above normal age level expectancy bilaterally; right (dominant) hand = 51.3 taps per 10 seconds, left (non-dominant) hand = 48.3 taps per 10 seconds.

Assessment of attention/level of concentration was carried out using the Test of Variables of Attention (TOVA). On this task, Moses was required to sustain attention for a period of 20 minutes during which he was requested to respond to target stimuli only. Analysis of Moses's performance indicates that he demonstrated average ability to sustain attention without significant evidence of impulsivity. Moses scored much lower during the first 10 minutes of the task than he did on the last 10 minutes, which is not the typical pattern of an individual with an attention deficit. Rather, it seems that Moses takes a little longer than most to settle down and concentrate on a task, but once he does this, his attention span is adequate. Further, Moses demonstrated an average reaction time in general without significant variability.

In order to assess learning and memory, Moses was administered the Children's Memory Scale (CMS). Analysis of Moses's performance on the subtests comprising the Attention/Concentration Index indicates that he is exhibiting focused attention/working memory skills that are in the low-average to average range commensurate with the average TOVA results and with his cognitive ability. Thus, Moses's ability to focus attention and hold material in working memory did not adversely affect his capability to learn and remember new material.

Comparison of Moses's mildly deficient General Memory Index (GMI = 67) with his best estimate of intellectual potential indicates that his ability to learn and remember is significantly below expectancy. However, more detailed analysis of Moses's performance indicates that he is demonstrating significant variability in his ability to learn and remember new material. Comparison of his auditory/verbal and visual/nonverbal index scores with his intellectual functioning as well as with each other indicates that Moses's overall visual memory is in the low-average range while his verbal memory is much lower, in the mildly deficient to borderline range. Within the visual subtests, Moses recalled visual content that is meaningful (pictures of faces) in the average range both immediately after presentation and after a 30-minute delay, while he struggled to recall a pattern of dots (spatial location), scoring in the borderline range on this task. Verbally, Moses demonstrated well-developed memory skills for organized, meaningful material, scoring in the average range when required to recall two stories that were read to him. In contrast, when required to learn and remember rote, unorganized material (a list of word pairs presented over three trials), Moses had extraordinary difficulty, scoring in the deficient range. Further, analysis of the learning trials indicates that Moses is very slow and inefficient when learning unorganized verbal material. In sum, Moses's learning and memory skills are quite variable, with a well-developed ability to learn and recall organized material contrasted by extreme difficulty learning and recalling rote, nonmeaningful material. This variability appears to be due to an inability to organize and encode material into memory and likely will translate into variability in his classroom and test-taking performance.

Academic Functioning

To assess Moses's reading and spelling skills, he was administered the Word Reading, Pseudoword Decoding, and Spelling subtests of the Wechsler Individual Achievement

Test, Second Edition (WIAT-II). On these subtests, he demonstrated average basic sight word knowledge, phonetic word attack skills, and spelling skills. As these tests measure reading recognition as opposed to reading comprehension, Moses was also administered the Gray Oral Reading Test, Fourth Edition (GORT-4). On this instrument, he was required to read stories aloud and then respond to multiple-choice questions related to the story content. The Fluency score assesses both reading speed and accuracy while the Comprehension score assesses understanding of what is read. Moses's reading rate and comprehension are both in the low-average range. However, his decoding accuracy is higher, in the average range.

In order to assess written expression, Moses was administered the Test of Written Language, Third Edition. On this instrument, he was required to write a story about a picture of a futuristic space scene. The story was then evaluated for development of a theme, vocabulary usage, punctuation and capitalization, style, spelling, and syntax. Moses's overall written expression score is in the low-average range. The content of Moses's story was well developed, in the average range, while his grammar and mechanics (use of punctuation, capitalization, etc.) were lower, in the low-average range.

Moses was also administered the math subtests of the WIAT-II. The Mathematical Reasoning subtest assesses the child's knowledge of concepts and ability to solve word problems while the Numerical Operations subtest assesses the child's computational abilities. Moses's math reasoning ability is low, in the borderline range, while his calculation skills are much higher, in the average range. Qualitatively, he was very slow to answer the questions on the Math Reasoning subtest.

Moses and his parents also completed a study skills questionnaire, in which they rated Moses's study habits and organizational skills. Analysis of this questionnaire indicates that Moses's study skills are fairly well developed. Areas that need improvement include note taking in class, organizing these notes in a notebook, double checking/proofreading work, and making to-do lists so he will not forget things.

Thus, academically, Moses demonstrates relative strengths in the areas of basic reading decoding, spelling, and mathematics calculation contrasted by relative weaknesses in the areas of reading rate/fluency, reading comprehension, mathematics reasoning, and written expression.

Social-Emotional and Behavioral Functioning

In order to assess behavioral/emotional functioning, the Behavior Assessment System for Children (BASC-II) and a behavior rating scale that reflects items related to the *DSM-IV* criteria for ADHD were completed by Moses's parents and one of his teachers. Analysis of the behavior rating scale data indicates that Moses is doing well in most areas assessed. However, his parents and his teacher rated him as somewhat more inattentive than most other children his age.

Summary and Diagnostic Impressions

In summary, the results of neuropsychological evaluation indicate that Moses currently is functioning within the low-average range of verbal intellectual ability. Additional assessment indicates that Moses demonstrates relative strengths in areas of nonverbal problem solving, most areas of receptive and expressive language, sustained attention, focused attention/working memory, and verbal and visual memory for organized and/or meaningful material. These strengths are contrasted by relative weaknesses in word finding/retrieval, complex comprehension skills, visual-motor/constructional skills involving motor planning, and learning/encoding of verbal and visual rote/unorganized material. Academically, Moses demonstrates relative strengths in basic reading decoding, spelling, and mathematics calculation contrasted by relative weaknesses in the areas of reading rate/fluency, reading comprehension, mathematics reasoning, and written expression. Organizational difficulties were reported during the parent interview and also on a study skills questionnaire. Behaviorally, Moses is well adjusted in most areas, although his parents and his teacher rated him as mildly inattentive. Moses's inattention does not appear to be due to an attention deficit disorder but likely results from the mental effort required to suppress his tics, taking away from his attention to tasks, and also due to side effects of his medication, particularly fatigue.

Taken together, this pattern of neuropsychological test performance is consistent with a diagnosis of Tourette syndrome in conjunction with mild executive functioning deficits and associated learning difficulties, particularly in the areas of mathematical reasoning, and poor handwriting/graphomotor skills. This pattern of weaknesses corresponds to the research findings frequently reported in students with Tourette syndrome and appears to be significantly impacting on Moses's educational performance. The disruptive nature of his tics, which affects his concentration on the task at hand, decreased attention due to tic suppression, and fatigue partially due to medication side effects further add to Moses's frustration and academic stress.

Recommendations

- It is recommended that Moses continue in his current 10th grade placement. Due to his increasing academic difficulties, Moses should be serviced within a special education resource/consultation setting designed for students with learning disabilities under the eligibility category of "Other Health Impaired" due to his Tourette syndrome, should his parents elect to continue placement within the public school system. Similar programs may be offered by the private schools in the area. Moses should attend the resource classroom during the last period of each day so that this placement is minimally intrusive to him. Resource services should focus on development of organizational and study skills, as described later in this section, including checking Moses's assignment book and notebooks to ensure that he has and understands homework assignments. Additionally, resource placement should focus on improving Moses's mathematics reasoning skills. The resource teacher could also help to keep his parents informed of his progress (daily or weekly progress reports), as well as facilitate communication between Moses's parents and his other teachers.
- Occupational therapy consultative services should be considered given Moses's poor handwriting, which affects his school performance.
- Behavioral considerations for Moses's tics include allowing him to leave class with permission when under high stress, giving him breaks to express tics (e.g., leaving class to get water, go to the bathroom), or going to the counselor's office when he feels a tic outburst or worsening of his tics. Just knowing that these options are available may reduce Moses's anxiety and thus decrease the severity of his tics. His teachers should be instructed with regard to Tourette syndrome and associated

learning and behavior difficulties, so that their reactions to Moses's behavior do not aggravate the situation.

- Formal study skills training will be warranted emphasizing such techniques as the appropriate outlining of lecture notes and how to study for tests. This training should be incorporated into Moses's resource time at school. A private tutor also could work with Moses to teach and improve these skills. He also will benefit from being taught how to take notes on text material and plan written reports using an outlining method. The resource teacher should teach Moses learning/memory strategies (memory devices) to help make unorganized material more meaningful. Moses also may require instruction on how to organize and plan his approach to novel tasks. This is particularly true for subject matter in which he is weaker, such as math and written expression. He also should be encouraged to double-check and proofread his work to avoid careless mistakes. In addition, direct instruction in basic organizational strategies will assist Moses in knowing what to do, when to do it, and how to do it. Specifically, he should be guided in the use of checklists and other organizational aids, such as a daily planner/assignment book. Additionally, teachers and tutors should help Moses to organize his notes within a notebook, and he should be instructed to keep a specific place for his homework. With help from teachers and parents, ideally he will plan each day of the week, including time after school. Finally, Moses should be provided with frequent review of previously learned as well as newly learned material in order to maximize learning and retention.
- Accommodations will be necessary to enhance Moses's ability to succeed in the classroom and should be included as part of his Individualized Education Plan. These accommodations should include preferential seating away from distracting stimuli. However, preferential seating should not be "front and center" in the classroom, where his tics would be noticed easily by the entire class. Instead, seating could be in the front and to the side of the classroom. As mentioned previously, correctly using his assignment book will be a very important modification, given his difficulties with organization and remembering assignments. Given his learning difficulties related to Tourette syndrome, a reduction in the amount, but not the difficulty level, of assignments may assist Moses in completing classroom tasks and homework in a timely manner. Moreover, whenever possible, he should be given additional time to complete assignments. Because of his poor handwriting and writing skills, tests should be in multiple choice/matching format instead of essay/short-answer format; additional time should be provided when necessary (in a resource room or counselor's office). Due to his poor graphomotor skills and motor tics that disrupt writing, Moses should not be required to produce handwritten work, such as copying material from the board or recording lecture notes. Instead, he should be provided with typed copies of teacher's notes or have a responsible student take notes on carbon paper so that Moses can have a copy of the student's notes. Finally, Moses should be allowed and encouraged to use various compensatory devices, such as a calculator and a computer with word processing capability.
- Moses would benefit from individual therapy to help him adjust to the frustrations of having Tourette syndrome as well as to aid with his current academic stress. Specifically, counseling should focus on reducing Moses's anxiety/stress along with enhancing his self-esteem and coping skills. Treatment also should

focus on relaxation training/stress management skills and may include behavioral interventions shown to be effective with children with Tourette syndrome, such as self-monitoring and habit reversal.

- Continued neurologic follow-up with Dr. Elliott is recommended.

Further Discussion of Case Study

The case of Moses illustrates several concepts discussed in this chapter. For example, Moses was first diagnosed with TS in early adolescence, and this was accompanied by increased problems in school, as appears to be typical (Leckman et al., 1998). Moses's specific neuropsychological profile indicated weaknesses in word finding/retrieval, verbal fluency, complex comprehension skills, visual-motor skills involving motor planning and handwriting, memory of unorganized material, organization, mathematics reasoning, and written expression. Consistent with research findings, Moses did not exhibit significant deficits in cognitive flexibility (as assessed with the WCST). Thus, although the research on neuropsychological functioning of children with TS has produced inconsistent results, Moses demonstrated some of the patterns identified in the literature. Because Moses did not appear to exhibit any comorbid diagnoses (which is rare among children with TS), it is hypothesized that his deficits in neuropsychological functioning are related to TS as opposed to ADHD, OCD, LD, or other comorbid conditions. This lack of comorbidity also probably accounts for the lack of significant deficits in most areas and normal emotional functioning, as Moses does not seem to have problems with social functioning or peer victimization, even though his tics are conspicuous and sometimes disruptive. Moses's case also demonstrates increasing frequency and severity of tics with stress. Finally, Moses illustrates one of the common difficulties of pharmacological treatment: Many of the medications are associated with adverse side effects. Moses used clonidine and Haldol at different times, both of which are common components of pharmacological treatment; however, the drowsiness caused by these medications was interfering with his performance in school.

Moses also illustrates the heterogeneity among children diagnosed with TS, as some of his symptoms and behaviors are inconsistent with what is often observed. For example, Moses exhibited coprolalia, even though this particular tic is thought to be relatively rare among children with TS (APA, 2000), and symptoms worsened as he got older instead of getting milder, which appears to be atypical of most children with TS (Leckman et al., 1998). Further, although Moses did show the VIQ > PIQ pattern often reported in the literature, the discrepancy was small.

CONCLUDING COMMENTS

Tourette syndrome represents one of the more complex childhood disorders, and one for which our current knowledge of neuropsychological functioning among children is limited. Research is especially limited by heterogeneous samples of individuals with TS, as many studies do not separate children with TS from adults with TS, thereby compromising our understanding of TS from a developmental perspective (Robertson & Baron-Cohen, 1996). Examining these groups separately may point to interventions that are particularly effective with children and adolescents (C. R. Cook & Blacher, 2007). Further, the TS phenotype is broadly defined, and research participants often are not grouped by presence of comorbid conditions, resulting in heterogeneity among TS subjects and inconsistent findings in studies of neuroanatomical differences and neuropsychological functioning (Scahill et al., 2001). Interestingly, in many studies, samples of TS plus some comorbid condition (most frequently ADHD or OCD) are larger than the TS-only group, suggesting that it is difficult to identify children with "pure" TS. At the same time, we must better account for the influence of comorbidity in studies of the etiology, treatment, and neuropsychological profiles of TS, as much of the social, behavioral, academic, and neuropsychological impairment observed among children with TS is likely the result of comorbid conditions, such as ADHD, OCD, and LD; more research is needed to show which deficits are related to TS alone (Robertson, 2000). Finally, the field is in need of more evaluation of long-term intervention effects, as many intervention studies have been short term.

Chapter 8

TRAUMATIC BRAIN INJURY

DEFINITION

Classification of Head Injuries

Head injuries or traumatic brain injuries (TBIs) are classified as either penetrating/open or closed head injuries (Zillmer, Spiers, & Culbertson, 2008). Penetrating head injury is said to occur when some object penetrates the skull and brain, as in the famous case of Phineas Gage (Macmillan, 2000) or as in a gunshot wound to the head. With a penetrating head injury, damage is a function of the location and the extent of the direct hit, including the path made in the process of the penetration and the amount of brain tissue damaged. With penetrating or open head injury there is also the potential for complications caused by infection and hemorrhage (Zillmer et al., 2008). In contrast, closed head injury is the result of a blow to the head (or the head impacting on a solid object) without penetration of the skull. With a closed head injury, the brain undergoes marked acceleration and/or deceleration (e.g., if you are moving quickly in a forward direction and run into a brick wall or if you are hit by a brick). This type of injury is more likely to result in diffuse injury and a wide range of neuropsychological deficits, because multiple areas of the brain are affected (Ewing-Cobbs, Barnes, & Fletcher, 2003). Physical effects occur at the point of impact (impact injury or coup) and/or its opposite pole (countercoup) due to the tearing and shearing of tissue with the "bouncing" action of the brain within the skull (Zillmer et al., 2008). Injuries that are most likely to result in this bouncing damage include motor vehicle accidents with whiplash or shaken baby syndrome. The bouncing can result in stretching, shearing, and tearing of tissue, including individual cells (most often in the frontal and temporal lobes) and diffuse axonal injury (M. P. Alexander, 1995). Diffuse injuries often lead to changes in the way neurotransmitters function in the brain, damage to axons and neurons, swelling and pressure, and microscopic lesions to and atrophy of the cerebral white matter (Ewing-Cobbs et al., 2003; Gennarelli, Thibault, & Graham, 1998). This type of damage limits the ability of neurons to transmit information, which in turn changes or limits the ability of different areas of the brain to communicate with one another (Joseph, 1996). Decreased activity of neurotransmitters (including dopamine, acetylcholine, and norepinephrine) has been found during the chronic phase of TBI (i.e., beginning roughly 24 hours postinjury), which follows a period of increased activity or excitation during the acute phase; this decreased activity during the chronic phase may be the cause of cognitive deficits (Kokiko & Hamm, 2007).

If the axon of a neuron is damaged, the axon may degenerate back to the cell body and result in cell death (retrograde degeneration). If the cell body (neuron) is damaged, this can result in degeneration of the axon or anterograde degeneration (Zillmer et al., 2008). Transneural degeneration occurs with the death of neurons that were innervated by damaged or destroyed neurons and are no longer being innervated. At the same time, this can lead to metabolic changes in the postsynaptic neuron and further cell death (a domino effect; Zillmer et al., 2008). In some cases, there may be new axonal sprouting that bypasses damaged areas; however, sometimes the new sprouting may form new connections that result in behavioral, emotional, or cognitive problems. Total brain volume also seems to decrease drastically immediately following TBI, followed by a more gradual and steady decrease in volume for approximately three years following TBI; these changes are indicative of rapid loss of neurons followed by a period of reorganization (Bigler, 1999). This loss of neurons, or changes in the way neurons function, is associated with cognitive deficits and changes in personality, emotion, and behavioral functioning (Royo, Shimizu, Schouten, Stover, & McIntosh, 2003). Areas of the brain most susceptible to injury include the frontal lobes, orbital gyri cortex, and inferior and lateral areas of the temporal lobes (Hanten et al., 2004). Damage to the frontal lobes often is associated with deficits in executive function and attention, while damage to the temporal lobes often results in deficits in learning and memory consolidation (Kehle, Clark, & Jenson, 1996; Levin, 1987).

Prevalence/Incidence

Researchers estimate that between 500,000 and 1.6 million people suffer TBIs in the United States every year; further, it is estimated that there are 20,000 children and adolescents per year who have persisting disabilities from TBIs (Ghajar, 2000; Ylvisaker et al., 2001). Causes of head injuries are motor vehicle accidents (MVAs), sports injury, falls, violence, and industrial accidents. Closed head (diffuse) injuries are more common among children than open head (focal) injuries (Ewing-Cobbs et al., 2003). Thus, among pediatric populations, more is known about the manifestation and outcomes of closed head injuries, which makes sense when we consider the differing causes of open and closed injuries.

For individuals under 45 years of age, head injuries cause more deaths and disabilities than any other neurological disorder (Bruns & Hauser, 2003). The highest incidence for TBI is between age 15 and 24 years, with males about two to four times more likely than females to sustain head injury (Thurman & Guerrero, 1999; Zillmer et al., 2008). Despite these statistics, it is estimated that only 0.2% of children in special education are classified as TBI (Ylvisaker et al., 2001). Under the Individuals with Disabilities Education Improvement Act (IDEIA), TBI is defined as an acquired injury to the brain that is caused by an external physical force and results in total or partial functional disability, or psychosocial impairment, or both, that affects the child's educational performance. In order to receive services under TBI, one or more deficits must be evidenced in cognition, language, sensory, perceptual, or motor skills. Deficits that result from congenital or degenerative disorders or brain injury caused by birth trauma are not included under TBI. Although not specifically noted, neither stroke nor brain surgery meet the definition of TBI. There are multiple problems in ascertaining "true" counts of children with TBI in schools (Ylvisaker et al., 2001). Notably, not all states use the TBI category in the same way, and the criteria for eligibility under TBI vary from state to state. In some instances, children may be served without formally going through the special education process or may be served under other categories (e.g., Other Health Impaired, Multiple Disabilities). Although it was once thought that only severe head injuries lead to permanent impairment, it is now known that mild head injuries can result in a variety of learning and mood disorders (R. Diamond, Barth, & Zillmer, 1988).

Severity of TBI

Severity of TBI is determined generally through the use of the Glasgow Coma Scale (GCS; Teasdale & Jennett, 1974; Zillmer et al., 2008). The GCS is used to assess the individual's symptoms in alertness (eye opening), verbal response, and motor response for a score ranging from 3 to 15; GCS usually is assessed within the first 24 hours and before sedation (Vallat-Azouvi, Weber, Legrand, & Azouvi, 2007). Scores of 13 or higher are indicative of mild confusion (i.e., mild TBI); scores between 9 and 12 are classified as moderate; and scores of 8 or lower are classified as severe (Kushner, 1998; Marik, Varon, & Trask, 2002). Thus, GCS scores over 8 generally are seen as indicative of more positive outcome while scores below 7 are more frequently associated with mortality and scores below 5 are suggestive of deep coma. Another indicator of potential outcome or prognosis is the number of days before the individual attains a GCS score of 15 (Zillmer et al., 2008). Although used widely, the reliability of the GCS can be impaired by the use of medications and the insertion of tubes that may impair the individual's ability to respond verbally or motorically.

Moderate to Severe TBI

It is estimated that about 10% of all head injuries are in the moderate to severe range (Levin, Benton, & Grossman, 1982). Complications of moderate to severe TBI include intracranial bleeding and hemorrhage, skull fractures, edema (swelling), and associated brain herniation (Zillmer et al., 2008). Edema and intracranial bleeding can produce increased intracranial pressure that results in diffuse damage to the brain. Increased intracranial pressure or swelling will affect blood flow and, as a result, the level of oxygenation (Ghajar, 2000). The increased pressure can result in movement of the brain in a downward direction (herniation). Hemorrhage can be subdural (i.e., the bleeding occurs between the dura and arachnoid space), which often occurs over the frontal and parietal lobes; extradural (i.e., between the skull and the dura) due to bleeding of the large meningeal artery; or epidural (i.e., between the meninges and the skull), which often is due to injury to an artery (Marik et al., 2002; Zillmer et al., 2008). Epidural and subdural hemorrhage are treated by drilling holes in the skull to drain the pocket of blood, which essentially "creates" an open head injury with increased likelihood of infection (Ghajar, 2000). Further, calcification or accumulation of large deposits of calcium at sites of neuronal degeneration may develop and be evident on brain scans; these deposits can obstruct normal blood flow, thus leading to increased intracranial pressure and obstructive hydrocephalus (Sun et al., 2008).

Mild Head Injury

The majority (i.e., 85% to 90%) of head injuries are classified as mild; among children and adolescents, most of these injuries are caused by bicycle accidents, sports injuries, falls, and MVAs (Bazarian et al., 2005). Mild head injuries often are characterized by symptoms such as headaches, dizziness, fatigue, and often limited or no loss of consciousness (Levin, Eisenberg, & Benton, 1989). Historically, because no significant "medical" issues were identified, less attention was paid to mild head injuries. Although most individuals recover from mild TBI within several months post injury, it is estimated that from 7% to 33% of people experience more persistent symptoms related to the TBI (Alexander, 1995; Belanger, Vanderploeg, Curtiss, & Warden, 2007). Thus, it is now understood that the same shearing, stretching, and tearing can occur in mild head injury with accompanied necrosis and that mild injuries also may result in difficulties with social relationships, daily functions, emotional functioning, and academic performance (Kushner, 1998). Further, it now is known that the effects can be cumulative (e.g., as in pugilistica dementia or in conjunction with other repeated sports injuries to the head; Erlanger, Kutner, Barth, & Barnes, 1999; Koh, Cassidy, & Watkinson, 2003).

COURSE AND PROGNOSIS

Recovery of Function

There is a complete devolution of behavior with TBI, followed by re-evolution (recovery) in rostral-caudal and proximal-distal order that parallels development and has been termed the *recapitulation of ontogeny* (see the work of Hughlings Jackson as described in Swash, 2005). For example, recovery of motor skills following TBI parallels the development of reaching and grasping responses with return of tendon and stretch reflexes. Rehabilitation includes interventions designed to regain any skills that have been lost as well as to identify compensatory skills that may be used in place of those skills that are not recoverable. There is enormous variation in the presenting problems as well as the extent of recovery from TBI. Complaints following TBI include memory problems, problems with attention and concentration, and alterations in mood and personality (e.g., in the case of Phineas Gage). With mild head injury, cognitive deficits may not be immediately evident in the hospital but become evident when the person returns to work/school. As such, it is recommended that a neuropsychological evaluation be completed prior to discharge to identify subtle deficits that may benefit from rehabilitation. Effects may be discrete (e.g., may impact language, executive function) or may be more diffuse and subtle, including overall reduced processing speed, inability to concentrate, and overall decreased cognitive efficiency (Lezak, 1995). Unless severe, the diffuse, subtle effects may not be evidenced on traditional IQ or achievement tests, so comprehensive neuropsychological assessment is needed.

Recovery depends on type, location, and extent of brain damage as well as the individual variation in brain organization. Premorbid functioning, as an indicator of brain organization, is often the best predictor of outcome (Catroppa & Anderson, 2007). In other words, those children who were functioning at a high level (intellectually, behaviorally, etc.) before the injury are likely to show the least severe deficits after the injury. Of course, we also must consider severity of injury, as numerous studies have demonstrated a dose–response relationship between severity and outcome, with severe TBI resulting in the most significant deficits in neuropsychological function followed by moderate and mild TBI (e.g., Catroppa & Anderson, 2007; Catroppa, Anderson, Morse, Haritou, & Rosenfeld, 2007, 2008; Wetherington & Hooper, 2006). In fact, in some cases, children with mild TBI are rather similar to control children (Farmer et al., 1999). Across different types of tasks, neuropsychological deficits are likely to be more conspicuous as task complexity and cognitive demands increase (Farmer et al., 1999; Ward, Shum, McKinlay, Baker, & Wallace, 2007). Thus, even a child who is well adjusted and performing at a high level pre-injury may show significant deficits following TBI if the injury is severe and task demands are high (Semrud-Clikeman, Kutz, & Strassner, 2005). Among children, TBI-related deficits are likely to influence functioning in school; adults are likely to manifest deficits in occupational contexts (Avesani, Salvi, Rigoli, & Gambini, 2005; Possl, Jurgensmeyer, Karlbauer, Wenz, & Goldenberg, 2001).

Recovery of function is a gradual process with rapid recovery in the first 6 months, followed by lesser degrees of improvement over the subsequent 12 to 18 months, and plateau (Ryan, LaMarche, Barth, & Boll, 1996). This means that neuropsychological assessment needs to be repeated to monitor the recovery process at 6-month intervals after medical stabilization and GCS of 15. Continued reassessment is critical to monitor recovery of function and ensure appropriate rehabilitation principles. Historically, the Kennard principle predominated; this was the idea that the earlier in development the injury occurred, the better the prognosis (K. Hart & Faust, 1988; Kennard, 1942). It is now known that this principle does not always apply and that the more neurodevelopmentally mature individual may have better prognosis, depending on variables such as type of injury and location of damage (Brink, Garrett, Hale, Woo-Sam, & Nickel, 1970; Dennis, 2000). In many cases, it appears that younger age at the time of injury is predictive of more negative outcomes (Catroppa et al., 2008; S. B. Chapman et al., 2004; Donders & Warschausky, 2007; Farmer et al., 1999). The child's age at the time of injury is also important in understanding deficits because different skills emerge at different points in development. Thus, clinicians and researchers need to know what skills (cognitive, language, etc.) the child had *before* the injury in order to determine whether postinjury deficits are due to the injury or rather to individual differences in development (i.e., did the child really lose these skills, or had she not yet developed them?).

Related to this is the concept of plasticity of function: If the injury occurs *before* a skill has been acquired (or while it is still developing), the acquisition of that skill may be more impeded over the long term (Catroppa et al., 2007, 2008; Dennis & Barnes, 2000). For example, if word decoding skills have been developed at the time of injury, they do not appear to be lost following the injury (Ewing-Cobbs & Barnes, 2002). While some degree of plasticity may be evidenced with focal, discrete deficits, this is not evident for more diffuse, subtle damage. Contributing to recovery of function is the notion that some functions are spared. *Sparing* is the process that allows certain behaviors or skills to survive the injury. Most critical to recovery of function is equipotentiality, which is the notion that multiple substructures in a given region of the brain mediate any given function; it is this redundancy of the functional system that allows for some recovery of function (A. S. Davis & Dean, 2005). Levin and Hanten (2005) presented an interactional model of recovery following TBI, with outcome dependent on interactions among preinjury factors (e.g., child factors, family factors), injury factors (e.g., severity), injury-related stress and depression, and postinjury factors (e.g., family environment, resources). Thus, recovery of function is thought to be multiply determined based on interactions among numerous pre- and postinjury factors, with variables such as coping strategies and social support having the potential to serve as protective factors (Dennis, 2000; Levin & Hanten, 2005; Tomberg, Toomela, Pulver, & Tikk, 2005).

In addition to the influence of variables such as type and location of injury on recovery, there is emerging evidence for genetic contributions to neuropsychological outcome. For example, Samatovicz (2000) reviewed evidence for the involvement of apolipoprotein E (apo E) in recovery from head injury. Apo E is a plasma lipoprotein that appears to play a role in transporting lipids to damaged neurons (e.g., those damaged by TBI) in order to facilitate their repair. Several recent studies suggest the APOE 4 genotype (a particular isoform of the apo E gene) may play a role in the severity of neurological deficits following TBI and may act as a genetic determinant of TBI outcome. For example, several studies found poorer outcomes among TBI patients with this genotype as compared to TBI patients without this genotype, suggesting the gene plays a role in how the brain recovers from injury. The APOE 4 genotype also has been identified as a genetic risk factor for Alzheimer's disease (Samatovicz, 2000).

Areas of Impairment

TBI is a multifaceted condition that may affect multiple functioning areas, including attention and executive function, memory and learning, psychosocial and behavioral functioning, intelligence, academics, and language (Semrud-Clikeman et al., 2005; Wetherington & Hooper, 2006). The next few sections briefly highlight these areas of functional impairment associated with pediatric TBI. Which of these areas become impaired, and the extent of such impairment, will vary with factors such as location, type, and severity of injury (Riccio & Reynolds, 1999). For example, localized injury to Broca's area is associated with expressive aphasia while damage to Wernicke's area is associated with receptive aphasia (A. S. Davis & Dean, 2005; Joseph, 1996). At the same time, since the developing brain is characterized by interactions among different regions with these regions working together to generate behavior and cognition (i.e., equipotentiality, as opposed to one isolated region being independently responsible for one behavior and another region independently responsible for a different behavior, etc.), it is often difficult to identify one-to-one correspondence between a region and a particular type of impairment (Johnson, 2003). With that said, *impaired communication* between specified regions may be identified as causing particular cognitive or behavioral deficits.

Attention and Executive Function

Attention problems are frequently associated with TBIs and likely are related to diffuse axonal injury with or without focal damage (Godefroy, Lhullier, & Rousseaux, 1996; Loken, Thornton, Otto, & Long, 1995; Stuss, Pogue, Buckle, & Bondar, 1994). For example, Loken et al. (1995) found that adults who had suffered a severe closed head injury exhibited slower response latencies on a continuous performance task as compared to a sample of matched controls; these results suggest deficits in sustained attention and vigilance following head injury. Given the involvement of networks among prefrontal subregions, posterior cortex, and subcortical structures in regulating executive function, damage to frontal and extrafrontal regions is likely to cause deficits in executive function due to disruption of these networks (Levin & Hanten, 2005). There is evidence for deficits in multiple areas, such as planning, inhibition, metacognitive skills, behavioral regulation, and shifting (Levin & Hanten, 2005).

A study of children's attentional and processing speed skills at 5 years post-TBI found deficits in these areas were long lasting, particularly when the injury was more severe and occurred in early childhood (Catroppa et al., 2007). Components of attention and extent affected varied depending on developmental level of attentional components at the time of injury, such that those abilities emerging at the time of injury were most likely to be affected long term. In another study, examination of executive function variables five years postinjury revealed persistent deficits among children with severe TBI but not among those with moderate or mild TBI (Nadebaum, Anderson, & Catroppa, 2007). Specific cognitive variables showing this pattern included divided attention, goal setting, and processing speed, and parent ratings on the Behavior Rating Inventory of Executive Function (BRIEF; Gioia, Isquith, Guy, & Kenworthy, 2000) indicated long-term deficits in behavioral manifestations of executive function. As found in research on other areas of impairment, the strongest predictor of executive function deficits was injury severity; executive skills that are thought to develop early in childhood were the least affected by TBI.

Memory and Learning

Overall, children with TBIs tend to show deficits in rate of learning, amount of acquired information, retrieval, and recognition (Ewing-Cobbs et al., 2003). Farmer et al. (1999) used the Wide Range Assessment of Memory and Learning (WRAML; Sheslow & Adams, 1990) to assess memory functioning among children with varying severity of TBI. Children with severe TBI performed worse on indexes of visual memory, general memory, learning, and recalling contextual verbal information as compared to those with mild to moderate TBI; no significant differences were found for overall verbal memory. These memory subskills may be those that are most susceptible to impairment following TBI and therefore may be the most important skills to consider when planning assessment of memory abilities.

In more recent research, children with TBI had poorer prospective memory performance than noninjured peers, particularly in situations of high cognitive demand (Ward et al., 2007). Differences in performance as a function of demand were most notable in adolescents and less notable in children. Age and injury effects were evident on the Self-Ordered Pointing Task (SOPT) and Stroop task, which implicated prefrontal regions (Ward et al., 2007). Individuals with severe TBI also demonstrated significant difficulty on executive aspects of working memory that required simultaneous storage and processing of information, dual-task processing, and updating (Vallat-Azouvi et al., 2007). No differences emerged on those tasks tapping into the phonological loop or visual sketchpad. Catroppa and Anderson (2007) found persistent deficits on memory, verbal learning, and visual learning tasks, especially among children with severe TBI; some of these deficits were observed up to 24 months postinjury. Even more notable, memory deficits have been found to persist for as many as 30 years postinjury (e.g., Himanen et al., 2005). It is likely that deficits in learning new information are related to memory impairment (Semrud-Clikeman et al., 2005).

Psychosocial and Behavioral Functioning

Common manifestations of psychosocial and behavioral difficulties following TBI include changes in personality, such as increased agitation, impulsivity, hyperactivity, emotional lability, irritability, aggression, anxiety, depression, motivation difficulties, conduct problems, low self-esteem, frustration over loss of skills, loneliness, and withdrawal from other people (Andrews, Rose, & Johnson, 1998; Kehle, Clark, & Jensen, 1996; McKinlay, Dalrymple-Alford, Horwood, & Fergusson, 2002; Semrud-Clikeman et al., 2005; Tateno, Jorge, & Robinson, 2003). A common outcome of TBI discussed in the literature is "frontal lobe syndrome," which results from injury to the frontal lobe and is characterized by significant personality change, such as increased impulsivity, lack of insight, behavioral disinhibition, and lack of motivation, in addition to changes in cognitive functioning (Lezak, 1995). Aggressive behavior following TBI has been associated with lesions to the frontal lobe, history of substance abuse, poor premorbid social functioning, and major depression (Tateno et al., 2003); individuals experiencing TBI are at increased risk of meeting criteria for psychiatric disorders and dysfunction (e.g., major depression, alcohol abuse, hostility, anxiety, personality disorders) as many as 30 years postinjury (Hoofien, Gilboa, Vakil, & Donovick, 2001; Koponen et al., 2002).

Children with TBIs are at increased risk of being diagnosed with psychiatric disorders such as Attention-Deficit/Hyperactivity Disorder (ADHD), mood disorders, and anxiety disorders (Nadebaum et al., 2007), and poor psychosocial outcomes appear to be more likely with severe cases of TBI (McKinlay et al., 2002). Catroppa et al. (2008) used a composite behavioral variable, including poor self-control, social incompetence, internalization, and somatic symptoms, to assess behavioral functioning over a 5-year period following TBI. No significant group differences in behavioral deficits were detected at 6-month follow-up, but by 30-month and 5-year follow-up, children with severe TBI were exhibiting significantly greater behavioral deficits than children with mild or moderate TBI. Thus, from a norm-referenced perspective, for children with severe TBI, deficits in behavioral functioning may not become pronounced until several years following the injury. Children with TBI also have demonstrated significant deficits in adaptive behaviors (Andrews et al., 1998; Levin et al., 2004). It has been speculated that younger children may be especially susceptible to psychosocial and behavioral deficits following TBI due to limited opportunities to develop coping skills as a function of their young age (Wetherington & Hooper, 2006), although behavioral symptoms may worsen with increasing age as academic and behavioral demands of school grow, thereby leading to increased frustration and acting-out behaviors (Ylvisaker et al., 2007). Clearly, the potential acute and chronic effects of TBI on psychosocial and behavioral functioning raise the likelihood that intervention programming will need to address emotional, behavioral, and social functioning.

Cognition

Semrud-Clikeman et al. (2005) identified several patterns in IQ scores among children with TBI. For example, on the Wechsler Intelligence Scale for Children, Third Edition (WISC-III; Wechsler, 1991), Performance IQ scores (including processing speed and perceptual organization) tend to show the most vulnerability to TBI at both acute and long-term assessment, while Verbal IQ often improves to premorbid level of functioning; thus, the Verbal IQ > Performance IQ profile is common among children with TBI and especially among those with severe TBI (Ewing-Cobbs et al., 2003). Further, IQ scores tend to show a dose–response relationship between severity and outcome, with severe TBI resulting in the most significant deficits in intellectual functioning. For example, Catroppa et al. (2007) assessed intellectual functioning among children with TBI 5 years postinjury using the WISC-III. With regard to Full Scale IQ, children with severe TBI (mean IQ = 84.5) scored significantly lower than children in the mild (mean IQ = 106.4), moderate (mean IQ = 100.0), and control (mean IQ = 114.1) groups; children in the severe group also scored lowest on the Index scales. Similar group differences in Full Scale IQ at the acute stage of TBI were reported by Catroppa and Anderson (2007) and Catroppa et al. (2008). Farmer et al. (1999) reported similar Verbal IQ between children with mild to moderate TBI (mean = 100.2) and children with severe TBI (mean = 95.7) but significant group differences for Performance IQ (mild to moderate mean = 96.8, severe mean = 85.0) and Full Scale IQ (mild to moderate mean = 98.2, severe mean = 89.5). Finally, young children with TBI are likely to have lower IQ scores than older children and adolescents with TBI (Ewing-Cobbs et al., 2003).

Achievement/Academic Skills

With measurement at acute, 6-, 12-, and 24-months post-TBI for severe, moderate, and mild groups of children, performance on academic measures varied depending on severity and task demands (Catroppa & Anderson, 2007). For example, children in the moderate

TBI group scored lower on reading and spelling measures as compared to children with mild and severe TBI while children in the severe group scored lower on the arithmetic and listening comprehension measures. Post-TBI academic performance was best predicted by pre-injury academic abilities as well as by verbal memory and verbal learning abilities. Interestingly, other studies also have found the greatest deficits in arithmetic (Catroppa & Anderson, 1999; Ewing-Cobbs, Fletcher, Levin, Iovino, & Miner, 1998). One study, however, found consistent deficits among children with severe TBIs across reading, spelling, and arithmetic subtests when compared to children in moderate, mild, and control groups (Catroppa et al., 2008).

Interestingly, one study demonstrated significant improvement in academic achievement scores (across reading, spelling, and arithmetic domains) at 6 months postinjury as compared to assessment shortly following the injury, with very little change occurring between this assessment and 2-year follow-up; in general, more severe injury was related to more severe deficits in achievement areas (Ewing-Cobbs et al., 1998). Further, most children were scoring in the average range on achievement tests (based on group means) by the 2-year follow-up, but many of the children with severe TBI had either repeated a grade or received services through the special education system. Thus, although many children with TBI score in the average range on norm-referenced achievement tests, these same children may struggle with classroom assignments because norm-referenced achievement tests are not sensitive enough to detect deficits in everyday academic functioning (Semrud-Clikeman et al., 2005). Curriculum-based assessments often are used to assess academic progress because of their sensitivity to change over time and because they can be developed to assess more discrete academic skills (Lezak, 1995).

Language

Three specific areas of language deficits following TBI have been studied extensively in the literature: word comprehension and production, discourse processes, and reading skills (Ewing-Cobbs & Barnes, 2002). Thus, children with TBI are likely to show impairment in:

- Expressive and receptive language
- Recognizing the intentions of others
- Detecting sarcasm and humor in communications with others
- Making inferences
- Understanding the nonliteral aspects of a story or conversation
- Using contextual variables in conversing with others in everyday situations
- Summarizing the gist of a story
- Interpreting ambiguous sentences
- Interpreting metaphors
- Word decoding speed
- Reading comprehension (Ewing-Cobbs & Barnes, 2002; Sullivan & Riccio, 2009)

These deficits in language skills seem to be most pronounced when the injury occurs at a young age and when the injury is more severe (S. B. Chapman, Levin, Wanek, Weyrauch, & Kufera, 1998; Dennis & Barnes, 2000, 2001). Some of these deficits in using language to communicate with others may lead to difficulty interpreting social situations.

Functional Impairment Across Environments

Given the multiple areas of impairment associated with TBIs, deficits are often observed across home, school, and community settings (Savage, Depompei, Tyler, & Lash, 2005). For example, if a child does not understand sarcasm or humor, she may make literal interpretations during conversations with others, thereby leading to misunderstandings, and changes in cognitive and psychosocial functioning may contribute to academic struggles and negative self-perceptions. Challenges for the student with TBI also might include physical limitations and developmental challenges (e.g., dealing with normal changes that occur with increasing age but with differing capabilities).

Issues of transition (from hospital to school, within school, and school to work) need to be addressed so that functional impairment is minimized (Ylvisaker et al., 2001). Further, family members likely will need support to deal with changes in their lives as a result of the TBI and subsequent changes in the child, and teachers and other professionals working with the child need to be educated about expectations and evolving abilities and recovery. For children with TBI, assessment needs to be conducted as soon as possible in order to institute appropriate interventions. In the year following the injury period, many students with TBI should receive extended school year services due to the need for continued rehabilitation until recovery has clearly reached a plateau.

Assessment of Functional Impairment over Time

No single assessment method for TBIs is used across settings or individuals. Due to the rapid changes that can occur following TBI, in order to document small changes in behavioral or psychological functioning over time, it may be necessary to supplement standardized norm-referenced measures that may require substantial improvement to demonstrate change over time due to item gradients with curriculum-based or criterion-referenced measures. In this section we briefly highlight some of the issues involved in assessment of functioning following TBI; for more thorough consideration of these issues, see Riccio and Reynolds (1999) and Semrud-Clikeman (2001).

Given the unique nature of TBI (e.g., deficits and symptoms vary with the nature and type of injury, resulting in a wide range of potential deficits and symptoms), the assessment process is more comprehensive than may be typical for other disorders or referral questions. That is, much variance exists within this diagnostic category, so that different children who have suffered TBI may exhibit quite different cognitive, behavioral, emotional, and other symptoms. For children with TBI, the primary assessment goal is not really to reach a diagnosis or classification but to establish postinjury baseline data, identify areas of strength and weakness, and continuously monitor change over time in neuropsychological and behavioral functioning (Riccio & Reynolds, 1999). This monitoring over time has been termed *developmental surveillance* (Wetherington & Hooper, 2006) and is necessary to detect unpredictable individual differences in recovery and change following TBI. Individual areas of strength and weakness should then drive the development of individualized interventions based on the child's unique needs. The assessment itself should be organized in such a manner that the majority of areas of functioning as well as the various contexts in which the child is expected to function are considered. Riccio and Reynolds (1999) identified a number of key features to the organization for neuropsychological assessment of children with TBI; these include:

- A comprehensive developmental history
- Estimate of premorbid functioning
- Assessment of cognitive skills and higher-order processes
- Sampling of right- and left-hemispheric functions
- Sampling of anterior and posterior functions
- Assessment of psychosocial and behavioral functioning
- Identification of specific deficits
- Identification of intact functional systems
- Determination of acuteness versus chronicity of deficits
- Consideration of environmental factors that may facilitate or hinder rehabilitation

Thus, neuropsychological assessment of children with TBIs should focus more directly on analysis of the functional concomitants and sequelae of injury as opposed to identification of neurological disorder, so that compensatory skills can be taught in order to overcome or remediate areas of impairment.

In light of the multiple areas of potential deficit, assessment of functioning and deficits following TBI should incorporate measures of intelligence, memory, attention and executive function, language skills, academic skills, and psychosocial and behavioral functioning (Ewing-Cobbs & Fletcher, 1987). In some cases, assessment also might include perceptual, motor, and sensory areas. Certainly, discrete tests often are used to assess these constructs separately (see Chapter 1 for examples), but comprehensive neuropsychological batteries are also used to tap into several of these domains of functioning. For example, the Halstead-Reitan Neuropsychological Battery (HRNB; Reitan & Davison, 1974; Reitan & Wolfson, 1985) and the Luria Nebraska Neuropsychological Battery—Children's Revision (LNNB-CR; Golden, 1984, 1997) often are used in neuropsychological assessment in conjunction with intelligence tests and provide a sampling of sensory and motor functions as well as additional information relating to left-/right-hemisphere differences and anterior/posterior differences. For example, the HRNB includes measures of concept formation, sensory abilities, attention/concentration, motor speed and dexterity, verbal abilities, and memory. Similarly, the LNNB-CR includes tasks that assess attention, motor, rhythm, tactile, visual, verbal (receptive and expressive), and memory functions.

Due to varying rates in recovery of function, the treatment plan or Individualized Educational Plan for a child with TBI needs to be reevaluated on a frequent basis using repeated assessments (formal or informal) of the child's progress in previously identified deficit areas in addition to ongoing consideration of new areas of concern (Ball & Zinner, 1994; Riccio & Reynolds, 1999). More specifically, it has been recommended that reassessment occur every 6 to 12 months in order to detect subtle changes in functioning (Boll & Stanford, 1997). This need for regular follow-up assessment points to the importance of curriculum-based measurement, especially for detecting subtle changes in academic skills that may not be detected with standardized, norm-referenced instruments (Shinn, 1989). Curriculum-based measures also may be more relevant for intervention development and planning. Curriculum-based measures are often timed in order to provide information about fluency (e.g., number of words read or math problems completed per minute), which contributes to the ecological validity of assessment since fluency is important to academic skills and learning (Riccio & Reynolds, 1999). Similarly, for skills such as speech comprehension, reading comprehension, and writing, the examiner may use informal methods, such as asking the child to follow simple verbal commands, follow written directions, or write sentences, in addition to more formal norm-referenced measures (Lezak, 1995).

In addition to estimating premorbid intellectual functioning (see Franzen, Burgess, & Smith-Seemiller, 1997; Reynolds, 1997), Riccio and Reynolds (1999) recommended establishing premorbid levels of psychological and behavioral functioning. For example, the clinician can have the child's parents and current teachers complete behavior rating scales, such as the Behavior Assessment System for Children, Second Edition (Reynolds & Kamphaus, 2004) and Conners' Rating Scales, Third Edition (Conners, 2008) based on the child's behavior for the 6 months prior to the injury. This approach will allow the clinician to compare current behavior against previous behavior and identify problems that appeared after the injury versus those that are more long-standing. Ideally, these retrospective ratings would be completed prior to the child's reentry into the home or school environment so that the ratings are not biased by postinjury functioning.

Assessment of language functioning should include measurement of verbal expression (expressive language skills, such as word fluency and naming), language comprehension (or receptive language), reading, writing, and pragmatic language (Hotz, Helm-Estabrooks, & Nelson, 2001). Pragmatic language assessment presents a good example of the importance of ecological validity in TBI assessment (Duff, Proctor, & Haley, 2002). *Ecological validity* refers to the notion that assessment should lead to an understanding of how the child is likely to function in everyday, real-world situations (e.g., academic and social settings). It is possible that standardized, objective language tests may miss some of the language deficits that are more apparent in everyday conversation (e.g., deficits in discourse processes) and deficits may not be apparent unless the child is observed in more complex settings (Morse et al., 1999). Thus, language assessment following TBI also should attempt to measure deficits in these more practical conversation skills in less structured settings (e.g., play or social settings). This issue of ecological validity is also important with assessment of academic skills, as a child could score in the average range on a standardized academic achievement test but still show functional impairment in the classroom. Again, curriculum-based measures may provide the best information about real-world academic functioning, and observations by clinicians, parents, and teachers likely will provide critical pieces of information.

Constructs such as learning skills, memory, attention, and executive function are critical to success in the classroom setting. Further, problems with memory, learning new information, and attention are the most common of all complaints following any type of central nervous system compromise and are often more subtle than other types of impairment (Gillberg, 1995; Reynolds & Bigler, 1997). Thus, these constructs should be assessed even with mild and moderate TBIs to identify possible deficits that can interfere with the acquisition of new learning.

Semrud-Clikeman et al. (2005) discussed the importance of social/family support as a variable that plays a role in recovery, with more support and resources associated with better recovery. Thus, the TBI assessment process should include consideration of environmental variables such as living conditions, socioeconomic status and resources, social support, family stress and adjustment to the TBI, and support and services available through the child's school (Riccio & Reynolds, 1999).

Initial evidence does not support the use of neuroimaging techniques to make predictions about neuropsychological outcome or performance on neuropsychological measures based on site (e.g., frontal vs. extrafrontal vs. generalized) or severity of injury

(Power, Catroppa, Coleman, Ditchfield, & Anderson, 2007), but this research with pediatric populations is just beginning. Further, the Power et al. study focused on attentional control and executive function variables; other constructs may be better predicted by lesion site. At the same time, since the developing brain is characterized by interactions among different regions, it may be difficult to identify one-to-one correspondence between a region and a particular behavioral or neuropsychological outcome (see Bigler, 1999; Johnson, 2003).

EVIDENCE-BASED INTERVENTIONS

Intervention for pediatric TBI is not a one-size-fits-all approach. Treatment will vary to some extent depending on the specific nature of the injury and deficits, with interventions focusing on clearly defined goals based on the specific symptoms unique to the child (e.g., S. S. Chapman, Ewing, & Mozzoni, 2005). For example, if emotional and behavioral symptoms are of concern, interventions are developed to address those specific symptoms. If the child demonstrates deficits in memory, the intervention might include repetition and drill of the skill area. In this way, rehabilitation includes interventions designed to regain any skills that have been lost as well as to identify compensatory skills that may be used in place of those skills that are not recoverable and to develop skills for coping with deficits.

Assessment of the child's unique needs should drive the development of individualized interventions to meet those needs (Bowen, 2005). Intervention programs should be based heavily on the information gathered during the assessment process; the more reliable data that are gathered through assessment, the more informed the interventions will be. Interventions are designed in a way that assists the child in moving from a more dependent, externally supported state to a more independent, internally supported and self-regulated state. Many interventions for pediatric TBI will be school based since most children with TBI return to school in general, special, or some combination of instructional settings (Bowen, 2005). Kehle et al. (1996) reminded clinicians to consider the cognitive deficits of children with TBI when designing individualized interventions to address behavioral deficits, as variations in cognitive functioning will impact which behavioral interventions are most appropriate (e.g., interventions that rely on metacognition, attention, or learning new information may need to be modified based on TBI-related deficits in these areas). For example, a behavioral intervention to address noncompliance might consider whether the noncompliance behaviors are due to a volitional desire to disobey the parent or teacher or are related to difficulty processing verbal instructions. In this way, conducting a functional behavior assessment may be especially helpful in identifying the antecedents and consequences of problem behaviors and determining how to structure the environment to decrease these behaviors and increase more adaptive behaviors.

It has been suggested that interventions for TBI must be multidimensional and incorporate not only academic, behavioral, and psychotherapeutic techniques but also include motivational, metacognitive, medical, and classroom management techniques (Riccio & Reynolds, 1999). Further, the selection of specific intervention strategies should be based on the individual's level of environmental dependency, the constellation of preserved and impaired functions, and level of awareness (Mateer, 1999). While treatment within the context of education generally consists of special education eligibility through IDEIA or Section 504, educational placement decisions, and the development of an educational plan, effective interventions for children with TBI also need to consider the myriad of psychosocial contexts in which the child functions, adjustment and coping issues, and environmental modifications that can ameliorate or reduce the behavioral effects of deficits (Batchelor, 1996; Teeter & Semrud-Clikeman, 1997). For example, parent training programs may help with behavioral difficulties at home, and education and support groups for families of children with TBI are often advocated in the literature as methods of easing the stress associated with raising a child with TBI. Environmental modifications that may facilitate the child's academic reintegration may include variations in the child's daily schedule if fatigue is an issue, modifications in time allowances for tasks if slowed processing is evident, or the use of any number of educational support materials (e.g., computers, calculators, tape recorders). Other examples include the use of devices (e.g., personal digital assistants, calendars, diaries) to compensate for deficits in memory and organization skills, which likely would necessitate instruction and monitoring in the use of these devices, especially with children (Glisky & Glisky, 2002). Environmental supports also can include labels, pictograms of what needs to be accomplished (e.g., as used with children with autism), or written instructions. For individuals with mild to moderate impairment, environmental supports such as these may be needed only at the onset of the treatment program and can gradually be faded. For those children with more severe impairment, the environmental cues may continue to be needed over time (Lee & Riccio, 2005). With the most rapid recovery from TBI evident within the first 6 months postinjury, the earlier the interventions are in place, the more effective they are likely to be.

Cognitive rehabilitation includes "interventions designed to promote the recovery of cognitive function and to reduce cognitive disability" (Cicerone et al., 2000, p. 1596). This rehabilitation involves identifying areas of strength and weakness and using this information to develop interventions that reinforce strength and remediate or compensate for areas of weakness. The goal may be seen as helping the child improve daily functioning so he or she can be more successful academically and socially and so the child can engage in activities of interest (Limond & Leeke, 2005). Cognitive rehabilitation may include a range of interventions targeting multiple skills, such as attention, memory, perception, speech and language, problem-solving skills, executive function, and combinations among these domains (other domains may include emotional and behavioral functioning when appropriate); which of these areas are targeted depends on the nature of the injury and subsequent deficits. Hence the importance of thorough assessment: The assessment process should identify areas of deficit and point the clinician in certain treatment directions to address these deficits.

Although there are numerous anecdotal and conceptual resources that provide guidance for intervention following TBI, especially psychosocial and psychoeducational intervention (e.g., Bowen, 2005; Savage et al., 2005), the empirically based literature is scarce with regard to applying interventions specifically to children and adolescents with TBIs (Bowen, 2005; Kehle et al., 1996). A number of evidence-based reviews have been published related to the effectiveness of interventions for TBI, but many of these reviews focus on TBI among adults (e.g., Cicerone et al., 2000; Comper, Bisschop, Carnide, & Tricco, 2005; M. R. T. Kennedy et al., 2008). Table 8.1 summarizes the few conclusions that have been reached with regard to evidence-based interventions for pediatric TBI. The large-scale Evidence-Based Review of Rehabilitation of Moderate to Severe Acquired Brain Injuries (ERABI; Teasell et al., 2007) provided conclusions on the evidence-based status of interventions targeting motor impairment, seizures, and cognitive variables following TBI, but most studies reviewed by this group included either adult-only samples

Table 8.1 Evidence-Based Status of Interventions for Children with TBI

Interventions	Target	Status
Family-centered rehabilitation programs (i.e., family members involved in planning and providing treatment)	Comprehensive	Positive practice (Laatsch et al., 2007)
Attention remediation programs (e.g., Amsterdam Memory and Training Program for Children)	Attention, memory, executive function, self-regulation	Positive practice (Laatsch et al., 2007)
Educational or informational interventions (e.g., using informational booklets about the effects and symptoms of TBI to facilitate the family's understanding of TBI)	Comprehensive	Promising practice (Laatsch et al., 2007)
Metacognitive Strategy Instruction (MSI)	Executive function, problem solving	Emerging with children (M. R. T. Kennedy et al., 2008; Limond & Leeke, 2005)
Methylphenidate (Ritalin, Concerta)	Attention, processing speed	Promising practice with children (Rees, Marshall, Hartridge, Mackie, & Weiser, 2007; Waldron-Perrine, Hanks, & Perrine, 2008)
General behavioral interventions (e.g., functional analysis of behavior, operant conditioning approaches, contingency management systems, positive behavior supports)	Disruptive behaviors, compliance, aggression, on-task behaviors	Positive practice (Gurdin, Huber, & Cochran, 2005; Ylvisaker et al., 2007)

or mixed child-adult samples. At the same time, the series of ERABI reviews (published online at www.abiebr.com, and in a special issue of *Brain Injury*; Teasell, 2007) provides a useful model for research on pediatric TBI to follow.

Limond and Leek (2005) reviewed the literature up to the year 2002 and found 11 studies meeting methodological criteria that investigated the effectiveness of interventions for attention, memory, and executive function deficits following TBIs. This review found no conclusive evidence to support the use of cognitive rehabilitation interventions with children due to a lack of randomized controlled trials, but the review examined cognitive variables only.

Laatsch et al. (2007) conducted a review of empirically supported treatment studies for deficits associated with pediatric TBIs, including deficits in language, attention, memory, behavior, and academics. The types of interventions and outcome variables were much more varied than those examined in the Limond and Leek (2005) review, and therefore a greater number of studies were identified by Laatsch et al. In all, 28 studies were identified that met methodological criteria, with search parameters including peer-reviewed journal articles published between 1980 and 2006. Of these 28 studies, 4 examined language or speech functioning as the outcome variables of primary interest, 8 examined attention or memory variables, 8 examined behavioral treatments, and 8 were comprehensive in nature (i.e., examined multiple cognitive or behavioral domains). Based on the review of these studies, only two interventions were recommended: (1) family-based approaches in which family members are involved in developing and implementing comprehensive interventions and (2) attention remediation programs. Information-based interventions also were identified as a promising approach for providing families with accurate information about TBI and alleviating some of the stress immediately following the injury. Note that educational interventions also have been identified as evidence-based interventions for adults with mild TBI (Comper et al., 2005). Interestingly, none of the interventions specifically targeting behavior or speech/language was identified as established or promising, suggesting that even though individual studies have found promising results, there has not yet been an adequate confluence across studies to recommend these interventions. Most of these studies are characterized by small sample sizes (ranging from 1 to 72, with many studies including fewer than 10 participants) and other methodological limitations (e.g., lack of control group, selection of measures), but they provide preliminary examples of interventions for deficits associated with TBIs. Further, many of the individual studies showed positive results (e.g., with family-centered approaches, metacognitive training, psychoeducational interventions, and instruction in problem-solving strategies), but replication with larger samples is necessary before these treatments can be recommended.

Rees et al. (2007) included pharmacological interventions in their evidence-based review of TBI treatments and concluded that there is strong evidence for the use of methylphenidate (Ritalin, Concerta) to improve attention among individuals with TBI. The review also found strong evidence for using external aids as a compensatory strategy for memory problems, and moderate evidence for dual-task training and goal management training; however, most of the studies included in this review sampled adults rather than children, making it difficult to determine whether these interventions are effective with children and adolescents with TBI (Rees et al., 2007).

Another evidence-based review focused only on pharmacological interventions for TBI. The position of the Kokiko and Hamm (2007) review is that if post-TBI cognitive deficits are related to decreased neuronal and neurotransmitter activity due to neuronal damage or death, it follows that using medications that act to increase neurotransmitter activity (i.e., "rehabilitative pharmacology") should result in improved cognitive functioning. While studies have supported the use of some medications (e.g., atomoxetine [Strattera], methylphenidate [Ritalin, Concerta], lithium [Eskalith, Lithobid]) for this purpose with injured rats, extant research with humans (and especially with children) with TBI does not allow for firm conclusions with regard to the evidence-based status of most medications. Similar conclusions were reached in a recent review of pharmacological treatments: Even though medications are commonly used in the treatment of TBI-related symptoms, few firm guidelines exist for their use for this specific purpose due to limited, inconsistent, and inconclusive research. Methylphenidate was identified as a promising treatment for improving attention and processing speed, but more methodologically sound research studies are needed to establish the effects of different medications on children with TBI. An additional interesting conclusion from the Waldron-Perrine et al. (2008) review stated:

> Given the paucity of research supporting the use of any specific drug for the treatment of neurobehavioral symptoms, nonpharmacological interventions such as environmental or behavioral modification should always be considered in the effort to control the target behavior and improve the quality of life of the patients and their families. (p. 437)

This notion of the importance of behavioral and/or environmental interventions leads to consideration of the empirical basis for these interventions. Gurdin et al. (2005) reviewed 20 empirical studies examining the effectiveness of behavioral interventions with children with TBI and concluded that, "with its emphasis on functional and measurable outcomes, applied behavior analysis can greatly enhance both rehabilitation and educational programs" (p. 15). Many studies reviewed employed functional behavior analysis and operant conditioning principles (e.g., manipulating antecedents and consequences of behaviors) to reduce disruptive behaviors, such as noncompliance and physical aggression, or to increase desirable behaviors, such as work completion. Similarly, Ylvisaker et al. (2007) reviewed 65 studies examining the use of behavioral interventions with children and adults with TBI and concluded that behavioral treatments were effective with a range of age groups and behavioral-dependent variables; behavioral treatments were classified as a "practice guideline" (i.e., moderate certainty of effectiveness to support the use of these interventions). Specific behavioral strategies found to be effective in at least one study included positive and negative reinforcement, extinction, response-cost procedures, providing choices and control, restructuring the environment, behavioral momentum procedures, and providing daily routines. At the same time, currently there is not sufficient evidence to firmly recommend *specific* behavioral treatment protocols for children with TBI; rather, behavioral treatments are recommended *generally* as a family of interventions until research provides more information regarding the effectiveness of specific interventions (Ylvisaker et al., 2007). Overall, although behavioral interventions have been supported through empirical research and represent a recommended approach with children who demonstrate behavioral difficulties following TBI, conclusions are still tentative due to a limited number of well-controlled studies, most of which employed small samples.

The Metacognitive Strategy Instruction (MSI) intervention listed in Table 8.1 involves training in problem-solving skills, planning, self-monitoring, self-evaluation, and organization (skills that collectively may be referred to as executive function or self-regulation). This intervention is a specific example of a family of interventions called metacognitive interventions, which often are used in cognitive rehabilitation programs (Lee & Riccio, 2005). The MSI intervention has been recommended for adults with TBI, but effectiveness with children is inconclusive due to limited research with pediatric samples (Kennedy et al., 2008).

Clinicians must keep in mind that deficits in some areas (e.g., executive function, memory) as a result of TBI also may contribute to deficits in other areas, such as language, and vice versa. Assessing function in all of these areas may help to understand how deficits in one area interact with and influence deficits in other areas related to TBI and also may facilitate appropriate intervention programming (Ewing-Cobbs & Barnes, 2002; Levin & Hanten, 2005). Additionally, changes in functioning may occur quickly among children with TBI, suggesting the importance of close monitoring and frequent reevaluation of functioning in order to assess changes related to development or recovery and to develop appropriate programming based on the child's individual needs (Wetherington & Hooper, 2006).

As compared to some of the other disorders discussed in this volume (e.g., ADHD), much less seems to be known about evidence-based interventions for TBI. This is likely due to the wide range of possible deficits, making it difficult to develop interventions that are equally appropriate for all or most children with TBI. A theme that emerges across the literature is that interventions resulting in significant effects on cognitive functioning domains are typically intense, requiring at least several hours of treatment per week over the course of several months or longer. Very few empirically based recommendations can be made due to the inconsistent findings across studies and methodological limitations of existing studies. These methodological limitations include lack of experimental control, heterogeneity among participants, small sample sizes, limited attention to developmental issues in recovery, and limitations of outcome measures used to assess dependent variables (Limond & Leeke, 2005). Finally, even when interventions are recommended in evidence-based reviews, they often are recommended with some hesitation due to the small number of available studies.

CASE STUDY: GAGE—TRAUMATIC BRAIN INJURY

The next report is from a hospital-based clinic. Identifying information, such as child and family name, teacher or physician name, and school information, has been altered or fictionalized to protect confidentiality.

Reason for Referral

Gage Smith is a 10-year-old young man who sustained a traumatic brain injury to the right frontal parietal region as a result of accidentally shooting himself with an arrow through his right orbit. Due to the injury, Gage has been left with a mild left hemiparesis and mild right ptosis. In addition, he also exhibits a short attention span for which he is taking atomoxetine (Strattera), 40 mg each morning. Since the beginning of the school year, Gage also has experienced considerable academic difficulty. At the request of his pediatrician, this neuropsychological evaluation was undertaken approximately one year postinjury in order to assess higher cortical functioning and make appropriate recommendations regarding school placement and the need for supportive therapies.

Assessment Procedures

In addition to the listed battery of assessment instruments, Gage's parents provided developmental history information via interview. For some of the comprehensive instruments listed, only selected subtests were administered in order to gain information about discrete domains of functioning.

Wechsler Intelligence Scale for Children, Fourth Edition (WISC-IV)
Kaufman Assessment Battery for Children, Second Edition (KABC-2)
Wide Range Achievement Test, Fourth Edition (WRAT-4)
Neuropsychological Assessment (NEPSY)
Peabody Picture Vocabulary Test, Third Edition (PPVT-III)
Clinical Evaluation of Language Fundamentals, Fourth Edition (CELF-IV)
Test of Written Language, Third Edition (TOWL-3)
Gray Oral Reading Test, Fourth Edition (GORT-4)
Detroit Tests of Learning Aptitude, Fourth Edition (DTLA-4)
Boston Naming Test (BNT)
Delis-Kaplan Executive Function System (D-KEFS)
Developmental Test of Visual-Motor Integration, Fifth Edition (DTVMI-V)
Children's Memory Scale (CMS)

Rey Complex Figure Test (RCFT)
Clock Face Drawing Test
Finger Oscillation Test
Behavior Assessment System for Children, Second Edition (BASC-2)

Background Information

Gage resides with his parents and his 15-year-old brother who is reported to be doing well in the tenth grade and in good health. Gage's father is 42 years of age, a high school and technical school graduate, who is currently employed as an operator at a power plant. Gage's mother is 41 years of age, a high school and technical school graduate, who is currently employed as a secretary at a local hospital. Both parents are reported to be in good health. Aside from a male paternal cousin with ADHD, the family history is negative for neurological and psychiatric disorder, including mental retardation.

Review of Gage's developmental and medical history indicates that he is the product of a normal 38-week gestation pregnancy and cesarean section delivery, weighing 8 pounds 11.5 ounces at birth. He did well as a newborn and went home with mother from the hospital on schedule. Gage attained his developmental motor milestones within normal limits with sitting up occurring at 6 months of age and walking at 12 months of age. Gage's mother was unable to recall Gage's exact developmental language milestones; however, she felt that he attained these within normal limits. Toilet training was fully accomplished at 2 years of age without difficulty. According to Mrs. Smith, Gage was in good general health until December 26, when he was taken by ambulance to a local hospital after an arrow pierced his right orbit and penetrated the brain. Gage removed the arrow himself. Gage's mother recalls that when the ambulance arrived at the home and during transport to the hospital, Gage was answering questions coherently. Upon arrival at the emergency room, Gage was taken for a computed tomography (CT) scan (see Figure 8.1), after which his condition deteriorated. He subsequently underwent an emergency craniotomy with removal of a bone flap. Once Gage was stabilized, he was transported to the pediatric intensive care unit (ICU) at the Children's Medical Center of Sherwood Forest. Gage was in the pediatric ICU for approximately two weeks where he was followed by

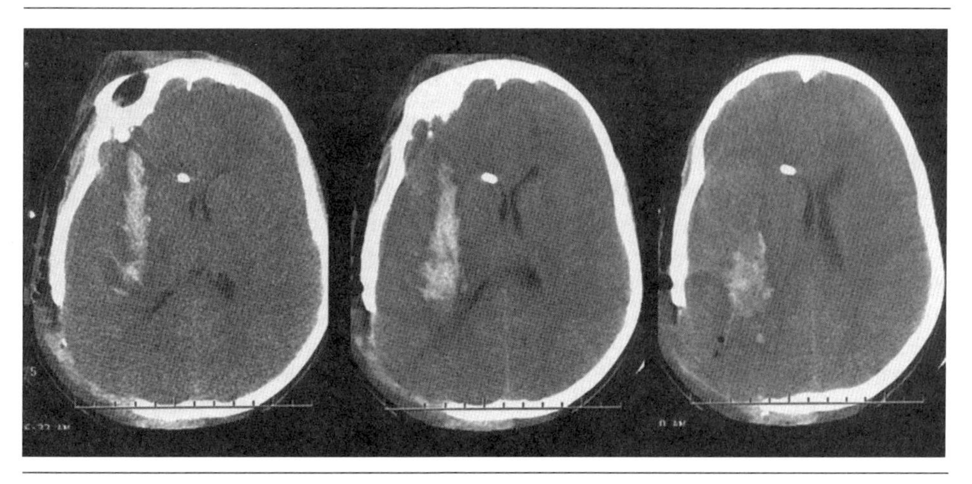

Figure 8.1 CT scan of Gage's injury showing damage from the arrow.

a pediatric neurosurgeon. After spending an additional week on the general pediatrics floor, Gage was discharged home. While in the hospital, he began receiving occupational, physical, and speech/language therapies. The occupational and physical therapies were continued on an outpatient basis and gradually decreased until they were discontinued in July.

On February 26 of the following year, Gage was readmitted to the Children's Medical Center, where he underwent cranioplasty for replacement of the bone flap. In addition to being followed by his neurosurgeon, Gage has also been followed as an outpatient by a rehabilitation medicine specialist who has treated the hemiparesis with Botox injections and casting of the left foot and leg. Medication therapy with Strattera was also initiated to assist in management of Gage's attention deficits. Mrs. Smith states that Gage's left hemiparesis has improved significantly and he no longer has to be reminded to use his left hand. He can now catch a football and hit a golf ball fairly well and has resumed many of his normal activities.

Review of academic history indicates that at 4 years of age, Gage began school in a prekindergarten program at North Sherwood Forest Elementary School. According to his mother, Gage continued to attend the same school through the fourth grade, where he was generally an A/B student making an occasional C. Following the TBI, which occurred during the Christmas break of the fourth grade, Gage began receiving homebound teacher services in February for one hour three times per week. He returned to school toward the end of March, attending half-days for approximately two weeks. After the spring break, Gage began attending full days. According to his mother, he began attending an Early Intervention Program (EIP) classroom for reading and mathematics (regular education program). During the summer, Gage's parents worked with him to improve his math skills without any extended school-year services provided by the school system.

At present, Gage is attending the fifth grade at South Sherwood Forest Elementary School. According to his mother, Gage continues to attend an EIP classroom for reading and mathematics; however, his regular education teacher does not feel he will continue to require these services for reading. With the start of the school year, Gage's teachers and his parents both noticed a significant problem with attention span at home as well as in the classroom. As a result, medication therapy with Strattera was begun toward the end of September. Mrs. Smith states that since initiation of the medication, Gage's attention span has improved significantly. However, Gage continues to experience academic difficulty in some areas. Review of his first report card issued on October 8 indicates that Gage earned an A in spelling, Bs in language arts and reading, Cs in English and social studies, and Fs in mathematics and science. In addition, he is having difficulty mastering cursive writing. Review of a school report form completed by his teacher indicates that she characterizes Gage as "a very polite boy. He likes to participate in class and tries. He is well liked by his peers and all of his teachers. He is very mild mannered."

Behavioral Observations

Gage presented himself for testing as a very pleasant, polite young man with blond hair and green eyes, who was dressed in a red baseball cap, a greenish/brown fishing T-shirt, and jeans. Gage separated from his parents easily and accompanied the examiners to the testing room without difficulty. Throughout the evaluation, which consisted of two sessions separated by a lunch break, Gage was able to relate appropriately toward the examiners with good eye contact and manners noted. In response to direct questions as well as when conversation was spontaneous, Gage's language usage was fluent and prosodic; however, at times he was observed to lose his train of thought. In addition, he often would repeat directions to himself in order to aid comprehension. During both the morning and afternoon testing sessions, Gage demonstrated an age-appropriate attention span and activity level with the benefit of his medication. When presented with difficult test items, Gage responded in a reflective manner and often would verbally mediate himself through the task. In general, Gage approached this evaluation in an enthusiastic manner with good task persistence noted. Lateral dominance is firmly established in the right hand. According to his mother, Gage's vision was last evaluated in January by his pediatric ophthalmologist at the Children's Medical Center of Sherwood Forest, and it was reported to be within normal limits. Hearing was last screened by the school system this past spring and also found to be normal. Given the adequacy of the testing conditions and Gage's general cooperation and effort toward the tasks, results of this evaluation should be considered a valid reflection of his current neuropsychological functioning.

Assessment Results and Interpretation

Individual subtest scores are presented in the Psychometric Summary (see Table 8.2). The results of cognitive and neuropsychological evaluation indicate that Gage currently is functioning within the borderline to low-average range of intellectual ability as measured by the Wechsler Intelligence Scale for Children, Fourth Edition. However, analysis of the Index scores indicates that Gage is exhibiting a significant discrepancy between his average verbal conceptual and his borderline nonverbal reasoning abilities. Further, Gage is exhibiting borderline ability in information processing speed. On additional neuropsychological assessment, Gage demonstrates relative strengths in areas of abstract verbal reasoning, expressive and receptive vocabulary development, phonological processing, and the ability to learn and recall (30 minutes later) auditory/verbal information. These strengths are contrasted by significant weaknesses in the areas of nonverbal problem solving/sequential planning, linguistic planning, visual-motor integration/construction, motor planning, fine motor functioning of the left (nondominant) hand, and the ability to learn and recall (30 minutes later) the spatial location of objects.

Academically, Gage is presently achieving at expectancy level (based on verbal reasoning ability) in the areas of word recognition/spelling, reading fluency, reading comprehension, and written expression. However, qualitative analysis of Gage's story on the Tests of Written Language, Third Edition revealed inconsistent spelling, poor punctuation (use of periods), and a story lacking in organization. Further, Gage made two careless errors on the numerical calculation section of the Wide Range Achievement Test, Fourth Edition. If these errors are controlled for, Gage's performance would fall within the average range.

Behaviorally, analysis of rating scales completed by Gage's mother and teacher indicates that he is not exhibiting significant emotional or behavioral difficulties at home or in the classroom at the present time, which is consistent with qualitative information provided by parents and teachers and with observations made during this assessment. Thus, it appears that medication therapy is having a positive effect on the short attention span that Gage began to exhibit following his traumatic brain injury. It is worth noting that behavioral ratings (especially those related to inattention) may have been more severe in the absence of medication treatment.

Summary and Diagnostic Impressions

Taken together, this pattern of neuropsychological test performance is consistent with a diagnosis of executive dysfunction, mild left hemiparesis, and ADHD by history that are

Table 8.2 Psychometric Summary for Gage

	Standard Score
Wechsler Intelligence Scale for Children, Fourth Edition (WISC-IV)	
Full Scale IQ	77
Verbal Comprehension Index	99
Similarities	105
Vocabulary	100
Comprehension	95
Perceptual Reasoning Index	77
Block Design	70
Picture Concepts	75
Matrix Reasoning	100
Working Memory Index	88
Digit Span	85
Letter-Number Sequencing	95
Processing Speed Index	78
Coding	75
Symbol Search	85
Neuropsychological Assessment (NEPSY)	
Tower	80
Phonological Processing	95
Arrows	85
Peabody Picture Vocabulary Test, Third Edition (PPVT-III)	95
Detroit Tests of Learning Aptitude, Fourth Edition (DTLA-4)	
Sentence Repetition	105
Clinical Evaluation of Language Fundamentals, Fourth Edition (CELF-IV)	
Concepts and Following Directions	90
Formulated Sentences	65
Boston Naming Test (BNT)	103
Delis-Kaplan Executive Function System (D-KEFS)	
Verbal Fluency Test	100
Kaufman Assessment Battery for Children, Second Edition (KABC-2)	
Gestalt Closure	105
Developmental Test of Visual Motor Integration, Fifth Edition (DTVMI-V)	77
Rey Complex Figure Copying Task (RCFT)	75
Clock Face Drawing	
Form	95
Time	109
Finger Oscillation Test	
Right (dominant) Hand	134
Left (nondominant) Hand	80
Children's Memory Scale (CMS)	
General Memory Index	85
Attention/Concentration Index	88
Numbers	100
Sequences	80
Picture Locations	85

Table 8.2 (*Continued*)

	Standard Score
Verbal Immediate Index	103
Stories	110
Word Pairs	95
Visual Immediate Index	75
Dot Locations	85
Faces	75
Verbal Delayed Index	97
Stories	105
Word Pairs	90
Visual Delayed Index	82
Dot Locations	75
Faces	95
Delayed Recognition Index	106
Stories	100
Word Pairs	110
Learning Index	82
Word Pairs	90
Dot Locations	80
Wide Range Achievement Test, Fourth Edition (WRAT-4)	
Reading	96
Spelling	107
Arithmetic	88
Gray Oral Reading Test, Fourth Edition (GORT-4)	
Fluency	105
Comprehension	100
Test of Written Language, Third Edition (TOWL-3)	
Written Language Quotient	94

Behavior Assessment System for Children, Second Edition (BASC-2)

	T-Scores	
	Parent	Teacher
Clinical Scales		
Hyperactivity	33	52
Aggression	39	44
Conduct Problems	37	51
Anxiety	36	59
Depression	34	41
Somatization	41	46
Atypicality	38	50
Withdrawal	44	39
Attention Problems	47	53
Adaptive Scales		
Adaptability	61	51
Social Skills	48	45
Leadership	44	51
Study Skills	NA	46

Note. NA = Not applicable.

secondary to right hemisphere dysfunction following TBI. It should be noted that these higher cortical deficits place Gage at significant risk for future academic difficulty, especially in the areas of higher-order mathematics and written expression. On a positive note, current medication treatment appears to be effective for treating inattention, and social-behavioral functioning represents an area of strength for Gage. His persistence will likely be an asset in the implementation of academic and cognitive interventions.

Recommendations

- It is recommended that Gage continue to receive Early Intervention Program classroom services for mathematics along with learning disability special education resource/consultative services under the "Traumatic Brain Injury" category in order to provide further academic support in the areas of mathematics and science as well as in the development of written expression skills.
- If Gage begins to exhibit distractability and a short attention span in school even with continuation of medication therapy, a behavior management program should be developed in order to improve on-task behavior as part of his Individual Educational Plan. As part of this plan, rules and expectations should be simply, clearly, and consistently presented and reviewed frequently. This plan should place an emphasis on consistently rewarding Gage's "good" behavior, such as working on classwork and following directions, rather than having a punitive system that primarily calls attention to his mistakes. In other words, he should have a high ratio of positive reinforcement to punishment (ratio = 5:1). Consequences for both appropriate and inappropriate behavior should be enforced on a consistent basis through positive reinforcement and response cost. This could be managed in the form of a contract system, given Gage's age and intellect. The behavioral plan should be coordinated with parents to ensure consistency between home and school with regard to target behaviors, reinforcers, and punishments.
- In order to enhance Gage's learning/retention, new material should be presented in an organized format that is meaningful to him. The material to be learned should be broken down into smaller components/steps and presented in a highly structured format with frequent repetition to facilitate learning.
- Gage would benefit greatly from being taught how to use mnemonic strategies when learning new material and studying for tests. These include but are not limited to:
  - Rehearsal—showing Gage how to repeat information verbally, write it, and look at it a finite number of times.
  - Transformation—showing him how to convert difficult information into simpler components that can be remembered more easily.
  - Elaboration—instructing Gage in how to identify key elements of new information and to create relationships or associations with previously learned material.
  - Visual imagery—showing him how to visualize and make a "mental picture" of information to be learned.
- When studying for several tests or doing multiple homework assignments on the same day, similar subject material should be separated in order to lessen interference.
- Gage should be provided with periodic review of previously learned material in order to enhance long-term retention.

Additional suggestions for the classroom and academic issues include:

- Accommodations will be necessary to enhance Gage's ability to succeed in the classroom, including preferential seating; a reduction in the amount, but not the difficulty level, of assignments; and additional time to complete assignments if necessary.
- Tests should be in multiple choice/matching/short-answer formats instead of essay format and should be administered individually if necessary, with additional time provided as needed.
- Gage should be allowed and encouraged to use various compensatory devices, such as a calculator to check written calculations and a computer with word processing capability.
- Study skills training will be warranted, emphasizing such techniques as the appropriate outlining of lecture notes and how to study for tests. Gage also will benefit from being taught how to take notes on text material and plan written reports using an outlining method.
- In a related vein, training in word processing is strongly encouraged.
- Gage also may require instruction on how to organize and plan his approach to novel tasks as executive functioning is an area of weakness for him. This is particularly true for subject matter in which he is weaker, such as written expression.
- In addition, direct instruction in basic organizational and self-regulation strategies will assist Gage in knowing what to do, when to do it, and how to do it. Specifically, he should be guided in the use of checklists and other organizational aids, such as a daily planner.
- Finally, Gage should continue to be followed by his rehabilitation medicine specialist for medical management of his improving left hemiparesis and ADHD. Periodic neuropsychological reevaluation also would be beneficial in order to monitor changes in higher cortical functioning as Gage progresses through middle and high school.

Further Discussion of Case Study

It is important to note that the range of types of case studies to illustrate pediatric TBI is essentially infinite due to the range of possible deficits based on differences in type, location, and severity of injury as well as the interaction of other variables, such as age, premorbid functioning, and environmental factors. This particular case dealt with deficits in academic functioning and executive and constructional skills, with relatively typical functioning in emotional and behavioral domains; differences also were observed between verbal memory (strength) and visual memory for spatial location (weakness). Other TBI cases may look very different depending on the nature of the injury; the injury may manifest as profound changes in emotional or behavioral functioning (e.g., severe irritability, impulsivity, depression, violent behaviors), which will require very different intervention approaches from those recommended for our case study. Our case study also demonstrates how functioning can change over time, in this case with improved academic functioning in reading but continued difficulty in math and science (with less severe difficulties in other academic subjects) as well as worsening attention problems, which improved with medication treatment. These changes postinjury suggest the importance of progress monitoring and regular follow-up assessment.

CONCLUDING COMMENTS

The study of deficits in pediatric TBI provides an excellent illustration of one of the core tenets of developmental psychopathology: In order to understand abnormal development, we must first understand normal development. Knowing the typical course of development during childhood provides researchers and clinicians with a map with which to detect the type and severity of cognitive, academic, emotional, behavioral, motor, and language deficits associated with TBI. These deficits can be identified only if we know what typical development in these areas looks like. Thus, advances in the study of normal development contribute to our knowledge of abnormal development and deficits following TBI.

Currently there is only limited information on empirically supported interventions with children with TBI (Bowen, 2005). Many studies are characterized by small sample sizes (often under 30 children with TBI) as well as statistical and methodological limitations, such as limited consideration of generalization and maintenance of treatment effects (Laatsch et al., 2007; Ylvisaker et al., 2007). Taylor (2004) identified the need for more research on the relationship between specific forms of neuropathology associated with TBI and neuropsychological outcomes, including outcomes related to language functioning and other cognitive and behavioral variables; he also articulated the need for studies to employ measures of discrete skills rather than global measures (e.g., IQ tests) in order to gain information about the more narrow abilities impacted by TBI. The TBI literature also is in great need of randomized controlled trials in order to provide a better research base for interventions following pediatric TBI (Teasell et al., 2007).

One of the more remarkable observations from the literature is the degree of variability in deficits, prognosis, and outcome among children and adolescents with TBI (Farmer et al., 1999; Haak & Livingston, 1997; Moran & Gillon, 2004; Stuss et al., 1994). That is, even when group differences in functioning are found between children with and without TBI, there is a wide range of variability among those with TBI, and this variability is seen across different areas of functioning. This variability is likely due to the fact that children with TBI are a heterogeneous group in terms of type, severity, and location of injury. Thus, interventions to address deficits following TBI should be based on the unique constellation of symptoms within the individual child, and understanding of these symptoms relies on comprehensive assessment. Finally, changes in functioning may occur quickly among children with TBI, suggesting the importance of close monitoring and frequent reevaluation of functioning in order to assess changes related to development or recovery and to develop appropriate programming based on the child's individual needs (Wetherington & Hooper, 2006).

Chapter 9

CHILDHOOD CANCER

DEFINITION

Childhood cancer is more common than many realize, occurring in 1 in 300 children under the age of 16 (Armstrong & Briery, 2004); only accidents cause more deaths in children from infancy to early adulthood (W. A. Bleyer, 1999). The types of cancer usually seen in children vary greatly from those in adults and include leukemias, brain and other nervous system tumors, lymphomas (lymph node cancers), bone cancers, soft tissue sarcomas, kidney cancers, eye cancers, and adrenal gland cancers (American Cancer Society [ACS], 2006). The most frequent types of cancers include the leukemias and particularly acute lymphocytic leukemia (ALL) (Pieters & Carroll, 2008) as well as solid tumors (e.g., gliomas, medulloblastomas, astrocytoma, neuroblastoma, and Wilms' tumor).

Leukemias

Leukemia is the most common form of cancer in children, accounting for almost one-third of all cancers in children under the age of 15 and one-fourth of cancers occurring before age 20 (ACS, 2006; Pui & Evans, 1998). *Leukemia* refers to a heterogeneous group of neoplastic diseases that are characterized by the proliferation of abnormal white cells (leukocytes) and their precursors (Berg & Linton, 1997). The large number of early-stage white cells blocks the production of normal white blood cells; this impedes the child's ability to fight infection.

Four main types of leukemia are classified according to whether they are chronic or acute. The most common types include two acute and two chronic: acute lymphocytic leukemia (ALL), acute myelogenous leukemia (AML), chronic lymphocytic leukemia (CLL), and chronic myelogenous leukemia (CML). ALL is the most common of these types; it accounts for about 75% to 95% of all childhood leukemias (ACS, 2006; Berg & Linton, 1997; Margolin, Steuber, & Poplack, 2002; R. W. Miller, Young, & Novakovic, 1995). Most often, ALL is diagnosed in young children, with diagnoses peaking in children aged 2 to 3 years. With ALL, there is abnormal growth and division of specific white cells that begin in the lymphoblasts in the bone marrow and spread through the rest of the body. AML usually is diagnosed within the first 2 years of life and is much less common in older children. The diagnosis of AML starts to pick up again during the teenage years, however, and is the most common leukemia in adulthood (ACS, 2006). ALL is slightly more common among Caucasian children than African

American and Asian American children; it occurs more with equal frequency across gender and ethnic groups.

Lymphoblastic lymphoma accounts for about 30% of lymphomas in children (ACS, 2006). Lymphoblastic lymphoma is most common in teenagers; boys are twice as likely as girls to have lymphoblastic lymphoma. Most cases of lymphoblastic lymphoma develop from a mass in the area behind the breast bone, which can interfere with breathing. Less often, lymphoblastic lymphoma may develop in the tonsils, lymph nodes of the neck, or other lymph nodes. It can spread very quickly to the bone marrow, other lymph nodes, the surface of the brain, and/or the membranes that surround the lungs and heart. The malignant cells of this lymphoma are the same as those in ALL in children. Thus, if more than 25% of the bone marrow is involved, the disease is reclassified as leukemia and treated as leukemia (ACS, 2006).

Staging is the method for classifying cancers in terms of their progression; however, leukemia is not staged like other forms of cancer because it starts in the bone marrow and blood. For leukemia, progression of disease is determined by the collection of cancer cells in other organs, such as the liver, spleen, or lymph nodes (ACS, 2006). Based on the presence of cancer cells in other locations, children with ALL and AML are divided into low-risk, standard-risk, high-risk, and very high-risk categories. Some of the signs and symptoms of leukemia may include fatigue, paleness of the skin, infection, easy bleeding or bruising, bone pain, swelling of the abdomen, swollen lymph nodes, enlargement of the thymus gland, headache, seizures, vomiting, rashes, gum problems, and/or weakness. Diagnosis is made on the basis of a combination of laboratory tests (e.g., blood smear, bone marrow aspiration and biopsy, spinal tap, lymph node biopsy) and imaging results (ACS, 2006).

Tumors

Brain tumors account for 15% to 20% of pediatric cancers (R. W. Butler & Mulhern, 2005). The most common types of tumors include medulloblastoma, ependymoma, gliomas, and gangliogliomas (R. W. Butler & Mulhern, 2005; Strother et al., 2002). Of these, medulloblastoma is the most frequent; medulloblastomas often are located in posterior fossa (Ries et al., 2005). Tumors are defined as atypical, uncontrolled growth of cells at the expense of healthy cells; these atypical cells do not serve any functional purpose (Zillmer et al., 2008). Infiltrating tumors are those tumors that invade neighboring areas of the brain and destroy surrounding tissue; most common are the gliomas (arise from glial cells). In contrast, noninfiltrating tumors are those tumors that are encapsulated, well differentiated, and noninvasive. Tumors also are classified as benign, metastic, or malignant. Benign tumors usually are surrounded by a capsule, are noninvasive, and pose low risk of regrowth. Metastic tumors are encapsulated but malignant tumors; these arise secondary to cancerous tumors that are in other parts of the body (e.g., in lungs, colon, pancreas). They are formed from cancerous cells that become detached and can travel throughout the body via the circulatory system. In contrast to the encapsulated tumors, the cells of malignant tumors invade other tissue, and there is usually regrowth even when the tumor is removed. Tumors are classified further by "grade" depending on the cell type and level of malignancy; if there is no malignancy, this is a grade 1 while a malignant tumor that has metastasized extensively is a grade 4. The classification of brain tumors is based on the premise that each type of tumor results from the abnormal growth of a specific cell type. To the extent that the behavior of a tumor correlates with basic cell type, tumor classification dictates the choice of therapy and predicts medical prognosis. Size and location as well as treatment are predictive of neurocognitive prognosis.

The most common of the malignant tumors is medulloblastoma, accounting for about two-thirds of all tumors in children. Medulloblastoma is a rapidly growing malignant tumor that is located in the inferior vermis (cerebellum) close to the fourth ventricle and the posterior fossa (Ries et al., 1999). Because of their location, medulloblastomas give rise to intracranial pressure and hydrocephalus. The initial presentation generally includes nonspecific symptoms of headache, lethargy, and vomiting; these are believed to be due to the increased intracranial pressure (Zillmer et al., 2008). The nonspecific nature of the symptoms may lead to delays in identification (Blaney et al., 2006). The location of medulloblastomas is associated with specific deficits in survivors of this type of childhood cancer.

Prevalence and Incidence

As one indication of the incidence of childhood cancer, in the United States in 2007, approximately 10,400 children under age 15 were diagnosed with cancer and about 1,545 children would die from the disease (ACS, 2006). Although this makes cancer the leading cause of death by disease among U.S. children 1 to 14 years of age, cancer is still relatively rare in this age group. On average, 1 to 2 children develop the disease each year for every 10,000 children in the United States (Ries et al., 2005). The incidence varies, however, by age and type of cancer. The incidence of childhood leukemia appeared to rise in the early 1980s, with rates increasing from 3.3 cases per 100,000 in 1975 to 4.6 cases per 100,000 in 1985. Rates in the succeeding years have shown no consistent upward or downward trend and have ranged from 3.7 to 4.9 cases per 100,000 (Ries et al., 2005). ALL and central nervous system tumors account for more than half of all cases newly identified (R. W. Butler & Haser, 2006). The incidence of ALL peaks in early childhood, at about 4 to 5 years of age, with 2,500 to 3,500 new cases identified each year (R. W. Butler & Mulhern, 2005). In contrast, the median age for diagnosis of AML is 9 years of age (ACS, 2006). ALL and other childhood cancers occur across ethnic groups with similar presentation and neurocognitive sequelae regardless of country (Petridou et al., 2008).

For childhood brain tumors, the overall incidence rose from 1975 through 2004, from 2.3 to 3.2 cases per 100,000 (Ries et al., 2005), with the greatest increase occurring from 1983 through 1986. This increase may reflect advances in medical technology that improved the diagnosis of brain tumors, changes in the classification of brain tumors, and improvements in neurosurgical techniques for biopsying brain tumors. Regardless of the explanation for the increase in incidence that occurred from 1983 to 1986, the incidence of childhood brain tumor has been essentially stable since the mid-1980s. The incidence of brain tumor is estimated at 3.3 to 4.03 per 100,000 (R. W. Butler & Mulhern, 2005). The peak incidence of medulloblastoma is 5 years of age; medulloblastoma occurs twice as often in boys as girls (Gottardo & Gajjar, 2006).

ETIOLOGY

No definitive cause has been identified for childhood cancers, particularly ALL (Mulhern & Butler, 2004). Genetic and environmental causes have been identified but do not account for the majority of childhood cancers. Certain genetic syndromes (e.g., LiFraumeni syndrome, neurofibromatosis, tuberous sclerosis, and Gorlin syndrome) have been linked to an increased risk of specific childhood cancers (Melean, Sestini, Ammannati, & Papi, 2004; Mulhern & Butler, 2004). In addition, children with Down syndrome (see Chapter 15) have an increased risk of developing leukemia (Mulhern & Butler, 2004). Additional genetic influences and environmental influences in conjunction with prognosis have been explored (Pieters & Carroll, 2008).

Genetic

For leukemias, the etiology is believed to involve multiple genetic alterations in preleukemic cells that begins in utero and is evident in the presence of TEL/AML1 gene fusion or hyperdiploidy in neonatal blood spots (Greaves, 2006). Hyperdiploidy is said to occur when there is a DNA index of 1.16 or more than 50 chromosomes per leukemia cell; hyperdiploidy is evident in about 50% of those with B-lineage ALL and is associated with a positive prognosis (Pieters & Carroll, 2008). The TEL/AML1 fusion is evident in about 25% of cases and reflects a fusion of the TEL gene on chromosome 12 with the AML1 gene on chromosome 21 (Ramakers-van Woerden et al., 2000). Although these preleukemia cells may be present at birth and are associated with more positive outcomes, the majority of these children do not develop leukemia so its utility for screening purposes is limited (Fischer et al., 2007). An additional genetic marker includes various abnormalities of the mixed lineage leukemia (MLL) gene at 11q23. The MLL marker is present in about 80% of infants with leukemia but in only about 2% of children who develop leukemia after the first year (Jansen et al., 2007; Pieters & Carroll, 2008). The translocation of the BCR gene on chromosome 22 with the ABL gene on chromosome 9 is less common in children but present in 25% of adults with leukemia and is associated with poorer outcome (Pieters & Carroll, 2008). T-cell ALL is another genetic component; prognosis is determined in part by most genetic markers, except in the case of T-cell (Pieters & Carroll, 2008).

The underlying mechanisms to the pathogenesis of brain tumors involve the increased expression for proto-oncogenes (i.e., growth-promoting factors) that precipitate uncontrolled cell growth and the inactivation of those tumor suppressor genes (i.e., those genes that act to suppress cell growth). It is the disruption of these normal restraints that allows for the cell proliferation that gives rise to tumors (Menkes & Till, 1995). Further, some tumors are congenital and result from an area of where neural development was disrupted (Menkes & Till, 1995).

Environmental

There are some indications that viruses may be responsible for the disruption of neural development that gives rise to congenital tumors (White, 2005). Other known risk factors include gender, with males being more susceptible; cured meat in the maternal diet during pregnancy; and family history of cancer (Gurney et al., 1999). Pesticides have been suspected to be involved in the development of certain forms of childhood cancer (Wigle et al., 2008); however, research to date has been equivocal (see Chapter 13). Similarly, a link between maternal cigarette smoking before pregnancy and childhood cancers has not been supported consistently. High levels of ionizing radiation from accidents or from radiotherapy have been linked with increased risk of some childhood cancers (Wigle et al., 2008). Children with cancer treated with chemotherapy and/or radiation therapy may be at increased risk for developing a second primary cancer (Gurney, 2007). For example, certain types of chemotherapy, including alkylating agents or topoisomerase II inhibitors (e.g., epipodophyllotoxins), can cause an increased risk of leukemia. Recent research has shown that children with AIDS (acquired immunodeficiency syndrome), like adults with AIDS, have an increased risk of developing certain cancers, predominantly non-Hodgkin lymphoma; however, little evidence has been found to link specific viruses or other infectious agents to the development of most types of childhood cancers. Some potential environmental factors have been eliminated; these include low levels of radiation exposure from indoor radon and exposure to ultrasound during pregnancy (Gurney, 2007).

COURSE AND PROGNOSIS

With significant advances in the treatment of these cancers, it is estimated that 60% to 90% of children with childhood cancer will survive 5 years or more (W. A. Bleyer, 1990; Ries et al., 2005). For children with ALL, the survival rate at 5 years is currently 70% with the majority of children with ALL living into adulthood; the comparable rate is 53% for children with AML (ACS, 2006). For children with tumors, the 5-year survival rate is estimated at 70% (Bleyer, 1999). Astrocytomas arise from astrocytes and grow more slowly than other tumors that arise from glial cells and typically affect cranial nerves V, VI, VII, and X. Because of their slower growth, astrocytomas are associated with a better prognosis than other infiltrating tumors (Zillmer et al., 2008).That said, because of the many different types of childhood cancer, the treatment protocol, prognosis, and other illness-related factors may vary considerably. With immaturity of preleukemia cells, leukemia in infancy has a poor prognosis, whereas the prognosis improves after the age of 1 and through about age 9, with variability due to genetic predisposition (L. K. Campbell et al., 2009; Pieters & Carroll, 2008). Because leukocytes, erythrocytes, and platelets are involved in fighting infection, clotting, and transporting oxygen, children with ALL are susceptible to infection, hemorrhage, and anemia. This susceptibility further compounds their risk for poorer outcomes.

Treatment effects rather than the disease process are implicated in the long-term course and prognosis. In many cases, treatment for brain tumor includes intrathecal (direct injection into the subarachnoid space) and intravenous injection of neurotoxins (e.g., methotrexate) in conjunction with 1,800 to 2,400 rad of cranial irradiation (Palmer et al., 2008). Treatment side effects have included significant memory and learning problems with some evidence of more right-hemisphere involvement than left (Copeland et al., 1988; Copeland, Moore, Francis, Jaffe, & Culbert, 1996; Moleski, 2000). Results of follow-up studies of children who survive cancer suggest that, regardless of the type of cancer, if it is diagnosed prior to age 5, there is a high probability of cognitive difficulties (Copeland et al., 1988, 1996). Regardless of type of cancer, central nervous system (CNS) irradiation results in general lowering of scores across tasks but particularly in nonlanguage skill areas. For survivors of childhood cancer, where the malignancy and/or treatment involved the CNS, there is often a consistent pattern of deficits (R. W. Butler, Copeland et al., 2008).

Outcome for children with cancer is directly related to the treatment received; options may include craniospinal radiation and chemotherapy (Mabbott, Penkman, Witol, Strother, & Bouffet, 2008). Surgery for tumors is an additional option and can have transient effects on speech and language skills due to connections between the cerebellum and frontal areas; surgery also may result in long-term deficits across domains of speech/language, visual-spatial, and problem solving/self-regulation (Aarsen, van Dongen, Paquier, van Mourik, & Catsman-Berrevoets, 2004; Beebe et al., 2005; Steinlin, 2008). Figure 9.1 is a postsurgical magnetic resonance image for a tumor that demonstrates the extent of brain tissue that may be excised in tumor removal. Despite some changes in the treatment protocols, over 30% of childhood cancer survivors demonstrate some degree of impairment (Mulhern & Butler, 2006). Among those with tumors, the incidence of some degree of impairment increases to 40% to 100% (Glauser & Packer, 1991; Mabbott et al., 2005), but it may be less apparent or severe. For example, with 31 children under 16 years of age who were diagnosed with astrocytoma, 21 of 31 survived beyond 5 years, and neurological sequelae were found in 43% (Zuzak et al., 2008). For those who also develop hydrocephalus, there are additional potential complications as a result of the shunting. Although cognitive deficits lead to significant school problems in 19% and behavioral and emotional adjustment disturbances in 27%, all individuals evidenced age-appropriate ability to perform daily life activities. Further, cancer survivors rated their health-related quality of life similar or higher than healthy controls (Zuzak et al., 2008).

Neurological Correlates

Neurological changes following chemotherapy and radiation have been identified, particularly in white matter (Mulhern et al., 1999; Reddick et al., 1998, 2005; Shan et al., 2006). Chemotherapy for ALL, for example, is associated with decreased white matter volume, particularly in the right prefrontal cortex (Carey et al., 2008; Reddick et al., 2006). For radiation, the mechanism of effects is believed to be through disruption of the developmental process of myelination (Coderre et al., 2006) as well as functioning of the main commissures of the brain (Palmer et al., 2002). Studies further suggest that neurocognitive dysfunction may be associated with the impairment of hippocampal neurogenesis (Fan et al., 2007). Subregions of the corpus callosum that normally are expected to have a high rate of growth in childhood (Giedd et al., 1999) are significantly smaller in childhood survivors treated with radiation (Palmer et al., 2002). Further, computed tomography findings indicate cerebral atrophy, focal and diffuse white matter lesions, and enlarged ventricles in children who have received radiation treatment (Constine, Konski, Ekholm, McDonald, & Rubin, 1988). White matter volume is, in turn, related to the extent of cognitive decline (Mulhern et al., 2004). In contrast, no difference in gray matter was found (Reddick et al., 1998).

Neurocognitive Correlates

Most important, neuropsychological deficits may not be evident immediately but may present over time; these deficits are believed to progress and persist over time as well (Mulhern & Butler, 2004; Palmer et al., 2003). Studies suggest the need for follow-up with nearly 40% of childhood cancer survivors evidencing late effects (Blaauwbroek, Groenier, Kamps, Meyboom-de Jong, & Postma, 2007). At the same time, these children are also at increased risk for deleterious effects on higher-order cognitive functioning and achievement, at least in part as a result of the treatments (Daly, Kral, & Brown, 2008). Similarly, with tumors, survivors evidence long-term cognitive, academic, and vocational impairments (Mabbott et al., 2005). These risks were compounded by factors of age, gender, with females at greater risk, lower level of educational attainment, and socioeconomic status. Similar risk indicators were suggestive of lower quality of life (Zeltzer et al., 2008). Multiple indicators (rate of marriage, college education, employment, functional impairment) suggest increased risk for survivors of childhood cancer in many areas of life

(Mody et al., 2008). Despite these findings, in many instances, childhood cancer survivors were found to be psychologically healthy (Patenaude & Kupst, 2005; Zeltzer et al., 2008); alternatively, other studies suggest that survivors of childhood cancer are significantly at risk for both medical and psychological problems in adulthood (Hudson et al., 2003). Most frequently, whether ALL or tumor, the neurocognitive deficits identified are in areas of memory, attention, processing speed, and fluid abilities (Mulhern & Butler, 2004), with collateral effects on general intellectual function and academic achievement (R. W. Butler & Haser, 2006; Palmer et al., 2001). Cerebellar tumors, for example, are most associated with deficits in visual-spatial, language, and memory functions (Mickelwright, King, Morris, & Morris, 2007; Steinlin, 2008).

In support of the notion that effects on cognition are collateral, up to 45% of variance in cognitive ability (IQ) was accounted for by working memory and processing speed in one study (Schatz, Kramer, Albin, & Matthay, 2000). There has also been some discussion of whether survivors of pediatric brain tumors exhibit a pattern of performance consistent with nonverbal learning disability (Carey, Barakat, Foley, Gyato, & Phillips, 2001; Espy et al., 2001; Reeb & Regan, 1998). Survivors of childhood cancer were more likely to report repeating a grade and having more school absences (Gerhardt et al., 2007). Further, Espy et al. (2001) found that childhood cancer survivors evidenced modest declines in arithmetic, visual-motor integration, and verbal fluency. In particular, intrathecal and systemic treatment was associated with poorer visual-motor integration and a faster rate of decline in visual-motor integration skills as compared to intrathecal treatment alone. Carey and colleagues (2001) found a trend for a positive association between nonverbal scores and social function, possibly related to white matter damage of the right hemisphere. Discussion of research findings by domain is presented next; specific deficits based on research associated with childhood cancer are detailed in Table 9.1.

Cognition

Follow-up of children treated for ALL indicated declines in IQ and less-than-expected achievement in both reading and mathematics (Peckham, 1991). Poor intellectual outcome is associated with higher radiation dosage, larger area, younger age, and medical complications (Ris, Packer, Goldwein, Jones-Wallace, & Boyett, 2001). The lower intellectual ability is believed to be associated with compromised white matter integrity (Khong et al., 2006; Mabbott, Noseworthy, Bouffet, Rockel, & Laughlin, 2006) as well as secondary to difficulties with attention, memory, and processing speed (Palmer, Reddick, & Gajjar, 2007). Further, a trend for better verbal skills compared to nonverbal skills was found using composite scores for one sample (Carey et al., 2001). Thus, the pattern of strengths and weaknesses associated with childhood cancer is more consistent with specific learning disabilities as opposed to diffuse lowering of abilities.

Learning and Memory

Memory deficits are reported to be the most frequent and severe delayed effect of radiation therapy (e.g., for brain tumor). Immediate effects, within two to three months after completion of treatment, tend to be mild and temporary. Later on, however, there are more severe impairments that are irreversible and may be progressive. Radiation selectively impairs verbal-semantic memory and particularly retrieval. As the end point of memory, retrieval requires reconstruction of information in consciousness with information stored in memory. Memory difficulties in verbal areas remain fairly stable; problems with visual memory get worse over time (Spiegler, Bouffet, Greenberg, Rutka, & Mabbott, 2004). The extent of memory deficit may depend on treatment protocol and timing. Alternatively,

Table 9.1 Deficits Following Treatment for Childhood Cancer

Domain	Status Following Treatment
Cognition	Not impaired initially but gradually declines Nonverbal reasoning may be affected
Auditory-linguistic/Language function	Generally, vocabulary and comprehension spared Naming fluency/retrieval impaired
Visual perception/Constructional praxis	Visual-perceptual ability impaired Visual-motor integration impaired Perceptual motor skills impaired Visual-motor/constructional skills impaired
Processing speed	Information processing speed/sluggish cognitive tempo
Learning and Memory	Short-term memory impaired Verbal memory impaired Nonverbal memory/visual memory impaired Working memory impaired Recognition skills tend to be spared
Attention/Concentration	Attention: focused, selective, and sustained tend to be impaired Attentional flexibility also impaired
Executive function	Sequencing impaired Fluid abilities and problem solving impaired Cognitive flexibility impaired
Achievement/Academic skills	Arithmetic achievement affected negatively Learning in general slowed
Emotional/Behavioral functioning	Difficulties with coping and emotion regulation evident in conjunction with executive function deficits

extent and type of memory deficit may depend on location for tumors. For example, tumors at the third ventricle are associated with deficits on list learning tasks for retrieval but not for recognition (Mickelwright et al., 2007).

Attention

Problems with sustained attention also are evident following treatment for brain tumor (Reeves et al., 2006); however, across studies, results relative to sustained attention are equivocal (Mabbott et al., 2008; Mulhern & Butler, 2004; Mulhern et al., 2004). Studies examining attention, inhibition, and processing speed using continuous performance tests (Mulhern et al., 2004; Reddick et al., 2006) consistently indicated impaired attention as well as decreased processing speed (increased latency).

Executive Function

With potential effects to the prefrontal cortex (Carey et al., 2008; Reddick et al., 2006), there tends to be executive function deficits; several studies have confirmed executive function deficits in children with a history of cancer and chemotherapy (V. Anderson, Godber, Smibert, & Ekert, 1997; L. K. Campbell et al., 2007; Carey et al., 2008). Children experienced difficulties in attention/concentration, memory, and sequencing. Consistent with these findings, impaired performance on working memory, behavioral inhibition, cognitive flexibility, and self-monitoring are frequent in children who have been treated for ALL; these impairments have been found to be associated with stress, behavior, and coping strategies that ultimately affect quality of life (L. K. Campbell et al., 2008).

Processing Speed

Slow processing speed has been associated with cranial radiation for ALL (Palmer et al., 2007; Reeves et al., 2007; Schatz et al., 2000). Decreased processing speed is further evident in studies of neurocognitive late effects associated with childhood cancer treatments (Askins & Moore, 2008).

Educational Implications

For children with childhood cancer, the longitudinal picture suggests that there is a slower rate of skill acquisition that ultimately creates a "Matthew effect" (Palmer et al., 2001). Academic difficulties are high and frequently are the impetus for neuropsychological evaluation; special education services may be indicated for those who are affected at younger ages and those who receive higher doses of cranial radiation (Mitby et al., 2003). Areas affected include reading decoding skills and spelling skills; those diagnosed prior to age 7 demonstrated the most significant effect. Survivors of tumors are much more likely to be retained; they are also less likely to finish high school (Mitby et al., 2003), which ultimately affects their capability to live independently (R. W. Butler & Mulhern, 2005).

A majority of medulloblastoma survivors continue to experience academic failure and significant learning delays (Palmer et al., 2007). Research suggests that 70% of brain tumor survivors who had received radiation therapy at age 6 or younger were receiving special education services (Mitby et al., 2003). For children with medulloblastomas or posterior fossa tumors, declines in academic areas continued to be evident across reading, math, and written expression for two or more years (Mabbott et al., 2005). The deficits among those with childhood cancer are not transient, and in fact, some studies indicate a continued decline in cognitive ability over time (Palmer et al., 2003; Ris et al., 2001; Speigler et al., 2004). Radiation is most likely to be associated with school problems (Bhat et al., 2005; Mitby et al., 2003). When treated with radiation, children are more likely to experience a decline in rate of skill acquisition (Palmer et al., 2001; Speigler et al., 2004). Because there is a slower rate of skill acquisition, these children tend to fall farther and farther behind, and this impacts their overall functioning (Mulhern et al., 2004; Palmer et al., 2007); they also are less likely to complete high school (Mitby et al., 2003).

One particular academic area impacted by survivors of childhood cancer is mathematics (Kaemingk, Carey, Moore, Herzer, & Hutter, 2004). Difficulties in math are the most frequently reported area of academic deficit in conjunction with ALL. Comparison of healthy controls matched for age and sex, as well as to normative levels, with a group of ALL survivors yielded converging evidence for math difficulties in the ALL group. The difficulties in math seemed to be related to memory function and psychomotor speed for the ALL group rather than basic reading skills and visual-motor integration (Kaemingk et al., 2004).

Emotional/Behavioral Implications

There is some indication of social-emotional and behavioral problems, including a number of symptoms associated with posttraumatic stress disorder (PTSD), among survivors of childhood cancer. Among tumor survivors, there are some indications of significant social deficits and a tendency for greater internalizing behavior problems

(Carey et al., 2001). Follow-up of children with tumors (n = 137) found that children with low-grade gliomas had the highest reported health-related quality of life (Bhat et al., 2005). Surprisingly, the children with the lowest health-related quality of life were those who received radiation therapy but no chemotherapy; those who received both radiation and chemotherapy had better reported health-related quality of life (Bhat et al., 2005).

Children with chronic illness, including those with childhood cancers, face a variety of stressful circumstances that require coping responses, indicating a need for preventive work (Kazak et al., 2007). Early findings indicate that certain functional areas may be affected by chronic illness, including social-emotional functioning and family functioning (Garrison & McQuiston, 1989). Childhood illness appears to function as a stressor that, in combination with other variables, may contribute to increased risk but is not the sole cause of adjustment difficulties. Despite the potential for psychopathology, findings from longitudinal studies indicated that most children demonstrate improvements in adjustment and functioning over time. A recent review of the research suggests that, across studies, survivors of childhood cancer are best described as demonstrating "hardiness," with rates of psychopathology below or equal to those found in the normal population (Noll & Kupst, 2007).

At the same time, there is a small subset of children with cancer who have serious psychological difficulties (Patenaude & Kupst, 2005; Stuber & Kazak, 1999). It has been suggested that differential coping and adjustment may depend on the child's developmental stage during diagnosis and treatment (Eiser, Hill, & Vance, 2000; Patenaude & Kupst, 2005). The problems often reported include anxiety, fear, depression, extreme dependency on parents, sleep disturbance, regression, anger, and withdrawal (Apter, Farbstein, & Yaniv, 2003; Van Dongen-Melman & Sanders-Woudstra, 1986). Distress in one area of life may occur despite generally good functioning in other areas (Patenaude & Kupst, 2005). Two main areas of functioning for the child with cancer that often are affected are social adjustment with peers and emotional well-being (Vannatta & Gerhardt, 2003). Parental ratings regarding the effects of treatment on their children included observed concerns of: social isolation, excitability, tendency to brood, concentration problems, aggression, and sleep disturbances (Noll & Kupst, 2007).

There remains controversy surrounding whether pediatric illness should be included as a stressor as delineated under PTSD (Noll & Kupst, 2007; Phipps, Long, Hudson, & Rai, 2005); subjective responses to diagnosis and treatment can include feelings of fear, horror, and helplessness (Stuber, 2006). A subset of children demonstrate symptoms reflective of the traumatic nature of cancer diagnosis and treatment (Kazak et al., 2001). Predominant studies have found rates of posttraumatic symptoms in 1.6% to 21% (Stuber, 2006) of childhood cancer survivors. These findings have indicated several factors that seem to increase the chances that PTSD concerns will arise in certain children, including age, female gender, family and social support, history of previous trauma, the child's level of anxiety, experience of painful or traumatic experiences during the treatment process, and his or her subjective appraisal of the threat of the illness (Apter et al., 2003; Stuber & Kazak, 1999). Consistent with Noll and Kupst's (2007) contention of hardiness, however, research suggests that survivors of childhood cancer demonstrate fewer PTSD symptoms than survivors of other stressful events (Phipps et al., 2005).

Most investigations of the psychological impact of cancer diagnosis and treatment on pediatric survivors have found that the majority of survivors are functioning well (Noll & Kupst, 2007; Stuber & Kazak, 1999). Within this group of children, several areas of psychosocial adjustment have been shown to be relatively resilient in the face of cancer diagnosis and treatment, including social development (Apter et al., 2003). Recent reviews of the literature have identified factors that seem to impact adjustment (Patenaude & Kupst, 2005). These factors include time since diagnosis, age at diagnosis, previous adjustment and functioning, degree of perceived stress, cognitive ability, family adaptability/cohesiveness, and associated family characteristics (Patenaude & Kupst, 2005). In other situations, an excess of problem behaviors has been found for childhood cancer survivors relative to healthy controls (Buizer, de Sonneville, van den Heuvel-Eibrink, & Veerman, 2006). The Children's Oncology Group Long-term Follow-up Guidelines Task Force on Neurocognitive/Behavioral Complications After Childhood Cancer developed guidelines related to the follow-up care of survivors of childhood cancer based on a comprehensive literature review and expert opinions (Nathan et al., 2007). Nathan et al. further provided additional recommendations for the screening and management of neurocognitive late effects as well as critical areas of school and legal advocacy that may be of interest for survivors of childhood cancer who have disabilities.

EVIDENCE-BASED INTERVENTIONS

As with all disorders, interventions to address neurocognitive deficits among children with cancer should draw on those neurocognitive domains that have been spared (Armstrong & Briery, 2004). Typically, auditory-linguistic domains are spared among childhood cancer survivors, while visual-motor, processing speed, and executive functions, including attention and memory, may be impaired (see Table 9.1). As such, a strong intervention program will emphasize language-based learning and decrease the emphasis on visual-motor learning and output (Daly et al., 2008). Interventions may take the form of medical approaches (e.g., medication), behavioral approaches, or cognitive approaches (see Table 9.2). The implementation of intervention training during treatment may be a proactive approach to minimizing the subsequent deficits, but this requires further study (Palmer et al., 2007).

Medication

The presence of many behaviors associated with attention deficit hyperactivity disorder (ADHD; see Chapter 6) and well-established research to support the use of stimulant medications to address these behaviors led to the consideration of stimulant medication to address the inattention problems that occur subsequent to treatment for ALL or brain tumor. Studies with clinical trials demonstrated both positive effects and no adverse effects (Conklin et al., 2007; Daly & Brown, 2007; Mulhern & Butler, 2004; S. J. Thompson et al., 2001).

Educational Interventions

One key component to successful school reentry and positive educational outcome is close collaboration among medical professionals, school staff, and family (Upton & Eiser, 2006). Research suggests that children who make a successful return to school following treatment of childhood cancer demonstrate a more positive outcome (Prevatt, Heffer, & Lowe, 2000). One of the most important aspects of intervention is the education of family members and educational professionals about the potential cognitive outcomes of

Table 9.2 Evidence-Based Status for Interventions with Childhood Cancer

Interventions	Target	Status
Stimulant medication	Attentional problems	Promising practice (Conklin et al., 2007; Daly & Brown, 2007; S. J. Thompson et al., 2001)
Attention Process Training (APT) in combination with brain injury rehabilitation	Vigilance and concentration	Emerging (R. W. Butler & Copeland, 2002)
Cognitive-behavioral therapy in a family systems context	Stress, trauma of diagnosis and treatment	Emerging (Kazak et al., 2004)
Teen Outreach Program (TOP)	Psychosocial effects	Emerging (Shama & Lucchetta, 2007)
Survivor Health and Resilience Education (SHARE)	Healthy lifestyle and prevention of late effects	Emerging (Donze & Tercyak, 2006; Tercyak, Donze, Prahlad, Mosher, & Shad, 2006)
Surviving Cancer Competently Intervention Program (SCCIP©)	Anxiety, depression	Emerging (Kazak, 2005; Kazak et al., 1999)
Cognitive Remediation Program (CRP)	Attention, academic achievement	Emerging (R. W. Butler & Copeland, 2002; R. W. Butler, Copeland et al., 2008; R. W. Butler, Sahler et al., 2008)
Social skills training	Social skills	Emerging (Barakat et al., 2003)
Response-shift therapy	Quality of life	Emerging (C. E. Schwartz, Feinberg, Jilinskaia, & Applegate, 1999)

childhood cancers (Daly et al., 2008). In particular, it is important for professionals within the schools to be aware of the need for frequent monitoring in order to detect late effects and intervene appropriately.

Accommodations and modifications for children returning to school include a shortened day or the option for resting in the nurse's office if fatigue is a problem. Classroom modifications to help with attention (see Chapter 6) also may be beneficial. Given the evidence suggesting decreased processing speed, modification of the workload or time constraints may be appropriate as well.

One avenue for academic intervention is through cognitive remediation. A randomized clinical trial of the Cognitive Remediation Program (CRP) was conducted with 161 participants, ages 6 to 17 years, at multiple sites nationwide (R. W. Butler, Copeland et al., 2008). Results indicated that the CRP yielded parent report of improved attention and statistically significant increases in academic achievement. The effect sizes found with the CRP were modest; however, they were comparable with those for other clinical trials (R. W. Butler, Copeland et al., 2008).

Emotional/Behavioral Interventions

Psychosocial interventions related to procedural pain and distress have strong empirical support (Kazak, 2005). Less is known about the efficacy of approaches to other sequelae.

Regardless of whether cancer constitutes a stressor as conceptualized in PTSD, providing some level of psychological support and services is now considered an important component of comprehensive cancer treatment (American Academy of Pediatrics, 1997). The majority of studies published relating to psychological services are preventive in nature rather than reactive to psychological distress (Pai, Drotar, Zebracki, Moore, & Youngstrom, 2006). These interventions tended to be of short duration (i.e., fewer than 10 weekly sessions) and may have been delivered to parents or the children themselves. The focus of these interventions tended to be on problem solving and stress inoculation for parents and social skills and school reintegration for children. Pai and colleagues identified nine clinical trials that used a standardized treatment manual. Outcome measures (parental distress, child distress) varied across studies. Notably, meta-analytic results indicated modest support for interventions targeting parent distress and parent adjustment, with minimal support for interventions for child distress (Pai et al., 2006).

Other studies have focused on the disruption that occurs in the developmental process for adolescents with cancer (Shama & Lucchetta, 2007). The Teen Outreach Program (TOP) was developed to help teens with cancer connect with each other as well as reconnect with their peers. The program does this by engaging them in typical adolescent activities; results indicate positive effects on psychosocial health (Shama & Lucchetta, 2007). Other approaches have included cognitive reframing and response shift (i.e., reframing what is "normal"), with some indications that there was a positive effect on perceived quality of life (C. E. Schwartz et al., 1999). In effect, response-shift intervention seemed to have normalized adolescent cancer survivors' conceptualization of quality of life so that it was similar to their age-matched cohort.

One specific area of intervention has been social skills. For example, a manual-based, social skills training group intervention on the social skills and social functioning of children treated for brain tumors was implemented with assessment of the impact of cognitive functioning on the effectiveness of the intervention (Barakat et al., 2003). Results indicated that social skills and social functioning variables improved with small to medium effect sizes. Cognitive factors moderated the effects with higher verbal and nonverbal functioning associated with greater improvement. Other areas of functioning addressed have included attitude to follow-up, increase self-efficacy or confidence to care for health, and raise awareness of possible vulnerability to future health issues among survivors of childhood cancer (Eiser, Hill, & Blacklay, 2000). The intervention enhanced awareness among childhood survivors about the importance of follow-up and need for vigilance in their healthcare. Similarly, the Survivor Health and Resilience Education (SHARE) program was designed to address lifestyle and behavioral factors that may place survivors at increased risk for secondary cancers and other chronic diseases (Donze & Tercyak, 2006). Initial data suggested that the intervention has a positive effect. A randomized controlled trial further suggested that participation in SHARE may help prevent and control the onset and severity of late effects related to cancer treatment (Tercyak et al., 2006). Another program, the Surviving Cancer Competently Intervention Program (SCCIP©) is a cognitive-behavioral and family therapy intervention to address psychological reactions for survivors and their parents (Kazak et al., 1999). This one-day family group intervention combines cognitive-behavioral and family therapy approaches. The goals of SCCIP are to reduce symptoms of distress and to improve family functioning and development. Program evaluation data indicated that all family members found the program to be helpful, with decreased symptoms of posttraumatic stress and anxiety at 6-month follow-up.

CASE STUDY: DAVID—LYMPHOCYTIC LEUKEMIA

The next report is from a hospital-based clinic. Identifying information, such as child and family name, teacher or physician name, and school information, has been altered or fictionalized to protect confidentiality.

Reason for Referral

David is a 10-year-old fourth grader who is being followed by his pediatric hematology/oncology team for a history of lymphocytic leukemia (b-cell). Following diagnosis, David received chemotherapy that included methotrexate (Trexall), and he is now in remission. Following the diagnosis, David received homebound teacher services for the majority of the third-grade school year, returning to school in the fourth grade; however, David is now repeating the fourth grade due to difficulty concentrating/short attention span and difficulty completing assignments, all of which have resulted in poor homework and test grades. As a result, his hematologist/oncologist requested neuropsychological evaluation in order to assess higher cortical functioning two years after diagnosis and make appropriate recommendations regarding school placement and the need for supportive therapies.

Assessment Procedures

Clinical interview (parent)

Behavioral observations

Wechsler Intelligence Scale for Children, Fourth Edition (WISC-IV)

Wisconsin Card Sorting Test (WCST)

Neuropsychological Assessment (NEPSY)/Neuropsychological Assessment, Second Edition (NEPSY-2; selected subtests)

Peabody Picture Vocabulary Test, Fourth Edition (PPVT-IV)

Boston Naming Test (BNT)

Clinical Evaluation of Language Fundamentals, Fourth Edition (CELF-IV; selected subtests)

Kaufman Assessment Battery for Children, Second Edition (KABC-2; selected subtests)

Finger Oscillation Test

Clock Face Drawing Test

Delis-Kaplan Executive Function Scale (D-KEFS; selected subtest)

Beery Developmental Test of Visual Motor Integration, Fifth Edition (DTVMI-V)

Children's Memory Scale (CMS)

Gray Oral Reading Test, Fourth Edition (GORT-4)

Wide Range Achievement Test, Fourth Edition (WRAT-4)

Test of Written Language, Third Edition (TOWL-3)

Behavior Assessment System for Children, Second Edition (BASC-2; Parent and Teacher Rating Scales)

DSM-IV ADHD Checklist (Parent and Teacher)

Background Information

David resides with his mother and twin (fraternal) brother who is characterized as an A/B student in the fifth grade and is in good health. David's parents separated approximately one year after David's diagnosis and have not reconciled. David's father is 41 years of age, a high school graduate, who is currently employed as a supervisor at a tire manufacturing plant. According to his mother, David's father has a history of academic difficulty in the fourth and fifth grades. The paternal family history is significant for a 17-year-old male cousin with a history of emotional/behavioral difficulty who was expelled from high school and has not earned a high school equivalency diploma. David's mother is 40 years of age, a high school graduate, who is currently employed as a senior deposit service specialist with a local area credit union. She is reported to be in good health. The maternal family history is significant for an aunt who dropped out of school in the eleventh grade and earned a general equivalency diploma, an 8-year-old cousin who is being evaluated for ADHD, and a 17-year-old cousin who is repeating the ninth grade for the second time. Finally, David's mother reported that her husband has weekend visitation with the boys every other weekend; however, the boys have voiced considerable displeasure about having to visit their father.

Review of David's developmental and medical history indicates that he is the product of a 38.5-week twin pregnancy and vaginal delivery, weighing 5 pounds 7.5 ounces at birth. Following delivery, David experienced some mild jaundice, which required brief phototherapy. The twins went home with their mother from the hospital after 3 days. According to his mother, David attained his developmental motor milestones within normal limits with sitting up occurring at 8 months of age and walking at 13 months of age. Language milestones were also felt to be normal, with first words coming at 8 months of age; however, as David's language development progressed, an articulation disorder was noted for which he began receiving therapy at school in the first and second grades. Toilet training was fully accomplished at 2.5 years of age without difficulty. David did exhibit bedwetting until 8 years of age. Aside from the usual childhood illnesses, David's past medical history is significant for the diagnosis of leukemia at 8 years 9 months of age. As noted earlier, David received chemotherapy that included methotrexate and is now in remission. According to his mother, David began to exhibit a short attention span in his third-grade classroom just prior to the diagnosis; this gradually escalated into a short frustration tolerance, temper tantrums, and aggression toward his brother. His mother feels that David's emotional/behavioral difficulty further escalated after the parents' separation.

Review of academic history indicates that David attended a kindergarten program for 4- and 5-year-olds at a private daycare; his mother indicated that he did fairly well with no major concerns voiced by his teacher. For first grade, David began attending the local public elementary school. According to his mother, David's grades varied from Cs to As, and it was during this year that he began receiving speech/language therapy for his articulation disorder. This continued through the second grade. In third grade, David began to exhibit evidence of a short attention span and poor academic performance as reflected in the grading report for the first six weeks. Following the diagnosis of leukemia in September, David began receiving homebound teacher services five hours per week with his third-grade teacher. According to his mother, David's behavior problems escalated during the second half of the school year, and he returned to his third grade classroom for the last two weeks of the year. David passed the end of the year achievement testing and, as a result, was promoted to the fourth grade.

In fourth grade, David's attention span problem escalated, and he also demonstrated evidence of poor organizational skills. Specifically, he did not write down assignments and forgot to bring his homework home. According to his mother, David experienced the greatest academic difficulty with reading, math, and science. She further stated that the guidance counselor informed her that David did not qualify for any extra assistance at school, even after his physicians wrote several letters requesting this. As a result, David currently is repeating the fourth grade. According to his mother, David earned grades of F in social studies, reading, and English on his first six-weeks report card, with C in math and spelling and A in health and science. As a result, David is scheduled to begin receiving after-school tutoring for one hour on Tuesdays and Thursdays.

Behavioral Observations

David presented himself for testing as a very pleasant, neatly groomed young man with dark brown hair and hazel eyes, who was casually dressed in a yellow T-shirt, jeans and a red Alabama jacket. He separated from his mother and accompanied the examiners to the testing room without difficulty. Throughout the evaluation, which consisted of two sessions separated by a lunch break, David was very pleasant and cooperative with good eye contact and manners noted. Further, his attention span and activity level were felt to be age appropriate. In response to direct questioning as well as when conversation was spontaneous, David's language usage was found to be fluent and prosodic, with a mild articulation disorder still in evidence. When confronted with difficult test items, David generally responded in a reflective manner with good frustration tolerance. Lateral dominance is firmly established in the right hand. Vision and hearing were not formally screened; however, they were felt to be functioning adequately for the purposes of this evaluation.

Assessment Results

Cognitive and Neuropsychological Functioning

The results of neuropsychological evaluation indicate that David currently is functioning within the low-average to average range of intellectual ability as measured by the Wechsler Intelligence Scale for Children, Fourth Edition; however, analysis of the Index scores indicates that there is a significant discrepancy between his average Verbal Comprehension Index and his borderline to low-average Perceptual Reasoning Index. Thus, it is recommended that David's Verbal Comprehension Index score be used as his best estimate of intellectual potential. This is further supported by David's average performance on the Working Memory and Processing Speed Indices of the WISC-IV (see Table 9.3).

Additional assessment indicates that David is demonstrating variable performance on measures of higher-order executive functions with average sequential reasoning and problem-solving capability noted on the Tower subtest of the NEPSY contrasted by low-average performance on the Wisconsin Card Sorting Test. David's performance on measures of expressive and receptive language domains are generally low-average to average range with a relative weakness noted on a measure of phonological processing/awareness. Visual-spatial perception and visual-motor integration are borderline to low average with poor motor planning noted. Fine motor tapping speed is above average bilaterally.

Analysis of David's performance on the Children's Memory Scale indicates that, at the present time, he is exhibiting significant variability in his ability to hold material in immediate auditory working memory in conjunction with borderline ability to hold spatial location in working memory. When asked to learn and remember newly

Table 9.3 Psychometric Summary for David

	Scaled Score	Standard Score
Wechsler Intelligence Scale for Children, Fourth Edition (WISC-IV)		
Full Scale IQ		87
Verbal Comprehension Index		93
Similarities	7	
Vocabulary	9	
Comprehension	10	
Perceptual Reasoning Index		75
Block Design	7	
Picture Concepts	8	
Matrix Reasoning	3	
Working Memory Index		94
Digit Span	9	
Letter-Number Sequencing	9	
Processing Speed Index		100
Coding	10	
Symbol Search	10	
Wisconsin Card Sorting Test (WCST)		
Categories Obtained (5/6)		86
Perseverative Errors		90
Failure to Maintain Set		110
Delis-Kaplan Executive Function System (D-KEFS)		
Verbal Fluency Test		80
Neuropsychological Assessment, Second Edition (NEPSY-2)		
Tower (NEPSY)		100
Phonological Processing		75
Comprehension of Instructions		90
Arrows		85
Peabody Picture Vocabulary Test, Fourth Edition (PPVT-IV)		85
Boston Naming Test (BNT)		83
Clinical Evaluation of Language Function, Fourth Edition (CELF-IV)		
Formulated Sentences		95
Finger Tapping Test		
Right (dominant) Hand (42.8 taps per 10 seconds)		125
Left (nondominant) Hand (37.0 taps per 10 seconds)		113
Rey Complex Figure Test (RCFT)		
Copy		88
Clock Face Drawing Test		
Form		95
Time (10:20)		66
Developmental Test of Visual Motor Integration, Fifth Edition (DTVMI-V)		77

(continued)

Table 9.3 (*Continued*)

	Scaled Score	Standard Score
Children's Memory Scale (CMS)		
General Memory Index		86
Attention/Concentration Index		91
Numbers	10	
Sequencing	7	
Picture Location	5	
Verbal Immediate Index		91
Stories	11	
Word Pairs	6	
Visual Immediate Index		85
Dot Locations	6	
Faces	9	
Verbal Delayed Index		100
Stories	10	
Word Pairs	10	
Visual Delayed Index		85
Dot Locations	5	
Faces	10	
Delayed Recognition Index		106
Stories	10	
Word Pairs	12	
Learning Index		72
Word Pairs	5	
Dot Locations	6	
Gray Oral Reading Test, Fourth Edition (GORT-4)		
Fluency		85
Comprehension		95
Wide Range Achievement Test, Fourth Edition (WRAT-4)		
Reading		93
Spelling		90
Arithmetic		100
Test of Written Language, Third Edition		
Written Language Quotient		74
Behavior Assessment System for Children, Second Edition (BASC-II)		
	T-Scores	
	Parent	Teacher
Clinical Scales		
Hyperactivity	73	57
Aggression	64	59
Conduct Problems	71	67
Anxiety	61	52
Depression	86	41
Somatization	71	90
Atypicality	76	53

(continued)

Table 9.3 *(Continued)*

	T-Scores	
	Parent	Teacher
Attention Problems	73	67
Learning Problems	NA	63
Adaptive Scales		
Adaptability	30	54
Social Skills	20	41
Leadership	30	42
Study Skills	NA	30
Activities of Daily Living	40	NA
Functional Communication	43	45
DSM-IV ADHD Checklist	**Raw Score**	
Inattention	24/27*	20/27
Hyperactivity/Impulsivity	21/27*	12/27

Note. NA = not applicable. Asterisk (*) denotes a significant score.

presented information, David experienced difficulty learning rote verbal material (a list of unrelated word pairs) over three highly structured learning trials; however, he was able to spontaneously recall the words he did learn after a 30-minute delay. Further, his recall was aided by the use of a recognition recall paradigm. In contrast, David demonstrated average ability to learn and recall stories that were read to him. Within the visual domain, David exhibited average ability to learn and recall a series of pictured human faces contrasted by borderline ability to learn and recall the spatial location of an array of dots presented over three highly structured learning trials. It also should be noted that David's delayed recall dot pattern was different from his product at immediate recall (same number correct), which served to artificially inflate his delayed recall standard score performance.

Academic Functioning

Academically, David demonstrates levels of performance in the areas of reading recognition/spelling, reading comprehension, and math calculation that are commensurate with what would be expected based on the Verbal Comprehension Index from the WISC-IV. This is contrasted by a significant weakness in the area of written expression that is of learning disability proportion. Further, David's reading fluency appears to be a relative weakness.

Emotional and Behavioral Functioning

Behaviorally, analysis of rating scales completed by David's mother and three of his teachers (as a group) indicates that David is exhibiting significant difficulty sustaining his attention along with poor conduct both at home and at school. In addition, David's mother endorsed significant concerns with regard to hyperactivity, depressed mood, poor socialization skills, and difficulty adapting to change.

Summary and Diagnostic Impressions

Taken together, this pattern of neuropsychological test performance indicates general sparing of verbal abilities in combination with deficits in nonverbal areas. Effects on memory and problem solving are somewhat variable, possibly compromised by attentional difficulties. In addition, these results are also consistent with a diagnosis of learning disability in the area of written expression. Finally, David also exhibits significant behaviors consistent with ADHD-inattentive type, and adjustment disorder with depressed mood.

Recommendations

As a result of these findings, it is recommended that David be considered for special education resource/inclusion services designed for children with learning disabilities under the eligibility categories of "Specific Learning Disability" or "Other Health Impaired." These services should be utilized to develop written expression skills and provide David with academic support as needed for other academics that require writing skill as a prerequisite. David also will benefit from a behavioral plan focused on enhancing his ability to focus and sustain attention, his listening skills, task completion, and self-concept as part of his Individual Educational Plan. As part of this plan, rules and expectations should be presented simply, clearly, and consistently and reviewed frequently. This plan should place a large emphasis on consistently rewarding David's "good" behavior, such as positive social interactions, working on classwork, and following directions rather than having a punitive system that primarily calls attention to his mistakes (i.e., emphasis on positive behavioral supports). In other words, he should have a high ratio of positive reinforcement (gaining points, tokens, etc.) to punishment (losing points, etc.) (ratio = 5:1). Consequences for both appropriate and inappropriate behavior should be enforced on a consistent basis through positive reinforcement and response cost. This could be managed in the form of a contracting system. The behavioral plan should be coordinated with David's mother to ensure consistency between home and school, including target behaviors, reinforcers, and punishments.

In order to enhance David's learning/retention, new material should be presented in an organized format that is meaningful to him. The material to be learned should be broken down into smaller components/steps and presented in a highly structured format with frequent repetition to facilitate learning. Instruction should be supplemented with visual aids, demonstrations, and experiential/procedural learning. Map learning tasks will prove extremely difficult for David and should be minimized. David would benefit greatly from being taught how to use mnemonic strategies when learning new material and studying for tests. These include but are not limited to these areas:

- Rehearsal—showing David how to repeat information verbally, to write it, and to look at it a finite number of times.
- Transformation—showing him how to convert difficult information into simpler components that can be remembered more easily.
- Elaboration—instructing David in how to identify key elements of new information and to create relationships or associations with previously learned material.
- Imagery—showing him how to visualize and make a "mental picture" of information to be learned.

When studying for tests or doing multiple homework assignments on the same day, similar subject material should be separated in order to lessen interference. Finally, David should be provided with periodic review of previously learned material in order to enhance long-term retention.

Accommodations will be necessary to enhance David's ability to succeed in the classroom, including preferential seating away from bulletin boards, doorways, windows, or other students, if necessary, where excessive stimuli might prove distracting. Instruction should be provided in small-group settings whenever possible, and efforts should be made to redirect his attention. Given his learning disabilities and ADHD, a reduction in the amount, but not the difficulty level, of assignments may assist David in completing classroom tasks and homework in a timely manner. Moreover, whenever possible, he should be given additional time to complete assignments. Tests should be in multiple-choice/matching/short answer formats instead of an essay format and should be administered individually, with additional time provided when necessary. Finally, David should be allowed and encouraged to use various compensatory devices, such as copies of classroom notes or a tape recorder to record lectures and a computer with word processing capability. Most word processing programs are equipped with spell checks and cut and paste and can be adapted for voice dictation if necessary. These capabilities will be increasingly valuable during David's education.

As David approaches middle school, study skills training will be warranted, emphasizing such techniques as the appropriate outlining of lecture notes and how to study for tests. He also will benefit from being taught how to take notes on text material and plan written reports using an outlining method. In a related vein, training in word processing is strongly encouraged. David also may require instruction on how to organize and plan his approach to novel tasks. This is particularly true for subject matter in which he is weaker, such as written expression. In addition, direct instruction in basic organizational strategies will assist David in knowing what to do, when to do it, and how to do it. Specifically, he should be guided in the use of checklists and other organizational aids such as a daily planner.

Finally, David and his family would benefit from therapy sessions designed to treat his depressed mood as it relates to his parents' separation and his ADHD. Specifically, therapy should focus on improving David's self-concept while helping David and his brother cope with his parents' marital difficulty. Treatment also should focus on improving his ability to self-monitor and regulate his behavior within the classroom and at home and should address potential influences of David's leukemia diagnosis and medical treatment on his emotional and behavioral functioning. If therapy, classroom accommodations, and a behavioral plan prove ineffective at managing his symptoms of inattention, consultation with his hematologist/oncologist regarding a trial of medication management should be considered.

Further Discussion of Case Study

The pattern of neuropsychological test performance David exhibits is fairly consistent with the findings reported in studies that have examined the cognitive outcome of ALL survivors treated with methotrexate without radiation therapy. In particular, he evidences significant deficits in attention as well as learning and memory. Notably, a standard psychoeducational assessment, which might not include the attention or memory domains, may not have identified these areas as in need of intervention. At present, these results are also consistent with a diagnosis of learning disability in the area of written expression. Finally, as frequently occurs, there are indications of adjustment issues and depressed mood that warrant attention as well, illustrating that psychosocial and family variables must be included in order to develop a comprehensive conceptualization of the child's functioning.

CASE STUDY: JAY—ASTROCYTOMA

The next report is from a hospital-based clinic. Identifying information, such as child and family name, teacher or physician name, and school information, has been altered or fictionalized to protect confidentiality.

Reason for Referral

Jay is an almost 13-year-old special needs sixth grader who is being initially evaluated by the pediatric neuropsychology service at the request of his neurologist and oncologist, who are following Jay for a history of brain tumor (pilocystic astrocytoma) that was diagnosed and surgically resected in July 2005; see Figure 9.1. His symptoms at the time of diagnosis were nausea, vomiting, headaches, and double vision. A magnetic resonance imaging scan of the brain revealed that the tumor involved the vermis and medial cerebellar hemispheres bilaterally. Following the surgery, Jay developed hydrocephalus, which required placement of a ventriculoperitoneal (VP) shunt in November that year. Due to the cerebellar involvement of the tumor, Jay has experienced significant difficulty with ataxia, which required extensive inpatient rehabilitation followed by outpatient occupational, physical, and speech/language therapy. Jay is also receiving extensive special education services. He requires the use of a walker and currently is using a wheelchair

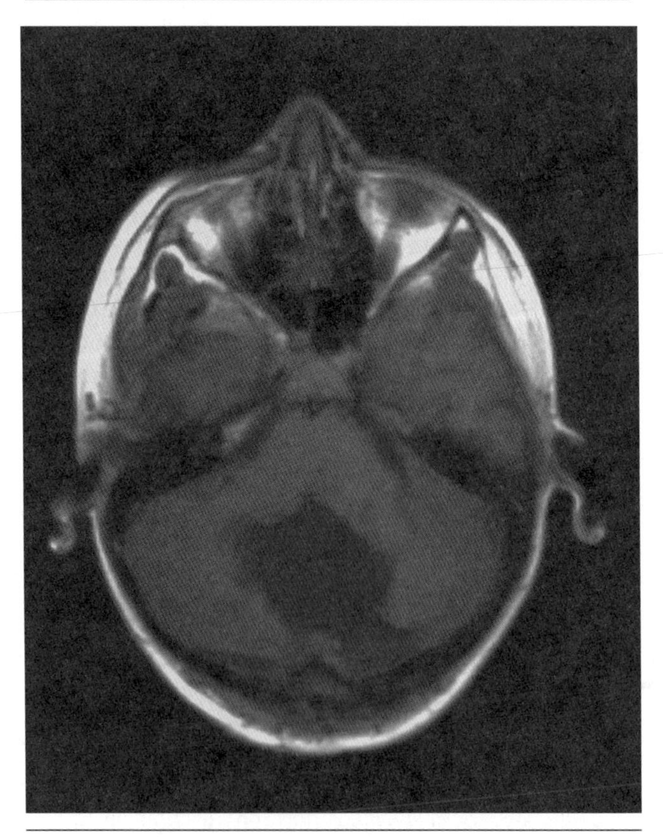

Figure 9.1 MRI two years status post gross total resection of a left cerebellar pilocystic astrocytoma.

due to a broken right foot. Finally, Jay is followed by a child psychiatrist for anxiety and depression for which he is currently prescribed sertraline (Zoloft). As a result, neuropsychological evaluation was undertaken in order to assess higher cortical functioning and make appropriate recommendations regarding school placement and the need for supportive therapies.

Assessment Procedures

Clinical interview (parent)

Behavioral observations

Wechsler Intelligence Scale for Children, Fourth Edition (WISC-IV)

Neuropsychological Assessment (NEPSY)/Neuropsychological Assessment, Second Edition (NEPSY-2; selected subtests)

Peabody Picture Vocabulary Test, Fourth Edition (PPVT-IV)

Boston Naming Test

Clinical Evaluation of Language Fundamentals, Fourth Edition (selected subtests)

Kaufman Assessment Battery for Children, Second Edition (KABC-2; selected subtests)

Finger Oscillation Test

Delis-Kaplan Executive Function Scale (D-KEFS; selected subtest)

Beery Developmental Test of Visual Motor Integration, Fifth Edition (DTVMI-V)

Children's Memory Scale (CMS)

Gray Oral Reading Test, Fourth Edition (GORT-4)

Wechsler Individual Achievement Test, Second Edition (WIAT-II)

Behavior Assessment System for Children, Second Edition (BASC-2; Parent and Teacher Rating Scales)

DSM-IV ADHD Checklist (Parent)

Background Information

Home

Jay resides with his parents. Jay's father is 40 years of age, has completed high school, and currently is employed as a plant shift supervisor. Jay's mother is 38 years of age, has a high school and technical school degree, and works as an IT support analyst at a bank. The paternal family history is significant for a female cousin with a "genetic disorder" who requires special education services in school. The maternal family history is significant for a brain aneurism in the grandmother, brain tumor in two great-uncles and a great-aunt, and migraine headache in the mother.

Medical History

Review of developmental and medical history with the mother indicates that Jay is the product of a 38-week-gestation pregnancy complicated by elevated blood pressure and toxemia. As a result, labor was induced; however, a cesarean section was performed. Jay weighed 8 pounds 15.5 ounces at birth. Aside from mild jaundice, which required brief phototherapy, Jay did well as a newborn and went home with his mother on day 4. Developmental motor milestones were obtained within normal limits with sitting up occurring at 5 months of age and walking at 11 months of age. Developmental language milestones also were attained within normal limits with first words at 13 months of age, short phrases at 15 months of age, and short sentences at 18 months of age. Toilet training was fully accomplished at 2 years of age during the day and by 4 years at night. Aside from the history of brain tumor and hydrocephalus, Jay's past medical history is also significant for short attention span and hyperactivity, which first became problematic in kindergarten. Jay was diagnosed with ADHD at the start of second grade by his pediatrician, who started him on dextroamphetamine (Adderall). According to the mother, this medication helped Jay focus and concentrate in class. The dosage was gradually increased, and by third grade, Jay was switched to Adderall XR (slow release) to assist with homework. During fourth grade, Jay's mother began to notice bilateral hand tremor and weight loss. As a result, she switched pediatricians. Jay was started on atomoxetine (Strattera) and later methylphenidate (Concerta). Since diagnosis of the brain tumor during the summer between fourth and fifth grades, Jay has remained off stimulant medications. Treatment for the tumor included gross total resection of a left cerebellar pilocystic astrocytoma (see Figure 9.1 earlier in the chapter).

Educational

Review of educational history indicates that Jay began attending a 4-year-old preschool program at a local daycare, where his teacher felt that he was very bright; however, his attention span was short and he was hyperactive. Jay went on to public school for kindergarten, where he remained through repetition of the fifth grade due to excessive absence as a result of the brain tumor. Due to Jay's short attention span and hyperactivity, a student support team (SST) was initiated in second grade along with his medication therapy.

Following inpatient rehabilitation, the SST referred Jay for psychological evaluation. This evaluation took place in the home due to Jay's severe ataxia, which appeared to worsen with fatigue. Intellectual function as assessed by the Reynolds Intellectual Assessment Scales was reported to be in the average range as measured by a Composite Intelligence score of 98. Academic assessment, with the Kaufman Test of Educational Achievement, Second Edition, revealed average word recognition skills, low-average reading comprehension and mathematical reasoning, and deficient mathematical computation. Based on the results of this assessment, Jay began receiving special education services toward the end of fifth grade. These included collaborative classes; a paraprofessional; and physical, occupational, and speech/language therapies as related services. Jay has continued to receive these services during repetition of fifth grade and now in sixth grade.

Behavioral Observations

Jay presented himself for testing as a very pleasant, neatly groomed youngster with blue eyes and blond hair who was casually dressed and seated in a wheelchair due to his broken right foot. It should be noted that Jay was able to ambulate short distances with assistance. Jay separated appropriately from his mother who assisted with manipulation of the wheelchair to the testing room. Jay exhibited good social eye contact and manners, and he related well toward the examiners with a broad range of affect noted. Throughout the evaluation, which consisted of two sessions separated by a lunch break, Jay's attention span and activity level were felt to be age appropriate. In response to direct questions as well as when conversation was spontaneous, Jay's use of language was slow and labored with mild word-finding difficulty and poor sentence formulation skills evident. When confronted with more challenging tasks, Jay typically responded in a reflective manner with excellent task persistence. Lateral dominance is firmly established in the right hand for paper-and-pencil manipulation with a bilateral tremor noted. Vision and hearing were not formally assessed; however, they appeared to be functioning adequately for the purposes of this evaluation.

Assessment Results

Cognitive and Neuropsychological Functioning

The results of neuropsychological evaluation indicate that Jay currently is functioning within the low-average to average range of intellectual ability as measured by the General Ability Index of the Wechsler Intelligence Scale for Children, Fourth Edition with fairly good consolidation noted across the Verbal Comprehension and Perceptual Reasoning Index scores. In contrast, Jay demonstrated a deficient Processing Speed Index score secondary to his bilateral motor ataxia. Additional assessment indicates that Jay exhibited low-average to average sequential reasoning/problem-solving capability. Jay's expressive and receptive language skills are generally in the low-average to average range with relative weaknesses noted in phonological processing, which appears to be a secondary manifestation of poor auditory working memory (see Table 9.4).

Visual-spatial perception and visual-motor integration/constructional skills were found to be variable, ranging from deficient to low average. Qualitative analysis of Jay's performance appears to indicate that his poor performance was the result of occulomotor scanning difficulty, hand tremor, and planning difficulty when drawing. Fine motor tapping speed is found to be bilaterally depressed as measured by the finger tapping test. Once again, Jay's tremor significantly impacted his performance.

Analysis of Jay's performance on the Children's Memory Scale indicates that, at the present time, he is exhibiting borderline to low-average ability to hold material in immediate/auditory working memory contrasted by visual working memory that is well within the average range. When asked to learn and remember (30 minutes later) newly presented material, Jay generally demonstrated low-average to average learning and recall capability with a relative strength noted in his ability to recall a list of rote word pairs presented over three structured learning trials (see Table 9.4).

Academic Functioning

Academically, Jay performed in the low-average to average range on measures of word recognition/spelling, pseudoword decoding, reading comprehension, and mathematical reasoning. In contrast, Jay demonstrated significant weaknesses in oral reading fluency, written expression, and mathematical calculation.

Emotional and Behavioral Functioning

Behaviorally, analysis of rating scales completed by Jay's mother and teachers indicates that, at the present time, Jay's mother endorsed significant concern with regard to inattention, hyperactivity, difficulty adapting to change in routine in conjunction with elevated anxiety, and depressed mood. In contrast, Jay's teachers did not endorse significant emotional or behavioral concerns at school.

Table 9.4 Psychometric Summary for Jay

	Scaled Score	Standard Score
Wechsler Intelligence Scale for Children, Fourth Edition (WISC-IV)		
Full Scale IQ		77
General Ability Index		89
Verbal Comprehension Index		87
Similarities	7	
Vocabulary	8	
Comprehension	8	
Perceptual Reasoning Index		92
Block Design	6	
Picture Concepts	11	
Matrix Reasoning	9	
Working Memory Index		88
Digit Span	6	
Letter-Number Sequencing	10	
Processing Speed Index		56
Coding	1	
Symbol Search	3	
Delis-Kaplan Executive Function System (D-KEFS)		
Verbal Fluency Test		100
Neuropsychological Assessment, Second Edition (NEPSY-2)		
Tower (NEPSY)		90
Phonological Processing		75
Comprehension of Instructions		85
Arrows		55
Peabody Picture Vocabulary Test, Fourth Edition (PPVT-IV)		102
Boston Naming Test (BNT)		82
Clinical Evaluation of Language Function, Fourth Edition (CELF-IV)		
Formulated Sentences		85
Kaufman Assessment Battery for Children, Second Edition		
Gestalt Closure		80
Clock Face Drawing Test		
Form		106
Time (10:20)		106
Developmental Test of Visual Motor Integration, Fifth Edition (DTVMI-V)		69
Children's Memory Scale		
General Memory Index		87
Attention/Concentration Index		72
Numbers	5	
Sequencing	6	
Picture Location	10	

(continued)

Table 9.4 (*Continued*)

	Scaled Score	Standard Score
Verbal Immediate Index		94
Stories	9	
Word Pairs	9	
Visual Immediate Index		82
Dot Locations	7	
Faces	7	
Verbal Delayed Index		100
Stories	8	
Word Pairs	12	
Visual Delayed Index		88
Dot Locations	8	
Faces	8	
Delayed Recognition Index		109
Stories	11	
Word Pairs	12	
Learning Index		85
Word Pairs	8	
Dot Locations	7	
Gray Oral Reading Test, Fourth Edition (GORT-4)		
Fluency		75
Rate		70
Accuracy		90
Comprehension		90
Wechsler Individual Achievement Test, Second Edition (WIAT-II)		
Word Reading		87
Pseudoword Decoding		93
Written Expression		76
Spelling		86
Mathematical Reasoning		85
Numerical Operations		78

Behavior Assessment System for Children, Second Edition (BASC-II)

	T-Scores			
	Parent	**Teachers**		
Clinical Scales				
Hyperactivity	80*	46	58	47
Aggression	56	46	48	46
Conduct Problems	60	43	45	43
Anxiety	70*	42	63	59
Depression	84*	53	59	45
Somatization	63	51	80*	63
Atypicality	57	58	54	44
Withdrawal	60	44	58	38
Attention Problems	63	54	52	49
Learning Problems	NA	59	57	59
Adaptive Scales				
Adaptability	33*	45	56	62

(continued)

Table 9.4 *(Continued)*

	T-Scores			
	Parent	Teachers		
Social Skills	39	46	59	70
Leadership	38	44	54	70
Study Skills	NA	46	50	51
Activities of Daily Living	22*	NA	NA	NA
Functional Communication	38	44	40	59
DSM-IV ADHD Checklist		Raw Score		
Inattention	21/27*	17/27*	11/27	14/27
Hyperactivity/Impulsivity	15/27*	3/27	11/27	1/27

Note. NA = not applicable. Asterisk (*) denotes a significant score.

Summary and Diagnostic Impressions

This pattern of neuropsychological test performance is consistent with a picture of a youngster with low-average to average intellectual ability who is experiencing significant cerebellar dysfunction characterized by oral-motor, ocular-motor, and motor apraxia. In addition, Jay is exhibiting executive functioning deficits (auditory working memory and motor planning) that may be related to his history of hydrocephalus and/or his prior history of ADHD. Taken together, these deficits have resulted in significant academic difficulty in the areas of reading fluency, written expression, and mathematical calculation. Finally, Jay continues to exhibit significant anxiety and depressed mood in the home setting, even with the benefit of medication therapy.

Recommendations

As a result, it is recommended that Jay continue to receive special education collaborative classroom services designed for children with learning disabilities under the eligibility category of "Other Health Impaired" in conjunction with continuation of physical, occupational, and language therapies as related services. Continuation of the paraprofessional is also strongly encouraged. The collaborative services should be provided in any classroom that requires reading, written expression, or mathematical calculation skills as a prerequisite. It may be beneficial for school-based physical therapy (PT) and occupational therapy (OT) to focus on the development of handwriting/note-taking skills and ambulation around campus. Private PT and OT should be geared toward development of strength and ambulation in the home environment along with development of fine motor and independent living skills. Language therapy should focus not only on articulation and fluency but also on the development of linguistic planning and auditory working memory skills. Jay should continue to receive oncology and neurological follow-up as well as psychiatric follow-up.

- In order to enhance Jay's learning/retention, new material should be presented in an organized format that is meaningful to him. The material to be learned should be pretaught, broken down into smaller components/steps, and presented in a highly structured format with frequent repetition to facilitate new learning.
- Instruction should be supplemented with visual aids and demonstrations.
- Jay would benefit greatly from being taught how to use mnemonic strategies when learning new material and studying for tests. These include but are not limited to:

- Rehearsal—showing Jay how to repeat information verbally, to write it, and look at it a finite number of times.
- Transformation—instructing Jay in how to convert difficult information into simpler components that can be remembered more easily.
- Elaboration—showing him how to identify key elements of new information and to create relationships or associations with previously learned material.
- Chunking—instructing Jay in how to group or pair down long strings of digits or different items into more manageable units and thereby facilitate encoding and retention.
- Imagery—showing Jay how to visualize and make a "mental picture" of information to be learned.

- When studying for tests or doing multiple homework assignments on the same day, similar subject material should be separated in order to lessen interference.
- Jay should be provided with periodic review of previously learned material in order to enhance long-term retention.

Additional suggestions for the classroom and academic issues include:

- Accommodations will be necessary to enhance Jay's ability to succeed in the classroom, including preferential seating, copies of classroom notes, a reduction in the amount, but not the difficulty level of written assignments, and additional time to complete assignments.
- Tests should be in multiple choice/matching/short answer formats instead of an essay format and should be administered individually/orally, with additional time provided when necessary.
- Jay also will benefit from the use of graph paper or different color highlighter pens to maintain place value when doing written calculation, having an outline of the steps necessary to complete multistep math problems available for reference, and the use of computer programs to solidify basic math facts.
- Jay should be allowed and encouraged to use various compensatory devices, such as textbooks on tape/reading pen, a calculator, and a computer with word processing capability. Most word processing programs are equipped with spell checks and cut and paste and can be adapted for voice dictation if Jay's motor difficulty does not allow for mastery of an adaptive keyboard.
- As Jay approaches middle school, study skills training will be warranted emphasizing such techniques as the appropriate outlining of lecture notes and how to study for tests. He will also benefit from being taught how to take notes on text material and plan written reports using an outlining method.
- In a related vein, Jay may also require instruction on how to organize and plan his approach to his studies, as executive functioning is an area of weakness for him.
- In addition, direct instruction in basic organizational strategies will assist Jay in knowing what to do, when to do it, and how to do it. Specifically, he should be guided in the use of checklists and other organizational aids, such as a daily planner. With help from teachers and parents, ideally he will plan each day of the week, including time after school.
- Jay and his parents would benefit from family therapy to assist with the management of Jay's emotional and behavioral difficulties reported by his mother in the home.

Identification and development of leisure activities and social outlets will be important as he progresses through adolescence.

Further Discussion of Case Study

In contrast to the case of David, Jay's presentation reflects greater compromise of brain function as might be expected with the combination treatment of surgery and shunting for hydrocephalus. Although overall cognitive ability is in the low-average range, Jay does not demonstrate the sparing of verbal abilities but evidences significant strengths (verbal memory) and weaknesses (processing speed) within and across areas. Jay demonstrated the attentional difficulties that often are noted as late effects early in the disease process with potential for these to continue to contribute to his functional and academic difficulties. Symptoms of anxiety and depression also likely contribute to, and may be exacerbated by, his functional and academic struggles. Related to both case studies, the research indicates that there is a continued need to monitor and track progress, with appropriate intervention at educational, vocational, and psychological levels as necessary for the individual.

CONCLUDING COMMENTS

Evidence suggests that survivors of childhood cancer make greater use of special education services than their nonaffected siblings (Haupt et al., 1994) and are at risk for academic difficulty across the academic areas. Early identification of late neurocognitive effects with appropriate accommodations and intervention is important for childhood cancer survivors (Daly et al., 2008). Survivors of childhood cancer pose additional issues in the sense that initially following treatment, they may be functioning at levels that do not reflect their at-risk status. Unlike other trauma survivors, the trajectory for survivors of childhood cancer is such that deficits and decline will become evident over time. This fact necessitates comprehensive assessment and intervention, with collaboration and monitoring across professionals and parents (Kazak et al., 2008). Further, it is not appropriate to wait until these children exhibit academic difficulty to consider such a comprehensive evaluation. Given what is known about the effect of the treatment protocols, best practice is to have comprehensive neuropsychological evaluation with an emphasis on attentional processes, memory, and processing speed prior to the child's return to school. Neurocognitive status will need to be monitored closely and additional supports provided as needed over time in order to account for late effects.

Psychological status is also an important consideration. While many childhood survivors exhibit hardiness, there is evidence that children with chronic illnesses are at risk for development of psychological problems but often do not present with clinically significant psychological disorders above what would be expected in the normative population (Kazak & Christakis, 1996; Noll & Kupst, 2007). Family support services and educational components may be helpful in preventing less positive outcomes. With increased survival rates, there is greater need for research related to quality of life for children with cancer (L. K. Campbell et al., 2008).

Chapter 10

EPILEPSY

DEFINITION

Epilepsy is a complex neurological disorder that affects individuals of all ages. The term *epilepsy* encompasses several different syndromes, but the underlying feature across the differing forms of epilepsy is a tendency to experience at least two unprovoked seizures. Another way to distinguish epilepsy is by the paroxysmal and noticeable changes in neuron firing that may or may not be accompanied by effects on consciousness or other functions (Neppe & Tucker, 1994). With epilepsy, the neuronal firing changes are initiated by internal processes. Initially these processes, however, may be triggered by an external occurrence (e.g., head injury). In contrast, a single seizure may be initiated by an internal or external process (e.g., tumor or head injury).

Another defining feature of epilepsy is that there is a tendency to experience at least two unprovoked seizures (Elger & Schmidt, 2008; R. S. Fisher et al., 2005). A seizure is defined as a sudden brief attack of motor, cognitive, sensory, or autonomic disturbances that are caused by abnormal and excessive neuronal activity in the brain (Zillmer, Spiers, & Culbertson, 2008). Seizures are changes in consciousness that occur suddenly during periods of expected wakefulness when neurons fire excessively in a synchronized pattern that may be up to six times faster than the normal rate (Zillmer et al., 2008). Seizures can present in myriad ways including staring spells, momentary disruption of the senses, short periods of unconsciousness, or convulsions (Hargis, 2008). The seizure itself is called an *ictal* event; the period preceding the seizure is referred to as preictal while the period following a seizure is referred to as postictal. Seizures may last from 1 second to 20 to 30 minutes. Seizure activity is measured using electroencephalography (EEG).

Classification of Epilepsy and Seizure Activity

There are multiple ways to differentiate the various forms of seizures and resulting epilepsy. The system used most frequently is one that was created by the International League Against Epilepsy and consists of three tiers related to seizure type, structural basis of the seizure, and specific syndrome (Fisher et al., 2005; MacAllister & Schaffer, 2007); within each tier, there is further delineation of differences. The first tier is related to the seizure type, including type of neuronal activity, and classifies the seizure in one of three ways: generalized, localization-related, or undetermined. For example, in partial seizures, the first observed EEG changes are limited to one area of the cerebral hemisphere. Complex partial seizures may begin as a partial seizure, but there is an alteration of consciousness such that there may be changes in mood, cognition, memory, or behavior. Temporal lobe epilepsy (TLE) is ascribed to the category of complex partial seizures localized to the temporal lobe; these may be associated with fear and rage, dissociative symptoms (period of confusion, impaired memory, and distorted sense of time), and other behavioral problems. Automatisms (lip smacking or other repetitive motor movements) may be associated with complex partial seizures regardless of the location. In addition, prodromal symptoms or aura may be associated with complex partial seizures; these include a sense of déjà-vu or olfactory hallucinations. Also characteristic of complex partial seizures, the person will generally be disoriented and will not recall the events that occurred once the seizure is over (Zillmer et al., 2008).

In contrast to partial complex seizures, primary generalized seizures are those where the first clinical signs occur in both hemispheres; any motor symptoms are bilateral. Tonic-clonic seizures are one type of generalized seizure; this type of seizure may present with or without warning or aura (J. M. Freeman et al., 1998). If there is an aura, it may take the form of abdominal discomfort, irritability, or dizziness; the individual may not recognize that it is an aura. With tonic-clonic seizures, there is loss of consciousness, rigidity with extension of extremities, and arching the back (tonic phase) followed by rhythmic contractions (clonic phase). For some partial and complex partial as well as tonic-clonic seizures, extended EEG monitoring may be needed to capture the abnormal pattern; this can be facilitated by sleep-deprived or ambulatory EEGs (Zillmer et al., 2008).

The second type of generalized seizure is absence seizures, which may appear as momentary lapses of attention; automatisms of lip smacking or head drooping may or may not be present (Ahmed & Varghese, 2006; Zillmer et al., 2008). The seizure can be as brief as 1 second, but usually lasts 5 to 10 seconds. There is no aura or warning; the individual usually is not aware anything has occurred. With absence seizures, there is often no accompanying motor activity, though eyelid flickering at a rate of 3 per second is common. This is consistent with the characteristic spike pattern (3 per second) that is fairly stable on EEG; it is not necessary for the individual to experience a seizure to demonstrate this pattern (Zillmer et al., 2008). There are also pseudoseizures or psychogenic seizures that appear to be epileptic in nature but are not accompanied by atypical electrical activity in the brain (J. M. Freeman, Kossoff, & Hartman, 2007). Finally, there are also nonepileptic events that are common in the children who have and do not have epilepsy (Pakalnis, Paolicchi, & Gilles, 2000; Paolicchi, 2002).

Second and Third Tiers

The second tier classifies seizures based on the detection of any brain lesions and whether the seizures are symptomatic, cryptogenic, or idiopathic (R. S. Fisher et al., 2005; MacAllister & Schaffer, 2007). Symptomatic seizures are epileptic syndromes that have a known cause, such as a developmental abnormality, fever, metabolic imbalance, and trauma. This type of seizure also is referred to as *reactive* or *provoked* when it is the result of a response to some damage to the brain, such as fever or trauma. The cause of this type seizure is either developmental or acquired. The second category of seizure disorders is cryptogenic seizures. This type of seizure has no clear cause but typically is related to another neurological or cognitive condition (Zillmer et al., 2008). Specific types of cryptogenic seizures include West syndrome, Lennox-Gastaut syndrome, epilepsy with myoclonic-astatic seizures, and epilepsy with myoclonic absences (MacAllister & Schaffer, 2007).

The third and final category is idiopathic seizures. Idiopathic generalized epilepsies (IGEs) comprise one of the most widely examined groups of epileptic disorders in children; these epilepsies affect approximately 1% of the population (R. S. Fisher et al., 2005). This type of seizure has no known cause, and there is no suspected brain abnormality. A child with this type of epilepsy appears normal with the exception of the seizures. Idiopathic seizures are presumed to be inherited and are defined in terms of age-related onset (Zillmer et al., 2008). Specific types of idiopathic seizures include benign neonatal convulsions, benign myoclonic epilepsy, juvenile absence epilepsy, and juvenile myoclonic epilepsy (Fisher et al., 2005; MacAllister & Schaffer, 2007). Individuals with IGE are a relatively homogeneous group with no brain lesion explaining the excessive neuronal activity (Hommet, Sauerwein, De Toffol, & Lassonde, 2005). EEG associated with IGE demonstrates that seizures have bilateral, synchronous, and symmetrical EEG spikes and waves or polyspike waves; the seizures occur throughout the cortex because of a generalized lowering of the seizure threshold (Elger & Schmidt, 2008).

The third tier classifies the specific syndrome. Although the classification system is multifaceted and subject to debate by researchers, it is beneficial for diagnosis and treatment because it can encompass the wide array of epileptic disorders, while differentiating by lesion detection (Elger & Schmidt, 2008).

Prevalence and Incidence

Seizure disorders comprise one of the most common and complex classes of neurological disorders that affect people of all ages; it has been estimated that in the United States, approximately 5% of children will experience a seizure before the age of 20 (Hauser, Annegers, & Rocca, 1996). Of these, about 25% will meet formal criteria for some form of epilepsy (Elger & Schmidt, 2008); the incidence of epilepsy is highest in the first year of life and increases again after the age of 60 (Elger & Schmidt, 2008). Approximately 75% of cases are identified prior to age 20; 30% have an initial seizure prior to age 5. In addition, single-episode febrile seizures occur at a rate of 29 per 100,000. The occurrence of seizures is frequent in infants, children, and adolescents. It is thought that nearly 8 out of every 1,000 children have experienced at least one seizure, and the prevalence rate of epileptic disorders ranges from 4% to 8% (Ho-Turner & Bennett, 1999). Occasionally, childhood seizure disorders will dissipate with time; however, over 80% of adults diagnosed with epilepsy were diagnosed as children (Ho-Turner & Bennett, 1999). Notably, the incidence of epilepsy is higher in children with other disorders.

ETIOLOGY

Epilepsy can be the result of diverse etiologies. The three major factors affecting the recurrence of seizures are genetics, age at onset, and environmental stressors (T. L. Bennett & Ho, 2009). The occurrence of specific types of seizures has been genetically linked (Hommet et al., 2005). In particular, there is a high co-occurrence of seizures with those genetic disorders associated with mental retardation (see Chapter 15) such that severity of mental retardation is correlated with the severity of epilepsy (Kumada et al., 2005). These disorders include Down syndrome, Angelman syndrome, Prader-Willi syndrome (see Chapter 15), and various other chromosomal abnormalities as well as tuberous sclerosis (see Chapter 16). Among nongenetic and identified causes is traumatic brain injury (TBI) (see Chapter 8). Epilepsy also occurs in the absence of these disorders, however, and is of varying and often unknown etiology.

Neurodevelopment

The seizure threshold for newborns is very high; therefore, the elicitation of a seizure is extremely difficult; however, this is not the case as children progress from infants to toddlers. From infancy through age 2 a child's seizure threshold is lowered, and, as a result, they become more vulnerable (T. L. Bennett & Ho, 2009). This is the time period when most childhood epilepsy syndromes begin; however, after the age of 2, the threshold increases until the child reaches adulthood. Finally, environmental stressors dramatically increase the instances of seizures. These stressors can include fever spiking, tiredness, excitement, and metabolism (T. L. Bennett & Ho, 2009). The occurrence of fever in children typically precipitates the actual seizure; the intensity and duration of the fever are related directly to the seizure onset and strength. It has been theorized that the cause of IGE is multifactorial with an interaction of environmental effects and genetic variations (J. S. Duncan, Sander, Sisodiya, & Walker, 2006; Elger & Schmidt, 2008).

Research has demonstrated that mutations in voltage-gated channels (potassium, sodium, and chloride) and ligand-gated receptors (acetylcholine [ACh] and gamma aminobutyric acid–A [GABA-A]) cause different forms of IGE (Elger & Schmidt, 2008). Research also has demonstrated that almost all IGE have an ion channel defect, but when examined alone, this defect accounts for only a minority number of cases. Even in typical benign rolandic epilepsy, the relation between rolandic epilepsy and learning disabilities is accounted for in part by epileptiform discharges during sleep and early age of onset (Piccinelli et al., 2008).

Generalized seizures involve both cortical hemispheres at onset whereas partial seizures are restricted to a specific area. Generalized seizures are characterized by a temporary lack of awareness. This type of seizure is illustrated by motor behavior that occurs in tonic (stiffening) and clonic (jerking) behaviors (Zillmer et al., 2008). During generalized seizures, a group of neurons within the thalamus, specifically those in the nucleus reticularis thalami (NRT), regulates the behavior of the thalamocortical loop and also has the ability to act on both hemispheres of the brain. The NRT is made up of GABAergic neurons that project to each other within other areas of the thalamus. The main function of these neurons is to control the cerebral excitability. Researchers indicate that the development of GABA-B receptors increases during childhood development and is pruned as the child reaches adult levels. It is theorized that an overabundance of this specific type of receptor causes an imbalance in the excitatory/inhibitory responses in the brain; a seizure disorder is the result (Zillmer et al., 2008). Partial seizures are divided into two subtypes: simple partial and complex partial. When simple partial seizures occur, the individual remains conscious; when complex partial seizures occur, consciousness is impaired. Partial and secondarily generalized seizures are the most likely to be localized because both the aura (symptoms such as nausea, dizziness, or numbness) and the behavior during a seizure can point to a seizure's site of occurrence (Zillmer et al., 2008).

COURSE AND PROGNOSIS

The appearance of epilepsy throughout different childhood developmental stages has varied characteristics, treatment interventions, and outcomes. There is a high likelihood of learning problems, with 51% to 57% identified as having a learning disorder (Jennekens-Schinkel & Oostrom, 2005; Oostrom et al., 2003; Sillanpää, 2004). Individuals with epilepsy have high prevalence of psychosocial problems, are less likely to marry, and evidence higher rates of social isolation (Camfield & Camfield, 2003; Kokkonen, Kokkenen, Saukkonen, & Pennanen, 1997; Parker & Asher, 1987). Further, individuals with epilepsy are less likely to be employed (Camfield & Camfield, 2003).

Neurocognitive Function

Age of onset has been found to be associated with poorer cognitive function (Bulteau et al., 2000; Mitchell, Chavez, Lee, & Guzman, 1991; O'Leary et al., 1983; Schoenfeld et al., 1999); however, the association is not always present (Sturniolo & Galletti, 1994). Various functional domains may be spared or impaired in children with seizure disorders, depending on seizure type, duration, age of onset, medication, and other variables. Home environment (e.g., level of organization and support) has been found to be a moderating variable of neurocognitive outcome in children with epilepsy (Fastenau et al., 2004; Thornton et al., 2008).

Neuropsychological correlates vary depending on the type of seizure and other factors (see Table 10.1). This is most evident in partial seizures, which, because of their specific seizure foci, are associated with circumscribed deficits. For example, frontal lobe partial seizures are likely to be associated with executive dysfunction or motor dysfunction (Hernandez et al., 2002) while temporal lobe seizures are likely to be associated with memory deficits (M. J. Cohen, 1992). Generalized seizures are less likely to be associated with focal deficits. Complex partial seizures occurring in the temporal lobe region of the brain produce more obvious behavior and cognitive changes than most of the other seizure types (Bortz, Prigatano, Blum, & Fisher, 1995). Studies of intellectual and neuropsychological functions in children with epilepsy, regardless of seizure type, indicate that onset of seizures early in life and a long duration of seizure disorder place children at higher risk for cognitive dysfunction (Bortz et al., 1995). Both groups of children with either partial or generalized seizures and an early seizure onset demonstrated poorer performance on neuropsychological measures than children whose seizures started at a later age (O'Leary et al., 1983). Secondary to the epilepsy, neurocognitive deficits (Ballantyne, Spilkin, Hesselink, & Trauner, 2008) can be exacerbated by anti-epileptic drugs, particularly in attentional and information processing domains (Meador, 2002a). Of note, it has been found that the presence of seizures limits plasticity such that not only is there significantly lower performance on intellectual and language measures, but the course of cognitive development is significantly altered (Ballantyne et al., 2008). Using structural equation modeling, a three-factor model of neuropsychological function was identified to predict academic difficulties in children with epilepsy (Fastenau et al., 2004). The three factors consisted of Verbal/Memory/Executive, Rapid Naming/Working Memory, and Psychomotor. The Psychomotor factor predicted only difficulties in writing; the other two predicted reading, writing, and math achievement.

Cognition

Effects on cognition also vary as a function of early age of onset of the seizure disorder, extent to which the individual has seizure control, duration of the seizure disorder, and whether the person demonstrates multiple seizure types or a single type (Besag, 1995, 2004; Dodrill, 1993; Kopp, Muzykewicz, Staley, Thiele, & Pulsifer, in press). As a group, however, many children with epilepsy do not differ from other children with regard to general cognitive functioning (Pascalicchio et al., 2007; Sonmez, Atakli, Sari, Atay, & Arpaci, 2004). When cognitive deficits do occur, children with epilepsy experience specific cognitive disabilities rather than a global deficit in general cognitive ability

Table 10.1 Neuropsychological Domains and Specific Deficits with Epilepsy

Domains	Specific Deficits
Cognition	Distribution of intelligence of children with epilepsy appears skewed toward lower values
Auditory-linguistic/ Language function	Language deficits often associated with temporal lobe epilepsy Benign rolandic epilepsy also associated with language deficits
Visual perception/ Constructional praxis	Visual-spatial functioning may be one area spared, except for in association with juvenile myoclonic epilepsy or absence seizures
Perceptual/Sensory perception	Somatosensory auras may be present
Learning and memory	Verbal and nonverbal memory may be impaired, particularly for long-term or delayed recall Short-term memory also may be impaired
Processing speed	Significant slowing of psychomotor speed, particularly in the presence of brain structure abnormalities
Executive function	Children with epilepsy (localized, TLE, or IGE) demonstrated impaired performance on executive function tasks Particular difficulties with cognitive flexibility and disinhibition noted
Attention/Concentration	Impaired attention associated with multiple forms of epilepsy
Motor function	Oromotor skills and articulation may be impaired Frontal epilepsy associated with motor difficulties Difficulty with sequential fine motor responses Difficulty in gross as well as fine motor functions
Achievement/Academic skills	Children with epilepsy at a greater risk than other children of demonstrating academic difficulties Benign rolandic epilepsy also associated with reading difficulties
Emotional/Behavioral functioning	Specific problems include immaturity, emotional lability, and disinhibition as well as difficulties with social integration and social adjustment

(Palade & Benga, 2007). In a study of 6-year-olds with epilepsy and a comparison group, no differences emerged in verbal ability; however, nonverbal abilities were impaired in the group with epilepsy (Selassie, Viggedal, Olsson, & Jennische, 2008). Further, although many children with epilepsy function in the average range (Bourgeois, 1998; Bourgeois, Prensky, Palkes, Talent, & Busch, 1983), the distribution of intelligence of children with epilepsy appears to be skewed toward lower values (Bailet & Turk, 2000; Chaix et al., 2006). Decreased cognitive ability is associated with comorbidity of other disorders (Kopp et al., in press). For example, comorbid conditions, such as tuberous sclerosis, affect the extent to which functional domains are compromised; nearly one-half of children with tuberous sclerosis complex are likely to demonstrate mental retardation (Kopp et al., in press).

Language

Effects on auditory/linguistic function also varies. Children with absence seizures generally do not demonstrate any deficits in verbal memory or language skills (Pavone et al.,

2001). Language disturbances often are associated with temporal lobe epilepsy (Bigel & Smith, 2001; Lendt, Helmstaedter, & Elger, 1999). Children with left temporal lobe epilepsy are likely to display difficulties with verbal fluency, verbal learning, verbal memory, and delayed recall of verbal learning (Guimaràes et al., 2007; Jambaqué et al., 2007). In addition, benign rolandic epilepsy is associated with deficient performance on tests of vocabulary, verbal fluency, and verbal memory (Croona, Kihlgren, Lundberg, Eeg-Olofsson, & Eeg-Olofsson, 1999; Gündüz, Demirbilek, & Korkmaz, 1999). Language deficits ultimately affect reading ability as well as social skills (T. L. Bennett & Ho, 2009).

Learning and Memory

Depending on the seizure classification, some children may demonstrate impaired verbal and visual immediate and working memory, attention, and processing speed (Pascalicchio et al., 2007; Sonmez et al., 2004); learning and memory deficits are particularly evident in conjunction with temporal lobe epilepsy (T. L. Bennett & Ho, 2009). Analysis of construct validity of the California Verbal Learning Test—Children's Version (CVLT-C) supports similar constructs of attention, learning, and recall (free and cued) in conjunction with pediatric epilepsy as with other groups (Griffiths et al., 2006). Younger age, family history of seizure activity, and experience with absence seizures were associated with greater levels of difficulty with verbal memory, general cognitive functioning, and short-term memory (Sonmez et al., 2004). Adults and children with focal seizures of the left temporal lobe generally have greater verbal than nonverbal deficits, whereas children with seizures emanating from the right temporal lobe have greater nonverbal than verbal deficits. Notably, long-term memory appears to be affected more significantly than short-term memory (Bortz et al., 1995; J. Williams et al., 2001b). It has been suggested that this may be due to similarities between the long-term potentiation model of memory and the kindling associated with seizure activity (Meador, 2007). In particular, verbal and nonverbal memory (e.g., immediate and working memory) appear to be impaired in children with idiopathic generalized, temporal lobe, and focal epilepsies (Henkin, Sadeh, & Gadoth, 2007; Prassouli, Katsarou, Attilakos, & Antoniadou, 2007). Focal epilepsy is associated with difficulty with auditory memory processing (Jocic-Jakubi & Jovic, 2006; Krause, Boman, Sillanmäki, Varho, & Holopainen, 2008) while TLE is associated with deficits in verbal and visual memory, delayed recall, and recognition (Guimaràes et al., 2007).

Comparing the differences in qualitative aspects of verbal memory between the left and right temporal foci and no seizure disorder, individuals with left temporal lobe seizures have more intrusion errors on delayed and free recall tasks and evidence response bias. Those with right temporal lobe seizures did not demonstrate any response bias (Bortz et al., 1995). This difference is most evident with consolidation of new materials and with difficulty in initial learning of verbal materials in conjunction with left temporal seizures. As a result, there is a deficit in the ability to recognize materials accurately (T. L. Bennett & Ho, 2009). For children with IGE, poor performance in initial learning resulted in retrieval difficulty, particularly with delay (M. Davidson, Dorris, O'Regan, & Zuberi, 2007). Age has been shown to be a contributing factor for children with benign epilepsy with centrotemporal spikes such that deficits in list learning recall and delay dissipated after age 10 (Vago, Bulgheroni, Franceschetti, Usilla, & Riva, 2008). There are some indications that deficits in auditory attention and memory are associated with decreased academic performance in children with epilepsy (J. Williams et al., 2001a).

Executive Function

In general, children with epilepsy (localized, TLE, or IGE) demonstrated impaired performance on executive function tasks (Parrish et al., 2007) with difficulties with cognitive flexibility, conceptualization, logical analysis, and disinhibition noted (T. L. Bennett & Ho, 2009; Deltour, Quaglino, Barathon, De Broca, & Berquin, 2007). Difficulty may be evidenced in resisting interference and shifting cognitive sets as well as in maintaining perseverance, fluency, and mental retrieval (Guimaràes et al., 2007; Pascalicchio et al., 2007; Sonmez et al., 2004). Across measures of executive function (Behavior Rating Inventory of Executive Function [BRIEF] and Delis-Kaplan Executive Function System [D-KEFS]), children with recent onset and well-controlled epilepsy have been found to exhibit significantly more difficulty than controls despite average mean cognitive ability (Parrish et al., 2007). These differences were significant for all subscales of the BRIEF; differences on the D-KEFS were significant for sorting and for inhibition but not on switching. Additionally, individuals with seizure disorders exhibit decreased reaction time and psychomotor speed. These deficits in executive functioning directly relate to their cognitive performance; further, executive function deficits influence the quality of life for children with epilepsy (Sherman, Slick, Connolly, & Eyrl, 2007). Research suggests that resting hypometabolism of the frontal lobes can be a useful predictor of executive dysfunction in patients with epilepsy (McDonald et al., 2006).

Visual Perception

Visual-spatial functioning may be one area that is spared, particularly if graphomotor and speed components are eliminated (Bender, Marks, Brown, Zach, & Zaroff, 2007). Children with juvenile myoclonic epilepsy may have difficulty with visual-spatial tasks (Sonmez et al., 2004), as may those with absence seizures (Pavone et al., 2001). Difficulties in visual-motor integration have been found, particularly with focal seizures, among children with epilepsy (T. L. Bennett & Ho, 2009).

Academic Implications

Children with epilepsy are at a greater risk than other children to demonstrate academic difficulties (Austin, Huberty, Huster, & Dunn, 1998; Bourgeois, 1998; Chaix et al., 2006; Fastenau, Shen, Dunn, & Austin, 2008; Fowler, Johnson, & Atkinson, 1985; Westbrook, Silver, Coupey, & Shinnar, 1991). Underachievement or low achievement is frequent among children with epilepsy, but no discernible connection between severity or duration of seizure disorder and achievement has been identified (Mitchell et al., 1991). Using an IQ-achievement discrepancy for specific learning disability (SLD), approximately one-half of children with epilepsy met criteria for SLD with the majority of difficulties in writing, followed by math and then reading (Fastenau et al, 2004, 2008); approximately one-third of children with epilepsy receive special education services (Zelnik, Sa'adi, Silman-Stolar, & Goikhman, 2001). Why this occurs is unknown, but the learning difficulties may be the result of brain damage/dysfunction, epilepsy may cause brain damage/dysfunction and subsequently lead to SLD, or epilepsy may cause SLD directly without any evident brain damage (Cornaggia & Gobbi, 2002). Alternatively, there are some indications that teachers underestimate the academic abilities of children they know to have epilepsy, potentially setting lower expectations and exacerbating their academic difficulties (Katzenstein, Fastenau, Dunn, & Austin, 2007). Further, there is the potential issue of chronic absences caused by the seizure disorders that in turn leads to underachievement. Ultimately, though, there is sufficient research to suggest that best practice would include screening for learning disability for any child who has epilepsy (Fastenau et al., 2008).

There are some indications of variability of risk by seizure type. Children with idiopathic epilepsy are at still greater risk for school failure and processing deficits than their healthy peers (Sturniolo & Galletti, 1994). Level of academic impairment may vary with type of seizure, age of onset, and duration of epilepsy (Chaix et al., 2006). For example, while some studies have suggested that children with generalized seizures are more at risk than those with partial seizures (Mandelbaum & Burack, 1997; Seidenberg, Beck, & Geisser, 1986), others have found no significant association between seizure type and academic outcome (Mitchell et al., 1991; Sturniolo & Galletti, 1994; J. Williams et al., 2001a). Further, temporal lobe epilepsy is associated with lower scores for reading speed and comprehension, particularly with left side focus (Chaix et al., 2006).

Emotional/Behavioral Correlates

Children with epilepsy are at risk for problems with school adaptation and emotional problems (Bailet & Turk, 2000; S. Davies, Heyman, & Goodman, 2003; Huberty, Austin, Huster, & Dunn, 2000); children with epilepsy are also at a greater risk of experiencing some form of psychological disorder with only recent recognition that psychiatric needs may not be addressed adequately (Ott et al., 2003; K. Smith et al., 2007). Components of both of the frequently used systems (e.g., Achenbach System of Empirically Based Assessment [ASEBA], Behavior Assessment System for Children, Second Edition [BASC-2]) for identification of problem behaviors have been found to be effective with children with epilepsy (Bender, Auciello, Morrison, MacAllister, & Zaroff, 2008). Psychiatric problems are estimated to co-occur in 37% to 77% of children with epilepsy (Plioplys, Dunn, & Caplan, 2007). Anxiety disorder or affective disorder are evident in 33% of pediatric epilepsy patients (Caplan et al., 2005). Depression has been found to occur in 36.5% of individuals with epilepsy in a community sample (Ettinger, Reed, & Cramer, 2004); 20% of children with pediatric epilepsy had suicidal ideation or plan (Caplan et al., 2005). Other studies have found that children with epilepsy have poorer social skills and are less assertive than typical peers (Tse, Hamiwka, Sherman, & Wirrell, 2007). They may demonstrate trends toward poorer peer relations and poorer interactions in the school environment (Yu, Lee, Wirrell, Sherman, & Hamiwka, 2008). It is not clear whether social stigma, neuropsychological functioning, or the interaction of these two factors accounts for the difficulty some children with epilepsy may face in the social arena.

The duration of the disease, age at onset, and polypsychopharmacological treatment are related to higher levels of interpersonal problems, ineffectiveness, negative self-esteem, and all-around greater depression level (Cushner-Weinstein et al., 2008). As with other areas of function, there is variability across seizure types. With complex partial epilepsy, the frequency of seizures in the past year is a strong predictor of behavioral difficulties (Schoenfeld et al., 1999). Absence seizures are associated with increased risk of school dropout, unplanned pregnancies, and substance abuse (Wirrell et al., 1997). In contrast TLE often is associated with depression, even when cognitive abilities are not impaired (Tracy et al., 2007). Depressive symptoms may be associated with external locus of control and sense of hopelessness (J. L. Wagner, Smith, Ferguson, Horton, & Wilson, 2009). For individuals over age 15, and controlling for a number of confounding factors, psychological comorbidity was evident in 35% of participants with juvenile myoclonic epilepsy (Trinka et al., 2006). The incidence of psychological impairment in these individuals was slightly higher than a representative community-based sample; however, it is difficult to tease out psychosocial and environmental effects associated with the epilepsy (Trinka et al., 2006).

Alternatively, when there is also developmental and cognitive delay, there is a higher likelihood of autistic-like behaviors and behaviors associated with Attention-Deficit/Hyperactivity Disorder (ADHD; Plioplys et al., 2007; Sherman et al., 2007). The prevalence of autism in children with epilepsy ranges from 5% to 38% (Danielsson, Gillberg, Billstedt, Gillberg, & Olsson, 2005; Rossi, Parmeggiani, Bach, Santucci, & Visconti, 1995; Tuchman & Rapin, 2002), and the likelihood increases if a child has severe mental retardation or cerebral palsy (Tuchman & Rapin, 2002). Similarly, parent reports suggest that children with epilepsy in conjunction with tuberous sclerosis complex exhibit clinically significant behavior problems with high rates of autistic-like behaviors, withdrawal, hyperactivity, and attention problems (Kopp et al., in press). Because of their difficulties with inattention and restlessness, children with epilepsy are likely to be diagnosed with ADHD (Hirshberg, Chui, & Frazier, 2005; Sherman et al., 2007).

EVIDENCE-BASED INTERVENTIONS

The choice of interventions depends on the targeted behavior, the desired outcome, and the needs of the individual child; however, in childhood epilepsy, the focus has been predominantly on reduction or control of the seizure frequency (see Table 10.2). The various treatments available for epilepsy include behavioral management, nutritional therapy, pharmacologic treatments, and neurosurgery; however, medication remains the most widely used form of treatment (Dichter, 1997). The occurrence of seizures themselves often is addressed through medical interventions—pharmacologically or surgically or both; educational and psychosocial effects may require more behavioral or ecological interventions, accommodations, or compensatory skills. It should be noted that the evidence base specific to outcomes with medical intervention generally focuses on the frequency of seizures following the intervention, with less information on functional or educational outcomes. An additional component of intervention that is often not addressed is ensuring that teachers working with children with epilepsy are aware of the associated issues with seizure disorders and the various medications that may be prescribed so as to avoid misattributions and dispel disease-related myths (Wodrich & Cunningham, 2008).

Pharmacology

From a medical perspective and with the goal of seizure control, medication is usually the initial approach (T. L. Bennett & Ho, 2009). An analysis of published, randomized trials of antiepilepsy drugs (AEDs) in children demonstrated equal efficacy with carbamazepine (Tegretol), oxcarbazepine (Trileptal), phenytoin (Dilantin), valproic acid (Depakote), clobazam (Frisium, Urbanol), primidone (Mysoline), ethosuximide (Zarontin), felbamate (Felbatol), gabapentin (Neurontin), lamotrigine (Lamictal), vigabatrin (Sabril), and phenobarbital (Phenobarbital) (T. L. Bennett & Ho, 2009; Camfield & Camfield, 2003). With regard to medication, the type of drug recommended depends on the type of seizure. Generalized tonic-clonic seizures often respond to anticonvulsants that prolong the inhibitory action of GABA in the brain. Absence seizures are treated by GABA-B antagonists such as ethosuximide (Zarontin) and valproic acid (Depakote). Partial seizures involving motor disturbances often are treated by clonazepam (Klonopin). While controlling the seizure disorder, the medications may affect current overall functioning as well as impact development over time (Ortinski & Meador, 2004). Effects of AEDs on neurocognitive functioning in children have not been studied extensively despite findings in the adult literature to suggest possible effects on learning and memory; some of the

Table 10.2 Evidence-Based Interventions for Pediatric Epilepsy

Intervention	Target/Goal	Level of Support
Antiepileptic drugs (AEDs)	Improve seizure control	Promising practice (Camfield & Camfield, 2003) but not without adverse effects (Freilinger et al., 2006)
Surgery	Improved seizure control for refractory seizures	Promising practice but not without adverse effects (Hakimi, Spanaki, Schuh, Smith, & Schultz, 2008)
Prednisolone (prednisone) in conjunction with AEDs	Improved seizure control	Emerging, particularly for cryptogenic epilepsies such as Landau-Kleffner, Lennox-Gastaut syndrome, Doose syndrome, Otahara syndrome (Yoo, Jung, Kim, Lee, & Kang, 2008)
Vagus nerve stimulation	Improved seizure control for refractory seizures	Emerging (Kwan & Brodie, 2005)
Ketogenic diet	Improved seizure control	Promising practice (J. M. Freeman et al., 1998; Henderson, Filloux, Alder, Lyon, & Caplin, 2006; Thiele, 2003)
Biofeedback	Improved seizure control for refractory seizures	Emerging (Hirshberg et al., 2005)
Antidepressant medications	Depression	Inconclusive (Mula, Schmitz, & Sander, 2008)
Progressive relaxation strategies	Control for refractory seizures	Emerging (J. L. Wagner & Smith, 2005)
Habituation training	Improved seizure control	Inconclusive (Noeker & Haverkamp, 2001)
Methylphenidate (Ritalin, Concerta), atomoxetine (Strattera)	Attention problems	Emerging (Torres, Whitney, & Gonzalez-Heydrich, 2008; Wernicke et al., 2007)

older AEDs are believed to compromise cognitive functioning, particularly processing speed and attention (Cornaggia & Gobbi, 2002; D. W. Loring & Meador, 2004; Prevey et al., 1996). Newer AEDs may not have the same negative effects as the older ones, but currently insufficient research is available; however, given the incidence of adverse effects of AEDs in the past, it has been suggested that monitoring for side effects be proactive, beginning with initiation of pharmacotherapy (Carreño et al., 2008). Across studies, there are indications of possible decline in cognitive ability as measured by IQ testing over time in association with the use of medications (T. L. Bennett & Ho, 2009); it is not known if these declines would have occurred in the absence of AEDs. It also should be noted that AED polypsychopharmacological treatment is associated with social problems, aggression, and inattention (Freilinger et al., 2006).

Surgery

In cases where seizures cannot be controlled by drugs, surgery as a treatment method has been used. If the area where the seizures occur can be identified, it is removed. Epilepsy surgery has been demonstrated to be a safe and effective treatment for refractory epilepsy and, compared to pharmacotherapy, is associated with decreased frequency of seizures (Hakimi et al., 2008) and improved cognitive functioning (Jambaqué et al., 2007). Follow-up study one year following anterior two-thirds corpus callosotomy for intractable epilepsy indicated that most of the individuals exhibited no significant change in cognitive functioning following surgery, even though about 40% demonstrated a beneficial effect with regard to seizure control and reduction in antiepileptic drugs (M. J. Cohen, Holmes, Campbell, Smith, & Flanigin, 1991). With temporal lobe epilepsy, temporal lobectomy is well established as a surgical procedure (Benifla, Rutka, Logan, & Donner, 2006). A retrospective review of 126 children indicated mean age of seizure onset was 5.6 years; the mean age at time of surgery was 13.5 years, suggesting that there is a significant delay from the onset of epilepsy to surgery (Benifla et al., 2006). Once the first AED fails, the chances of control with a second drug trial is about 14%. This number decreases with each subsequent trial; however, more than one-third of the neurologists indicated that failure on four monotherapy AED trials was needed for consideration for epilepsy surgery (Kwan & Brodie, 2000). Alternatively, seizure frequency emerged as the key determinant in whether to refer a person for surgery (Hakimi et al., 2008). At the same time, it has been suggested that for surgical intervention to be considered appropriate, this avenue for intervention must occur before the duration and frequency of the seizures cause irreversible consequences (Shevell et al., 2003).

Vagus Nerve Stimulation

Another form of nonpharmacological treatment for medically intractable epilepsy is vagus nerve stimulation (VNS; Amar, 2007; Kossoff, Pyzik et al., 2007). The vagus nerve originates in the medulla; stimulation of the vagus nerve has been shown to affect brain activity (Howland, 2006). The vagus nerve stimulator is made up of a signal generator that is programmed and implanted under the skin in the child's left upper chest. The stimulator is powered by a battery; the system delivers intermittent electrical stimulation to the left vagus nerve in the neck through a connecting lead. It is believed that VNS affects blood flow to regions of the brain that are associated with seizure activity (Howland, 2006). Alternatively, VNS may stimulate neurons that are involved in the modulation of cortical excitation (Li & Mogul, 2007). VNS has demonstrated efficacy against partial onset and generalized seizures, although few individuals have become seizure-free as a result of VNS (Ardesch, Buschman, Wagener-Schimmel, van der Aa, & Hageman, 2007; McHugh et al., 2007; Saneto et al., 2006). For example, in a study of 43 children with generalized, mixed, and partial epilepsy, 37% had at least 90% reduction in seizure frequency with VNS (Saneto et al., 2006). It is generally well tolerated, and the process is not technically demanding (Kwan & Brodie, 2005). Some problems with infection and coughing have been identified (Khurana et al., 2007).

Ketogenic Diet

Dietary treatment called the ketogenic diet (initially developed in the 1920s) mimics the effects of biochemical changes that occur during fasting (acidosis, dehydration, and ketosis). The ketogenic diet is a low-carbohydrate diet, based on an intake of fats and proteins (Bergqvist, Schall, Gallagher, Cnaan, & Stallings, 2005; Kossoff, Pyzik et al., 2007). This treatment generally is used when seizures are difficult to control and when the patient is unresponsive to medications, or when the drugs are not tolerated well. This type of diet has demonstrated effectiveness in children and had positive results in adults as well (Henderson et al., 2006; Vining, 1999; Vining et al., 2002). Recent studies have demonstrated a 90% reduction rate of seizures for 37% of patients (J. M. Freeman et al.,

1998); additionally, 30% attain reductions ranging from 50% to 90% (Thiele, 2003). One major problem in the use of the ketogenic diet is the need for adherence to the restrictive dietary regimen (Benbadis, Tatum, & William, 2001; J. M. Freeman et al., 2007). It is important for the whole family to become involved, and close collaboration among the child, family, pediatrician, and dietician are essential to successful implementation. While the ketogenic diet does not have the tranquilizing and negative cognitive effects of antiepileptic drugs, there are some potential concerns regarding its effects on growth in children (Benbadis et al., 2001).

Behavioral Approaches

Behavioral approaches have been used to address some components of seizure disorders, with some success across studies (Efron, 1957; Pritchard, Holmstrom, & Giacinto, 1985); however, no agreement has been reached due to the lack of available studies and the limited control in the experimental designs. Specific techniques vary and the type, duration, and severity of the seizure disorders of study participants vary. For those individuals who experience an aura or identifiable trigger to the seizure, one behavioral component may include habituation training (Noeker & Haverkamp, 2001). Alternatively, it may help to make individuals aware of their auras in order to stop the escalation of neuronal activity before the seizure occurs (J. L. Wagner & Smith, 2005). Sensory auras, such as smell, touch, and taste, appear to be most successful using this type of intervention. This technique is done by strongly stimulating the part most threatened by the seizure. For example, tactile auras have been remediated by using tickling and squeezing methods (J. L. Wagner & Smith, 2005).

In addition to these techniques, the use of stress reduction measures and biofeedback have been examined (Bortz et al., 1995; J. L. Wagner & Smith, 2005). Progressive relaxation strategies have been used with some effectiveness (J. L. Wagner & Smith, 2005). This technique involves the tightening and relaxing of certain muscle groups and the application of this strategy when confronted by stressful situations and feelings that are associated with high risk for seizure activity. In addition to stress, sudden changes in arousal may be associated with instances of seizure occurrence. As a result, a technique called countermeasures has been used to fight the initial stages of the seizures (Hirshberg et al., 2005). The goal of this behavioral approach is to change the arousal level. For example, if seizures are triggered by feelings of drowsiness, the goal of the countermeasure approach is to teach the individual to attain a state of hyperarousal to prevent the progression of the seizure.

Biofeedback is another method that has been used to gain seizure reduction for those who do not respond to medications (Sterman & Egner, 2006). Individuals are trained to understand their brain and mind states using operant conditioning principles to direct brain activity. With children, it is typically done by presenting the child with a reward for movement of brain signals in the desired direction and by presenting their brain activity in a creative way. A recent meta-analysis indicated that 82% of patients demonstrated more than 30% reduction of seizures, with an average of more than a 50% reduction (Sterman, 2000). In general, biofeedback for the treatment of epilepsy has demonstrated positive results; however, no consensus has been reached as to which variation of this feedback works best due to the limited studies available. Additionally the studies that do exist come from varying populations with a lack of control in the designs (Hirshberg et al., 2005). Further, participants in these studies were nonresponsive to medication treatment; for many, the only other alternative was surgery.

Educational Modifications and Accommodations

Research on specific academic interventions for children with epilepsy was not identified. With potential side effects of medications and seizure disorder both impacting on speed of processing as well as fatigue, it is important to consider modification of time allowances or reduction of workload for students with seizure disorders. Many parents, particularly those from higher socioeconomic levels, express concern with the lack of appropriate knowledge and educational services (K. N. Wu et al., 2008). In-service or educational information for staff, teachers, and students who work and interact with a child with a seizure disorder, as well as for the child and family members, may increase their level of comfort and ease, ultimately improving the outcome for the child. A study of the effects of an epilepsy education program indicated that children who participated in the educational intervention demonstrated an increase in knowledge and positive attitude about epilepsy as compared to control counterparts (Martinuik, Speechley, Seeco, Campbell, & Donner, 2007). For many individuals, changes may be needed in level of intervention or type of intervention as physiological changes occur. For this reason, frequent monitoring of progress and data-based decision making are needed whenever an intervention (medical, psychological, or educational) is instituted due to potential changes in functioning over time.

Psychosocial Interventions

Research suggests that often the mental health needs of children with seizure disorders are not identified or, when identified, are unmet (Austin & Caplan, in press; Austin et al., 1998; K. N. Wu et al., 2008). Survey and educational sessions with various groups of professionals indicated that pediatricians often do not consider mental health issues while mental health professionals may not be comfortable or feel competent to work with children with epilepsy (K. Smith et al., 2007). With approximately 23% of children with epilepsy also evidencing depression (Cushner-Weinstein et al., 2008), screening for possible depression may be appropriate. Enhancing a more positive attitude toward having epilepsy might help improve problems with poor self-concept or behavior problems but might not influence social competence (Tse et al., 2007). Further, family supports are also important in improving outcomes of children with epilepsy. It has been suggested that parent training programs that address epilepsy education, include skills in behavior management, foster social support networks, and modify inadequate parental coping behaviors may be beneficial (Rodenburg, Meijer, Dekoic, & Aldenkamp, 2007). Finally, consideration of parental comfort level with their child's diagnosis and acceptance of the treatments also may need to be addressed.

Medications for Comorbid Conditions

Co-occurring ADHD in children with epilepsy is common; first-line treatment for ADHD is often the initiation of medication therapy (see Chapter 6). There has been some evidence, based on case reports, of increased or recurring seizure activity when stimulant medications such as methylphenidate (Ritalin, Concerta) have been used to address the ADHD symptoms (Baptista-Neto et al., 2008). Based on an extensive review of what is known about the most frequently prescribed medications, methylphenidate has shown high response rates and no increase in seizures in small trials; however, further study with larger samples and over longer periods of time are needed to determine if there is an associated risk of increased seizure activity (Torres et al., 2008). Similar findings with small studies have been found with the use of atomoxetine (Strattera) (Wernicke et al., 2007). Taken together, the evidence available at this time best supports consideration of the joint vulnerability of ADHD and epilepsy, with use of medication for the treatment of ADHD as part of a comprehensive treatment plan when attentional issues have not been amenable to changes in antiepileptic drugs or improvements in seizure control (Torres et al., 2008; Wernicke et al., 2007). Similarly, although depression is not uncommon in those individuals with epilepsy, little data are available on the use of antidepressants and interactions with AEDs for individuals with epilepsy (Mula et al., 2008).

CASE STUDY: ZOEY—COMPLEX PARTIAL SEIZURES WITH TEMPORAL LOBE ORIGIN

The next report is from a hospital-based clinic. Identifying information, such as child and family name, teacher or physician name, and school information, has been altered or fictionalized to protect confidentiality.

Reason for Referral

Zoey is an 11-year 10-month-old repeating fourth grader who is being followed by her pediatric neurologist for a history of complex partial seizure disorder that began at approximately 1 to 2 years of age. Initially, Zoey's seizures were febrile in nature; however, at approximately 2 to 3 years of age, she began having seizures without fever. The seizures were characterized by an aura described by Zoey as "It feels like it's coming up from my stomach." This was followed by staring, loss of consciousness, right arm posturing, and lip smacking, after which Zoey might fall to the floor if she was not seated. The seizures typically lasted 10 to 15 seconds, and she was averaging three to four every 2 weeks with multiple anti-epileptic medications (carbamazepine [Tegretol] and topiramate [Topamax]). Initial magnetic resonance imaging (MRI) scan of the brain was reported as normal; however, a repeat MRI of the brain (see Figure 10.1) was reported to be significant for left mesial temporal (hippocampal) sclerosis. Video EEG monitoring (see Figure 10.2) was reported to be significant for epileptiform discharges from the left temporal area consistent with the MRI findings. Finally, a positron emission tomography scan was reported to be significant for decreased accumulation within the anterior left temporal lobe. As result, Zoey underwent epilepsy surgery (left temporal lobectomy with removal of the hippocampus and amygdala). Since the surgery, Zoey's mother reports that Zoey has not experienced any actual seizures; however, she does report auras approximately three times a week. The auras are characterized by similar feelings from her stomach that emanate to her head. She may then see black for a few seconds after which she returns to normal. At present, Zoey continues taking Topamax for seizure control. In addition, she takes amitriptyline (Elavil) for management of migraine headaches. At her neurologist's request, postoperative neuropsychological evaluation was undertaken in order to monitor higher cortical functioning approximately four years after her surgery in accordance with the Pediatric Epilepsy Surgery Protocol.

Tests Administered

Clinical interview

Wechsler Intelligence Scale for Children, Fourth Edition (WISC-IV)

Peabody Picture Vocabulary Test, Fourth Edition (PPVT-IV)

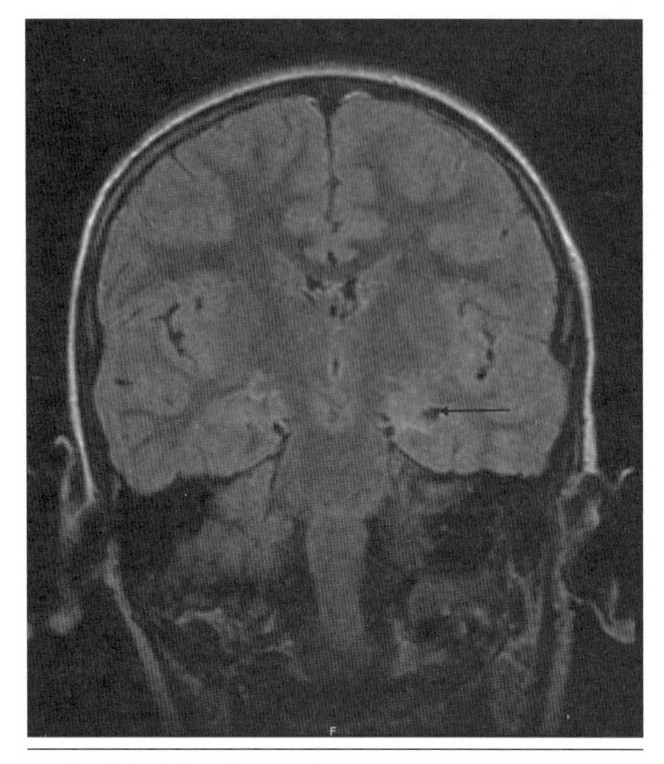

Figure 10.1 MRI of Zoey's brain.

Boston Naming Test (BNT)

Neuropsychological Assessment (NEPSY)/Neuropsychological Assessment, Second Edition (NEPSY-2; selected subtests)

Dichotic Listening Test

Kaufman Assessment Battery for Children, Second Edition (KABC-2; selected subtests)

Clinical Evaluation of Language Fundamentals, Fourth Edition (CELF-IV; selected subtests)

Beery Developmental Test of Visual Motor Integration, Fifth Edition (DTVMI-V)

Finger Tapping Test

Children's Memory Scale (CMS)

Gray Oral Reading Test, Fourth Edition (GORT-4)

Wide Range Achievement Test, Fourth Edition (WRAT-4)

Study Skills Questionnaire

Behavior Assessment Scale for Children, Second Edition (BASC-2; Parent and Teacher Rating Scales)

Background Information

Zoey continues to reside with her mother and stepfather. In addition, Zoey has two older sisters who are also living in the home. Jane, age 21, is a high school graduate who is

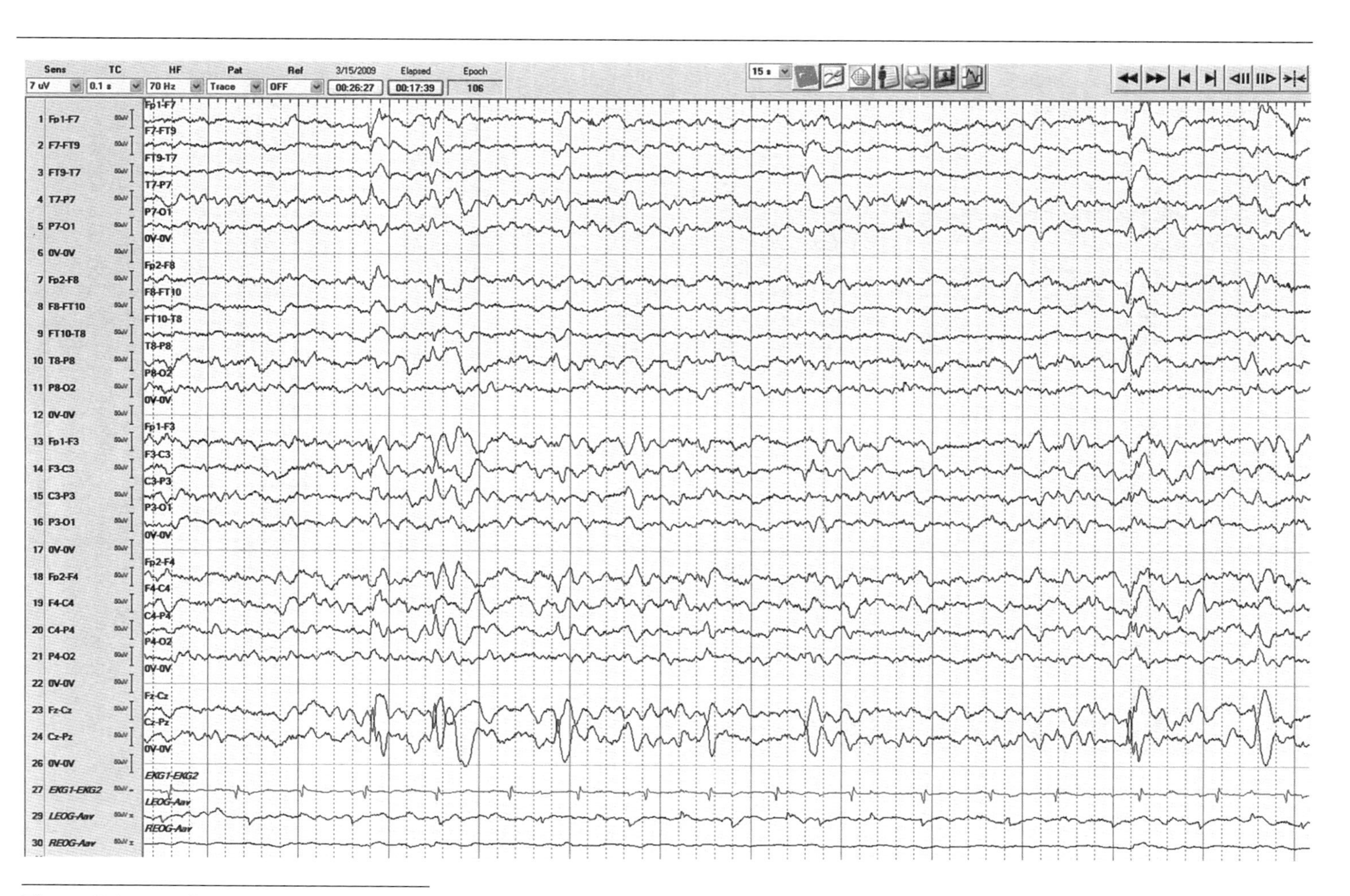

Figure 10.2 Zoey's Video EEG Monitoring.

attending technical school to earn a registered nursing degree. Jessica, age 13, is an A student in the seventh grade. She too has a history of migraine headache. Zoey also has three older brothers who are living outside of the home, only one of whom is a high school graduate. Zoey's natural parents divorced when she was 6 years of age. Her father dropped out of school in the tenth grade and was employed in the area of construction prior to being incarcerated for multiple offenses. He was adopted, and, as a result, nothing is known about the paternal family history. Zoey's mother is a high school graduate with two years of college coursework, who is currently employed at a local hospital. The maternal family history is significant for a brain tumor and seizures in the grandmother, who is now deceased.

Review of Zoey's developmental and medical history with her mother indicates that Zoey is the product of a full-term pregnancy complicated by physical and emotional spousal abuse. Delivery was vaginal and reported to be within normal limits. Zoey was reported to weigh 6 pounds 8 ounces at birth. She did well as a newborn and went home with her mother from the hospital after two days; however, her mother recalled that Zoey would often "jerk in her sleep" as a newborn. Zoey attained her developmental motor milestones within normal limits, with sitting up occurring at 6 months of age and walking at 8 months of age. Language milestones also were attained within normal limits; however, her mother was unable to recall exact dates. Toilet training was accomplished at 2 years of age without difficulty. Aside from the usual childhood illnesses, Zoey's past medical history is significant for the above-mentioned seizure disorder and migraine headaches, which have worsened since the surgery. Since her surgery, Zoey has been in good general health. She enjoys a normal appetite and sleep pattern; however, Zoey's mother reports that Zoey is easily distracted at school.

Review of academic history indicates that Zoey began attending a prekindergarten program at 4 years of age. According to her mother, she experienced mild hyperactivity in this setting; however, this resolved when Zoey's father left the home. At 5 years of age, Zoey attended kindergarten, where she began to experience difficulty with phonics. As a result, her teacher recommended retention. The following year, Zoey repeated kindergarten and then went on to first grade.

In March of the first-grade year, Zoey underwent preoperative neuropsychological evaluation by this service. The results indicated that Zoey was functioning within the borderline to low-average range of intellectual ability as measured by her Full Scale IQ of the WISC-IV; however, analysis of the Index scores indicated that Zoey was exhibiting a significant discrepancy between her deficient Verbal Comprehension Index and her average Perceptual Reasoning Index. A significant discrepancy also was noted between Zoey's low-average Working Memory Index and her average Processing Speed Index. Due to the significant deficits in verbal reasoning and auditory working memory, it was recommended that the Perceptual Reasoning Index be used as the best estimate of intellectual potential when making academic placement decisions for Zoey. Additional neuropsychological assessment demonstrated that Zoey was exhibiting relative strengths in areas of nonverbal reasoning, visual-spatial construction, and in her ability to learn and recall (30 minutes) the spatial location of visual objects (where). These were contrasted by relative weaknesses in abstract verbal reasoning, expressive and receptive language, auditory working memory, and in the ability to learn and recall auditory/verbal material. The results of a dichotic listening test for consonant vowel syllables appeared to indicate that language was lateralized in the left cerebral hemisphere with a relative suppression in right ear performance consistent with dysfunction involving the left geniculo-temporal pathway. Fine motor tapping speed was found to be within normal limits bilaterally with a relative depression noted in right (dominant) hand performance. Academically, Zoey demonstrated average word recognition/spelling, reading fluency, and numerical calculation skills consistent with nonverbal intellectual expectancy. In contrast, significant weaknesses were noted in the areas of reading comprehension and written expression that were of learning disability proportion. Behaviorally, analysis of rating scale data appeared to indicate that Zoey was not exhibiting significant evidence of emotional/behavioral difficulty in the home. In contrast, Zoey's teacher endorsed mild concern with regard to features of depressed mood in the classroom. Taken together, this pattern of neuropsychological test performance was felt to be consistent with a diagnosis of specific language impairment (mixed type) and learning disability in the areas of reading comprehension and written expression were secondary to left hemisphere dysfunction and Zoey's history of left temporal complex partial seizures.

As a result, it was recommended that Zoey be considered for special education services within a resource classroom setting designed for students with learning disabilities under the eligibility categories of "Specific Learning Disability" and/or "Other Health Impaired." Resource placement was recommended for language arts as well as considered for other academics that place heavy demands on reading comprehension and written expression (i.e., any class that requires the reading of a textbook or essay/report writing). Language therapy was recommended as a related service in order to improve expressive and receptive language. A behavioral plan also was recommended in order to enhance Zoey's self-concept.

Following her surgery, Zoey returned to her classroom after one week at home without any special education programming in place. In second grade, Zoey's mother reported that Zoey earned mostly Bs; however, Zoey was reported to daydream in class, and she frequently forgot her homework assignments. As a result, Zoey's third-grade teacher wrote down the assignments and dates of tests for her mother to keep track of them. In fourth grade, her mother stated that Zoey had a "very negative teacher"; this teacher caused Zoey to shut down in class when criticized. She began experiencing difficulty in reading and language arts, and her grades fell to "Cs across the board." This year, Zoey is repeating the fourth grade, and her mother states that Zoey earned As and Bs on her first 9-week report card. Zoey continues to daydream in class, and a family member must check to make sure she has the correct homework assignments and books before leaving the school.

Behavioral Observations

Zoey presented herself for testing as a pleasant, neatly groomed young lady with blue-green eyes and blond hair, who was casually dressed and somewhat overweight. She separated from her mother and accompanied the examiners to the testing room without difficulty, and she related well toward the examiners with good eye contact and a broad range of affect noted. In response to direct questions as well as when conversation was spontaneous, Zoey's language usage was fluent and prosodic with word-finding ("I know it but not how to say it") and sentence formulation difficulties noted. Her comprehension of directions was felt to be poor as well, and she frequently required repetition of directions when permissible. Throughout the evaluation, which consisted of two sessions separated by a lunch break, Zoey demonstrated an age-appropriate attention span and activity level. When confronted with difficult test items, Zoey typically responded in a reflective manner, and she responded well to praise and encouragement from the examiners. Lateral dominance is firmly established in the right hand for paper-and-pencil manipulation. Vision and hearing were screened at the health department and reported to be normal.

Test Results

The results of neuropsychological evaluation indicate that Zoey continues to function within the low-average range of intellectual ability as measured by the Full Scale IQ score of the Wechsler Intelligence Scale for Children, Fourth Edition (WISC-IV); however, analysis of the Index scores once again indicates that Zoey is exhibiting a significant discrepancy between her borderline Verbal Comprehension Index and her average Perceptual Reasoning Index (see Table 10.3). A significant discrepancy also is noted between Zoey's deficient Working Memory Index and her average Processing Speed Index. Thus, the results of intelligence testing indicate that Zoey continues to exhibit deficient to borderline verbal reasoning and auditory working memory contrasted by average nonverbal reasoning and information processing speed. Additional assessment indicates that Zoey is now exhibiting significant improvement in her sequential/nonverbal reasoning ability on the Tower subtest of the NEPSY; now her scores are in the high-average range. Expressive and receptive language are generally in the deficient to borderline range with significant word-finding difficulty still in evidence, consistent with the finding of specific language disorder on preoperative assessment. The results of a dichotic listening test for consonant vowel syllables continue to reveal suppression in right ear performance consistent with dysfunction involving the left geniculo-temporal pathway. Visual-spatial perception and construction are now elevated into the average range with mild motor planning difficulty still in evidence qualitatively. Fine motor tapping speed continues to be depressed in the right (dominant) hand.

Assessment of learning and memory with the Children's Memory Scale (CMS) revealed that Zoey continues to exhibit difficulty holding material in immediate auditory working memory contrasted by a significant improvement in visual working memory. When asked to learn and remember (30 minutes later) newly presented material, Zoey is now demonstrating further decline (deficient) in her ability to learn and recall auditory/verbal information contrasted by average visual/nonverbal learning and memory; however, it should be noted that within the visual domain, Zoey exhibited above-average ability to recall spatial location (where) contrasted by borderline recall of a series of pictured human faces (what she sees) consistent with preoperative assessment. Academically, Zoey demonstrated low-average to average word recognition/spelling and reading fluency. Her written expression standard score improved into the low-average range; however, qualitative analysis of her writing continues to reveal a performance that is well below intellectual expectancy. Reading comprehension continues to be significantly below expectancy, and numerical calculation skills are now deficient to borderline, well below preoperative testing. As compared with nonverbal intellectual ability, the deficiencies in reading comprehension, written expression, and numerical calculation are all of learning disability proportion. Behaviorally, analysis of rating scales completed by Zoey's mother and teacher indicates that, at home, Zoey is now exhibiting significant evidence of short attention span. In addition to concerns about short attention span, Zoey's teacher endorsed concern with regard to conduct, anxiety/depressed mood, poor social skills, and academic difficulty.

Table 10.3 Psychometric Summary for Zoey

	Preoperative Standard Scores	4 Years Postoperative Standard Scores
Wechsler Intelligence Scale for Children, Fourth Edition		
Full Scale IQ	80	84
Verbal Comprehension Index	61	77
Similarities	55	75
Vocabulary	70	75
Comprehension	75	90
Perceptual Reasoning Index	98	104
Block Design	100	100
Picture Concepts	100	110
Matrix Reasoning	95	100
Working Memory Index	83	65
Digit Span	80	75
Letter-Number Sequencing	90	65
Processing Speed Index	100	100
Coding	85	100
Symbol Search	115	100
Neuropsychological Assessment, Second Edition (NEPSY-2)		
Tower (NEPSY)	80	110
Phonological Processing	70	70
Sentence Repetition	80	70
Verbal Fluency	75	90
Arrows	85	105
Peabody Picture Vocabulary Test, Fourth Edition (PPVT-IV)	77	70
Boston Naming Test (BNT)	<40	<40
Clinical Evaluation of Language Fundamentals, Fourth Edition (CELF-IV)		
Formulated Sentences	65	70
Concepts and Following Directions	65	65
Dichotic Listening	**Number Correct (Pre)**	**Number Correct (Post)**
Left Ear	12/30	13/30
Right Ear	11/30	9/30
	Standard Score	**Standard Score**
Gestalt Closure (KABC-2)	80	95
Developmental Test of Visual-Motor Integration –Fifth Edition (DTVMI-V)	90	83
Clock Face Drawing		
Form	87	108
Time (10:20)	—	107
Finger Tapping Test		
Right (dominant) Hand	104	83
Left (nondominant) Hand	105	95

(continued)

Table 10.3 ***(Continued)***

	Preoperative Standard Scores	4 Years Postoperative Standard Scores
Children's Memory Scale		
Attention/Concentration Index	82	78
Numbers	75	70
Sequences	95	95
Picture Locations	105	135
General Memory Index	80	67
Verbal Immediate Index	72	54
Stories	80	60
Word Pairs	75	65
Visual Immediate Index	106	106
Dot Locations	110	110
Faces	100	100
Verbal Delayed Index	75	54
Stories	70	55
Word Pairs	90	70
Visual Delayed Index	91	94
Dot Locations	105	115
Faces	80	75
Delayed Recognition Index	85	50
Stories	80	55
Word Pairs	95	60
Learning Index	88	91
Word Pairs	75	70
Dot Locations	110	115
Gray Oral Reading Test, Fourth Edition (GORT-4)		
Fluency	90	95
Comprehension	70	65
Wide Range Achievement Test, Fourth Edition (WRAT-4)		
Reading	104	91
Spelling	99	93
Arithmetic	92	76
Test of Written Language, Third Edition (TOWL-3)		
Written Language Quotient	74	87
Behavior Assessment System for Children, Second Edition (Current Ratings)		
	T-Scores	
	Parent	Teacher
Clinical Scales		
Hyperactivity	61	63
Aggression	55	59
Conduct	54	66
Anxiety	57	72
Depression	60	82

(continued)

Table 10.3 *(Continued)*

	T-Scores	
	Parent	Teacher
Somatization	84	58
Atypical	49	82
Withdrawal	42	63
Attention	64	64
Learning Problems	NA	66
Adaptive Scales		
Adaptability	41	41
Social Skills	56	36
Leadership	59	44
Study Skills	NA	34
Activities of Daily Living	49	NA
Functional Communication	45	41

Notes. NA = not applicable.

Summary and Diagnostic Impressions

Zoey is an 11-year-old girl who is encountering difficulty in academic areas, as well as with attention. She has a history of seizures, has undergone epilepsy surgery (temporal lobectomy), and continues on seizure medication. Taken together, the current pattern of neuropsychological test performance continues to be consistent with a picture of left-hemisphere dysfunction and a diagnosis of specific language impairment mixed type, with learning disability in the areas of reading comprehension, written expression and now mathematical calculation. Finally, Zoey is now exhibiting significant difficulty with attention regulation at home and school; she is also experiencing significant emotional and behavioral difficulty at school due to a lack of support services since her surgery.

Recommendations

As a result, it is again recommended that Zoey be considered for resource/inclusion special education services designed for students with learning disabilities under the eligibility categories of "Specific Learning Disability" and/or "Other Health Impaired." Resource placement should be utilized for remediation of reading comprehension, written expression, and now mathematical reasoning/calculation skills. Inclusion services should be provided as needed to ensure that Zoey has support in the regular education setting as needed. Language therapy should be provided as a related service in order to improve expressive and receptive language. Zoey also would benefit from a behavioral plan at school that is focused on enhancing her ability to regulate her attention, improve her self-concept, listening skills, and task completion as part of her Individualized Education Plan.

In order to enhance Zoey's learning/retention, new material should be presented in an organized format that is meaningful to her. The material to be learned should be broken down into smaller components/steps and presented in a highly structured format with frequent repetition to facilitate learning. Instruction should be supplemented with visual aids, demonstrations, and experiential/procedural learning whenever possible. When studying for tests or doing multiple homework assignments on the same day, similar subject material should be separated in order to lessen interference. Finally, Zoey should be provided with periodic review of previously learned material in order to enhance long-term retention.

Accommodations will be necessary to enhance Zoey's ability to succeed in the classroom, including preferential seating away from bulletin boards, doorways, windows, or other students, if necessary, where excessive stimuli might prove distracting. Instruction should be provided in small-group settings whenever possible. Given her learning disabilities, a reduction in the amount, but not the difficulty level, of assignments may assist Zoey in completing classroom tasks and homework in a timely manner. Moreover, whenever possible, she should be given additional time to complete assignments. Tests should be in multiple choice/matching/short answer formats instead of essay format and should be administered individually, with additional time provided when necessary. Finally, Zoey should be allowed and encouraged to use various compensatory devices, such as textbooks on tape, a calculator to check written calculations, and a computer with word processing capability. Most word processing programs are equipped with spell checks and cut and paste and can be adapted for voice dictation if necessary. This will be increasingly valuable during Zoey's education.

Zoey should continue to be followed by her neurologist for management of her seizure disorder. Finally, Zoey's mother may wish to consult with him regarding a trial of medication therapy to improve Zoey's attention span.

Further Discussion of Case Study

As with traumatic brain injury, it is important to consider the need for proactive programming immediately following epilepsy surgery in order to maximize positive outcome and rehabilitation. In this case, although surgery was successful in attaining seizure control, there has been an increase in migraines and attentional issues. At the same time, while some supports were provided, these were minimal, and did not address Zoey's preoperative deficits in language areas, which continue to be evident. As discussed in conjunction with language and reading deficits, over time, the effects of these impairments generalize and begin affecting all areas of functioning. For Zoey and other children who undergo epilepsy surgery, it is important that interventions be in place quickly and be of sufficient intensity to address the preoperative deficits as well as any additional deficits that emerge postoperatively.

CASE STUDY: LANE—LANDAU-KLEFFNER SYNDROME (EPILEPTIC APHASIA)

The next report is from a hospital-based clinic. Identifying information, such as child and family name, teacher or physician name, and school information, has been altered or fictionalized to protect confidentiality.

Referral and Background Information

Lane is a 10-year 6-month old boy who is being followed by his pediatric neurologist for a history of benign rolandic epilepsy with continuous spike and wave activity during sleep (CSWS) and Landau-Kleffner syndrome (epileptic aphasia). Lane's seizure disorder remained refractory to conventional medication therapy as well as treatment with prednisone and intravenous immune globulin. As a result, Lane underwent a left frontotemporal craniotomy and subdural grid placement for phase II epilepsy monitoring. Based on the monitoring results, Lane underwent epilepsy surgery (left anterior inferior frontal resection with left inferior frontal multiple subpial transaction). Lane did well for the first 6 weeks following surgery, after which he developed obsessive/bizarre thoughts and mental confusion. Lane began seeing a child psychiatrist who initiated trials of medication therapy with sertraline (Zoloft) followed by risperidone (Risperdal) without success. Three months after epilepsy surgery, Lane began exhibiting daytime staring episodes and on 4 or 5 occasions he would awaken in the morning "wet and confused." As a result, his neurologist restarted phenytoin (Dilantin) along with the lamotrigine (Lamictal) that Lane was already taking. Following the addition of Dilantin, Lane's obsessive/bizarre thoughts stopped and his behavior normalized. At present, Lane continues to take Lamictal (200 mg twice a day) and Dilantin (300 mg at bedtime) for seizure management. At the request of his neurologist, neuropsychological reevaluation was undertaken in order to monitor higher cortical functioning 6 months postsurgery and make appropriate recommendations regarding school placement and the need for supportive therapies.

Lane continues to reside with his parents and his 13-year-old sister, who is currently an A student in the eighth grade. She is followed by a child psychiatrist for cyclothymia and ADHD. Lane's father is a high school and college graduate, who is currently employed as a manager at a nuclear reactor site. He is in good general health; however, he is being treated for anxiety attacks. The paternal family history is significant for seizures in a distant female relative, who also has a son who recently began having seizures. Lane's mother is a high school graduate, who is currently a full-time homemaker after being employed as a paraprofessional in the local school system. She is reported to be in good general health and currently is being treated for cyclothymia. The maternal family history is significant for cyclothymia in the grandmother, academic difficulty and anxiety attacks in an aunt, as well as ADHD and learning disability in a male and female cousin. Lane's mother also has two half siblings; one has a history of ADHD and the other has a history of global learning disability.

Review of Lane's developmental and medical history indicates that he is the product of a normal, full-term pregnancy and vaginal delivery, weighing 9 pounds 1 ounce at birth. Apgar scores were reported to be 8 at 1 minute and 9 at 5 minutes, respectively. Lane did well as a newborn and went home with his mother from the hospital on schedule. Lane attained his developmental motor milestones at an accelerated rate, with sitting up occurring at 4.5 months of age and walking at 9.5 months of age. Language milestones also were felt to be accelerated, with first words at 5 to 6 months of age and short sentences at 18 months of age. Toilet training was fully accomplished at 2 years of age without difficulty. The parents report that Lane had always been a very active youngster: however, Lane did not exhibit evidence of short attention span until after he began experiencing seizures. Specifically, his parents report that since seizure onset, he is more forgetful about following through with chores as well as fun activities, he is less patient, and has a "shorter fuse." Lane's first observed seizure occurred when he was 8 years, 2 months of age, while he was going to sleep. His second seizure occurred two months later in the early morning just prior to awakening. Initially, Lane's neurologist started him on oxcarbazepine (Trileptal). Lane's initial EEG was felt to be consistent with benign rolandic epilepsy. On Trileptal, his parents reported that Lane became lethargic and was not his active self. In addition, they observed a slight drop in his academic performance. At nine months postonset, Lane experienced his first daytime seizure, which involved jerking of the right arm and face with an associated loss of speech lasting approximately 25 minutes. After the seizure, Lane experienced a right Todd's paralysis for the remainder of the day. In addition, he continued to have difficulty talking. Following this seizure, his neurologist increased the dosage of Trileptal; thereafter, the parents reported a more noticeable drop in his academic performance as well as his activity level. At 11 months postonset, Lane experienced his first seizure at school, which involved eye twitching and unresponsiveness.

At that point, Lane was admitted to the pediatric epilepsy monitoring unit for video EEG monitoring. When awake, his EEG was significant for bilateral independent spike and wave activity from the central temporal region consistent with benign rolandic epilepsy. During sleep, Lane's EEG demonstrated continuous spike and wave activity with REM sleep suppression (CSWS; see Figure 10.3). MRI scan of the brain was reported to be normal. Based on the EEG findings, Lane's neurologist elected to begin Lane on Lamictal. On Lamictal, his parents report that "Lane got his legs back." Specifically, he was more active, thinking more clearly, and his attention span seemed to be improved. Three months later, Lane again began experiencing seizure activity with a decline in academic functioning. As a result, initial neuropsychological evaluation was conducted.

The results of neuropsychological evaluation indicated that Lane was functioning within the average to high-average range of intellectual ability as measured by the General Ability Index of the Wechsler Intelligence Scale for Children, Fourth Edition. It was felt that this represented the best estimate of Lane's intellectual potential, given the significant weaknesses noted on the Working Memory and Processing Speed indices. Additional assessment indicated that Lane demonstrated relative strengths in the areas of expressive and receptive vocabulary development and abstract verbal reasoning, phonological processing, visual-spatial perception/closure, and in his ability to learn and recall (30 minutes later) pictures of human faces (what he sees). These were contrasted by relative weaknesses in Lane's higher-order problem solving capability when he was not provided with the solution he is working toward. Relative weaknesses also were noted in linguistic planning/sentence formulation and in Lane's fine motor tapping speed in the right (dominant) hand as compared to the left. The results of a Dichotic Listening test appeared to indicate that language was lateralized in the left cerebral hemisphere as evidenced by a right ear advantage in Lane's ability to report consonant vowel syllables simultaneously to each ear. Academically, Lane appeared to be developing basic reading, reading comprehension, written expression, and math calculation/reasoning skills at levels that were generally commensurate with to above intellectual expectancy. A relative weakness was noted in Lane's written expression as compared with the other areas assessed. Behaviorally, analysis of rating scales completed by Lane's mother and teacher indicated that, at that time, Lane was not exhibiting significant emotional or behavioral difficulty at home or in the classroom.

Taken together, this pattern of neuropsychological test performance was felt to be consistent with a picture of dysfunction involving the more anterior aspects of the left cerebral hemisphere, placing Lane at risk for development of a language disorder and language-based learning disability in the future should he continue to experience periodic episodes of poor seizure control or a pattern of intractable epilepsy and Landau-Kleffner syndrome.

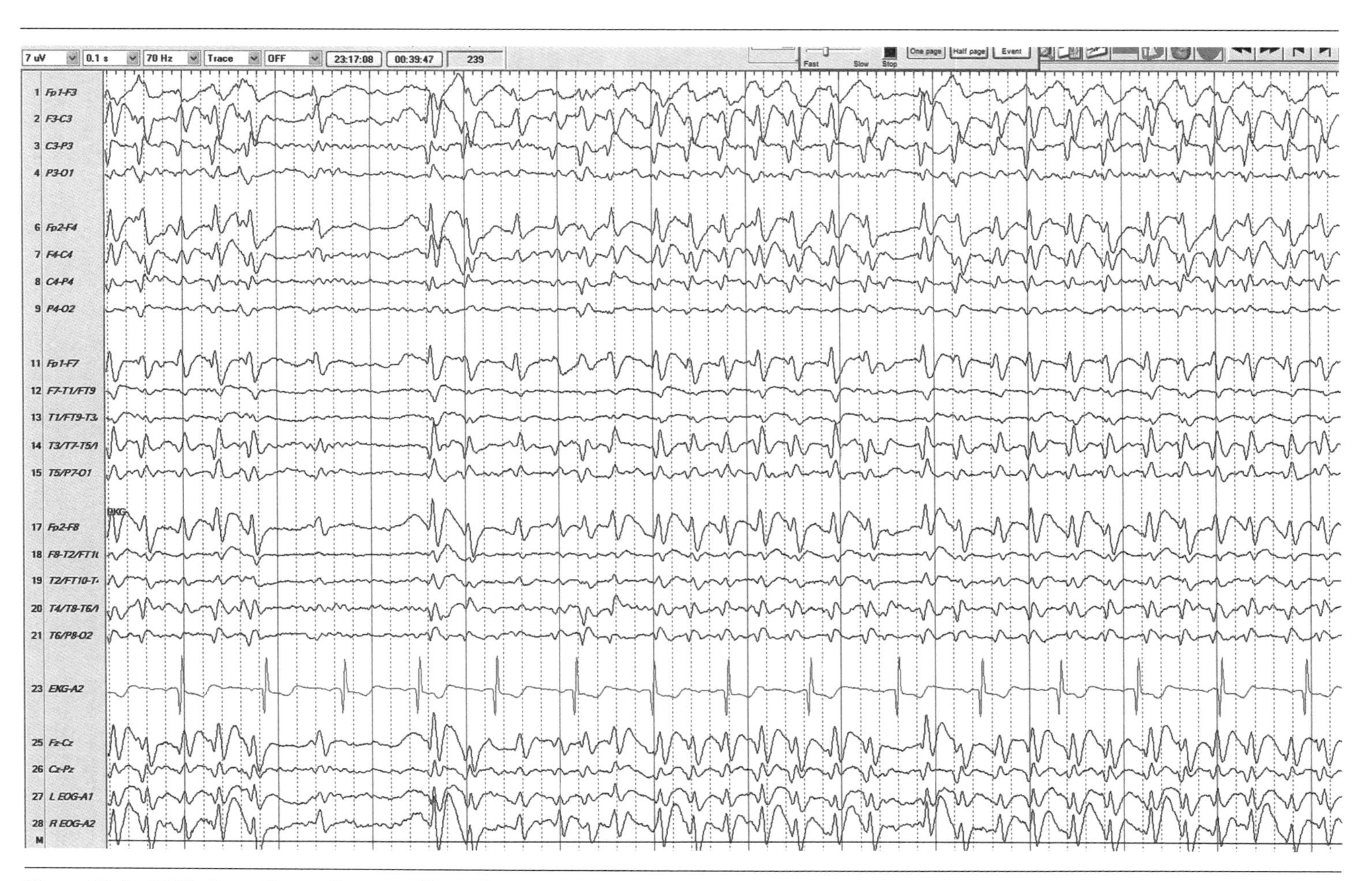

Figure 10.3 EEG shows the continuous spike and wave activity in sleep for Lane.

As a result, Lane's neurologist began him on a course of steroids due to a concern regarding Landau-Kleffner syndrome. Lane was readmitted to the pediatric epilepsy monitoring unit, and his EEG continued to be consistent with a picture of CSWS. During this admission, a repeat screening of language and memory functions was performed that revealed a significant decline in performance on the immediate and delayed recall portions of the Stories subtest of the CMS. In contrast, language and visual memory skills remain stable. Lane was discharged on Lamictal, Dilantin, and Prednisone. It was recommended that Lane receive homebound teacher services while he recuperated at home. It was further recommended that a student support team be convened with a referral made for special education inclusion services designed for students with learning disabilities under the eligibility category of "Other Health Impaired" should Lane continue to experience language/verbal memory deficits upon return to school. Language therapy as a related service also was recommended.

After approximately one month of steroid therapy, Lane's seizure frequency improved, and repeat neuropsychological screening of language and memory was once again carried out (see Table 10.4). The results indicated that on steroids, Lane demonstrated stable performance on language assessment with stable to improved verbal and visual memory, taking practice effects into account. Lane continued to do well with seizure control for almost three months, after which he relapsed. As a result, he was readmitted to the pediatric epilepsy monitoring unit, and immunoglobulin therapy was initiated. After discharge, neuropsychological screening of language and memory was carried out once again. The results indicated that Lane was exhibiting significant difficulty comprehending multipart directions. In addition, he continued to exhibit difficulty processing/encoding large amounts of verbal material into long-term memory. Visual learning and memory continued to be a relative strength although well below prior assessment levels.

Lane's seizure disorder remained refractory to conventional anticonvulsant therapy, as well as treatment with Prednisone and intravenous immune globulin. As a result, Lane underwent a left frontotemporal craniotomy and subdural grid placement for phase II epilepsy monitoring. Based on these monitoring results, Lane underwent epilepsy surgery (left anterior inferior frontal resection with left inferior frontal multiple subpial transection). Lane did well for the first 6 weeks following surgery, after which he developed obsessive/bizarre thoughts and mental confusion. Lane began seeing a child psychiatrist, who initiated trials of medication therapy with sertraline (Zoloft) followed by risperidone (Risperdal) without success. Three months after epilepsy surgery, Lane began exhibiting daytime staring episodes and on four or five occasions he would awaken in the morning "wet and confused." As a result, his neurologist restarted phenytoin (Dilantin) along with the Lamictal that Lane was already taking. Following the addition of Dilantin, Lane's obsessive/bizarre thoughts stopped and his behavior normalized. At present, Lane continues to take lamotrigine (Lamictal), 200 mg twice a day, and Dilantin, 300 mg at bedtime for seizure management.

Review of Lane's academic history indicates that his first formal school experience was kindergarten at 5 years of age. According to his parents, he did extremely well academically, even though he missed a lot of school. Lane continued to do well academically in first and second grades; however, toward the end of second grade, his teacher began to voice some concern about variability in his classroom performance around the time he had his first identified seizure. In the third grade, Lane's parents observed a noticeable decline in his grades while he was on Trileptal. Review of a school report form completed by Lane's third grade teacher indicated that she characterized Lane as

Table 10.4 Monitoring with Differing Treatments

Measure	Initial Evaluation	Steroids	Immunoglobulin Therapy (pre)	Immunoglobulin Therapy (post)
Sentence Repetition (Neuropsychological Assessment [NEPSY]/CELF-IV)	85	80		105
Concepts and Directions (CELF-IV)	105		115	60
Boston Naming Test (BNT)	117	114		104
Formulated Sentences (CELF-IV)	105		105	90
Stories (Children's Memory Scale [CMS])				
Immediate	90	75		70
Delayed	90	70		75
Word Pairs (CMS)				
Immediate	100		115	
Delayed	100		105	
Faces (CMS)				
Immediate	120	130		105
Delayed	110	120		95
Dot Locations				
Immediate	85		100	
Delayed	90		110	

> a friendly child. He is well liked by his peers. He has a good imagination. He gets along with others and has a wide variety of friends. Lane can be outgoing at times and seems to enjoy being at school. Lane is a great reader; he enjoys writing stories and drawing. Lane has a great vocabulary and his spelling is above average. Lane enjoys science activities in the classroom.

She went on to estimate that he was reading at an above average level for grade placement with average performance in arithmetic. After approximately 1.5 weeks into the fourth-grade year, Lane's seizure frequency escalated. As a result, he began receiving homebound teacher services. Following epilepsy surgery, Lane continued to receive homebound teacher services until he returned to school in May for the last two weeks. During the summer, his mother worked almost daily with Lane in the areas of reading, language arts, and mathematics; however, she reported that after the seizures returned, "It was like he forgot everything."

At present, Lane is attending the fifth grade. Review of his most recent Individualized Education Plan (IEP) indicates that he is receiving special education collaborative services in his regular education classroom under the "Other Health Impaired" category. This includes support during reading class with monitoring of his progress in other subjects. In addition, Lane has an auditory trainer in order to help minimize distractibility in the classroom; however, it is used inconsistently. Lane has an additional set of textbooks for use at home and is afforded several accommodations including preferential seating, a computer to supplement instruction, a note taker, extra time, simplified/shortened instructional sets, reduced copying tasks/copies of notes and board work, study guides, and is allowed to retake examinations. His mother reports that Lane's teachers are concerned that his learning is "spotty and inconsistent" and it is "difficult to predict when he is on or off." Lane's mother also reports that she is spending 1.5 hours per night with Lane trying to get homework done. During these sessions, she has to provide frequent redirection and "leading" to keep Lane on task and meeting with success. During the first grading period, Lane earned an A in spelling; Bs in reading, social studies, language arts, and science; a C in English; and an F in mathematics.

General Observations and Impressions

Lane presented for testing as a very pleasant, neatly groomed youngster with blue eyes and brown hair who was casually dressed in a striped polo shirt, jeans, and sneakers. He separated from his mother and accompanied the examiners to the testing room without difficulty. Throughout the evaluation, which consisted of two sessions separated by a lunch break, Lane related well toward the examiners with good eye contact, a broad range of affect, appropriate use of humor, and good manners noted. It should be noted that his mother reported that Lane was having "an average to above-average day" with regard to his level of alertness and mental awareness. In response to direct questioning, as well as when conversation was spontaneous, Lane's language usage was fluent and prosodic with good comprehension of task demands noted. Lane's attention span and activity level were felt to be age appropriate, and he appeared to put forth a good effort on all tasks presented. When confronted with difficult test items, Lane typically responded in a reflective manner with good task persistence. Lateral dominance continues to be firmly established in the right hand for paper-and-pencil manipulation. Vision and hearing were not formally screened; however, Lane wore his glasses for reading.

Tests Administered

Clinical interview
Wechsler Intelligence Scale for Children, Fourth Edition (WISC-IV)
Wisconsin Card Sorting Test (WCST)
Peabody Picture Vocabulary Test, Fourth Edition (PPVT-IV)
Boston Naming Test (BNT)
Neuropsychological Assessment (NEPSY)/Neuropsychological Assessment, Second Edition (NEPSY-2; selected subtests)
Dichotic Listening Test
Kaufman Assessment Battery for Children, Second Edition (KABC-2; selected subtests)
Clinical Evaluation of Language Fundamentals, Fourth Edition (CELF-IV; selected subtests)
Beery Developmental Test of Visual Motor Integration (DTVMI-V)
Finger Tapping Test
Children's Memory Scale
Gray Oral Reading Test, Fourth Edition (GORT-4)
Test of Written Language, Third Edition (TOWL-3)

Wide Range Achievement Test, Fourth Edition (WRAT-4)
Behavior Assessment System for Children, Second Edition (BASC-2; Parent and Teacher Rating Scales)

Test Results

The results of neuropsychological evaluation indicate that Lane continues to function within the average range of intellectual ability as measured by the Full Scale IQ score and the General Ability Index of the Wechsler Intelligence Scale for Children, Fourth Edition (see Table 10.5). Analysis of the various Index scores reveals that although Lane is demonstrating a slight decline in his verbal conceptual abilities as compared with his initial assessment (8 points), he is now exhibiting improved auditory working memory (17 points) and processing speed (6 points), which are both in the average range. Additional assessment indicates that Lane is demonstrating significantly improved higher-order problem-solving capability, which is now in the average to high-average range. Both receptive and expressive language areas are in the average to high-average range with a marked improvement in sentence formulation/linguistic planning noted. The results of a Dichotic Listening Test continue to indicate that language is lateralized in the left cerebral hemisphere as evidenced by a right ear advantage in Lane's ability to report CV syllables simultaneously to each ear. Lane continues to demonstrate high-average visual-perceptual skills along with average visual-motor/constructional ability. Fine motor tapping speed continues to be above average with a relative weakness noted in right (dominant) hand performance still in evidence.

Analysis of Lane's performance on the Children's Memory Scale (CMS) indicates that he is exhibiting average ability to hold auditory/verbal material in immediate working memory contrasted by superior visual/nonverbal working memory. Lane also demonstrated average ability to learn and remember (30 minutes later) auditory/verbal material contrasted by superior visual learning and recall. Further, it should be noted that Lane's verbal recall ability was significantly aided with the use of a cued recall paradigm, indicating difficulty with retrieval of previously learned verbal material.

Academically, while Lane continues to achieve at levels that are commensurate with/above his current level of intellectual functioning, he is demonstrating a plateauing in skill development (based on raw score comparisons) in the areas of oral reading fluency, reading comprehension, written expression, and mathematical calculation as compared with his prior assessment.

Behaviorally, analysis of rating scales completed by Lane's mother and teachers appears to indicate that, at the present time, Lane's mother endorsed significant concern with regard to his level of anxiety and social/emotional immaturity. Lane's teachers currently are not endorsing significant concerns with regard to Lane's behavior in the classroom.

Summary and Diagnostic Impressions

Lane is a 10-year 6-month-old who is being evaluated 6 months post epilepsy surgery for treatment of Landau Kleffner syndrome. He has been followed through this service for the past two years, including a prior comprehensive neuropsychological evaluation following initial presentation of his seizure disorder. Taken together with his extensive history, the current pattern of neuropsychological test performance continues to be consistent with

Table 10.5 Psychometric Summary for Lane

	Scaled Scores	Standard Scores
Wechsler Intelligence Scale for Children, Fourth Edition (WISC-IV)		
Full Scale IQ		99
General Ability Index		102
Verbal Comprehension Index		104
Similarities	10	
Vocabulary	13	
Comprehension	10	
Perceptual Reasoning Index		98
Block Design	10	
Picture Concepts	9	
Matrix Reasoning	10	
Working Memory Index		97
Digit Span	12	
Letter-Number Sequencing	7	
Processing Speed Index		94
Coding	9	
Symbol Search	9	
Wisconsin Card Sorting Test (WCST)		
Categories Obtained (6/6)		106
Perseverative Errors		104
Failure to Maintain Set		91
Neuropsychological Assessment, Second Edition (NEPSY-2)		
Tower (NEPSY)		115
Phonological Processing		105
Sentence Repetition		85
Verbal Fluency		100
Arrows		115
Peabody Picture Vocabulary Test, Fourth Edition (PPVT-IV)		112
Boston Naming Test (BNT)		92
Clinical Evaluation of Language Fundamentals, Fourth Edition (CELF-4)		
Formulated Sentences		115
Concepts and Following Directions		95
Dichotic Listening	**Number Correct**	
Left Ear	11/30	
Right Ear	15/30	
		Standard Score
Gestalt Closure (KABC-2)		110
Developmental Test of Visual-Motor Integration, Fifth Edition (DTVMI-V)		116
Clock Face Drawing		
Form		95
Time (10:20)		109
Finger Tapping	**Taps/10 sec.**	**Standard Score**
Right (dominant) Hand	40.3	118
Left (nondominant) Hand	42.0	128

Table 10.5 (*Continued*)

	Scaled Scores	Standard Scores
Children's Memory Scale (CMS)		
Attention/Concentration Index		109
Numbers	13	
Sequences	10	
Picture Locations	13	
General Memory Index		119
Verbal Immediate Index		97
Stories	0	
Word Pairs	10	
Visual Immediate Index		125
Dot Locations	13	
Faces	15	
Verbal Delayed Index		94
Stories	10	
Word Pairs	8	
Visual Delayed Index		134
Dot Locations	14	
Faces	17	
Delayed Recognition Index		112
Stories	11	
Word Pairs	11	
Learning Index		106
Word Pairs	10	
Dot Locations	12	
Gray Oral Reading Test, Fourth Edition (GORT-4)		
Fluency		105
Comprehension		100
Wide Range Achievement Test, Fourth Edition (WRAT-4)		
Reading		127
Spelling		125
Arithmetic		96
Test of Written Language, Third Edition (TOWL-3)		
Written Language Quotient		100
Behavior Assessment System for Children, Second Edition (BASC-2)		
	T-Scores	
	Parent Rating Scale	Teacher Rating Scale (Teacher 1/ Teacher 2)
Clinical Scales		
Hyperactivity	50	41/46
Aggression	40	43/43
Conduct	40	42/42
Anxiety	72	45/52
Depression	57	45/50
Somatization	59	43/92
Atypical	75	50/53
Withdrawal	49	47/47
Attention	53	42/61

(continued)

Table 10.5 ***(Continued)***

	T-Scores	
	Parent Rating Scale	Teacher Rating Scale (Teacher 1/ Teacher 2)
Learning Problems	NA	58/54
Adaptive Scales		
Adaptability	57	56/56
Social Skills	52	61/65
Leadership	44	42/56
Study Skills	NA	53/49
Activities of Daily Living	49	NA/NA
Functional Communication	33	—/49

Note. NA = Not applicable.

a picture of relative dysfunction involving the more anterior aspects of the left cerebral hemisphere, although significant improvement in functioning is very much in evidence as compared with initial neuropsychological assessment. Given that Lane continues to experience seizure activity following epilepsy surgery and he is exhibiting a plateauing in skill development in the areas of oral reading fluency, reading comprehension, written expression, and mathematical calculation as compared with his preoperative assessment, he continues to be at significant risk for development of a language disorder and a language-based learning disability in the future.

Recommendations

As a result, it is recommended that Lane continue to receive special education resource/ inclusion services under the "Other Health Impaired" category. These services should be directed at providing support in the regular education setting as needed along with a time at the end of the school day during which Lane can receive one-to-one instruction to review and reinforce newly presented material, organize his homework, and take/finish examinations. In the event that Lane's seizure disorder worsens, a one-to-one teacher aide may be necessary to assist Lane in the regular classroom.

Given his pattern of strengths and weaknesses, it is once again recommended that academic instruction emphasize multisensory approaches. In order to enhance Lane's learning/retention, new material should be presented in an organized format that is meaningful to him. The material to be learned should be broken down into smaller components/steps and presented in a highly structured format with frequent repetition to facilitate learning. Instruction should be supplemented with visual aids, demonstrations, and experiential/procedural learning whenever possible. Lane would benefit greatly from being taught how to use mnemonic strategies when learning new material and studying for tests. These include but are not limited to:

- Rehearsal—showing Lane how to repeat information verbally, to write it, and look at it a finite number of times.
- Transformation—showing Lane how to convert difficult information into simpler components that can be remembered more easily.

- Elaboration—instructing Lane in how to identify key elements of new information and to create relationships or associations with previously learned material.
- Imagery—showing Lane how to visualize and make a "mental picture" of information to be learned.

When studying for tests or doing multiple homework assignments on the same day, similar subject material should be separated in order to lessen interference. Finally, Lane should be provided with periodic review of previously learned material in order to enhance long-term retention.

Accommodations will continue to be necessary to enhance Lane's ability to succeed in the classroom, including but not limited to preferential seating away from bulletin boards, doorways, windows, or other students, if necessary, where excessive stimuli might prove distracting. Instruction should be provided in small-group settings, and efforts should be made to redirect his attention if necessary. A reduction in the amount, but not the difficulty level, of assignments may assist Lane in completing classroom tasks and homework in a timely manner. Copying from the board should be minimized, and Lane should be provided with a copy of teacher notes or notes from another student so that he can better focus on teacher instruction without having to worry about note taking. Whenever possible, Lane should be given additional time to complete assignments. Tests should be in multiple choice/matching/short-answer formats instead of an essay format and should be administered individually/orally, with additional time provided when necessary. Finally, Lane should be allowed and encouraged to use various compensatory devices, such as a calculator to check written calculations. Instruction in keyboarding and the use of a computer with word processing capability also will be helpful with lengthy written assignments. Most word processing programs are equipped with spell checks and cut and paste, and can be adapted for voice dictation if necessary.

Lane should continue to be followed by his neurologist for medical management of his epilepsy. Given that Lane continues to have "good days and bad days," it may be helpful to have him return for a screening evaluation by this examiner when he is having a bad day in order to document his declining performance on a "bad day." Finally, Lane should be formally reevaluated by this service in approximately one year in accordance with the pediatric epilepsy surgery protocol.

Further Discussion of Case Study

Landau Kleffner is one of the epilepsy syndromes that, if not treated early with medication, can result in significant cognitive decline (Arts & Geerts, 2009). In this case, Lane has been treated, and although some may consider his treatment (antiepileptic medications and surgery) to be somewhat aggressive over a short period of time, he is not demonstrating the cognitive decline that likely would be associated with more a more conservative wait-and-see approach. In previous studies of individuals with Landau Kleffner syndrome, some participants experienced some remission of the associated language disturbance, as in the case of Lane, while others experienced long-term problems with aphasia and agnosia that negatively affected their quality of life (Duran, Guimarães, Medeiros, & Guerreiro, 2009). With the potential for further difficulties with language and associated academic and social issues, it will be important for Lane's progress to be monitored and interventions implemented to address any emerging needs over time.

CONCLUDING COMMENTS

In general, a neuropsychological evaluation is not part of the determination of whether the child has epilepsy, but rather in what way(s) the epilepsy is affecting higher cortical functioning. In particular, neuropsychological evaluation is often useful in differentiating epileptic from psychogenic seizures (Fargo et al., 2008). Using an analog format and four scenarios, Fargo and colleagues found that the accuracy of neuropsychologically based classification was equivalent to, if not better than, statistical prediction. Neuropsychological evaluation may provide supportive information when there are lesions that are too small or located such that they are not detected easily on standard MRI or the individual may not experience a full range of seizure activity during the electrophysiology evaluation. Further, specific patterns of performance on neuropsychological evaluation are believed to be predictive of the seizure classification (Fargo et al., 2008). Neuropsychological evaluation has a role, however, in translating the medical (EEG) information into the day-to-day activities encountered by the child. Because the focus or foci of the epilepsy may differ, individuals with the same classification may have different levels of difficulty or strength yet still evidence the same general pattern. Comprehensive evaluation allows for identification of subtle deficits and documents those domains that are spared or impaired.

Chapter 11

CEREBROVASCULAR DISEASE: FOCUS ON SICKLE CELL DISEASE

DEFINITION

Cerebrovascular disease describes a group of vascular disorders that result in brain injury. In general, the blood vessels to or within the brain are damaged, resulting in decreased blood flow within the brain. Cerebrovascular disease may be a blockage, bleeding, or constriction that affects the flow of blood (and therefore oxygenation); this can result in dead or dying brain tissue. Not all cerebrovascular disorders result in stroke, but often cerebrovascular diseases are referred to as cerebrovascular accident (CVA) or stroke. Technically, the term *stroke* is best reserved for those occasions when neuronal death occurs (Zillmer, Spiers, & Culbertson, 2008).

There are multiple types of cerebrovascular disorders. In childhood, risk factors for cerebrovascular disease or arterial ischemic stroke are not the same as for adults. In childhood, stroke is associated with cerebral arteriopathies, congenital heart defects, infection, trauma, prothrombotic abnormalities, and sickle cell anemia (L. Bernard, Muldoon, Hasan, O'Brien, & Steward, 2008).

Migraine is a very common form of cerebrovascular disorder but is less likely to progress to full-blown stroke. The trigeminal nerve is implicated in migraines in adults and children (Zillmer et al., 2008). Studies examining the characteristics of migraine in children have indicated that common features include dizziness and duration of migraine as well as occurrence of an aura (Eidlitz-Markus, Gorali, Haimi-Cohen, & Zeharia, 2008). Vomiting was the single most significant parameter in younger children. Vomiting and duration were correlated with the occurrence of an aura. Frequency of migraine was seen to increase with age, possibly due to changes in brain structure with development. Notably, the same criteria as indicated for adults were not found to be typical for children with migraine, and it was suggested that family history be included in pediatric criteria (Eidlitz-Markus et al., 2008). Migraines may be associated with transient ischemic attacks (TIAs), which arise from insufficient blood supply to specific structures with short lasting or transient deficits (Zillmer et al., 2008).

In contrast to the transient nature of TIAs, an infarction is a blockage of an artery that causes more permanent damage to specific cells and results in more lasting neuropsychological deficits that usually are localized. The blockage may be the result of an embolism (i.e., clot or "plug" that travels from somewhere else in the body and lodges in the arteries of the brain). Thrombosis, however, is an occlusion in which the clot forms at the site of the blockage. Another indication of cerebrovascular disease is the presence of aneurysms or weak areas in the walls of an artery that may result in hemorrhage, or severe bleeding and displacement of brain tissue that arises from that bleeding; in its most severe form, hemorrhage causes permanent brain damage or death.

Stroke in Children

Prenatal or perinatal stroke occurs any time from 28 weeks' gestation to 28 days after birth (Ballantyne, Spilkin, & Trauner, 2007). Perinatal stroke occurs in 1 of 2,300 to 5,000 live births and is probably an underidentified cause of significant long-term disabilities and neurological impairment (Barnette & Inder, 2009). Other terms for perinatal stroke include in utero stroke or neonatal stroke. Perinatal stroke involves poorly understood neurological events affecting the fetus and the newborn with a potential for serious neurological outcome. For example, perinatal arterial ischemic stroke is the most common known cause of cerebral palsy in term and near-term infants; perinatal stroke accounts for 50% to 70% of cases of congenital hemiplegic cerebral palsy (Kirton & deVeber, 2006). The pathophysiology of perinatal or prenatal stroke is complex and involves maternal, fetal, placental, and neonatal factors (Barnette & Inder, 2009). Perinatal stroke is 17 times more common than pediatric stroke beyond the newborn period. Notably, with unilateral perinatal stroke, there is no evidence of decline in cognitive function over time in children with perinatal unilateral brain damage (Ballantyne, Spilkin, Hesselink, & Trauner, 2008). These findings were interpreted to suggest that sufficient ongoing plasticity in the developing brain following early focal damage allows for stability of cognitive functions over time, particularly if there is no co-occurring epilepsy (see Chapter 10). Thus, with infarct early in brain development, cerebral functional reorganization can intercede to sustain a stable rate of development over time (Ballantyne et al., 2008). Following the perinatal period, the effects are more significant. Stroke is one of the top 10 reasons for death in children; 10% of children who have a stroke will die each year, 20% to 35% of infant stroke survivors will go on to have another stroke, and more than two-thirds of survivors will have neurological deficits or seizures (Ballantyne et al., 2008).

ETIOLOGY

A number of risk factors are associated with infant or childhood stroke. These include a number of cardiac disorders (e.g., congenital heart disease), infection, specific maternal conditions (e.g., autoimmune disorders, coagulation disorders), in utero exposure to cocaine, placental disorders (e.g., placental thrombosis), dehydration, and various blood disorders. In some cases, the cause of the stroke is unknown. Among the blood disorders that are associated with childhood stroke are those that result in deficiencies or mutations in coagulation factors and hyperviscosity, increasing the likelihood that the blood will clot or hemorrhage. Other blood disorders include polycythaemia, disseminated intravascular coagulopathy, factor-V Leiden mutation, protein-S deficiency, protein-C deficiency, prothrombin mutation, homocysteine, lipoprotein (a), and factor VIII; however, one of the more common blood disorders associated with childhood stroke is that of sickle cell disease.

Sickle Cell Disease

Sickle cell disease is actually a group of genetically transmitted blood disorders. Sickle cell disease results from production of abnormal hemoglobin or red blood cells. It is an autosomal recessive disorder that may be homozygous (HbSS) or, less frequently, may be heterozygous with a C-type hemoglobin and a variety of other variants (Schatz & McClellan, 2006). Sickle cell is most frequent among people of African descent with an incidence of 1 in every 350 births; it also occurs in individuals of Caribbean, Asian, Middle Eastern, and Mediterranean descent but with less frequency (Angastiniotis & Modell, 1998). The primary result of sickle cell disease is that of chronic anemia. Complications associated with sickle cell include infarction of major cerebral arteries, silent infarcts, chronic anemia, and low oxygenation (anoxia) due to poor pulmonary functioning and oxygen saturation; 5% to 10% of children under age 15 years with sickle cell are at risk for infarct (R. T. Brown, Armstrong, & Eckman, 1993; Schatz & McClellan, 2006; Wang, 2007). In addition, 16% to 22% evidence silent infarct on radiology (Hindmarsh et al., 1977; Pavlakis et al., 1988; Pegalow, Macklin, Moser, & Names, 2002; Wang et al., 2001). Based on autopsy results, histological findings indicate stenosis of the large cerebral arteries (Koshy, Thomas, & Goodwin, 1990); infarcts predominantly occur in the anterior brain regions (Pavlakis et al., 1988). In effect, the infarction is most likely to occur in the areas supplied by the distal branches of the internal carotid artery. Silent infarcts can be identified due to the diffuse scars in the deep white matter and cerebral gray matter; they likely represent lesions in the smaller arteries. Some of the mechanisms by which sickle cell disease increases the likelihood of infarct have been identified. First, the sickle cells, by virtue of their shape, are likely to stick together and adhere to the endothelial cells. It is believed that this is in conjunction with impaired nitric oxide production and increased consumption that leads to cycles of hypoxia and reoxygenation (Kaul, Liu, Fabry, & Nagel, 2000). A second mechanism implicated is the coagulation system with increased surface-dependent coagulation reactions (Kuypers et al., 1996) and elevated platelet levels (R. B. Francis, Jr., 1991). It has been suggested that the increased cell adhesion and increased stress due to anemia initiates the injury to the endothelial cells of the cerebral arteries, setting the stage for the infarct (Hillery & Panepinto, 2004). At the same time, there are oxidative fluctuations, vasodilation and increased perfusion as a result of the anemia, and increased likelihood of infarct in both large and small vessels. In addition to the illness-related consequences of sickle cell disease, environment and socioeconomic status also contribute to the variance in outcome (Tarazi, Grant, Ely, & Barakat, 2007).

COURSE AND PROGNOSIS

The "clinical" picture associated with cerebrovascular disease and stroke may take time to develop or may change over time; one means of evaluating neurological outcome is through the Pediatric Stroke Outcome Measure (deVeber, MacGregor, Curtis, & Mayank, 2000), a standardized evaluation for children. Factors involved include the type of damage or lesion, general health of the cerebrovascular system (i.e., are there sufficient other paths for blood flow?), location and size of lesion, and premorbid functioning of the individual. Significant functional and cognitive impairments can result; these vary depending on the factors just listed as well as the individual's age, how soon rehabilitation can be started, nature of the stroke, past medical history, and likelihood of additional strokes. Perinatal stroke is associated with language delays regardless of hemisphere involved (Bates et al., 2001; Nass & Trauner, 2004). Left-hemisphere perinatal stroke is most likely to be associated with expressive language deficits; right-hemisphere lesions are more likely associated with receptive language deficits (Bates et al., 2001). With perinatal stroke, regardless of hemisphere affected, the child can develop functional communication by age 5 (Bates et al., 1997). Among effects that may be precipitated by prenatal or perinatal stroke are epilepsy (seizures), hemiplegia, hemiparesis, hypotonia, speech and language difficulties, vision deficits, and learning disabilities. Affected children may require speech therapy, occupational therapy, medications, special education, and related services. Finally, significantly reduced health-related quality of life, as compared to normative data of healthy children, was found based on parent and child report (Friefeld, Yeboah, Jones, & de Veber, 2004). Of greatest concern for both parents and children was the effect of stroke on school functioning, followed by its impact on emotional and social functions. Physical concerns were less notable than psychosocial concerns. Results of multivariate analysis indicated that neurological deficits following stroke significantly accounted for lower health-related quality of life (Friefeld et al., 2004).

Of the cardiovascular diseases, sickle cell disease has both direct and indirect effects on brain development and function; it affects all aspects of life (Ballas, 2002). Some of the effects occur as a result of decreased oxygenation due to anemia and clumping of cells. Early on (12 to 24 months of age), there is a decline in overall cognitive functioning with increased risk of decline associated with the phenotype (HbSS or HbSC) of the child as well as psychosocial stressors and biomedical risk (R. Thompson, Gustafson, Bonner, & Ware, 2002). These children evidence subtle cognitive and academic delays (C. C. Peterson, Palermo, Swift, Beebe, & Drotar, 2005), most notably in areas of visual-motor integration, attention and concentration, and memory (Fowler et al., 1988). In relation to silent infarcts with sickle cell, neurocognitive compromise has been found to be associated with level of neurological injury and location of the infarct with deficits in attentional and executive dysfunction predominating (Berkelhammer et al., 2007). Findings such as these have prompted "preventive" medical intervention to offset the effects of poor oxygenation over time. Children with sickle cell also may have MoyaMoya syndrome, which may complicate the effects of sickle cell due to the increased stenosis of the internal carotid arteries, resulting in cumulative neurological insult (Hogan, Kirkham, Isaacs, Wade, & Vargha-Khadem, 2005).

Neurocognitive Effects of Sickle Cell Disease

Cognitive deficits are identified most readily in those children who have overt strokes, but the effects may be as significant for the child who has a silent infarct (Schatz, Puffer, Sanchez, Stancil, & Roberts, 2009). There is evidence of compromised cognitive functioning for overall ability (Full Scale IQ), verbal ability, and/or nonverbal ability (Armstrong et al., 1996; R. Thompson et al., 2003; Wang et al., 2001; K. E. Watkins et al., 1998). Effects of the infarct also may depend on the hemisphere affected. For example, children with left cortical infarct are more likely to be impaired across verbal and nonverbal areas while those with right cortical infarct are more likely to evidence impairment in nonverbal areas but not in verbal areas (M. J. Cohen, Branch, McKie, & Adams, 1994). Cognitive deficits are evident not only in those with infarcts, however. Subtle changes may occur at the cellular level or as a result of the low oxygenation that are not evident on magnetic resonance imaging (MRI); studies of children with normal MRIs and no evidence of overt or silent infarct suggest that children with sickle cell obtain lower scores on cognitive measures (Full Scale IQ) as compared to same-age and same-race peers (Steen et al., 2005; Steen, Xiong, Mulhern, Langston, & Wang, 1999). Other domains are also affected; these effects are summarized in Table 11.1.

Table 11.1 Neuropsychological Domains and Specific Deficits with Sickle Cell Disease

Domains	Specific Deficits
Cognition	Some generalized impairment but varies depending on location and size of infarct
Auditory-linguistic/Language function	Language delays evident, particularly for those with overt infarct to left hemisphere
Visual perception/Constructional praxis	Problems with visual orientation and visual-spatial tasks contralateral to lesion but are task and lesion-location dependent
Learning and memory	Working memory deficits Overt infarct associated with deficits in verbal and visual short-term memory Anterior infarcts associated with deficits in short-term and long-term memory
Executive function	Deficits in planning and problem solving
Attention/Concentration	Deficits evident in attention
Motor function	Motor skills may be affected with or without overt infarct Mild overall motor deficits and fine motor impairment with infarct
Achievement/Academic skills	Deficits in academic areas common
Emotional/Behavioral functioning	Internalizing and externalizing behavior problems and symptoms Decreased self-efficacy

Language

As noted, verbal abilities may be impaired in conjunction with sickle cell and infarct, particularly if the left hemisphere is affected. Specific to language development, children with sickle cell and infarct tend to demonstrate language levels below expectancy (Hariman, Griffith, Hurtig, & Keehn, 1991), with more difficulty noted in association with overt evidence of stroke (R. T. Brown et al., 2000). With overt and silent infarct, the volume and lateralization of the infarct was associated with effects on language such that lesion size was moderately related to language abilities or deficits (Schatz et al., 1999). Further, children with left cortical infarct evidenced more language deficits than those with right cortical infarct (M. J. Cohen et al., 1994). It has been suggested, therefore, that language deficits are related to size and location of the infarct; however, the cumulative effect of the infarct and general effects of sickle cell disease may contribute to more language deficits in children with sickle cell than previously considered (Berkelhammer et al., 2007). Further, it has been suggested that the language deficits are likely to occur across semantic, syntactic, and phonological components of language rather than only vocabulary (Schatz et al., 2009).

Visual Perception

The results of studies examining the visual-spatial domain in children with sickle cell are equivocal. One study examined visual-spatial deficits in children with stroke ($n = 33$) and children without stroke ($n = 43$) (Schatz, Craft, Koby, & DeBaun, 2004). Children with unilateral left ($n = 14$) or right ($n = 7$) injury showed less efficient visual search for the visual field contralateral to their injury. In addition, right-hemisphere injury was associated with impaired processing globally; left-hemisphere injury was associated with focal strengths and deficits. As expected, bilateral injury ($n = 12$) resulted in disruption of visual search across visual fields as well as relative deficits in global-level processing. Certain visual-spatial functions typically mediated by the left hemisphere appeared to be less vulnerable to disruption (Schatz, Craft et al., 2004). Alternatively, others have reported average visual spatial abilities and average visual-motor skills in those children without infarct (Grueneich et al., 2004) and regardless of infarct status (R. T. Brown et al., 2000).

Visual orientation also has emerged as a deficit area following cerebrovascular injury (Schatz, Craft et al., 2000). Contralateral lesions including the parietal lobe and middle frontal gyrus were associated with larger validity effects on an orienting task, suggesting difficulties disengaging attention; in contrast, contralateral basal ganglia injury was associated with less facilitation of attention. Thus, there is variability in the type of visual orienting deficits as a function of the specific location of lesions (Schatz, Craft et al., 2000).

Attention and Executive Function

In comparing children with silent infarct, overt infarct, and no infarct, measures from the attention and executive domains were the most useful for identifying children with silent cerebral infarct (DeBaun et al., 1998; Schatz et al., 2001). The neuropsychological profile associated with sickle cell and infarct in 28 children, mean age of 12.4 years, revealed that sickle cell groups performed significantly worse than sibling controls on measures of attention/executive function and spatial domains but not on language or memory (Schatz et al., 1999). Further, the anterior infarct and diffuse groups had poorer scores on Tower of Hanoi number correct and greater response variability on the Test of Variables of Attention (TOVA). The anterior infarct group had more rule-breaking errors on the Tower task while the diffuse group performed worse on all spatial tasks (Schatz et al., 1999). Children with sickle cell evidenced difficulty on cancellation tasks (R. T. Brown et al., 2000) as well as card-sorting tasks (K. E. Watkins et al., 1998) and continuous performance tests (DeBaun et al., 1998; Schatz et al., 1999). Of the executive measures used, the TOVA was the most robust measure, yielding a sensitivity rate of 86% and a specificity rate of 81%; the TOVA also showed a sensitivity rate of 95% in identifying overt stroke (DeBaun et al., 1998).

Memory

In conjunction with deficits in attention and executive function, studies of children with sickle cell disease consistently indicate working memory deficits as well as deficits in short- and long-term memory that are associated with frontal infarct (Brandling-Bennett, White, Armstrong, Christ, & DeBaun, 2003). Working memory deficits have been identified across studies regardless of whether the infarct is overt or silent (M. J. Cohen et al., 1994; Craft, Schatz, Glauser, Lee, & DeBaun, 1993; Wang et al., 2001). In contrast, children with overt infarcts were more likely to demonstrate verbal and visual short-term memory deficits as compared to those with silent infarcts, no infarcts, or siblings; no group differences emerged, however, for recall of prose (K. E. Watkins et al., 1998). There were also no differences between children with overt or silent infarcts on measures of delayed cued recall or recognition recall (Brandling-Bennett et al., 2003).

Academic Achievement

Of children with sickle cell disease, many are retained in grade or placed in special education or both; approximately one-fourth to one-third evidence academic deficits

(Schatz et al., 2001). Sickle cell disease and infarct were associated with reading difficulties relative to those with normal MRI (Armstrong et al., 1996; Wang et al., 2001). Mathematics achievement emerged as a deficit in conjunction with overt infarct in some studies but not in others (Armstrong et al., 1996; Wang et al., 2001). In particular, left-hemisphere infarct was associated with academic deficits in reading comprehension, spelling, and math computation, while right-hemisphere infarct was associated only with math deficits (M. J. Cohen et al., 1994).

Emotional/Behavioral Implications

Children with cerebrovascular diseases such as sickle cell are at increased risk for psychological and emotional difficulties (Kelch-Oliver, Smith, Diaz, & Collins, 2007). Some studies have suggested that behavioral problems, poor social competence, and disturbances of body image frequently are associated with sickle cell disease (R. T. Brown, Armstrong et al., 1993). At the same time, there are indications of "hardiness" in children with sickle cell such that they are described as being less aggressive and more prosocial (Noll, Reiter-Purtill, Vannatta, & Gerhardt, 2007). There are some indications that, over the long term, the chronicity of the disease, fewer friends, and higher rates of absenteeism may take a toll on psychosocial functioning (Palermo, Schwartz, Drotar, & McGowan, 2002; R. Thompson et al., 2003). Of the psychological disorders, children with sickle cell may be more prone to experiencing depression or other internalizing disorders as compared to healthy peers or peers with other chronic illnesses (R. T. Brown, Doepke, & Kaslow, 1993; S. A. Morgan & Jackson, 1986). Issues with self-efficacy are also frequent (Clay & Telfair, 2007). There are some indications that risk of psychological problems may be mediated by gender or socioeconomic status (Barbarin, Whitten, & Bonds, 1994; Hurtig & White, 1986; Schatz & McClellan, 2006). Indications are that additional biomedical factors as well as family factors and social supports contribute to the adjustment status for the individual with sickle cell disease (Kelch-Oliver et al., 2007; Schatz, Finke, & Roberts, 2004).

EVIDENCE-BASED INTERVENTIONS

With sickle cell disease, intervention tends to be predominantly in ongoing management and support, with additional intervention in reaction to adverse events, such as stroke (Ballas, 2002). Therapeutic management of stroke in children is similar to that in adults, predominantly because of the paucity of evidence from pediatric observational studies and clinical trials (S. Bernard et al., 2008). Although cognitive rehabilitation therapy in childhood stroke has great potential for meaningful improvements in long-term outcomes, especially given the plasticity of the young brain, currently there is insufficient research in this area. What we know about intervention for sickle cell is summarized in Table 11.2.

Medical Management and Sickle Cell Disease

Medical management generally includes monitoring and follow-up of all crises, transfusions, and various approaches to pain management. Some preventive behaviors that are recommended, for example, include maintenance of adequate hydration, folic acid supplements, proper diet, and a regular sleep routine (S. A. Jensen et al., 2005). Educational materials to improve knowledge about stroke in relation to sickle cell disease may be an important strategy to increase completion of stroke screening tests and follow-up by caregivers, particularly with children under the age of 11 (S. A. Jensen et al., 2005;

Table 11.2 Evidence-Based Status of Interventions for Sickle Cell Disease

Interventions	Target	Status
Transfusions	Decrease likelihood of stroke	Promising practice but may require chelation if exchange transfusion not used (Ballas, 2002)
Bone marrow or cord blood transplant	Curative approach	Inconclusive (Ballas, 2002; Eggleston et al., 2007)
Medical management of diet, vitamins, hydration	Decrease likelihood of stroke and decrease pain	Promising practice (Ballas, 2002)
Caregiver education	Medical management and screening	Emerging (S. A. Jensen et al., 2005; M. L. Katz, Smith-Whitley, Ruzek, & Ohene-Frempong, 2002)
Diary self-reports	Monitoring and management of pain episodes	Emerging (Dampier, Ely, Brodecki, & O'Neal, 2002)
Biofeedback and relaxation training	Pain management	Emerging (M. Collins, Kaslow, Doepke, Eckman, & Johnson, 1998; Cozzi, Tryon, & Sedlacek, 1987)
Self-hypnosis	Pain management	Emerging (Argargün, Öner, & Akbayram, 2001; M. Collins et al., 1998; Dinges et al., 1997)

M. L. Katz et al., 2002). Pain management needs to be individualized and incorporate appropriate use of analgesics (Ballas, 2002). Transfusions need to be matched for a variety of antigens and exchange transfusions used to avoid or delay the onset of iron overload and the need for chelation therapy (see Chapter 13). Preventive therapy also may include prophylactic penicillin or the use of hydroxyurea. Curative approaches of bone marrow and cord blood transplantation have been successful in some children, but more research is needed to determine appropriate candidates (Ballas, 2002). One newer approach involves cellular rehydration, but research is limited thus far.

Nonpharmacological Interventions

Specifically with regard to pain management, a number of differing approaches have been studied with children with sickle cell disease, including the use of biofeedback, relaxation training, and self-hypnosis (M. Collins et al., 1998). The majority of research available on these methods has been promising; however, few studies included children (Argargün et al., 2001; Cozzi et al., 1987). Also related to pain management, and the potential for dependency on medications, is the use of behavioral contracting to decrease reliance on medication and hospitalization (M. Collins et al., 1998). Sufficient empirical evidence to support this approach is not yet available; evidence is limited to case studies (Walco & Dampier, 1987).

Educational Interventions

Because sickle cell is associated with increased risk of neurocognitive deficits, early intervention and screening, particularly in language areas, has been recommended

(Schatz, McClellan, Puffer, Johnson, & Roberts, 2008). Comprehensive studies, and even case studies, with children with sickle cell that target educational outcomes are not readily available in published research. As a result, initial efforts at academic intervention for children with sickle cell most likely will follow the approaches identified in Chapters 2 and 3 for reading and math respectively. Research with regard to the efficacy of specific interventions with this population is needed.

Psychological Interventions

Cognitive-behavioral approaches and coping skills training (Gil et al., 1996) have been suggested and studied with individuals with sickle cell (M. Collins et al., 1998). Cognitive-behavioral methods also have been used to address pain management with results indicating a positive response (L. A. Schwartz, 2007). As with educational interventions, little research has directly addressed interventions for the psychosocial stressors associated with sickle cell.

CASE STUDY: LANIA—SICKLE CELL DISEASE WITHOUT STROKE

The next report is from a hospital-based clinic. Identifying information, such as child and family name, teacher or physician name, and school information, has been altered or fictionalized to protect confidentiality.

Reason for Referral

Lania is an 11-year-old African American female who has hemoglobin sickle cell disease and frequent vaso-occlusive pain crises. She was referred for a comprehensive neuropsychological evaluation by her hematologist due to problems with attention and concentration and increasing difficulty with retention of previously learned information. Additional difficulty with achievement in mathematics and science also was noted.

Assessment Procedures

In order to gain historical information about Lania, multiple sources of information were consulted. Her mother provided comprehensive educational records. Medical records were reviewed in the online medical record at the hospital where she receives her ongoing treatment for sickle cell and also was participating in this neuropsychological evaluation. Interviews were conducted individually and collaboratively with Lania and her mother to gain additional information about Lania's current level of functioning. Direct information from one of her teachers also was obtained via completion of questionnaires. Additionally, these assessment measures were utilized during the comprehensive neuropsychological evaluation:

- Behavioral observations
- Wechsler Intelligence Scale for Children, Fourth Edition (WISC-IV)
- Woodcock-Johnson Tests of Achievement, Third Edition (WJ III)
- Test of Everyday Attention for Children (TEA-Ch)
- Delis-Kaplan Executive Function System (D-KEFS)
- Peabody Picture Vocabulary Test, Fourth Edition (PPVT-IV)

Expressive Vocabulary Test, Second Edition (EVT-II)
California Verbal Learning Test—Children's Version (CVLT-C)
Purdue Pegboard Test
Beery Developmental Test of Visual-Motor Integration, Fifth Edition (DTVMI-V)
Behavior Assessment System for Children, Second Edition (BASC-2; Parent, Teacher, and Self-Report)
Behavior Rating Inventory of Executive Function (BRIEF; Parent and Teacher Report)

Background Information

Home

Lania lives in a rural town with her mother and her stepfather; they have been married for approximately four years. Lania's half brother, her mother's 16-year-old son, Demetric, also lives in the home. Lania's mother obtained a high school diploma and attended a vocational school; she currently works part time as a hair stylist. She is in good general health at the present time but has a history of treatment for depression and anxiety. Lania's stepfather is also a high school graduate and is employed as a sales manager. Demetric is in the eleventh grade and obtains mostly Bs. He is in good general health and does not have any significant difficulty with learning or behavior. He plays football and basketball on the varsity teams at school.

Lania's father and mother were never married. Her father lives in an urban city about 45 miles from Lania and her mother. He lives with his wife and their 15-year-old son, Daniel (Lania's half brother). The father suffers from hypertension and migraines. He obtained an associate's degree and works as an account manager in the advertising industry. Lania's stepmother obtained her high school diploma and works at a daycare; she is in good general health but struggled throughout her education. Daniel is in the tenth grade and receives special education assistance for a learning disability in reading comprehension. He is in good general health but has been diagnosed with Attention-Deficit/Hyperactivity Disorder—combined type (ADHD-CT), for which he receives methylphenidate (Concerta).

Lania's mother has primary physical and legal custody of Lania. Lania's father has infrequent contact with Lania, calling approximately once every two months. In addition to her mother and stepfather, with whom she reportedly has a good relationship, Lania also has numerous other outside supports, including a maternal aunt and the church pastor. There are no other known psychiatric or learning disorders within the family history besides the aforementioned history of anxiety, depression, learning disability in reading, ADHD-CT, migraines, and hypertension.

Medical History

Lania's mother provided information about Lania's gestational, developmental, and medical history. Her pregnancy with Lania was free of complications and she was born at normal gestational age via normal vertex procedure, weighing 7 pounds 8 ounces. She did not experience any neonatal difficulties and was discharged home after two days; Lania was diagnosed with sickle cell disease following a newborn screening. As an infant and toddler, Lania's mother described Lania as normal with regard to activity level and temperament. She achieved language and motor developmental milestones slightly earlier than expected, with independent walking occurring at 10 months of age and use of single words at almost 8 months of age.

Lania had an uneventful early childhood, with no chronic ear infections, head injuries, or seizures. At 5 years of age, Lania experienced her first acute chest syndrome. She subsequently was placed on chronic transfusion (every 6 weeks) but has continued to experience multiple vaso-occlusive crises, most of which require hospitalization for pain management. She has also experienced two additional episodes of acute chest syndrome, the last of which occurred approximately one month prior to the present evaluation. As needed for pain, she receives ibuprofen (mild pain), codeine (moderate pain), or hydrocodone (severe pain). According to recent MRI and diffusion tensor imaging (DTI) of her brain, there is no indication of previous silent or overt strokes.

In addition to the course of her sickle cell symptoms, Lania suffers from allergic rhinitis and asthma, for which she receives fluticasone/salmeterol (Advair) and albuterol (Ventolin, Proventil). There were no concerns noted with her vision or hearing. Although she does not have difficulty with sleep onset or maintenance, morning arousal is very difficult for her, and Lania often complains of physical and cognitive fatigue throughout each day. Her appetite varies depending on her level of fatigue and pain; Lania's mother stated that Lania does not have any appetite when she is experiencing moderate to severe pain.

Educational History

Lania is in the fifth grade at the local intermediate school; she has never been retained and maintains a B/C average, although she struggles greatly with mathematics and science. During the past year, Lania successfully passed the reading portion of the state-mandated assessment; she failed to pass the mathematics and science portions of these tests. Lania's mother shared that Lania has frequent absences due to pain crises and for transfusion and that she is unable to complete all of the work that is sent home with her. In fact, Lania's mother indicated that Lania often feels "overwhelmed" by the amount of work she is given and has trouble keeping up with the curriculum.

Lania is receiving special education services under the eligibility category of "Other Health Impairment." She attends all classes in the general education environment. According to reports from her teachers, they are concerned that Lania often fails to turn in assignments. Additional comments from her teachers indicate that Lania has problems with organization and sometimes shows poor effort. According to the most recent Individualized Education Plan (IEP), instructional accommodations included oral administration of tests and reduced assignments or extended time on assignments.

Psychosocial

Lania's mother reported that her primary concern is Lania's concentration. That is, she stated that her daughter seems to have her mind "somewhere else" when she is being spoken to; her teachers denied concerns with attention and concentration. Lania's mother denied concerns with hyperactivity, impulsivity, or aggression for her daughter either at home or in the school setting. At school, Lania's teachers noted that she is not overly active and in fact often appears tired. Her teachers also denied impulsive behaviors; conversely, they stated that she does not initiate work without assistance.

With regard to emotional functioning, Lania's mother indicated that she does not seem to have excessive levels of anxiety, withdrawal, or depression. However, she is sometimes cranky and irritable, although these issues are not chronic. Her teachers reported that Lania sometimes appears sad but does not cry easily, is not easily frustrated, and does not appear fearful. Chronic stressors for Lania include the "stress of dying" due to complications from sickle cell disease. Lania's mother also stated that Lania wants very much to be independent, and this is a stressor because there are limits to what she can do independently at her age. In her free time, Lania enjoys reading, listening to music, playing with Barbie dolls, and drawing.

Socially, Lania's mother related that Lania seeks friendships with her peers and sometimes is sought out by others for interaction. She interacts with children of all ages but has a very close friend, who is also her "protector." Specifically, Lania's mother stated that this friend reminds Lania to remain hydrated by drinking a lot of water. Unfortunately, Lania's mother described several issues that have made the current school year "awful," including several unprovoked physical assaults (i.e., kicking) by female students who reportedly kicked Lania when she was on crutches for a problem with her ankle. While on the bus to and from school, other students tease and bully Lania. Lania's mother stated that she is teased because of her illness. Although Lania's teachers reported that she expresses some anger and frustration with peers, she reportedly gets along well with other students, does not isolate herself, has several friends in class, and works cooperatively.

Behavioral Observations

Lania was accompanied to the evaluation by her mother. She was casually dressed and appropriately groomed. She greeted the psychologist appropriately and easily separated from her mother. Rapport was quickly established and easily maintained. Lania was cooperative throughout testing and demonstrated good motivation and perseverance throughout the evaluation. She did not appear to experience any pain or excessive fatigue during the assessment.

Lania's mood and affect were positive throughout the testing. She appeared comfortable with the examiner, was responsive to questions, and appeared to enjoy conversation with the examiner. Lania spoke with appropriate intonation and prosody. Her speech occasionally required clarification for very similar-sounding words (e.g., "can" or "can't"), but it was generally easy to understand. Lania was able to work for long periods of time and was not fidgety or restless. Occasionally her attention drifted from the task, but she was easily redirected. On more difficult tasks, Lania often began a response and looked to the psychologist as if to get a hint of whether her answer was correct before proceeding. Lania was generally conscientious in her responses, pausing briefly to think before answering.

With regard to motor skills, Lania was right-handed and demonstrated a tripod pencil grip. Although she wrote slowly, Lania did not exhibit any observable difficulty with writing or fine motor skills. Overall, Lania exhibited adequate rates of attention and concentration as well as excellent motivation, task perseverance, and cooperation. Therefore, the test results should be considered a valid estimate of Lania's neuropsychological functioning.

Assessment

The results of neuropsychological evaluation indicate that Lania currently is functioning within the average range of general intellectual ability as measured by the Wechsler Intelligence Scale for Children, Fourth Edition (WISC-IV). Comparatively, significant weaknesses were noted in areas measuring her cognitive processing speed and auditory working memory. Lania's standard scores on the cognitive measure are listed in Table 11.3.

Table 11.3 Psychometric Summary for Lania

	Scaled Score	Standard Score
Wechsler Intelligence Scale for Children, Fourth Edition (WISC-IV)		
Verbal Comprehension Index		102
Similarities	10	
Vocabulary	11	
Comprehension	11	
Perceptual Reasoning Index		100
Block Design	8	
Picture Concepts	12	
Matrix Reasoning	10	
Working Memory Index		68
Digit Span	5	
Letter-Number Sequencing	4	
Processing Speed Index		78
Coding	6	
Symbol Search	6	
Delis-Kaplan Executive Function System (D-KEFS)		
Trail Making Test		
Visual Scanning	9	
Number Sequencing	8	
Letter Sequencing	12	
Number-Letter Sequencing	5	
Motor Speed	4	
Verbal Fluency Test		
Letter Fluency	7	
Category Fluency	6	
Category Switching Total	11	
Color-Word Interference		
Color Naming	5	
Word Reading	8	
Inhibition	8	
Inhibition/Switching	9	
Tower		
Total Achievement Score	6	
Mean First-Move Time	7	
Time-Per-Move Ratio	7	
Move Accuracy Ratio	12	
Rule-Violations-Per-Item Ratio	7	
Test of Everyday Attention for Children (TEA-Ch)		
Sky Search		
Correctly Identified Targets	8	
Time	1	
Attention Score	6	
Score!	13	
Sky Search Dual Task	9	
Score Dual Task	7	

(continued)

Table 11.3 *(Continued)*

	Standard Score	
Peabody Picture Vocabulary Test, Fourth Edition (PPVT-IV)	93	
Expressive Vocabulary Test, Second Edition (EVT-II)	87	
Purdue Pegboard Test		
Dominant (right) hand	70	
Nondominant hand	77	
Both hands	51	
Developmental Test of Visual-Motor Integration, Fifth Edition (DTVMI-V)		
Visual-Motor Integration	77	
Visual Perception	100	
Motor Coordination	88	
California Verbal Learning Test—Children's Version (CVLT-C)	**T-Score**	
List A Trial 1	70	
List A Trial 5	50	
List A Trials 1–5	60	
List B Free Recall	55	
List A Short-Delay Free Recall	55	
List A Short-Delay Cued Recall	55	
List A Long Delay Free Recall	55	
List A Long Delay Cued Recall	60	
Learning Slope	35	
Correct Recognition Hits	60	
False Positives	60	
List A Trial 1	70	
List A Trial 5	50	
Behavior Rating Inventory of Executive Function (BRIEF)		
	T-Scores	
Clinical Scales	Parent	Teacher
Inhibit	44	57
Shift	45	61
Emotional Control	49	69
Initiate	40	65
Working Memory	55	65
Plan/Organize	45	77
Organization of Materials	52	69
Monitor	46	77
Behavioral Regulation Index	47	74
Metacognition Index	47	72
General Executive Composite	44	57

(continued)

Table 11.3 *(Continued)*

	Standard Score	
Woodcock-Johnson Tests of Achievement, Third Edition (WJ III)		
Letter-Word Identification	99	
Reading Fluency	93	
Calculation	101	
Math Fluency	70	
Spelling	101	
Passage Comprehension	92	
Applied Problems	82	
Writing Samples	103	
Behavior Assessment System for Children, Second Edition (BASC-2), (Self-Report)		
Clinical Scales	**T-Score**	
Attitude to School	52	
Attitude to Teachers	40	
Atypicality	52	
Locus of Control	46	
Social Stress	43	
Anxiety	47	
Depression	45	
Sense of Inadequacy	41	
Attention Problems	49	
Hyperactivity	58	
Adaptive Scales		
Relations with Parents	58	
Interpersonal Relations	44	
Self-Esteem	58	
Self-Reliance	47	
Composites		
School Problems	45	
Internalizing Problems	45	
Inattention/Hyperactivity	54	
Emotional Symptoms Index	44	
Personal Adjustment	52	
Behavior Assessment System for Children, Second Edition (BASC-2)		
	T-Scores	
Clinical Scales	Parent	Teacher
Hyperactivity	41	47
Aggression	46	63
Conduct Problems	48	57
Anxiety	45	72

(continued)

Table 11.3 *(Continued)*

	T-Scores	
	Parent	Teacher
Depression	55	69
Somatization	84	100
Atypicality	52	50
Withdrawal	47	63
Attention Problems	56	51
School Problems	NA	56
Adaptive Scales		
Adaptability	50	43
Social Skills	63	47
Leadership	51	42
Activities of Daily Living	55	NA
Functional Communication	40	47
Study Skills	NA	42
Composites		
Externalizing Problems	44	56
Internalizing Problems	64	88
Behavioral Symptoms Index	49	59
Adaptive Skills	52	43
School Problems	NA	54

Note. NA = Not applicable.

Lania's attention and concentration were also evaluated based on her performance on selected subtests of the Test of Everyday Attention for Children (TEA-Ch) and Delis-Kaplan Executive Function System (D-KEFS); see specific scores in Table 11.3. On the first simple visual attention task, when she was asked to find a specified number that was embedded in a group of other numbers, she performed in the average range with regard to speed and accuracy. She did not make any errors of omission or commission (i.e., mistakenly identifying a nontarget), indicating good inhibition and visual scanning. On the second task of visual attention during which she was asked to locate pairs of objects embedded in visually similar distracters, she performed in the borderline range overall; although she demonstrated accuracy within the low-average range, her speed of completion was extremely slow. During a sustained auditory attention task during which Lania was asked to count sounds from a CD player, she performed in the high-average range; she correctly responded to all of the items.

Two additional tasks were administered to Lania to assess her ability to divide her attention between two competing stimuli. The first task required her to perform a visual and auditory attention task simultaneously, on which she performed in the average range. On the second task, Lania was asked to listen to a story while counting the number of sounds from a CD player. She performed in the low-average range on this task, having slightly greater difficulty with these two competing stimuli.

On tasks measuring Lania's executive functioning skills (see specific scores in Table 11.3), her performance was somewhat variable. Specifically, she performed generally within the average range on tasks measuring her nonverbal sequencing skills. However, her demonstration of cognitive flexibility on similar sequencing tasks fell in the borderline range. On tasks measuring Lania's verbal fluency skills, she performed in the low-average to borderline range, with average performance on the verbal switching tasks. On rapid-naming tasks, Lania obtained a score in the borderline range when she was asked to name colors quickly; she did so without error but certainly completed them much more slowly than expected for her age. When asked to read color words quickly, she performed in the low-average range, again without error. On more complex tasks when she was asked to inhibit natural responses, she completed them slightly slower than expected, obtaining a score in the low-average range; she made only two errors, which indicates accuracy in the high-average range. When asked to inhibit natural responses and respond according to two competing rules, she completed the task within an average range, demonstrated six total errors and a low-average accuracy level. Overall, Lania's performance indicates good inhibition and adaptation to rules.

Lania was administered a Tower task to assess her planning and problem-solving skills when presented with novel problems. On this task, Lania had a low-average first-move time, indicating that she started the task a little more slowly than her same-age peers. In completing the tasks, although Lania took slightly longer to make each move, she demonstrated accuracy within the high-average range. However, she incurred seven rule violations, which is in the low-average range and indicates that Lania may have been experiencing mild difficulty keeping the rules in mind while completing each tower. In general, Lania has more than expected levels of difficulty completing complex problems with efficiency.

Furthermore, Lania's mother and Lania's teacher completed a questionnaire detailing their perceptions of Lania's executive functioning abilities; their responses were not overly negative or inconsistent, resulting in a valid profile (see scores in Table 11.3). Based on their responses, there were no concerns identified with regard to Lania's ability to inhibit impulsive behavior. In fact, Lania's mother denied concerns in any of the measured areas. Conversely, Lania's teacher indicated mild concern with her ability to demonstrate cognitive flexibility and significant concern in all of the remaining measured areas. These include concerns with Lania's ability to control her emotions, monitor her behavior, initiate problem solving, maintain working memory, plan and organize problem solving, and organize her environment.

Although Lania's conversational skills appeared appropriate, given her mild word-finding difficulties noted on the D-KEFS, measures of receptive and expressive vocabulary were administered to her. The specific scores can be found in Table 11.3. On the Peabody Picture Vocabulary Test, Fourth Edition (PPVT-IV), Lania performed in the average range. She had slightly more difficulty on the Expressive Vocabulary Test, Second Edition (EVT-II), on which she performed in the low-average range.

In order to identify problems in Lania's ability to learn, recall, and recognize newly learned information, the California Verbal Learning Test—Children's Version (CVLT-C) was administered to Lania. On this task, she was asked to learn a list of 15 words. She recalled 10 words of the 15-word list after it was read to her the first time, suggesting a very superior initial attention span for auditory-verbal information. After the first list was read to her five times and she had the opportunity to recall words after each trial, she demonstrated a learning slope in the borderline range; however, this simply reflects the fact that her initial retention of the information (i.e., 10 words) did not increase significantly over time. When presented with a second word list, she recalled seven words (average range), exhibiting more than expected levels of proactive interference (i.e., previous learning interferes with new learning), meaning that she did not recall as many words during the first trial of List B as she did during the first trial of List A. When asked to recall the first list after she was presented with the second list and again after a 20-minute delay, she recalled 12 and 11 words, respectively. Compared to her recall of 11 words during Trial 5, Lania demonstrated no impact from retroactive interference (i.e., learning new information interferes with recall of old information). Furthermore, when given the opportunity to recognize words from the list among distracters, she performed in the high-average range, identifying all of the 15 words as part of the original list; she did not misidentify any non-targets, which is also in the high-average range, suggesting adequate ability in discriminating relevant from irrelevant responses when trying to recognize verbal information. For specific scores on this measure, please refer to Table 11.3.

On tasks that measured Lania's visual-motor and visual-perceptual skills, she demonstrated a tripod pencil grip with her right hand. On tasks measuring her fine motor dexterity, she performed in the borderline range with her right and left hands independently. Specifically, she placed 12 pegs with her right hand and 11 pegs with her left hand, which does not indicate a significant lateralizing difference between hands. She performed in the moderately impaired range when asked to complete the task with both hands simultaneously, placing only 6 pairs of pegs during the 30-second time limit. Lania's ability to copy increasingly complex geometric figures fell in the borderline range. Conversely, on a non-motor visual-perceptual measure during which she was asked to match geometric figures, she performed in the average range, completing 28 of the items during the three-minute time limit. On tasks measuring speeded visuomotor accuracy and precision, her performance fell in the low-average range. Specific scores for these tasks can be found in Table 11.3.

Academic Functioning

The Woodcock-Johnson Tests of Achievement, Third Edition (WJ III) was administered as a measure of academic achievement. Based on her performance, she obtained scores in the average range with regard to basic academic skills; Lania performed in the low-average range on applied academic tasks. With regard to reading skills, Lania performed in the average range on tasks measuring her ability to read single words and understand simple sentences; her ability to complete reading fluency tasks also fell in the average range. On measures of writing, Lania performed in the average range on tasks of spelling and written expression. With regard to mathematics ability, Lania performed in the average range on basic paper-and-pencil numerical operations. Her ability to complete applied math (i.e., word) problems fell in the low-average range. Notably, her speeded math ability fell in the borderline range. Compared to her average general intellectual ability, her academic performance is commensurate with where she would be expected to perform. However, the significant weakness in math fluency and greater than expected weakness in applied mathematics is a concern and certainly can impact her academic performance. Lania's standard scores on the WJ III subtests are listed in Table 11.3.

Social-Emotional and Behavioral Functioning

Lania and her mother each completed a questionnaire to gain additional information about her emotional and behavioral functioning. Lania's responses were all within the average range without significant concern for anxiety, depression, interpersonal difficulties, inattention, or hyperactivity. On the contrary, significant levels of somatization were noted by her mother and teacher, which is not surprising, given Lania's complex medical history and frequent pain crises. Although her mother denied concerns with aggression, Lania's teacher indicated that this was an area of mild concern. Specifically, her teacher noted that Lania sometimes threatens to hurt others, loses her temper too easily, defies teachers, bullies others, seeks revenge on others, calls other children names, annoys others on purpose, hits other children, and teases others. Similarly, although Lania's mother denied concerns with anxiety, depression, or social withdrawal, Lania's teacher indicated concerns in these areas.

With regard to adaptive skills, there were no concerns with adaptability, social skills, leadership abilities, or daily living skills. Lania's teacher did not indicate concerns with functional communication, but her mother's responses led to very mild concerns in this area. A review of the profiles obtained by Lania and her caregivers can be seen in Table 11.3.

During the individual clinical interview with Lania, she reported that she "almost always" has pain and has gone to the hospital approximately twice a week for some time for pain-related treatment. She denied symptoms of anxiety or depression, stating that she mostly feels "happy." However, when asked about school, Lania shared that she does not like attending school because of how she is treated by her teachers and other students. Lania related that, fortunately, she has several close friends and enjoys interacting with other children at her church on a regular basis.

Summary and Diagnostic Impressions

Based on the present neuropsychological evaluation, Lania's profile was somewhat variable. Her general cognitive ability fell in the average range. Mild weaknesses were noted in areas of applied mathematics, word finding, verbal fluency, and problem solving. More significant weaknesses in her neuropsychological profile were found in math fluency, working memory, processing speed, visual-motor abilities, and fine motor skills. Other areas of weakness were noted in Lania's cognitive flexibility.

Probably the most significant issue impacting Lania is her difficulty with general executive functioning skills. Despite the fact that her mother did not indicate concerns with these skills, problems in these areas were evident during the evaluation and reported by her teacher. Cognitive flexibility was an area of weakness for Lania and evident on tasks requiring varied or multiple problem-solving strategies, during which Lania seems to perseverate on her initial understanding of the problem, which limits her ability to incorporate new information or to correct earlier mistakes. She may persist in an activity after being redirected or may not be able to incorporate increasingly complex steps to solving problems due to this inability to shift focus. This difficulty also may be reflected in Lania's vulnerability to proactive interference.

A second area of relative weakness is Lania's difficulty maintaining auditory attention and working memory. Although Lania seems to be performing at an average level with regard to visual attention, her performance on auditory attention tasks was varied. She performed in the high-average range on tasks requiring attention to a single auditory cue without distraction. When required to listen for multiple pieces of overlapping information, however, Lania performed in the low-average range. Although this discrepancy does not reflect a significant difficulty, it may reflect small lapses in her ability to attend to auditory information when additional auditory distractions are present (e.g., receiving verbal directions from a teacher while other students are talking in the background). In a real-world setting, auditory attention and working memory can be even more difficult to manage, and demonstration of adequate skills is impacted by an individual's current medical and psychological state as well as by environmental issues (e.g., noise, rate of presentation of material). Specifically for Lania, poor working memory skills may impact task initiation greatly. Although her general receptive language skills (i.e., language comprehension) are within the average range, if complex directions are provided to the class as a whole and involve more than two steps, Lania may not fully grasp all that she is being asked to do. Other children with similar weaknesses find it difficult to hold all of the information in their mind from multiple-step directions. As a result, they may follow only part of the directions given to them, not out of forgetfulness or oppositionality, but due to the inability to complete tasks in a stepwise order and in a timely manner so that other information does not fall by the wayside.

Finally, given the aforementioned difficulty in solving applied math problems, which creates a significant discrepancy between her general intelligence and performance in applied mathematics, Lania meets criteria for a learning disability in the area of mathematics reasoning. Further complicating her performance is Lania's slow processing speed, which will affect her ability to complete any task within a restricted time limit; this was seen very clearly on the math fluency task. Despite the fact that Lania performed in the average range on reading fluency tasks, when asked to read during class or complete tests or other assignments, it is likely that she will struggle to finish in the same amount of time as other students.

In addition to the neurocognitive weaknesses that have been detailed, Lania is also struggling with social relationships and managing her pain. Children with significant medical issues often find themselves feeling different from other children their age. Emotional difficulties may impact Lania's ability to cope with daily stressors of the school and home environments. Although she did not indicate feeling out of control, chronic pain can lead to feelings of helplessness. Chronic fatigue and physical complaints may exacerbate emotional difficulties and affect her feelings of confidence with regard to academic tasks and social relationships. Despite the fact that she does not demonstrate significant levels of anxiety or depression, these issues should be monitored, especially with the level of social difficulties she experiences at school. It appears that her family and extended support networks have maintained her current level of emotional functioning. Accommodations designed for children with similar difficulties will be beneficial to Lania, and she should continue participating in individual therapy to facilitate the best possible outcome for her.

Given that Lania has been hospitalized multiple times for vaso-occlusive crises and multiple episodes of acute chest syndrome, it is not surprising that relative weaknesses in sustained attention, working memory, processing speed, and fine motor coordination were noted in her neurocognitive profile. Children with sickle cell disease, even those without a history of overt or silent stroke, are at greater risk for cognitive, learning, and behavioral difficulties compared to children without sickle cell disease and its related complications.

Recommendations

Considering Lania's current level of functioning, especially in light of her significant weaknesses in cognitive processing speed and working memory, additional modifications and accommodations need to be provided to her. Although the current modifications are indeed appropriate, additions to her instructional supports are necessary. Some of the most salient recommendations to benefit Lania's educational performance include:

- With regard to completion of assignments, it will be necessary to provide additional accommodations. First, due to the large number of absences Lania may incur due to her medical status, provisions should be made for missed assignments, tests, and homework. Both classwork and homework should not be expected. Instead, a sampling of Lania's learning based on content (not quantity) should be expected. Missed assignments should not be tacked on top of new work. Also, given that the speed at which Lania is able to understand, initiate, and complete tasks may impede her ability to complete the task within a timely manner, she should be allowed extra time to complete tests, homework assignments, or other classroom tasks. Assignments should be shortened in order that Lania may complete them within a given time period. Accuracy should be encouraged over speed.

- With regard to her attention and working memory, these recommendations are offered:
  - Caregivers should not have Lania continue working on a task while the next activity or task is explained since she has difficulty with multitasking. Instead, allow Lania to stop what she is doing to attend fully to the instruction or directions being given. That way, she will be more likely to comply and follow through with directions.
  - In the classroom, she should be seated next to a student who will encourage her on-task behavior rather than distract her by talking.
  - Placing her seat near the teacher provides greater opportunity to observe when she is adequately focused and when she is fatiguing, and redirection or breaks can be implemented more easily.
  - It may be necessary to provide Lania with a study carrel or desk away from other students when taking tests or completing other important assignments.
  - Frequent but brief breaks may be necessary to alleviate the drain on her focus and ameliorate her working memory capacity.
- With regard to problem solving, encourage Lania to be flexible when it comes to solving academic tasks. For instance, although she may have been taught to complete a math problem in a certain way by her teacher, this may not be the only way to solve it. Her parents may solve one of the problems for her, showing her that an answer can be obtained through other ways than the one taught at school. Doing this will help to increase her cognitive flexibility.

Consideration of Lania's current social and psychological functioning is also important for her development, especially given the significant difficulty she has experienced with peers at school over the past year. These recommendations are offered as methods to increase confidence and the use of appropriate coping mechanisms:

- Because of her medical issues, Lania may be at risk for teasing and stigmatization.
  - Lessons in individual differences provided by the classroom teacher may be helpful for other students to be more sympathetic toward others' differences.
  - Providing increased supervision during times that students are more at risk for teasing also would be helpful.
  - Also, when groups are being formed in the general education classroom or for other activities (e.g., sports), the groups should be assigned so as to limit the social isolation Lania may feel by being chosen last for a group.
  - It may be necessary to place her in a group with peers who will not be critical of her but who will encourage her active participation in the group.
  - To encourage Lania's self-esteem and social skills with same-age peers, she should be given the opportunity to participate in activities with other children. An example of such an activity is the church youth group in which Lania is involved. She expressed that this is a positive peer group, and her continued participation is encouraged.
- Due to her frequent pain crises, it may be helpful for Lania to participate in individual psychotherapy with a pediatric psychologist who is familiar with sickle cell disease. Therapy should focus on learning additional coping mechanisms, especially when she is in uncomfortable social situations. Relaxation techniques and imagery also should be discussed as effective methods to reducing Lania's perceived level of pain. Due to her level of cognitive ability, cognitive-behavioral therapy would likely be beneficial for Lania.

Further Discussion of Case Study

Despite the fact that Lania has not experienced an overt or silent stroke, the effects of chronic and acute pain, in addition to the cumulative effects of multiple acute chest syndromes, play a significant role in her current neuropsychological profile. Not all children without stroke will have such a chronic series of vaso-occlusive crises, but those who do may be at risk for increased levels of dysfunction in neurocognitive, behavioral, and emotional functioning. Notably, psychological issues associated with the chronic history further exacerbate Lania's difficulties. Lania's case illustrates the potentially wide-ranging neuropsychological and emotional implications of sickle cell and its medical management, pointing to the importance of a comprehensive assessment in order to determine appropriate educational interventions.

CASE STUDY: JED—SICKLE CELL DISEASE WITH STROKE

The next report is from a hospital-based clinic. Identifying information, such as child and family name, teacher or physician name, and school information, has been altered or fictionalized to protect confidentiality.

Reason for Referral

Jed is a 15-year-old African American male who was referred for evaluation by his hematologist due to increasing problems with attention, concentration, and organization. Jed has hemoglobin sickle cell disease and experienced an overt stroke at 7 years of age.

Assessment Procedures

In order to gain historical information about Jed, multiple sources of information were consulted. His mother provided comprehensive educational records. Medical records were reviewed in the online medical record at the hospital where he receives his ongoing treatment for sickle cell and also was participating in the present neuropsychological evaluation. Interviews were conducted individually and collaboratively with Jed and his mother to gain additional information about Jed's current level of functioning. Direct information from teachers was unavailable as the evaluation was conducted during the summer. Additionally, these assessment measures were utilized during the comprehensive neuropsychological evaluation:

Wechsler Intelligence Scale for Children, Fourth Edition (WISC-IV)
Woodcock-Johnson Tests of Achievement, Third Edition (WJ III)
Delis-Kaplan Executive Function System (D-KEFS)
Peabody Picture Vocabulary Test, Fourth Edition (PPVT-IV)
Expressive Vocabulary Test, Second Edition (EVT-II)
Children's Memory Scale (CMS)
California Verbal Learning Test, Children's Version (CVLT-C)
Beery Developmental Test of Visual-Motor Integration, Fifth Edition (DTVMI-V)
Behavior Assessment System for Children, Second Edition (BASC-2; Parent and Self-Report)
Behavior Rating Inventory of Executive Function (BRIEF; Parent Report)

Background Information

Home Environment

Jed lives in a suburban city with his mother. His mother is in good general health. Jed is the only child of his mother and father. His parents were never married, and Jed has always lived with his mother, with sporadic contact with his father. His father died in a motor vehicle collision when Jed was 9 years old. Prior to that time, he suffered from hypertension. His mother is a high school graduate and works in retail. His father received his general education diploma and was working as an auto mechanic prior to his death. In addition to the aforementioned hypertension, there is a history of migraines and coronary artery disease within the extended family. There are no known psychiatric or learning disorders within the family history.

Medical History

Jed's mother provided information about Jed's gestational, developmental, and medical history. Her pregnancy with Jed was reportedly without complications, and he was born at normal gestational age via normal vertex procedure, weighing approximately 7 pounds. He did not experience any neonatal difficulties but was diagnosed with sickle cell disease following a newborn screening. As an infant and toddler, she described Jed as easily distracted but otherwise normal in activity level and temperament. Jed achieved language and motor developmental milestones at appropriate ages, with independent walking occurring at 11 months of age. He began using single words at slightly over 8 months of age.

At 7 years of age, Jed experienced an overt stroke in the region of the left middle cerebral artery. There is very little information about this event as Jed was not receiving his medical care at the current pediatric facility and records were not available. Jed's mother recalled that Jed was hospitalized for several days following the stroke and received outpatient speech-language, occupational, and physical therapies for several months. He also was placed on a chronic transfusion protocol at that time. When he was 13 years old, Jed's care was transferred to the current pediatric facility. Based on the sickle cell clinic standard protocol, a computed tomography scan of his head revealed mild generalized atrophy; an MRI of his brain was also completed, which revealed encephalomalacia of the left frontal region. The chronic transfusion protocol had been discontinued for approximately one year prior to this imaging. One year later, Jed was admitted to the hospital for abdominal pain, which led to a diagnosis of biliary pancreatitis and cholelithiasis (i.e., gallstones), for which he underwent gall bladder removal. Approximately 6 months prior to the present evaluation, a repeat MRI of Jed's brain was completed, which revealed dilation of the anterior horn of the left lateral ventricle and thinning of the genu and body of the corpus callosum. The aforementioned encephalomalacia had remained stable. Jed receives two medications on a daily basis, including deferasirox (Exjade) and hydroxyurea (Hydrea); he receives hydrocodone bitartrate and acetaminophen (Norco) as needed for pain. There have not been any recent pain crises or acute chest syndromes.

Educational History

Jed recently completed ninth grade; he has never been retained. During ninth grade, his mother reported that her son passed every class except for mathematics; he is currently in summer school to make up the course credits in order to enroll in 10th-grade mathematics courses in the fall. Besides math, his lowest grade was in science (he received a 72); his other grades were Bs. According to Jed, his class schedule was changed in the middle of the year so that his math class was in the morning; he was reportedly having significant difficulty concentrating during math when it was in the afternoon. Generally, Jed's mother shared that her son "often misses the details in his assignments" but related that he is able to catch his mistakes if he remembers to double-check his work. Additionally, Jed's mother reported that he needs a lot of direction with regard to organization, especially with turning in his completed homework. Many times he has failed to turn in his homework because he has misplaced it.

According to the most recent Individualized Education Plan, Jed was receiving special education services under the eligibility categories of "Other Health Impairment" and "Learning Disability" (reading, written language, and math). He receives all of his instruction in the general education classroom, with content mastery support. A major area of concern noted in the IEP was Jed's difficulty with sustained attention. Instructional accommodations included allowing for retesting; using a math facts chart, calculator, and formula cards for math and science; breaking tests into smaller segments; checking for understanding; extending testing time up to one class period; limiting the number of possible answers on multiple-choice tests; providing annotated notes and reviews; and sitting near the teacher.

Psychosocial

Socially, Jed's mother reported that Jed seeks friendships with both older and younger adolescents; however, others do not consistently seek him out for friendship. She also stated that Jed seems to interact easily with adults. He also occasionally withdraws from social situations, perhaps due to parent reports that he has difficulty relating to his peers in certain situations.

With regard to his general emotional functioning, Jed expressed a desire to find a counselor with whom he could discuss some of the significant issues in his life, including the death of his father. He denied symptoms of depression or anxiety but admitted that he sometimes has difficulty dealing with "all of the stress."

Behavioral Observations

Jed was accompanied by his mother to the assessment. He is somewhat tall in stature and was casually dressed and well groomed, appropriate for the evaluation and the weather. When the psychologist first introduced himself to Jed, he responded appropriately. He separated easily from his mother, and rapport was quickly and easily developed and maintained throughout the evaluation session. Even during times when Jed expressed fatigue, he demonstrated good motivation and perseverance. He attempted all tasks and responded well to additional encouragement on tasks he perceived as unappealing or difficult.

Jed's mood and affect were appropriate, and he appeared at ease and comfortable with the psychologist. He did not appear to have difficulty understanding instructions or directions, and he did not require excessive repetition or clarification. Jed was usually quiet and did not engage the psychologist in much spontaneous conversation. Nevertheless, when asked questions, he was able to express his answers without significant difficulty. He did not demonstrate any articulation or phonetic errors, substitutions, or dysfluencies.

Jed did not demonstrate difficulty with sustained attention or concentration beyond what would be expected for his age. However, he was noted to experience significant levels of cognitive fatigue after work periods, and he appeared to benefit from breaks and change of tasks. In addition, Jed did not demonstrate difficulty with general behavioral regulation. He was not fidgety or restless and waited until instructions were completed prior to providing his answer. Brief moments of impulsivity were evidenced when he was asked to read words orally. For the most part, Jed took longer to complete tasks than would be expected for his age.

With regard to motor skills, Jed ambulated independently without difficulty or need for assistance. He used his left hand for writing and drawing and demonstrated a thumb-wrap pencil grip. Overall, Jed exhibited adequate rates of attention, concentration, motivation, task perseverance, and cooperation. Therefore, the next test results should be considered a valid estimate of Jed's neuropsychological functioning.

Assessment Results

Cognitive and Neuropsychological Functioning

The results of neuropsychological evaluation indicate that Jed currently is functioning within the average range of general intellectual ability as measured by the Wechsler Intelligence Scale for Children, Fourth Edition (WISC-IV). Comparatively, relative weaknesses were noted in areas measuring his auditory working memory, with significant weaknesses in cognitive processing speed. Jed's standard scores on the cognitive measure are listed in Table 11.4.

On tasks measuring Jed's executive functioning skills, he demonstrated better performance on nonverbal tasks than he did on tasks requiring verbal responses (see specific scores in Table 11.4). Specifically, he performed in the average range on tasks measuring his nonverbal sequencing skills. However, his demonstration of cognitive flexibility on similar sequencing tasks fell in the borderline range. On tasks measuring Jed's verbal fluency skills, he performed in the borderline to low-average range, again with difficulties on the cognitive flexibility tasks. On rapid-naming tasks, he demonstrated generally impaired (i.e., slow) performance despite being quite accurate; similar tasks that measured cognitive inhibition and flexibility also revealed significant slowness of cognitive processing.

Jed also was administered a tower task that measures an individual's ability to quickly and efficiently solve novel tasks. On this task, Jed had a faster-than-average first-move time. He demonstrated a low-average time per move, likely due to the fact that he failed to take more time prior to initiating the task and therefore was trying to solve the problem while under time pressure. Although Jed was able to complete the tasks as expected for his age, his move accuracy fell in the borderline range, suggesting slightly greater than expected problems with efficient problem solving despite arriving at the correct result in the end.

Furthermore, his mother completed a questionnaire detailing her perceptions of Jed's executive functioning abilities; her responses were not overly negative or inconsistent, resulting in a valid profile. Overall, her responses indicated diffuse difficulty across areas. That is, she views significant difficulties with Jed's ability to demonstrate cognitive flexibility, control his emotions, initiate problem solving or activity, sustain working memory, plan and organize problem-solving approaches, and monitor his behavior. Somewhat milder concerns were noted with regard to Jed's ability to inhibit impulsive responses. Despite her report during the clinical interview that Jed often cannot find his homework, his mother's responses did not indicate concerns with Jed's ability to organize his environment.

Although Jed's conversational skills appeared appropriate, given the location of his stroke, measures of receptive and expressive vocabulary were administered to him. The specific scores can be found in Table 11.4. On the Peabody Picture Vocabulary Test, Fourth Edition (PPVT-IV), Jed performed in the average range. He had slightly more difficulty on

Table 11.4 Psychometric Summary for Jed

	Scaled Score	Standard Score
Wechsler Intelligence Scale for Children, Fourth Edition (WISC-IV)		
General Intellectual Ability		98
Verbal Comprehension Index		95
Similarities	8	
Vocabulary	9	
Comprehension	10	
Perceptual Reasoning Index		102
Block Design	11	
Picture Concepts	7	
Matrix Reasoning	13	
Working Memory Index		80
Digit Span	6	
Letter-Number Sequencing	7	
Processing Speed Index		68
Coding	1	
Symbol Search	7	
Delis-Kaplan Executive Function System (D-KEFS)		
Trail Making Test		
Visual Scanning	10	
Number Sequencing	9	
Letter Sequencing	9	
Number-Letter Sequencing	6	
Motor Speed	11	
Verbal Fluency Test		
Letter Fluency	6	
Category Fluency	8	
Category Switching Total	6	
Color-Word Interference		
Color Naming	4	
Word Reading	1	
Inhibition	1	
Inhibition/Switching	2	
Tower		
Total Achievement Score	10	
Mean First-Move Time	12	
Time-Per-Move Ratio	8	
Move Accuracy Ratio	6	
Rule-Violations-Per-Item Ratio	9	
Peabody Picture Vocabulary Test, Fourth Edition (PPVT-IV)		94
Expressive Vocabulary Test, Second Edition (EVT-II)		78

(continued)

Table 11.4 *(Continued)*

	Scaled Score	Standard Score
Developmental Test of Visual-Motor Integration, Fifth Edition (DTVMI-V)		
Visual-Motor Integration		93
Visual-Perception		95
Motor Coordination		88
Children's Memory Scale (CMS)		
Dot Locations		
Learning	11	
Total Score	12	
Long Delay	12	
Stories		
Immediate	14	
Delayed	14	
Delayed Recognition	12	
Faces		
I Recognition	10	
II Recognition	12	
California Verbal Learning Test—Children's Version (CVLT-C)		
		T-Score
List A Trial 1		50
List A Trial 5		45
List A Trials 1–5		51
List B Free Recall		55
List A Short-Delay Free Recall		55
List A Short-Delay Cued Recall		55
List A Long Delay Free Recall		55
List A Long Delay Cued Recall		60
Learning Slope		45
Correct Recognition Hits		45
False Positives		40
List A Trial 1		50
List A Trial 5		45
Behavior Rating Inventory of Executive Function (BRIEF), (Parent Form)		
Clinical Scales		
Inhibit		63
Shift		76
Emotional Control		65
Initiate		66
Working Memory		77
Plan/Organize		66
Organization of Materials		55
Monitor		73
Indices		
Behavioral Regulation Index		70
Metacognition Index		70
General Executive Composite		72

(continued)

Table 11.4 *(Continued)*

Woodcock-Johnson Tests of Achievement, Third Edition (WJ III)	**Standard Score**
Letter-Word Identification	90
Reading Fluency	77
Calculation	78
Math Fluency	68
Spelling	84
Passage Comprehension	74
Applied Problems	94
Writing Samples	86
Behavior Assessment System for Children, Second Edition (BASC-2) (Self-Report)	
Clinical Scales	**T-Score**
Attitude to School	45
Attitude to Teachers	70
Sensation Seeking	56
Atypicality	50
Locus of Control	69
Social Stress	69
Anxiety	45
Depression	55
Sense of Inadequacy	56
Somatization	53
Attention Problems	54
Hyperactivity	54
Adaptive Scales	
Relations with Parents	45
Interpersonal Relations	36
Self-Esteem	55
Self-Reliance	50
Composites	
School Problems	58
Internalizing Problems	59
Inattention/Hyperactivity	55
Emotional Symptoms Index	54
Personal Adjustment	45
Behavior Assessment System for Children, Second Edition (BASC-2) (Parent Report)	
Clinical Scales	
Hyperactivity	54
Aggression	50
Conduct Problems	48
Anxiety	72
Depression	87
Somatization	41
Atypicality	70
Withdrawal	69

(continued)

Table 11.4 *(Continued)*

	T-Score
Attention Problems	61
Adaptive Scales	
Adaptability	52
Social Skills	60
Leadership	54
Activities of Daily Living	27
Functional Communication	45
Composites	
Externalizing Problems	51
Internalizing Problems	70
Behavioral Symptoms Index	70
Adaptive Skills	47

the Expressive Vocabulary Test, Second Edition (EVT-II), on which he performed in the borderline range. Analysis of Jed's performance on the Children's Memory Scale (CMS; see results in Table 11.4) indicates that, at the present time, he is exhibiting average or better ability to learn and recall visual and auditory information. When he was asked to remember the location of dots, he performed in the average range after three trials and in the high-average range after an interference trial. After a 30-minute delay, Jed performed in the high-average range, correctly placing all eight dots on the grid. When presented with photographs of faces to remember, he performed in the average range after their initial presentation and in the high-average range after a delay, correctly recognizing one more face during the delay than he was able to during the immediate trial. His performance indicated age-appropriate consolidation and retention of visual stimuli.

Additionally, Jed's ability to learn and recall two stories was in the superior range immediately after they were read and after a 30-minute delay. After the delayed recall, Jed was asked to answer yes/no questions about the two stories. He performed in the high-average range on this recognition task. Of the three questions he answered incorrectly, he had not been able to provide the correct information previously for two of the questions, indicating that he probably did not initially encode the information.

Jed also was asked to learn a list of 15 words. He recalled 7 words of the list after it was read to him the first time, suggesting an average initial attention span for auditory information. After the first list was read to him five times and he had the opportunity to recall words after each trial, he demonstrated a learning slope in the average range, increasing the amount of information recalled across the trials at an expected rate. When presented with a second word list, he recalled 8 words (average range), exhibiting no vulnerability to proactive interference (i.e., previous learning interferes with new learning). When asked to recall the first list after he was presented with the second list and again after a 20-minute delay, he recalled 10 and 13 words, respectively. Compared to his recall of 12 words during Trial 5, Jed demonstrated little to no impact from retroactive interference (i.e., learning new information interferes with recall of old information). In fact, additional time allowed him to consolidate the previous learning further. Furthermore, when given the opportunity to recognize words from the list among distracters, he performed in the average range, identifying 14 of the 15 words as part of the original list; he misidentified 2 nontargets, which is in the low-average range, suggesting very mild difficulty in discriminating relevant from irrelevant responses when trying to recognize verbal information.

On tasks that measured Jed's visual-motor and visual-perceptual skills, he demonstrated a thumb-wrap pencil grip with his left hand. His ability to copy increasingly complex geometric figures fell in the average range. On a nonmotor visual-perceptual measure during which Jed was asked to match geometric figures, he performed in the average range during the three-minute time limit. On tasks measuring speeded visual-motor accuracy and precision, his performance fell in the low-average range. Specific scores for these tasks can be found in Table 11.4.

Academic Functioning

The Woodcock-Johnson Tests of Achievement, Third Edition (WJ III) was administered as a measure of academic achievement. Based on his performance, Jed appears to have somewhat dampened performance across academic areas compared to his level of cognitive functioning. On applied math tasks, Jed performed in the average range despite borderline performance on paper-and-pencil tasks and impaired math fluency skills. His spelling and writing abilities fell in the average range. Compared to average performance on a word-reading task, Jed's reading comprehension and fluency were in the borderline range. Compared to his average general intellectual ability, his global academic performance is much lower than where he would be expected to perform. Jed's standard scores on the WJ-III subtests are listed in Table 11.4.

Social-Emotional and Behavioral Functioning

Jed and his mother each completed a questionnaire to gain additional information about his emotional and behavioral functioning. In perusing the results, Jed's responses led to poor attitudes toward teachers. In addition, mild levels of social stress and difficulties with interpersonal relationships plus a somewhat external locus of control were also reported. Jed's responses did not lead to elevated levels of internalizing problems (i.e., anxiety, depression) or other concerns. On the contrary, his mother's responses indicated significant concerns with anxiety and depression and mildly increased levels of withdrawal and atypical behaviors. She denied the presence of externalizing problems, such as aggression or conduct problems. With regard to adaptive functioning, Jed's mother reported mild concerns with his ability to complete activities of daily living. However, he reportedly has age-appropriate skills in the areas of adaptability, social skills, leadership abilities, and functional communication. A review of the profiles obtained by Jed and his mother can be seen in Table 11.4.

During the individual clinical interview with Jed, he denied symptoms of anxiety or depression although he reiterated that he would like to have a counselor with whom he could talk on a regular basis. When asked about his social relationships, Jed indicated that he is occasionally teased by other students because he is "trying to be white," reporting that he works hard and studies, qualities that other African American students reportedly attribute to "white kids."

Summary and Diagnostic Impressions

Based on the present neuropsychological evaluation, Jed's profile was somewhat variable. His general cognitive ability fell in the average range. Compared to his intelligence, Jed's reading comprehension and math calculation abilities fell far below the expected level. As a result, he meets criteria for a learning disability in the areas of reading comprehension and mathematics calculation. Furthermore, his inability to complete academic tasks quickly will significantly impact his performance in the classroom and on timed academic tasks. Notably, Jed's writing skills are only slightly below his cognitive abilities and do not represent a significant area of weakness. Commensurate with his intellectual ability,

Jed performed in the average or better range on tasks measuring his nonverbal sequencing, planning and organization, auditory and visual memory, visual-motor skills, and visual-perception skills. Relative weaknesses in working memory, cognitive processing speed, verbal fluency, rapid naming, cognitive flexibility, and efficiency of problem solving were noted. Additionally, significant weaknesses in a variety of executive functioning skills (i.e., cognitive flexibility, emotional control, task initiation, working memory, planning and organization, behavioral monitoring) also were noted by Jed's mother.

Children with significant medical issues, such as those experienced by Jed, may be at greater risk for neurocognitive difficulties. However, even if there are significant risk factors, positive environmental influences, such as a consistent home environment and supportive caregivers, have the potential to mitigate the development and impact of such difficulties. As can be noted from Jed's overall neuropsychological profile, poor executive functioning (i.e., impulsive task initiation when thoughtfulness is best, slow processing speed, poor working memory, difficulty with organization) was revealed through direct evaluation and from information gained from his mother. His medical history is significant for sickle cell disease and other health issues, including overt stroke. In addition to overt strokes, children with sickle cell disease are at risk for experiencing covert infarcts that are not detected based on behavioral observation. As previously mentioned, imaging of his brain indicated encephalomalacia in the left frontal region of his brain, mild generalized atrophy, dilation of the anterior horn of the left lateral ventricle, and thinning of the genu and the body of the corpus callosum. Damage or interference in the left frontal region of the brain can result in some difficulties with executive functioning, such as slower processing speed and relatively weaker working memory skills, as well as problems with expressive language. Also, the corpus callosum, which is the bundle of fibers that connects the two hemispheres of the brain, promotes efficient communication of information between the many cortical and subcortical regions of the brain. Thinning or atrophy may result again in less efficient processing speed and problem solving. Therefore, the select neurocognitive weaknesses that Jed demonstrates are not surprising.

In addition to the neurocognitive weaknesses discovered, children and adolescents with significant medical issues often find themselves feeling different from others their age. Emotional difficulties may impact Jed's ability to cope with daily stressors of the school and home environments. Although his mother endorsed symptoms of anxiety and depression, Jed did not. However, social stress, difficulties with interpersonal relationships, and feelings of lack of control may exacerbate any predisposition to such difficulties. Given his generally average cognitive skills, Jed has insight into his learning difficulties and likely perceives that he should be achieving at a higher level or at a faster rate. Also, his family situation should be taken into consideration as far as its impact on his current functioning. Although he does not meet the criteria for a diagnosis of a mood or anxiety disorder at the present time, accommodations and interventions designed for children with similar difficulties will be beneficial to Jed, and he should participate in individual therapy to facilitate the best possible outcome for him. Overall, his mother in particular should be cautious of significant emotional triggers that may exacerbate his symptoms, which may include familial discord, academic failure, or peer relationship issues.

Recommendations

Considering the data from this evaluation and in review of Jed's performance at school during the previous year, it appears that Jed's current special education accommodations and modifications are appropriate. Given his current difficulty with mathematics and science, in addition to his general difficulty with organization and planning, additional modifications may be warranted. Some of the most salient recommendations to benefit Jed's educational performance include:

- The right fit between teacher and student is very important in Jed's case. Although he has average cognitive skills, his ability to apply this knowledge to academic tasks is greatly compromised. In concert with these weaknesses, very slow processing speed and poor working memory inhibit Jed from achieving at the same rate as his peers. Teachers must be cautious of getting frustrated with Jed if he needs directions clarified or reiterated. Slow processing speed is not the result of a lack of motivation and should not be interpreted as such. Therefore, he must not be pressured by strict time limits. He should be allowed extra time to complete tests, homework assignments, or other classroom tasks. *Accuracy should be encouraged over speed.* Additionally, he may be asked to complete only the odd or even problems, so that the same content area is sampled, but he does not spend an extended amount of time on any one task. Instead, a sampling of his learning based on content (and not quantity) should be expected.
- Children with sickle cell disease may experience slightly greater levels of cognitive fatigue. As a result, he may require longer or more frequent breaks than other peers. Placing Jed where he can feel more "in the middle" of activity may help increase his arousal and help with sustained focus. Use hands-on or interactive activities when possible to engage Jed in the task. Also, changing tasks more frequently may alleviate some of the drain on sustained working memory for Jed.

Consideration of Jed's current psychological functioning is also important for his development. Provision of supports ideally will result in better emotional coping and a greater sense of confidence. As a result, these recommendations are offered:

- In order to buffer him from negative social interactions, do not have students grade each other's papers. So Jed's academic difficulties will not be made known to other students. Continued participation in preferred activities will help further increase his self-esteem. Offer him opportunities to engage with other adolescents in a supervised environment so that caregivers can monitor his interaction with others and provide support, encouragement, and direction if necessary.
- As he requested, it would greatly benefit Jed to participate in individual psychotherapy with a pediatric psychologist who is familiar with the issues that accompany sickle cell disease. Therapy should focus on learning additional coping mechanisms and decreasing the symptoms of anxiety or depression observed by his mother. Therapy also should address Jed's external locus of control, which probably results from experiencing medical issues from a young age that were beyond his control. Due to his level of cognitive ability and insight into his own needs, cognitive-behavioral therapy likely would be beneficial for Jed.
- Because Jed may experience frustration in certain circumstances, teachers should be aware that he may need extra encouragement and support to complete tasks. To reduce the likelihood of further escalation, allow Jed time for breaks if it appears that he is becoming emotionally overwhelmed by the situation. Given his propensity toward greater fluctuations in mood at home, Jed's mother should be conscious of his lowered ability to control his emotions as well as other adolescents his age. When these mood swings occur, Jed should be given a break to recover from the incident that may have initiated the emotion.

Further Discussion of Case Study

The neurocognitive, physical, emotional, and behavioral effects of an overt stroke are widely variable. As with Jed, children and adolescents with infarct in the left hemisphere likely will experience at least some degree of language difficulty. Conversely, children with infarct in the right hemisphere may experience greater levels of nonverbal dysfunction. Both groups may have physical weakness in the extremities contralateral to the stroke location. Children with infarct in any region of the brain may demonstrate changes in their mood and behavior, including increased aggression, impulsivity, and hyperactivity, or dampened mood and psychomotor responses. Overall, this case study was presented in order to elucidate some of the common findings for individuals with overt stroke in the left hemisphere and the impact of the stroke on neurocognitive skills, especially executive functions, numerous years after the incident.

CONCLUDING COMMENTS

Although globally about cerebrovascular disorders, this chapter has focused on sickle cell disease, as it is the most prevalent genetic cerebrovascular disorder and the most frequent of the cerebrovascular disorders affecting children and adolescents. Most states conduct screening for sickle cell at birth, but many times the importance of the results is not evident until there are complications or stroke; children often are lost to medical follow-up as families move from place to place or change physicians. In these cases, inaccurate attributions may be made about the causes of the inattention (i.e., presuming the child has ADHD); alternatively, reports of pain may be ignored or not taken seriously (i.e., assumed to be psychosomatic and unfounded). With the high incidence of sickle cell disease, there is a need for increased awareness of the disease and its impact on functioning and child outcomes (Schatz & McClellan, 2006). Sickle cell disease is associated with multiple risk factors, biological as well as environmental and social, that need to be incorporated into the case conceptualization of a child or adolescent with this disorder (Schatz, Finke et al., 2004).

Research findings support the need for periodic neuropsychological evaluation following stroke to identify patterns of higher cortical dysfunction and assist in the development of appropriate rehabilitation and special education programs (M. J. Cohen et al., 1994). The usefulness of pediatric neuropsychological evaluation for a child with sickle cell disease has not been established but may be warranted if learning problems are evidenced. Many individuals with sickle cell disease present with cognitive, academic, and functional difficulties; universal screening may promote earlier detection and appropriate psychoeducational intervention (C. C. Peterson et al., 2005). As can be seen from the case studies presented here, consideration of social-emotional effects of sickle cell is also important. At the same time, multicenter cohort study efforts, and ultimately devoted pediatric clinical trials, are needed to establish comprehensive evidence-based guidelines for the treatment of childhood stroke.

Chapter 12

LOW BIRTH WEIGHT

DEFINITION

Low birth weight (LBW) typically is defined as birth weight less than 2,500 grams, or less than 5 pounds 8 ounces. Very low birth weight (VLBW) is defined as birth weight less than 1,500 grams, or less than 3 pounds 5 ounces (Taylor, Klein, & Hack, 2000), and extremely low birth weight (ELBW) is defined as birth weight less than 1,000 grams, or less than 2 pounds 3 ounces (G. P. Aylward, 2002; Saigal et al., 2006). The majority of infants with LBW are considered to have "moderate" LBW, or birth weight between 1,500 and 2,499 grams (J. A. Martin et al., 2005). With advances in medical technology and care, many more infants with all categories of LBW survive than was the case in the early 1900s, although mortality rates remain high for infants weighing less than 600 grams at birth (Lemons et al., 2001; Taylor, Klein, & Hack 2000). Many infants with LBW continue to show deficits in multiple areas of development into childhood, adolescence, and young adulthood (Saigal et al., 2006). As survival rates have increased, so has our understanding of the developmental outcomes associated with LBW.

Prevalence/Incidence

It is estimated that approximately 7% to 8% of infants born in the United States are LBW (J. A. Martin et al., 2005; Taylor, Klein, & Hack, 2000), with about 1.5% classified as VLBW (B. S. Peterson et al., 2000). Lower birth weight (i.e., VLBW and ELBW) is associated with higher mortality rates; thus, most surviving infants with LBW have the moderate classification (Mathews & MacDorman, 2006). LBW appears to be more common among African American infants (J. A. Martin et al., 2005; Mathews & MacDorman, 2006), and abnormal behavioral, cognitive, and academic outcomes tend to be more common and severe among males with LBW as compared to females (G. P. Aylward, 2002).

ETIOLOGY

Two primary causes of LBW have been identified: preterm delivery of the infant (i.e., delivery at less than 37 weeks' gestation) (Slattery & Morrison, 2002) and growth retardation of the infant while in the uterus when the infant is delivered full term (Taylor, Klein, & Hack, 2000). Preterm delivery is the most typical cause of LBW; preterm delivery is associated with African American ethnicity, low socioeconomic status (SES), substance use, and poor maternal nutrition (Paneth, 1995; Shiono & Behrman, 1995; Slattery & Morrison, 2002) and appears to be related to a range of biological complications surrounding pregnancy, such as multiple pregnancy (Slattery & Morrison, 2002). There is limited evidence suggesting that women who are physically, emotionally, or sexually abused during pregnancy are slightly more likely than nonabused women to give birth to LBW infants, but the interaction between abuse and other variables (e.g., maternal ethnicity, SES, age, marital status, health factors) in predicting LBW is not yet understood (C. C. Murphy, Schei, Myhr, & Du Mont, 2001). Maternal periodontal disease also has been identified as a risk factor for LBW, although such disease likely is related to additional health and nutrition factors (N. J. Lopez, Smith, & Gutierrez, 2002). Maternal exposure to air pollution (e.g., carbon monoxide, nitrogen dioxide, sulfur dioxide) during pregnancy is considered an environmental risk factor for LBW (Ha et al., 2001; Ritz & Yu, 1999), and maternal distress and cigarette smoking also have been identified as predictors of LBW and preterm birth (Lobel et al., 2008; Rondo et al., 2003).

Neuroanatomical Substrates

Due to the vulnerability of the premature brain and deficits in the regulation of cerebral blood flow, infants with LBW are at increased risk for brain injury during labor and delivery (Taylor, Klein, & Hack, 2000; Zillmer et al., 2008). Injuries to the brain are a major complication for infants with LBW and contribute to the neuropsychological sequelae observed as children with LBW mature. These insults include germinal matrix intraventricular hemorrhage (sometimes leading to progressive hydrocephalus), periventricular leukomalacia (which involves focal and diffuse necrosis of white matter and formation of cysts), ventricular dilatation, and brain abnormalities (e.g., reduction in white matter volume, cortical atrophy, and lesions in various regions) (Hack et al., 2005; Taylor, Klein, & Hack, 2000). Periventricular leukomalacia is the most common manifestation of brain insult among LBW children and is responsible for much of the impairment experienced by these children, as periventricular leukomalacia appears to be related to restriction of blood supply to the cerebral white matter (Volpe, 2001). Germinal matrix intraventricular hemorrhage also is common and is defined using a four-point grading system of increasing severity, with grade I = hemorrhage confined to the germinal layer, grade II = intraventricular hemorrhage without ventricular dilatation, grade III = intraventricular hemorrhage with ventricular dilatation, and grade IV = parenchymal hemorrhage or periventricular hemorrhagic infarction (Baumert et al., 2008; Patra, Wilson-Costello, Taylor, Mercuri-Minich, & Hack, 2006). All grades of germinal matrix intraventricular hemorrhage appear to predict worse neurodevelopmental outcomes among LBW children due to destruction of glial cells and reductions of cortical gray matter (Patra et al., 2006).

B. S. Peterson et al. (2000) examined magnetic resonance imaging (MRI) scans of 25 preterm children at 8 years of age and found that compared to control children, preterm children had reduced brain volumes. The most pronounced differences were found in the sensorimotor, premotor, midtemporal, parieto-occipital, and subgenual regions. Specific structures showing reduced volume included the corpus callosum (including rostrum/genu, anterior body, midbody, isthmus, and splenium), cerebellum, basal ganglia (including caudate, putamen, and globus pallidus), amygdala, and hippocampus. Further, positive correlations were found between brain volume and Full Scale, Verbal, and Performance IQ scores. Thus, even at 8 years of age, preterm children continued to exhibit significant differences in brain volume compared to control children; these abnormalities likely contribute to neuropsychological and motor deficits observed in children with LBW.

Similarly, an MRI study indicated that LBW children who showed abnormal myelination in the central occipital white matter and the centrum semiovale at age 1 continued to show abnormalities at age 6, presenting as delayed myelination or gliosis, which are indicative of periventricular leukomalacia (Skranes, Nilsen, Smevik, Vik, & Brubakk, 1998). These results were confirmed using MRI to show higher rates of ventricular dilatation, reduction in white matter, thinning of the corpus callosum, and gliosis among a sample of adolescents with VLBW who were assessed at 14 to 15 years of age; these brain abnormalities were significantly more frequent among VLBW adolescents as compared to controls (Indredavik et al., 2005). Martinussen et al. (2005) also found lower cortical surface area and lower cortical volume among a sample of VLBW adolescents; these two cortical variables also were positively and significantly correlated with IQ scores, but only among the VLBW adolescents. Further, significant cortical thinning was observed in the parietal and temporal lobes, and cortical thickening was observed in the frontal lobe, circular insula superior sulcus, and occipital superior gyrus (Martinussen et al., 2005).

An additional study assessed adults (mean age = 23 years) who were VLBW at birth and found that as compared to sibling controls, the VLBW adults had a 46% increase in ventricular volume and a 17% decrease in volume of the posterior corpus callosum; there were no significant differences in volumes of the hippocampus, cerebral gray matter, or total brain (Fearon et al., 2004). Isaacs et al. (2000), in contrast, did observe significantly reduced hippocampal volume (and commensurate memory deficits) among a sample of VLBW adolescents. However, the VLBW sample included only 11 adolescents. Finally, Nosarti et al. (2002) followed a sample of preterm infants to adolescence (age = 14–15 years) and found, compared to controls, 42% increase in ventricular volume, 6% reduction in total brain volume, 11.8% reduction in gray matter volume, 15.6% reduction in right hippocampal volume, and 12.1% reduction in left hippocampal volume (all statistically significant). In all, these studies provide evidence that brain abnormalities associated with LBW persist over time.

COURSE AND PROGNOSIS

The literature on LBW often distinguishes between short-term (through elementary school age) and long-term (from middle school age and up) consequences or outcomes of LBW. A large body of research has been amassed on both immediate and later consequences. Table 12.1 summarizes the neuropsychological deficits associated with LBW based on some of the findings in the research literature.

Short-Term Consequences

Consequences of LBW at the time the child has reached elementary school age include effects on health status, overall cognitive ability, academic achievement, and behavior (Saigal & Doyle, 2008; Taylor, Klein, & Hack, 2000). For example, physical health consequences include cerebral palsy, hydrocephalus, seizures, asthma, infections, chronic lung disease, vision and hearing impairments, frequent nose and throat infections, injuries, higher systolic blood pressure, and reduced height and weight, in addition to increased hospitalization rates, dependency, and functional limitations in daily activities due to these issues (Chen & Millar, 1999; Hack, Schluchter, Cartar, & Rahman, 2005; Hack, Taylor, et al., 2005; Lemons et al., 2001; Saigal et al., 2006; Taylor, Klein, & Hack, 2000), although recent research indicates that the prevalence of cerebral palsy

Table 12.1 Neuropsychological Deficits Associated with Low Birth Weight

Global Domain	Specific Deficits
Cognition	General intelligence Verbal ability Reasoning/nonverbal ability Processing speed
Executive function	Organizational skills Planning Attention
Learning and Memory	Recalling complex figures Verbal working memory Verbal list learning Delayed recall Errors in recall Learning efficiency
Auditory-linguistic/Language function	Oral directions Recalling sentences Speed of number naming Expressive language Communication skills
Achievement/Academic skills	Math Reading Spelling Grade retention Learning disabilities Special education placement (speech-language impairment, developmental disabilities, low-incidence disabilities)
Visual perception/ Constructional Praxis	Copying tasks Spatial-constructional skills Coordination Vision Hearing Fine motor skills Gross motor skills Visual-motor integration Visual-spatial abilities Balance Locomotion Nonlocomotion Receipt and propulsion
Emotional/Behavioral functioning	Adaptive behaviors Attention deficit hyperactivity disorder symptoms Withdrawal Thought problems Social skills/interaction Parent-rated internalizing problems (depression, anxiety) Parent-rated externalizing problems (hyperactivity, oppositional-defiant behaviors)

among children with LBW has decreased over the last several decades (Platt et al., 2007). Interestingly, the combination of preterm birth *and* LBW appears to be especially significant, as infants with this combination are at increased risk for poor health outcomes as compared to either full-term children with LBW or preterm children with normal birth weight (Chen & Millar, 1999).

Longitudinal data indicate evidence for a dose-response relationship between birth weight and outcome, such that children with birth weight less than 750 grams show worse outcomes than children with birth weight between 750 and 1,499 grams, who in turn show worse outcomes than control children (Taylor, Klein, & Hack, 2000). Thus, children with ELBW and VLBW tend to have greater likelihood of physical, developmental, and learning problems, and more severe problems, than children with LBW, with significant correlations between birth weight and scores on cognitive tests (G. P. Aylward, 2002; Bhutta, Cleves, Casey, Cradock, & Anand, 2002; Kono, Mishina, Sato, Watanabe, & Honma, 2008; Saigal, Hoult, Streiner, Stoskopf, & Rosenbaum, 2000). Similarly, lower gestational age at birth is associated with higher mortality and more severe problems, such as cerebral palsy and neuromotor dysfunction; rates of these problems become progressively lower as gestational age at birth increases (Hille et al., 2007; Saigal & Doyle, 2008). It is worth noting that many differences between children with and without LBW are still apparent even when controlling for global cognitive ability (Taylor, Burant, Holding, Klein, & Hack, 2002).

Cognitive consequences are manifest on measures of infant intelligence, motor skills, memory, delayed memory, planning, and math skills (Litt et al., 2005; Taylor, Klein, & Hack, 2000). Taylor, Hack, and Klein (1998) found that children with LBW performed more poorly on a continuous performance test of attention than control children even when covarying for intelligence, and risk for attention problems was associated with degree of LBW. At the same time, no group differences were observed for other attention measures or parent and teacher ratings when IQ was used as a covariate. At 11 years of age, a sample of children with LBW was rated by mothers and teachers as having more attention problems than control children, but this pattern across raters held only for LBW children living in urban settings (Breslau & Chilcoat, 2000). Further, there were higher rates of externalizing problems among LBW children, but these problems were explained largely by maternal smoking during pregnancy.

At follow-up at age 5 years, a cohort of children with ELBW in Finland were assessed with the Wechsler Preschool and Primary Scale of Intelligence—Revised (WPPSI-R) and the Neuropsychological Assessment (NEPSY) (Mikkola et al., 2005). Overall rates of cognitive impairment and cerebral palsy among children with ELBW were 9% and 14%, respectively; problems with vision associated with retinopathy of prematurity also were common. Mean NEPSY scores suggested norm-referenced deficits in language, attention, visual-spatial, sensorimotor, and verbal memory functioning. About 26% of the cohort was classified as "normal," meaning there were no indications of neuropsychological impairment or abnormal functioning. Thus, about 74% of children in the ELBW cohort exhibited some sort of neurodevelopmental abnormality at 5 years of age, with about 20% exhibiting major disabilities. Similarly, another study that assessed a group of ELBW children at 5 years of age found that as compared to their full-term siblings, these children exhibited lower IQ scores as assessed by the Stanford-Binet and lower scores on measures of spelling and motor skills (i.e., balance, locomotion, nonlocomotion, receipt and propulsion; Kilbride, Thorstad, & Daily, 2004).

With regard to verbal memory, one study used the California Verbal Learning Test—Children's Version to compare functioning between children with LBW and controls

(Taylor, Klein, Minich, & Hack, 2000b). Significant group differences (with LBW children performing more poorly than controls) were found for list learning, delayed recall, learning efficiency, rate and improvement of learning over time, and inaccurate recall. Group differences in rate of learning remained even when controlling for IQ, vocabulary, and neurosensory disorders.

Language and social skills also may be affected, including fewer speech acts, fewer attempts at initiating interactions, inappropriate responses to social interactions, and less developed expressive language skills (Taylor, Klein, & Hack, 2000). Physical and motor problems associated with LBW may restrict participation in social and academic activities with peers, thereby leading to peer interaction difficulties and possible emotional problems (G. P. Aylward, 2002).

Preterm birth and LBW appear to be related to deficits in fine motor skills, gross motor skills, total motor skills, and visual-motor integration at 4 years of age, with the greatest impairment in these areas among preterm children with neurological illness (e.g., seizures, hydrocephalus, intraventricular hemorrhage; M. C. Sullivan & McGrath, 2003). Motor skills deficits typically involve the legs and trunk, depending on the degree of hemorrhage into the descending white matter tracks. There also is evidence to suggest that children with LBW are at much higher risk for developmental coordination disorder than normal children; in one study, about 50% of ELBW children assessed at 9 years of age met diagnostic criteria for this disorder (Holsti, Grunau, & Whitfield, 2002).

In light of these multiple constructs implicated with LBW, it is not surprising to see higher rates of learning disabilities and academic difficulties among LBW children when compared with full-term children; higher rates have been observed for reading disabilities, math disabilities, and combined reading/math disabilities (Litt, Taylor, Klein, & Hack, 2005). In a subsample of preterm children with neurological illness, about 45% received speech-language services and about 25% received special education services for learning disabilities by age 8 (M. C. Sullivan & McGrath, 2003). Given the fine motor skill component required for academic tasks involving handwriting, it will be important for future research to explore the role that motor skills deficits play in math and spelling difficulties.

In sum, with regard to research on the short-term consequences of LBW, there is much inconsistency in findings due to methodological limitations of existing studies (e.g., small heterogeneous samples of children with LBW, different designs and measures used in different studies). Some of the more consistent cognitive and behavioral outcomes across studies, based on differences when compared to control groups, include lower scores on intelligence tests (with an average of about 11 points lower than controls), increased prevalence of externalizing (e.g., hyperactivity, oppositional-defiant behaviors) and internalizing (e.g., depression, anxiety) behaviors, and increased risk for developing attention problems or Attention-Deficit/Hyperactivity Disorder (ADHD) (Bhutta et al., 2002). These cognitive and behavioral problems, in conjunction with the physical health problems often experienced by children with LBW, may contribute to increased parental and family stress, especially during the first few years of the child's life (Bhutta et al., 2002; Saigal & Doyle, 2008), which may in turn lead to more negative long-term outcomes for the child.

Long-Term Consequences

Research following children with LBW into middle school age and beyond suggests that for many children, the deficits just described are long lasting (Taylor, Klein, Minich, &

Hack, 2000a). The smaller physical size associated with LBW appears to persist into later childhood and adolescence, with LBW children and adolescents showing significantly lower weight, height, and head circumference than full-term adolescents (Kilbride et al., 2004; Knops et al., 2005; M. Rogers, Fay, Whitfield, Tomlinson, & Grunau, 2005). At the same time, physical growth is characterized by a great deal of heterogeneity, with many LBW children "catching up" with their peers' height over time (Brandt, Sticker, Gausche, & Lentze, 2005); females appear to be more likely to catch up with peers by young adulthood than males (Hack et al., 2003), and some studies find differences in height and weight but not for head circumference (Van Baar, Ultee, Gunning, Soepatmi, & de Leeuw, 2006). Additional research will be necessary to identify variables that may explain or predict which LBW children will continue to show smaller physical size and which will catch up with their peers.

Several studies have examined the long-term impact of LBW on neuropsychological functioning in adolescence and young adulthood, and a sample of these studies will be described here. For example, a series of studies with adolescents who had LBW as infants found that as compared to control groups, these adolescents showed much higher rates of neurosensory impairment (e.g., cerebral palsy, microcephaly, hydrocephalus, mental retardation, vision or hearing impairment), lower Wechsler IQ scores, and lower scores on reading, spelling, and math achievement (Saigal et al., 2000). These adolescents also exhibited greater symptoms of depression and ADHD based on parent report, in addition to increased likelihood of being rated as clumsy, of failing a grade in school, and of being rated below average in sports; LBW adolescents did not exhibit significantly greater psychopathology than controls, based only on self-report, and were similar to controls on social competence and relationship variables (Saigal, Pinelli, Hoult, Kim, & Boyle, 2003). Adolescents with LBW generally did not report significantly lower self-esteem than control adolescents, with the exception of the domain of athletic competence, which may be related to motor skills impairment among adolescents with LBW (Saigal, Lambert, Russ, & Hoult, 2002).

Hille et al. (2007) followed a large sample of Dutch infants with LBW into young adulthood (follow-up assessment occurred at approximately 19 years of age) and found that these young adults demonstrated: moderate to severe problems in cognitive functioning, including verbal skills, numerical skills, memory, reasoning, and processing speed (4.3%); deficits in neuromotor functioning, including hand function, coordination, walking, and posture (8.1%); deficits in hearing (1.8%); and vision problems (1.9%). Further, previous participation in special education occurred at a rate of 24%, and 7.6% reported being either unemployed or not enrolled in an educational program. With the exception of vision problems, these rates were much higher than those for the general Dutch population, suggesting that the consequences of LBW persist into young adulthood. In a similar study, Saigal et al. (2006) followed a sample of infants with ELBW through adolescence and young adulthood (22–25 years of age), and compared their functioning to a control group. Functional outcomes were indicators of transition into young adulthood, including educational attainment, employment, independence, marriage, and parenthood. Interestingly, significant group differences were *not* observed for these outcomes; the ELBW and control groups performed similarly in terms of graduating from high school, enrollment in postsecondary education programs, employment status, living independently from parents, getting married or cohabitating, and having children, and both groups achieved these milestones at a similar age. Thus, based on these indicators of adjustment and transition into adulthood, many young adults with ELBW were functioning similar to normal-birth-weight young adults.

A study of ELBW adolescents without significant sensorimotor or cognitive impairment at approximately 17 years of age found that, compared to controls, these adolescents scored lower on the Vocabulary, Block Design, and Coding subtests of the WAIS-III and the Reading and Arithmetic subtests of the WRAT-3; the largest group difference by far was observed for the Arithmetic subtest (Grunau, Whitfield, & Fay, 2004). Adolescents with ELBW also had lower self-ratings of competence along academic, athletic, romantic, and occupational dimensions, and higher levels of parent-rated problems with internalizing and externalizing behaviors (with specific behaviors including withdrawal, social problems, thought problems, inattention, and aggressive and delinquent behaviors). Hack et al. (2002) assessed a sample of VLBW children at 20 years of age. As compared to a control group, the sample of VLBW children was characterized by lower high school graduation rates, higher rates of grade repetition, lower Full Scale IQ, lower scores on a test of academic achievement, and higher rates of neurosensory impairment. At the same time, the VLBW sample reported lower rates of alcohol and drug use, which may be related to greater parental monitoring or less interaction with peers among young adults with VLBW (unfortunately, peer interaction and social competence variables were not examined in this study).

Taylor, Minich, Klein, and Hack (2004) followed a cohort of children with VLBW from about age 7 to about age 14 years, with four follow-up assessments occurring after the initial assessment. At follow-up assessments, children with VLBW showed deficits in language processing, verbal list learning, perceptual-motor skills, and organization; these deficits (as compared to controls) remained when controlling for IQ. Perhaps of greater importance is that children with VLBW also showed slower rates of development on perceptual-motor and executive function measures, suggesting that for these constructs, VLBW children do not catch up with their peers over time. Further, the problems with memory observed among adolescents with LBW are consistent with MRI studies showing smaller hippocampal volume among LBW adolescents (Isaacs et al., 2000; Nosarti et al., 2002). LBW children assessed at approximately 16 years of age also demonstrated deficits in motor skills including oral, fine, and gross skills; neonatal white matter abnormality predicted both motor problems and lower Full Scale IQ scores (Whitaker et al., 2006). In another study examining motor skills, a group of unimpaired adolescents who were ELBW at birth demonstrated significant deficits in physical and motor variables such as grip strength, leg strength, aerobic capacity, vertical jump, flexibility, abdominal strength, number of push-ups, and maintenance of rhythm (Rogers et al., 2005). Adolescents in the ELBW group also reported less participation in sports, lower activity level, and lower physical coordination. Thus, even among LBW adolescents who do not exhibit neurosensory impairment (e.g., cognitive deficits, cerebral palsy, hearing or vision impairment), differences in motor skills are apparent when compared to full-term adolescents.

Evidence suggests that young adults with VLBW reported similar overall satisfaction with their health and well-being as controls and actually reported higher work performance and risk avoidance (e.g., avoidance of alcohol and drug use, sexual activity, violence; Hack, Cartar, Schluchter, Klein, & Forrest, 2007); however, the young adults with VLBW reported less resilience and adaptability related to physical activity (i.e., less involvement in physical activity) and family involvement (i.e., less perceived family support) and greater likelihood of chronic medical and psychosocial problems. Overall, research suggests that for many young adults, the consequences of LBW are long lasting, but there also is a sizable group who are able to make a successful transition into young adulthood based on this limited set of outcome variables.

Research on increased risk for psychiatric problems has been mixed. A Norwegian study found that as compared to controls, children with VLBW (assessed at 14 years of age) reported more psychiatric symptoms and more psychiatric disorders, with especially higher prevalence of anxiety and attention problems (Indredavik et al., 2004). Hack et al. (2004) assessed a sample of LBW infants at 20 years of age and examined psychopathology by gender, based on self- and parent report. Males with LBW self-reported significantly fewer delinquent behaviors and less excessive alcohol use as compared to controls; parents of males with LBW rated significantly more thought problems and inattention and higher rates of clinically significant withdrawal behaviors. Similar to the males, females with LBW self-reported fewer delinquent behaviors and less excessive alcohol use as compared to controls but reported higher withdrawal, more internalizing problems, having fewer friends, and having less positive family relationships. Parents of females with LBW rated significantly more anxiety/depression, withdrawal, and attention problems among their children in addition to higher rates of clinically significant thought problems. Similarly, Dahl et al. (2006) studied a sample of Norwegian VLBW adolescents and assessed emotional, behavioral, social, and academic outcomes using the Child Behavior Checklist and Youth Self-Report. Compared to the normative sample, male adolescents self-reported less internalizing, externalizing, thought, and attention problems while parents reported more problems with social competence, school competence, and inattention. For females, the adolescents self-reported less externalizing, social, thought, and attention problems while parents reported more problems with internalizing behaviors, anxiety/depression, social interaction, inattention, and school competence. Thus, there were discrepancies between adolescents' and parents' perceptions, with parents reporting more problems than the adolescents and adolescents presenting as relatively well adjusted. Much research has *not* found significant differences between children with LBW and full-term children for depression, feelings of competence, or social skills (Taylor, Klein, Minich, & Hack, 2000a). Interestingly, preterm children in Van Baar et al.'s (2006) sample demonstrated more externalizing behaviors than full-term children when assessed at ages 4 and 5, but this difference was no longer present when the children were assessed at 10 years of age; this developmental change indicates the need to monitor psychiatric symptoms over time.

A confluence of evidence indicates a pattern on IQ tests such that children and adolescents with LBW score lower on performance (nonverbal) subtests than on verbal subtests; this pattern is supported by research demonstrating greater deficits on measures of motor skills, memory, and visual-perceptual reasoning as compared to measures of language (Taylor, Klein, & Hack, 2000). This pattern is similar to the common Verbal IQ > Performance IQ profile noted among children with traumatic brain injuries (TBI; see Chapter 8). Longitudinal data on IQ and achievement indicated that LBW children actually demonstrated declining scores over time, thereby suggesting that LBW continues to affect cognitive development and academic performance from infancy into young childhood (Kalmar, 1996; Taylor, Klein, Minich, et al., 2000a). It is likely that LBW contributes to long-term deficits by interfering with the ability to self-regulate and learn new information (Taylor, Klein, & Hack, 2000). Thus, over time, the discrepancy between children with LBW and children with normal birth weight may get wider and wider (Saigal et al., 2000). At the same time, Ment et al. (2003) found that LBW children's picture vocabulary, Full Scale IQ, and verbal IQ scores increased with age, but this was *not* the case for LBW children with early-onset intraventricular hemorrhage and central nervous system injury, whose picture vocabulary scores decreased over time. LBW status alone may not be a sufficient predictor of cognitive ability; information about related complications likely will be needed in order to explain or predict deficits.

Finally, and similar to research on short-term consequences of LBW, children with LBW are much more likely to have learning difficulties, receive special education services, and repeat a grade by middle school (Hack et al., 1994; O'Keeffe, O'Callaghan, Williams, Najman, & Bor, 2003; Saigal et al., 2000; Taylor, Klein, Minich, et al., 2000a; Van Baar et al., 2006). The short- and long-term physical and neuropsychological consequences of LBW, therefore, seem to have an influence on academic outcomes in middle school and beyond.

Predicting Course and Prognosis

In light of the somewhat inconsistent findings across studies (i.e., some studies find more negative outcomes than others), it seems important to examine potential factors that may explain why some children with LBW experience severe developmental deficits and others do not. Several researchers (e.g., Taylor, Klein, & Hack, 2000; Taylor et al., 2002, 2004) have identified characteristics found to associate with poorer developmental and behavioral outcomes among children with LBW. These predictors include degree of LBW (lower birth weight associated with poorer outcomes), cerebral insult or damage (especially hemorrhage, periventricular leukomalacia, and brain abnormalities, as described earlier), small head circumference, bacteria in the blood, lung disease, length of neonatal hospitalization, low SES or limited resources, parental or family distress, male sex, and ethnic minority status; further, achievement scores in reading and math are predicted by neuropsychological constructs (e.g., planning, verbal list learning, verbal working memory) among children with LBW.

With regard to social factors, Hille et al. (2007) found that SES (as measured by parental education level) was strongly correlated with number of problems in functioning among young adults who had LBW as infants. Similarly, Weiss and Seed (2002) found that parent-rated emotional and behavioral problems among children with LBW at 2 years of age were predicted by family environment variables such as low SES, poor family adaptability and cohesion, maternal mental health, and insecure infant-mother attachment; these environmental factors were more predictive than infant characteristics such as birth weight, cognitive ability, and social competence.

With regard to biological factors, the presence of neonatal neurological compromise (e.g., intraventricular hemorrhage) is an important predictor of future functioning in cognitive ability and academic achievement, with more severe neurological compromise associated with poorer outcomes (McGrath, Sullivan, Lester, & Oh, 2000). Children with LBW who had additional developmental problems, such as failure to thrive and small size for gestational age status, were especially likely to experience the least physical growth and lowest scores on cognitive, achievement, and visual-motor integration measures at 8 years of age (Casey, Whiteside-Mansell, Barrett, Bradley, & Gargus, 2006). Thus, children with this combination of growth problems should be monitored especially closely, as these issues seem to have an interactive effect with LBW. There also is evidence to suggest that preterm children (gestational age less than 32 weeks) with less severe neonatal difficulties and with more typical cognitive and motor development are less likely to exhibit school difficulties in early childhood (Van Baar et al., 2006).

The medical or biological complications associated with LBW may be more powerful predictors of long-term outcome than social factors such as SES (Taylor, Klein, & Hack, 2000), with biological factors especially more predictive of perceptual-motor skills and planning, and social or family environment variables more predictive of behavior problems, knowledge, and language skills (Boyce, Saylor, & Price, 2004; Taylor et al., 2002). Thus, outcomes for children with LBW likely are determined by a combination of biological and environmental factors.

Assessment Issues

It should be noted that the findings just reported are trends, as outcomes among children with LBW range from no or very mild deficits to severe deficits across multiple areas of functioning. Many people who were born LBW and who demonstrated neuropsychological or physical struggles as children are well-functioning adults capable of living independently (Saigal & Doyle, 2008). Thus, knowing that a child was born with LBW allows the clinician to make hypotheses about areas of deficit and long-term outcomes, but not with a reasonable degree of certainty because children with LBW vary so widely. Similar to the case of TBI (see Chapter 8), clinicians must conduct a comprehensive assessment in order to gain understanding of the child's unique pattern of strengths and weaknesses, and this assessment information then should lead to the development of individualized interventions. Assessment also should employ a team approach due to the multiple domains that need to be assessed, address criterion-related functioning rather than focusing solely on norm-referenced interpretation, and lead to very specific functional goals and objectives to address identified areas of deficit (Xu & Filler, 2005). Further, children with LBW should be reevaluated on a regular basis in order to monitor changes in functioning and to identify any changes that need to be made to intervention programs; this is especially important in light of research suggesting that deficits may change and become more pronounced over time (G. P. Aylward, 2002; Taylor, Klein, Minich, et al., 2000a).

Constructs identified as important in the assessment process include executive function, memory, learning, intelligence, academic skills, attention, perceptual-motor skills, visual-spatial processing, complex language skills, family functioning and environmental variables, and behavioral or psychosocial adjustment (G. P. Aylward, 2002; Taylor, Klein, & Hack, 2000). Assessment of these constructs is likely to provide the clinician with sufficient data to identify specific areas of weakness, form goals, and develop appropriate interventions. In light of structural differences in the brain associated with LBW, neuroimaging methods often are used to detect brain lesions among infants with LBW within the first 2 weeks of life in order to predict neuropsychological functioning and develop plans for managing areas of deficit (Ment et al., 2002). At the same time, there is currently insufficient evidence to support the use of MRI to make firm predictions about developmental outcome based on brain abnormalities among children with LBW, which also points to the importance of monitoring and frequent follow-up assessment (Hart, Whitby, Griffiths, & Smith, 2008).

EVIDENCE-BASED INTERVENTIONS

Given the sometimes critical and immediate needs of infants with LBW, many interventions are designed to address medical needs such as breathing, feeding, and risk for lung disease and infection (e.g., C. T. Collins et al., 2004; S. E. Jacobs, Sokol, & Ohlsson, 2002; O'Shea, Washburn, Nixon, & Goldstein, 2007; Sinn, Ward, & Henderson-Smart, 2002). Further, in light of the enormous costs of LBW for families, schools, and the health system due to the need for services such as special education and repeated hospitalizations

(Petrou, Sach, & Davidson, 2001), in addition to the impact on neuropsychological and psychosocial functioning described previously, many efforts have focused on prevention of LBW (e.g., psychosocial interventions, social support, educational approaches; Lu, Lu, & Schetter, 2005). As opposed to medical treatments and preventive approaches, this review considers interventions that target neuropsychological and psychosocial variables following the infant's birth. Table 12.2 summarizes the evidence-based status of interventions for LBW; these interventions are described in more detail next.

As a general statement, intervention programs for children with LBW should be comprehensive, given the multiple domains affected. Further, it has been suggested that intervention occur early in development due to neural plasticity (Malekpour, 2004). In light of this need for comprehensive and early intervention, approaches have included methods of building positive parent-child interactions, parent support approaches, information-based interventions, and specialized infant care approaches (Taylor, Klein, & Hack, 2000).

The cognitive, behavioral, and physical health problems often experienced by children with LBW may contribute to increased parental and family stress (Bhutta et al., 2002; Saigal & Doyle, 2008), which in turn may lead to negative parent-child interactions and more negative outcomes for the child. Thus, many interventions focus on improving mother-infant interactions, with the idea that more positive and effective relationships will

Table 12.2 Evidence-Based Status of Interventions for Children with LBW

Interventions	Target	Status
Home visit interventions	Comprehensive (parenting skills, mother-child interactions, cognitive and motor skills)	Positive practice (Meeks Gardner, Walker, Powell, & Grantham-McGregor, 2003; Walker, Chang, Powell, and Grantham-McGregor, 2004)
Infant health and development program	Comprehensive (cognitive development, behavior problems, mother-child interactions)	Positive practice (McCormick et al., 2006; McCormick, McCarton, Brooks-Gunn, Belt, & Gross, 1998)
Information-based interventions	Knowledge of infant behavioral cues	Emerging practice (Maguire, Bruil, Wit, & Walther, 2007)
Parent training programs	Caregiving skills, parent-child interactions	Promising practice (Achenbach, Howell, Aoki, & Rauh, 1993; Patteson & Barnard, 1990)
Parent support groups	Parental emotional responses	Emerging practice (Patteson & Barnard, 1990)
Developmental handling	Motor organization	Promising practice (Becker, Grunwald, & Brazy, 1999)
Individualized developmental care (Newborn Individualized Developmental Care and Assessment program)	Comprehensive (medical, neurodevelopmental, and family function outcomes)	Promising practice (Als et al., 2003)
Creating Opportunities for Parent Empowerment (COPE) program	Cognitive development, maternal coping, mother-infant interactions	Emerging practice (Melnyk et al., 2001)

enhance the infant's emotional, social, cognitive, and language development (Malekpour, 2004) and will facilitate the infant's development of trust in the parent (Xu & Filler, 2005). These interventions often include efforts to help the mother recognize the meaning (e.g., distress, hunger, desire for interaction) of various cues from the infant and to respond appropriately to these cues (Achenbach et al. 1993). For example, Melnyk et al. (2001) conducted a randomized clinical trial evaluating the Creating Opportunities for Parent Empowerment (COPE) program, which was used with LBW infants and their parents in the neonatal intensive care unit (NICU). The intervention included information about the NICU and about premature infants and their behaviors and activities to help mothers recognize cues, respond to their infants' needs, and foster cognitive development. Follow-up at 3 and 6 months of age showed large and significant differences between the intervention and control groups on a measure of cognitive development, with infants in the intervention group scoring much higher than controls; intervention mothers also reported less stress related to the NICU and stronger beliefs in their ability to understand their infants' behaviors. The authors theorized that infant outcomes were the result of the mothers' reduced stress and enhanced self-efficacy, which led to more positive mother–infant verbal interactions that facilitated cognitive development; however, additional research with larger samples will be necessary as this was only a pilot study, and the long-term impact of the early intervention is unknown.

Given the contributions of family environment to the development of emotional and behavioral problems among children with LBW (S. J. Weiss & Seed, 2002), several intervention approaches have used home visits as a context for providing parent training in caregiving skills, such as responding to the infant and using positive reinforcement (Barrera, Rosenbaum, & Cunningham, 1986). Further, by helping parents feel more confident and competent, these interventions attempt to improve infant outcomes by enhancing the knowledge and skills of caregivers; this may be especially important for parents of LBW infants as the circumstances surrounding the birth may be especially distressing, and LBW infants may be less responsive to attempts at interaction with parents (Malekpour, 2004; Patteson & Barnard, 1990). Home visit interventions have been effective with parents of both typically developing and at-risk children (Kendrick et al., 2000), and recent evidence suggests the efficacy of these programs with families of LBW infants. Walker and colleagues (Meeks Gardner et al., 2003; Walker et al., 2004) conducted a randomized trial evaluating a psychosocial intervention for children with LBW. The first phase of the intervention consisted of weekly home visits by community health workers, who used established curricula to train mothers how to respond to their LBW infants (e.g., talking to the infant, showing affection, responding to the infant's cues). The second phase was similar, with home visits focusing on parenting skills and mother-child interactions (e.g., playing with the child, using praise). The intervention began in infancy and lasted until the children were approximately 2 years of age. Compared to LBW children who did not receive the intervention, children in the intervention group performed better on early problem-solving tasks (e.g., intentional toy retrieval tasks), were more cooperative, had a higher mean developmental quotient, and had home environments that were characterized by greater maternal involvement and less use of punishment. Further, not only did LBW children in the intervention group outperform LBW children in the control group; they also performed similarly to children of normal birth weight across dependent variables. Nevertheless, more long-term follow-up is needed to determine effects beyond 2 years of age.

Other parent training interventions focus on providing information and knowledge of child development and behavioral cues, without assessing skill acquisition. For example,

Maguire et al. (2007) found that parents' knowledge of infant behavioral cues improved following a four-session, hospital-based intervention that involved brief teaching sessions to increase knowledge of their infant's behaviors. However, parents in the intervention group did not show significant improvement in their caregiving confidence following the intervention.

Several characteristics of effective parent-training interventions for parents of LBW infants have been identified, including regular long-term contact with parents, developing a relationship with parents, providing support and empowerment to parents, responding to the individual needs of families, and encouraging parents' active involvement in the intervention (Patteson & Barnard, 1990; Zahr, 2000). Further, some home-based interventions have not been effective consistently with Latino families with low SES, suggesting the need for more research examining ethnic group differences in intervention outcomes and the possibility of differentiating the interventions for different groups (Zahr, 2000).

Perhaps the most recognized LBW intervention program, and one that has received considerable attention in the research literature, is the Infant Health and Development Program (IHDP), which is a longitudinal, multisite, randomized controlled trial examining the effectiveness of an educational intervention designed for infants with LBW (Bradley et al., 1994; Brooks-Gunn, Klebanov, Liaw, & Spiker, 1993; Hill, Brooks-Gunn, & Waldfogel, 2003; Klebanov, Brooks-Gunn, & McCormick, 2001; McCormick et al., 1998, 2006). The IHDP intervention included (a) home visits (weekly for the first year, every other week for the second and third year) conducted by professionals trained in a well-established curriculum designed to encourage participation in developmental activities among parents and children and also to teach parents problem-solving skills; (b) center-based developmental education (i.e., daycare 5 days per week), which was an extension of the curriculum used during the home visits; and (c) parent support groups that met every other month. The center-based education and parent support groups began when the child was approximately 1 year of age. LBW children were grouped into heavier LBW (between 2,001 and 2,499 grams) and lighter LBW (less than 2,001 grams), and children receiving the intervention were compared to children receiving standard care. Initially, outcomes were measured at 36 months of age, and additional follow-up assessments have occurred at 5, 8, and 18 years of age in order to assess long-term effects of the intervention. At 36 months, children in the intervention group scored significantly higher on measures of cognitive development and significantly lower on measures of behavior problems. However, these groups became much more similar on the behavioral measures at the 5- and 8-year follow-up, and the intervention group differences in cognitive functioning remained only for heavier LBW children. Thus, the intervention effects appeared to dissipate over time, especially for the lighter LBW children (McCormick et al., 1998). Further, the intervention did not seem to influence other variables, such as health status or number of hospitalizations, but was positively associated with more positive mother-infant interactions and subsequent availability of learning materials in the home, and the intervention may produce stronger effects for low SES families (McCormick et al., 1998). Data also suggest that mothers in the intervention group reported lower levels of distress following the intervention compared with mothers in the standard care group, and this was especially true for mothers with less education (Klebanov et al., 2001). LBW infants characterized by more negative emotionality at 12 months of age also showed the largest treatment effects at the 36-month assessment on cognitive and behavioral measures, suggesting the intervention may be especially impactful for this group of LBW infants (Blair, 2002).

More recently (McCormick et al., 2006), children in the IHDP studies were followed up at 18 years of age, with continued differences between children of heavier LBW and lighter LBW. For heavier LBW children, participants in the intervention group performed significantly more favorably on measures of math achievement, receptive vocabulary, and risk-taking behaviors compared to children in the standard care group. Inconsistent with expectations, for the lighter LBW children, participants in the standard care group scored higher on a measure of reading achievement than participants in the intervention group. Thus, the long-term benefits of the intervention were seen only in the group of heavier LBW children, suggesting that lighter LBW children (i.e., VLBW and ELBW) need longer or more intense intervention in order to produce more long-term effects. Across the IHDP studies, factors associated with more favorable outcomes included the mother's knowledge of child development, the mother's intellectual ability, involvement of the father, and high rates of participation in the intervention program (Hill et al., 2003; McCormick et al., 1998).

A similar intervention was evaluated by Achenbach et al. (1993). After receiving seven in-hospital sessions and four in-home sessions (all occurring within 90 days after discharge from the hospital) during which a trained nurse assisted mothers with adapting to and interacting with their LBW infants, LBW infants were compared to a control group of LBW infants and also to a group of normal-birth-weight infants. When followed up at 9 years of age, LBW children who received the intervention performed better than control LBW children on measures of cognitive ability, school achievement, and problem behaviors. Further, at follow-up, the LBW children receiving intervention performed similarly to the normal-birth-weight children. This pattern of results was similar to what was observed at follow-up at 3, 4, and 7 years; the LBW groups did not differ at 1 year of age but progressively diverged over time, with the intervention group gradually performing better than the control LBW group and much closer to the normal-birth-weight group. More recently, a modified form of this intervention seemed to have a positive impact on LBW infants' initiating and responding to social interactions (Olafsen et al., 2006).

Thus, the IHDP studies reported significant short-term effects but more limited long-term effects (a pattern that has been observed in other intervention studies as well; S. Johnson, Ring, Anderson, & Marlow, 2005), while the Achenbach study reported limited short-term effects but progressively more pronounced long-term effects. These interventions seem to be having an effect, but the extent to which the effects are immediate or sustained (or perhaps delayed) varies across studies and interventions.

Other interventions focus primarily on developmental care of the infant rather than on parent-infant interactions. Becker et al. (1999) conducted a quasi-experimental crossover study to evaluate the effects of a developmental handling intervention on VLBW infants' motor organization. The "developmental handling" intervention involved providing individualized care during medical and feeding procedures in which caregivers' actions were based on the infant's cues and needs. Methods of support included aids for self-regulation, containment to reduce excess movement, maintaining flexed posture, providing surfaces for stability, and using time-out procedures to calm the infants when they became disorganized or destabilized. Observers noted that during the intervention (as compared to the traditional, task-driven condition, which involves minimal handling), infants demonstrated increases in number of organized movements (e.g., hand to face, hand grasping) and decreases in number of disorganized movements (e.g., jerks, twitches). Thus, developmental handling interventions may help to limit mild motor deficits among infants with LBW.

A similar individualized developmental care intervention, the Newborn Individualized Developmental Care and Assessment Program, was evaluated by Als et al. (2003) using a randomized, controlled trial design. Like the IHDP program, the intervention was multifaceted, involving education, support, and environmental adaptations to care based on the infant's individualized strengths and needs. Multiple outcome variables were measured, suggesting favorable short-term outcomes for infants receiving the intervention; for example, these infants showed improved physical growth, enhanced attention and self-regulation, and better motor organization, and intervention parents reported lower stress. Infants receiving the intervention also had better medical outcomes. Although these results are promising, more long-term follow-up is needed to assess sustained benefits of the intervention. An occupational therapy intervention (60 minutes per week from 6 to 12 months of age) also showed slight beneficial effects for ELBW children on measures of verbal intelligence and attachment at age 4 (Sajaniemi et al., 2001). However, the intervention also included parent training, support, and educational components, thereby making it difficult to determine whether the occupational therapy component was in fact the active ingredient or if the other components were responsible for the treatment effects.

Finally, Spittle, Orton, Doyle, and Boyd (2007) conducted a meta-analysis using 16 studies evaluating intervention programs (including the IHDP program just described) that targeted motor and cognitive skills among preterm and LBW infants. All interventions addressed the parent-infant relationship, the infant's development, or both of these broad targets, often using educational approaches to enhance parents' knowledge and skills in interacting with their infant. All 16 studies were randomized or quasi-randomized controlled trials evaluating early interventions that were implemented within the first 12 months of the preterm infants' lives. Overall findings indicated that interventions improved cognitive skills during infancy and preschool age but not at school age (i.e., 5 to 17 years). Motor skills interventions were not supported at any age, but more long-term follow-up data are needed. Further, the cognitive and motor skills interventions varied widely in terms of content and implementation, thereby preventing broad conclusions on the effectiveness of early developmental intervention programs. This meta-analysis does suggest the importance of focusing on the *combination* of enhancing (a) the parent-infant relationship *and* (b) the infant's neuropsychological functioning; this notion has been expressed by others as well (e.g., McCarton, Wallace, & Bennett, 1996).

CASE STUDY: EMILY—EXTREMELY LOW BIRTH WEIGHT

The next report is from a hospital-based clinic. Identifying information, such as child and family name, teacher or physician name, and school information, has been altered or fictionalized to protect confidentiality.

Reason for Referral

Emily is a 6-year-old White female in the first grade, who is being evaluated by the pediatric neuropsychology service at the request of Dr. Parker, M.D., pediatrician, and Dr. Duncan, M.D., neonatologist, who have been following Emily for a history of prematurity and developmental delay. As a result, a neuropsychological evaluation was undertaken in order to monitor higher cortical functioning and make appropriate recommendations regarding school placement and the continued need for supportive therapies.

Assessment Procedures

In addition to the next battery of assessment instruments, Emily's mother provided developmental history information via interview, and information regarding previous psychoeducational evaluations and special education services was gathered via extensive review of educational, psychological, and medical records. Further, for some of the comprehensive instruments listed, only selected subtests were administered in order to gain information about discrete domains of functioning.

Differential Ability Scales, Second Edition, School Age Level (DAS-II)
Kaufman Assessment Battery for Children, Second Edition (KABC-II)
Wide Range Achievement Test, Fourth Edition (WRAT-4)
Neuropsychological Assessment (NEPSY)/Neuropsychological Assessment, Second Edition (NEPSY-2)
Peabody Picture Vocabulary Test, Third Edition (PPVT-III)
Expressive One-Word Picture Vocabulary Test—Revised (EOWPVT-R)
Developmental Test of Visual-Motor Integration, Fifth Edition (DTVMI-V)
Bracken Basic Concept Scale—Expressive
Finger Oscillation Test
Children's Memory Scale (CMS)
Adaptive Behavior Assessment System, Second Edition (ABAS-2)
Behavior Assessment System for Children, Second Edition (BASC-2)
DSM-IV ADHD Checklist

Background Information

Home

Emily resides with her mother, Norma. Emily's parents were never married. Her father is 31 years old and in active duty with the Air Force. He is reported to have a high school degree with some college coursework, and is in good health. According to the mother, he does keep visitation around his military schedule and calls Emily frequently. Emily's mother is 30 years old, a high school graduate with two years of college, who is currently employed on the security force of a local telecommunications company. She is also in good health. The maternal family history is significant for a brain tumor and a stroke in a great-aunt, and ADHD in a female cousin.

Medical and Developmental History

Review of developmental and medical history indicates that Emily is the product of a preterm pregnancy (estimated gestational age of 25 weeks) and cesarean section delivery, weighing 600 grams at birth. Additional diagnoses included chronic lung disease, anemia of prematurity, tricuspid valve insufficiency with murmur, gastric reflux, and retinopathy of prematurity. Emily remained in the neonatal intensive care unit until the age of 3 months 24 days. She underwent laser surgery prior to discharge and passed an audiology screen bilaterally. Emily was referred to the NICU follow-up program and has been followed by various pediatricians and specialists. Emily is also followed by a pediatric ophthalmologist, for bilateral amblyopia (left > right) and nearsightedness for which she currently wears prescription eyeglasses and a patch on her right eye. According to her mother, Emily's motor and language milestones were delayed. As a result, she began receiving occupational therapy, physical therapy, and speech/language therapy at 9 months of age until recently with good progress.

At age 2 years 9 months, Emily underwent initial psychological evaluation by the pediatric neuropsychology service. At that time, she was administered the Differential Ability Scales—Lower Preschool Level and found to be functioning within the borderline range of intellectual ability (General Conceptual Ability = 74) with a relative strength noted on nonverbal tasks. At that time, Emily demonstrated weaknesses in expressive and receptive language as well as adaptive skills per mother's report. Taken together, Emily's pattern of test performance continued to be consistent with a diagnosis of significant developmental delay. As a result, special education preschool classroom services were recommended beginning at 3 years of age. Continued occupational, physical, and speech/language therapies also were recommended as related services. Given her energy level and curiosity, development of a behavior management program was encouraged along with continued NICU follow-up and reevaluation in one year. Formal audiological evaluation conducted on the same day reported that speech awareness thresholds of 5 decibels suggested that hearing was normal in at least the better ear.

Educational

When Emily turned 3 years of age, she began receiving one hour per week of in-home preschool special education services provided by the local school system. At 4 years of age, Emily attended a regular prekindergarten classroom. Review of Emily's Individualized Education Plan (IEP) from that time revealed that she received 2 hours of preschool special education services per week because she continued "to meet state eligibility criteria for Significant Developmental Delay (SDD) in the areas of Personal-Social, Adaptive, Motor, and Communication." Emily experienced significant behavioral difficulty in the classroom, and her mother frequently was called to come to school during naptime to aid with Emily's compliance. In addition, Emily was sent home one day for disruptive behavior. As a result, another IEP meeting was convened; review of the addendum indicates that Emily's regular education teacher discussed her concerns regarding Emily's inappropriate behaviors within structured and unstructured settings. The special education teacher stated that Emily did well with one-on-one instruction. Emily's mother also expressed concerns regarding her behavior. The school occupational therapist stated that occupational therapy probably would be a disadvantage. However, she suggested that a vision specialist probably would be an advantage to her. The special education teacher also recommended increasing the SDD service hours and having a person shadow Emily during "peak" times of the day. All participants agreed to a behavioral intervention plan for the regular prekindergarten classroom along with an increase in SDD/team collaboration service from 2 to 3 hours per week.

Approximately one month after this IEP meeting, Emily underwent psychological reevaluation. The results of the evaluation indicate that Emily was functioning within the mildly deficient to borderline range of intellectual ability as measured by the Differential Ability Scales—Lower Preschool Level (General Conceptual Ability = 63). However, it was felt that this represented an underestimate of her true ability, given her language delay and her extremely short attention span. Emily continued to exhibit relative strengths on nonverbal tasks as well as improvement in receptive vocabulary. Emily's preschool readiness and adaptive functioning were also significant strengths. In contrast, Emily's expressive language and her ability to comprehend multipart instructions continued to be significant weaknesses for her. Review of rating scales completed by Emily's mother and regular education teacher indicate that she was exhibiting significant levels of hyperactivity, inattention, and social-emotional difficulties, which were also evident during this evaluation. Taken together, this pattern of test performance was felt to be consistent with a diagnosis of significant developmental delay. In addition, Emily met formal criteria for a diagnosis of ADHD, combined type. As a result, it was recommended that Emily continue to receive special education preschool services with an increase in one-to-one instruction time, as recommended by her special education teacher during the IEP addendum meeting. The additional recommendation for a one-to-one teacher's aide also was felt to be reasonable. Given that significant language deficits continued to be evident on testing and per her mother's and her teacher's reports, continued individual language therapy also was recommended at school. Specific changes to the behavioral plan at school were provided as well.

During the previous school year, Emily attended a regular kindergarten classroom with continuation of SDD preschool special education inclusion services and a behavioral plan. It should be noted that during the year, Dr. Parker also initiated stimulant medication therapy due to Emily's persistent difficulty with attention span and activity level. However, Emily is responding less well to the generic version of this medication. At present, Emily is attending a regular first grade setting with continuation of SDD preschool special education inclusion services and the behavioral plan.

Behavioral Observations

Emily presented herself for testing as an energetic and playful youngster who was in no apparent physical distress. She separated without difficulty from her mother. Emily made good social eye contact and related appropriately toward this examiner throughout the testing session, which consisted of two sessions separated by a lunch break. In response to direct questions, as well as when conversation was spontaneous, Emily's use of language was somewhat limited and consisted of one- to three-word phrases. Her attention span, activity level, and impulsivity within the context of this one-to-one assessment were somewhat problematic by the afternoon session. As a result, the examiner had to institute many more breaks than normal during the afternoon testing session as Emily became resistant to working on more challenging items. During the afternoon session, Emily also began to perseverate on a bear in a clinic window that she had seen during her lunch break. On particular tasks, Emily seemed to be confused by the directions and therefore was not successful in completing these tasks. When Emily became frustrated due to difficulty completing items or poor comprehension of directions, she no longer responded when asked questions by the examiner. She would sit silently, seemingly ignoring the examiner's questions. With regard to laterality, dominance is firmly established in the right hand and foot. Vision was not formally screened; however, Ms. Bennett reported that it had been evaluated in the past year by Dr. Bowen. Emily wore her glasses as well as a patch over her right eye during the evaluation. Hearing has been formally evaluated at this hospital in the past and reported to be normal.

Assessment Results and Interpretation

Cognitive and Neuropsychological Functioning

Individual subtest and composite scores for all measures are presented in the Psychometric Summary (see Table 12.3). Intellectual functioning was measured with the Differential Ability Scales, Second Edition, School Age Level (DAS-II). This instrument provides

Table 12.3 Psychometric Summary for Emily

	Standard Score
Differential Ability Scales, Second Edition (DAS-II) (School-Age Level)	
General Conceptual Ability	81
Verbal Cluster	92
Word Definitions	98
Similarities	91
Nonverbal Cluster	89
Matrices	90
Sequential & Quantitative Reasoning	91
Spatial Cluster	70
Recall of Designs	84
Pattern Construction	65
Neuropsychological Assessment, Second Edition (NEPSY-2)	
Tower (NEPSY)	85
Phonological Processing	85
Sentence Imitation	100
Comprehension of Instructions	85
Word Generation	80
Peabody Picture Vocabulary Test, Third Edition (PPVT-III)	90
Expressive One-Word Picture Vocabulary Test, Revised (EOWPVT-R)	95
Kaufman Assessment Battery for Children, Second Edition (KABC-2)	
Gestalt Closure	70
Developmental Test of Visual-Motor Integration, Fifth Edition (DTVMI-V)	
Visual Motor Integration	85
Finger Oscillation Test	
Right (dominant) Hand	<40
Left (nondominant) Hand	<40
Children's Memory Scale (CMS)	
General Memory Index	—
Attention/Concentration Index	94
Numbers	105
Sequences	85
Picture Locations	80
Verbal Immediate Index	78
Stories	100
Word Pairs	65
Visual Immediate Index	—
Dot Locations	NV
Faces	105
Verbal Delayed Index	82
Stories	105
Word Pairs	65
Visual Delayed Index	—
Dot Locations	NV
Faces	80
Delayed Recognition Index	75

(continued)

Table 12.3 *(Continued)*

	Standard Score	
Stories	95	
Word Pairs	65	
Learning Index	72	
Word Pairs	60	
Dot Locations	NV	
Wide Range Achievement Test, Fourth Edition (WRAT-4)		
Reading	92	
Spelling	86	
Arithmetic	79	
Bracken Basic Concept Scale—Expressive		
School Readiness Composite	83	
Adaptive Behavior Assessment System, Second Edition (ABAS-2)		
General Adaptive Composite	81	
Communication	80	
Community Use	70	
Functional Pre-Academics	90	
Home Living	95	
Health and Safety	70	
Leisure	90	
Self-Care	80	
Self-Direction	100	
Social	80	
Behavior Assessment System for Children, Second Edition (BASC-2)		
	T-Scores	
	Parent	Teacher
Clinical Scales		
Hyperactivity	79	61
Conduct Problems	88	49
Anxiety	45	70
Depression	57	56
Somatization	56	42
Atypicality	82	66
Withdrawal	58	66
Attention Problems	73	60
Learning Problems	NA	60
Adaptive Scales		
Adaptability	37	43
Social Skills	34	42
Leadership	29	38
Study Skills	NA	35
Activities of Daily Living	26	NA
Functional Communication	33	38
DSM-IV ADHD Checklist	Raw Score	
Inattention	26/27	10/27
Hyperactivity/Impulsivity	27/27	5/27

Notes. NA = Not applicable. NV = Not valid.

an assessment of reasoning and conceptual abilities. Emily's General Conceptual Ability (GCA) was found to be in the low-average range as evidenced by a standard score of 81 (Average Score = 100 ± 15; 95% confidence interval = 76–87). Emily demonstrated average performance on the Verbal Cluster, low-average to average performance on the Nonverbal Cluster, and mildly deficient to borderline performance on the Spatial Cluster. Emily's performance on the Verbal and Nonverbal clusters was relatively consistent yet both discrepant from her Spatial cluster. This suggests that the overall score (GCA = 81) is likely not representative of Emily's cognitive abilities; instead, the Verbal Cluster may provide a better estimate of her ability.

In order to assess higher-order executive functions such as problem solving ability and mental flexibility, Emily was administered the Tower subtest of the Neuropsychological Assessment (NEPSY). On this task, she had to move three colored balls to target positions on three pegs in a prescribed number of moves. In addition, Emily was given specific rules and time constraints that increased task difficulty, therefore requiring planning. Her score was in the low-average range, indicating that Emily has planning/problem-solving ability that is inconsistent with her intellectual functioning when her Verbal Cluster performance is used as the best estimate of her ability.

Assessment of linguistic functioning was conducted in order to evaluate receptive and expressive language development. Analysis of Emily's performance indicates that her receptive vocabulary, sentence imitation skills, phonological processing ability, and comprehension of instructions are all in the low-average to average range. Emily's expressive language, as measured by her expressive vocabulary development and confrontational picture-naming ability, were in the average range; however, qualitative assessment of Emily's language was significant for echolalia, which appeared to be employed to assist with comprehension, syntax and grammatical errors, word-finding difficulty, and poor pragmatics.

In order to assess visual-spatial perception/discrimination ability without a motor component, Emily was administered the Gestalt Closure subtest of the Kaufman Assessment Battery for Children, Second Edition (KABC-II) and the Arrows subtest from the NEPSY. It is important to note that her performance on the Arrows subtest is not reported here; results from this test were felt to be invalid due to perseverative responding. Analysis of her performance on the Gestalt Closure subtest indicates that Emily's visual-perceptual functioning is in the mildly deficient to borderline range.

Constructional praxis, as measured by the Developmental Test of Visual Motor Integration (DTVMI), was in the low-average range. This result taken together with Emily's performance on the Pattern Construction subtest of the DAS-II indicates that her performance on measures of visual-motor functioning is highly variable ranging from deficient to low average. Fine motor finger oscillation as measured by a manual finger tapper is found to be significantly depressed bilaterally; right (dominant) hand = 7.3 taps per 10 seconds, left (nondominant) hand = 5.7 taps per 10 seconds.

In order to assess learning and memory, Emily was administered the Children's Memory Scale (CMS). Analysis of her performance on the subtests comprising the Attention/Concentration Index indicates that Emily is exhibiting focused attention/working memory skills commensurate with the obtained DAS-II results. Emily performed within the average range when minimal auditory attention was required to retain and reproduce a string of numbers. When she was required to reverse a sequence of numbers given to her, she also performed within normal limits. However, her performance was significantly discrepant on more complex working memory tasks when she was required to both generate and manipulate information based on prior learning (Sequences). On more complex items of the Sequences task, she frequently demonstrated loss-of-set errors when she was required to reverse material. That is, she was able to focus her attention within normal limits for limited amounts of information that did not require simultaneous processing of prior knowledge. Thus, Emily's ability to focus attention and hold material in working memory could have adversely affected her capability to learn and remember.

When asked to learn and remember (30 minutes later) newly presented information, Emily demonstrated significant variability in her ability to learn and recall verbal material. Specifically, she exhibited average ability when asked to recall organized/meaningful information, such as stories that were read to her. In contrast, she performed within the deficient range when the material was rote and unorganized, such as a list of 10 word pairs presented over three structured learning trials. Within the visual domain, Emily demonstrated average immediate recall of a series of pictured human faces contrasted by borderline to low-average delayed recall. It should be noted that due to poor comprehension of task demands, the Dot Locations subtest was deemed invalid.

Academic Functioning

In order to assess word recognition, spelling, and numerical calculation skills, Emily was administered the Wide Range Achievement Test, Fourth Edition. She successfully printed her first name and 12 of 13 letters to dictation. She recognized 15 of 15 letters of the alphabet, read 2 sight words, identified single-digit numbers, and performed a basic subtraction word problem (3 pennies spend 1 = 2).

To further assess academic readiness, Emily was administered the School Readiness Composite section of the Bracken Basic Concept Scale—Expressive. She was able to identify basic colors, shapes, letters, and numbers but demonstrated little understanding of size and comparative concepts beyond very basic categories (i.e., small/big, short/long). Perhaps her vocabulary limited her from recognizing more complex comparisons (e.g., shallow/deep). In addition, she was unable to produce blended sounds, was unable to identify two-digit numbers (she read them incorrectly, or with reference to only one number), and struggled to identify more complex shapes. Instead, she labeled them as the objects that they resembled (e.g., Cube-square, pyramid-tent). Thus, academically, Emily demonstrates relative weaknesses in spelling, two-digit number identification, basic arithmetic, and mastery of complex comparisons.

Social-Emotional and Behavioral Functioning

Adaptive behavior was measured using the Adaptive Behavior Assessment System, Second Edition, with mother serving as the informant. Results indicate that Emily's overall adaptive behavior falls within the borderline to low-average range as evidenced by a General Adaptive Composite score of 81 ± 4. In order to assess behavioral/emotional functioning, the Behavior Assessment System for Children, Second Edition, and a behavior rating scale that reflects items related to the *DSM-IV* criteria for ADHD were completed by Emily's mother and teachers. Analysis of these scales indicates that, at this time, Emily is experiencing significant emotional/behavioral concerns at home related to her problems with inattention, hyperactivity, conduct problems, social/emotional immaturity, and poor social skills. She also has significant impairments in performing activities of daily living (e.g., following regular routines, trouble fastening buttons on clothing, organizing chores or other tasks well), functional communication, and leadership. In contrast,

Emily's teacher indicated significant problems only with anxiety, social/emotional immaturity, withdrawal, and study skills.

Summary and Diagnostic Impressions

In summary, the results of this neuropsychological evaluation indicate that Emily currently is functioning within the low-average to average range of intellectual ability. Emily demonstrates relative weaknesses in visual-spatial perception/construction, fine motor function bilaterally (including handwriting), variable performance on measures of working memory, and difficulty in her ability to learn and recall rote/unorganized verbal material as well as in her ability to recall a series of pictured human faces. Academically, Emily demonstrates relative strengths in letter/word recognition contrasted by relative weaknesses in spelling and arithmetic. Behaviorally, Emily is experiencing significant emotional/behavioral concerns at home related to her problems with inattention, hyperactivity, conduct problems, social/emotional immaturity, and poor social skills. At school, these behaviors appear to be less problematic, indicating that she is responding to her medication therapy and academic/behavioral support.

Taken together, this pattern of performance is consistent with a continued diagnosis of ADHD, combined type with mild executive and learning/memory deficits that are impacting academics as well as behavior. In addition, Emily meets diagnostic criteria for developmental coordination disorder, and her conversational language is characterized by poor grammar and syntax, mild comprehension difficulty, and poor pragmatics consistent with her history of specific language impairment.

Recommendations

- It is recommended that Emily receive resource and inclusion special education services under the "Other Health Impaired" category due to the fact that her ADHD is impacting her ability to learn and perform in the classroom. Emily continues to have residual speech/language delays; thus, a formal speech/language evaluation and therapy is recommended to remediate these impairments. An occupational therapy evaluation also is warranted because of persistent difficulties with visual-spatial material. In addition, occupational therapy will be beneficial in assisting with Emily's fine motor impairments as they impact on her classroom performance (e.g., handwriting). Emily also will require various compensatory strategies, such as extra time and assessment techniques that employ the use of recognition paradigms, such as true/false, matching, and multiple choice, administered orally as opposed to essay and fill-in-the-blank formats.
- Given the significant problems with conduct, inattention, and hyperactivity indicated by Ms. Bennett and observed during the current evaluation, it also will be important to develop a behavior management program in the classroom designed to improve Emily's attention span/level of concentration, listening skills, and on-task behavior. Emily already may be in a classroom that provides many good strategies for decreasing inattention and problematic behavior. However, she may benefit from the following recommendations as she continues her education:
  - A consistent daily routine.
  - Clear transitions between activities.

- An environment that is as distraction-free as possible. This may involve moving her seat away from distractions (e.g., pencil sharpener, shared space), including distracting peers, and removing unnecessary items from her workspace.
- Preferential seating in the front, right side of the classroom due to her eye patch. This placement also should facilitate monitoring and early detection of off-task behaviors and daydreaming.
- Frequent and immediate feedback and praise for good behavior and good academic effort or performance along with prompt redirection when she is off task.
- Break assignments into smaller manageable chunks.
- A daily report card that identifies several behavioral goals (e.g., paying attention in class, completing assignments in a timely fashion, and other behaviors that Emily may need to work on). Columns may be used to convey information across different subject areas throughout the day.

- Systematic work on social skills to foster increased prosocial behavior with other children and adults is especially important for Emily. Ideally, this social skills training would be combined with a school-based intervention that would allow Emily to implement the skills she is learning in the school setting. This recommendation should be clearly stated as part of her Individualized Educational Plan. As part of this plan, rules and expectations should be presented simply, clearly, and consistently and reviewed frequently. Consequences for both appropriate and inappropriate behavior should be enforced on a consistent basis through positive reinforcement and response-cost systems. This could be managed in the form of a token economy, given Emily's age. In addition, the behavior management program should focus on improving eye contact, socialization skills as well as adaptive skills in general. The behavioral plan also should be coordinated with Emily's mother to ensure consistency between parent and teachers, including target behaviors to be addressed, appropriate reinforcers, and appropriate punishment/response cost (e.g., time out). To facilitate this behavior plan and institute behavioral training where necessary, it is recommended that Emily and Emily's mother attend behavioral family counseling. A behavior-focused family counselor will ensure institution of a behavior management program that is consistent across school and home environments. A successful behavior modification program would be designed to reward all of Emily's efforts toward prosocial communication and social skills. Emily's mother may wish to pursue a fun tutorial after-school program or extracurricular group activity in order to facilitate the development of new social skills and to decrease Emily's oppositional behavior.
- Additionally, in light of the observation that Emily maintained on-task behavior with minimal structure during the morning portion of the evaluation, compared to later in the day (in part, because her medication was no longer active), it will be important for her pediatrician to prescribe the nongeneric extended release form of dextroamphetamine (Adderall XR) to allow Emily to be well managed on her medication throughout her school day as well as during homework time.

Further Discussion of Case Study

This assessment was comprehensive in nature due to the wide-ranging implications of LBW (Xu & Filler, 2005), and these multiple pieces of information were necessary in order to develop a complete understanding of Emily's specific areas of strength and weakness. Based on the definitions provided at the beginning of this chapter, Emily would be considered ELBW, and in light of the dose-response relationships between birth weight and neuropsychological performance described previously, Emily's deficits may have been less severe if she were VLBW or above. In addition to chronic and multiple deficits in neuropsychological functioning, Emily exhibited some of the neonatal medical issues associated with LBW, such as chronic lung disease and retinopathy of prematurity. Emily's neuropsychological deficits (e.g., related to attention, coordination, executive function, language, learning/memory, adaptive behavior) contributed to her academic struggles, resulting in the need for long-term special education services and behavioral interventions in the school setting. As seen throughout this chapter, children with LBW commonly experience more difficulty in school as compared to their full-term peers, and Emily is an example of how these difficulties are related to deficits across a range of neuropsychological and behavioral domains. Emily also provides a useful example of the importance of a team-based approach to treatment, as she had an extensive history of occupational therapy, physical therapy, and speech/language services in addition to academic and behavioral interventions; the ability of multiple professionals to work together is critical for children such as Emily due to their many areas of need.

CONCLUDING COMMENTS

As eloquently noted by Boyce et al. (2004), "There is presently no magical way to know which of the children who have experienced...LBW will develop disabilities. Consequently . . . there should be more concern about missing those infants who need services than with including those who may not need services" (p. 273). Indeed, research has highlighted a wide range of variability in prognosis and outcome among children with LBW (Taylor, Klein, & Hack, 2000), similar to children with TBI; hence the need for frequent follow-up assessment to monitor development and identify deficits as they arise, so that interventions can be implemented or modified as needed. It is thought that some of this variability in outcome may be accounted for by methodological inconsistencies across research studies, although some variability appears to be related to true sources of variance, such as differences in type of brain abnormalities or insults and degree of LBW (Taylor et al., 2002). Studies of children with LBW typically reveal a subsample of LBW children who do not demonstrate significant deficits in neuropsychological, academic, or psychosocial functioning (Van Baar et al., 2006). The implication is that some children with LBW will have no deficits in neuropsychological functioning while others may have severe deficits in addition to physical problems. Comprehensive assessment approaches are necessary in order to identify strengths and weaknesses in neuropsychological functioning and develop appropriate interventions based on assessment results.

At this time, intervention studies are limited by methodological issues, such as small or restricted samples, heterogeneous samples, limitations of measures used to assess treatment outcomes, lack of attention to possible environmental influences on treatment outcome, lack of longitudinal designs, and the use of different measures, norms, and definitions by different research teams (G. P. Aylward, 2002; Taylor, Klein, & Hack, 2000). In addition to these issues, research needs to pay more attention to the neuropathology associated with different developmental and behavioral consequences of LBW, the interactions among biological and environmental variables, and prevention of LBW (Taylor, Klein, & Hack, 2000). Intervention studies also should focus more on specific targets of the interventions and the impact of specific components of interventions on these more discrete targets; these studies also should address the limited long-term effectiveness of many treatment programs, as even the most promising interventions often produce minimal sustained effects. Finally, the field is in need of additional meta-analytic work in order to synthesize the findings of intervention studies, which would help shape practice and future research on infants with LBW.

Chapter 13

ENVIRONMENTAL TOXIN EXPOSURE

DEFINITION AND ETIOLOGY

Issues related to teratogenic effects of environmental substances have received increased attention with the passage of an executive order (Clinton, 1997) as well as Healthy People 2010 (U.S. Department of Health and Human Services, n.d.). Toxic exposure comprises exposure to a large range of substances—environmental toxins, prescribed medications, and recreational substances—that ultimately are poisonous to one or more aspects of the neural system (J. H. G. Williams & Ross, 2007). Exposure may be in the form of direct interaction, as in the case of a child who chews on a toy that has been finished with lead paint; alternatively, effects on an unborn child are indirect and occur through maternal contact or ingestion of the toxin. Neurodevelopmental toxicity of various chemicals or metals, such as lead, mercury, and pesticides, constitute an important public health concern (Buck, 1996); these toxins can have both indirect and direct effects on children across their lifetime. Many of these toxins occur naturally in the environment; others are man-made. In many ways, children may be more susceptible than adults to the effects of toxins, such as pesticides or lead, due to their developmental status (Dietrich et al., 2005; Lidsky, Heaney, Schneider, & Rosen, 2007). Other toxins, such as prescribed medications or recreational substances, introduced prenatally may be time limited in terms of exposure but have lifelong effects as well. The effects of environmental toxins (i.e., pesticides, lead, mercury) are discussed in this chapter; alcohol, medications, and other substances together with their related disorders are discussed in Chapter 14.

Pesticides

Of the various environmental toxins, pesticides are toxic chemicals that are introduced intentionally into the environment to reduce some nuisance species (Colosio, Tiramani, & Maroni, 2003). Unfortunately, the same toxicity that makes pesticides effective in eliminating certain species may pose significant risks to humans. The organophosphates (OPs) and carbamates, for example, inhibit acetyl cholinesterase (AChE); this increases the level of acetylcholine (ACh) at the synapse, overactivating the cholinergic pathways (Aldridge, Meyer, Seidler, & Slotkin, 2005). The cholinergic system is related directly to habituation, attention, and activity level. Effects may be acute, but there also may be delayed onset effects resulting from permanent changes or inhibition of specific enzymes (Aldridge et al., 2005). Other pesticides bind to hormone receptor sites, altering hormonal balance and potentially impacting early brain development, sexual development, and gender-related behaviors (Garry, Holland, Erickson, & Burroughs, 2003; Pierik, Burdorf, Deddens, Juttmann, & Weber, 2004). Most of the organochlorine pesticides (OCs) have been banned in the United States but continue to be used in other countries, including Mexico. OCs are fat soluble; they are absorbed into water sediments that can contaminate marine mammals as well as affect dairy products. Children can be exposed to them in utero or through breast milk (Centers for Disease Control [CDC], 2003) as well as through other means postnatally, depending on their environments. Many pesticides have been shown to have effects on varying components of the central nervous system (CNS) depending on the dose and duration of exposure. It is, in part, through this mechanism that pesticides achieve their intended objective for the target species. The primary uses of pesticides are for control of insect populations in homes and in agricultural settings; however, consistent research suggests an association between even low levels of pesticide exposure and neurobehavioral deficits (Rothlein et al., 2006).

Although the use of some organochlorines (e.g., dichlorodiphenyltrichloroethane [DDT]) has been prohibited, other pesticides have taken their place, including pyrethoids and organophosphorus insecticides. The OPs account for about half of all pesticides used; they act against a broad range of insects (Lizardi, O'Rourke, & Morris, 2008). The OPs, for example, break down into a number of metabolites (Heudorf, Angerer, & Drexler, 2004) including the dialkyl phosphate metabolites. Of the OPs, parathion use was banned as of 2003 in the United States. Another OP, chlorpyrifos, is believed to act on the serotonergic system and the 5-HT receptors, transporters, and signal transduction (Aldridge et al., 2005; Aldridge, Seidler, Meyer, Thillai, & Slotkin, 2003) as well as on the dopaminergic system (Aldridge et al., 2005). Although chlorpyrifos accounted for one-fifth of the insecticides used in 1997, it is expected that its use will decrease with the increased restrictions of the Food Quality and Protection Act of 1996 (CDC, 2003). Diazinon and malathion, however, continue to be used extensively. Guidelines for evaluation of pesticide neurotoxicity are limited in that they do not include assessment of effects at various periods of vulnerability or of effects that may become evident only over time (Claudio, Kiva, Russell, & Wallinga, 2000).

Thus far, the majority of studies examining neurotoxic effects of pesticides have focused on the workers who have direct, identified contact with the pesticides. Effects vary depending on whether the metabolite or pyrethroid is inhaled, ingested, or if contact is dermal in nature (CDC, 2003; Heudorf et al., 2004). In general, results indicate that exposure by workers to pesticides such as diazinon result in lowered performance overall (Maizlish, Schenker, Weisskopf, Seiber, & Samuels, 1987). Depending on the study, however, specific deficits (e.g., in processing speed, vigilance, working memory, inhibition, visual-motor processing, constructional abilities, and psychiatric) have or have not emerged (Bazylewicz-Walckzak, Majkzakova, & Szymczak, 1999; Després et al., 2005; Fiedler, Kipen, Kelly-McNeil, & Fenske, 1997; London, Myers, Neil, Taylor, & Thompson, 1997; Maizlish et al., 1987; Roland-Tapia et al., 2006). Unfortunately, many of the studies have not included biomarkers for pesticide exposure (Quandt et al., 2006).

Exposure to children comes from multiple sources (Curl et al., 2002; Lambert et al., 2005; Quandt et al., 2006). Residential contamination has been found at farms, from children's exposure when they visited their parents in the fields, from drift associated with spraying, or from soil that is tracked into or blown into the home (Lambert et al., 2005; Moses et al., 1993; Mott, 1995; Zahm & Ward, 1998). In agricultural communities, there is a far greater risk for children's exposure to pesticides than in the general population (Curl et al., 2002; Fenske et al., 2000; Lu & Fenske, 1999; Lu, Fenske, Simcox, & Kalman, 2000). Exposure of children to pesticides may result from internal and external residential use of pesticides (Carrillo-Zuniga et al., 2004; Simcox, Fenske, Wolz, Lee, & Kalman, 1995). The use of pesticides in homes is widespread (J. R. Davis, Brownson, & Garcia, 1992) and elevated levels of pesticide residue is common. These levels may be exacerbated in those residences that are located either within or directly adjacent to agricultural fields. The distal and proximal causes of exposure are further mediated by home practices, such as hand washing, as well as workplace practices, including the types of fabrics worn in the workplace (Quandt et al., 2006).

A recent study of agricultural settings along the Texas–Mexico border examined the level of childhood exposure to OCs and OPs by sampling house dust and hand-rinse samples for 45 children between 5 and 36 months of age (Carrillo-Zuniga et al., 2004). The climate in the area, combined with the lower socioeconomic status of the communities, results in windows being open most of the year and no air filtration system in the homes. Results indicated that OPs were detected at higher levels than OCs but that concentrations did not correspond to the proximity of the home to the agricultural setting using the pesticide. While the level of toxicity is much lower in the home than in the workplace, the lower levels over time may have similar negative effects CNS function. In a study of children in an agricultural region of Italy (Aprea, Strambi, Novelli, Lunghini, & Bozzi, 2000), levels of dimethylthiophosphate (DMTP, as one metabolite of OPs) were found to be five times that expected based on the National Health and Nutrition Examination Study (NHANES) 1999–2000 subsample of similarly aged children (CDC, 2003). Elevated levels of dimethylphosphate also were found. Notably, the urinary output of the alkylphosphates in the children sampled was significantly higher than the output of adults living in the same province. A study of children in Washington state examined levels of pesticide exposure and found seasonal differences, but no relation to parental work, contact age, or proximity of the home to the farmland (Koch, Lu, Fisker-Andersen, Jolley, & Fenske, 2002). This finding suggests that potential sources of pesticide exposure vary.

Previous studies have established that children in the *colonia* (i.e., agricultural communities) of Rio Bravo in the Rio Grande Valley are exposed to pesticides (Carrillo-Zuniga et al., 2004; Shalat et al., 2001, 2003). Shalat et al. (2003) found that OPs were detected in more than 60% of household dust samples collected. Based on Carrillo-Zuniga et al., the median level of OP detected in the urine of children ages 6 months to 4 years was comparable to or exceeded the 90th percentile level of the NHANES study (National Center for Environmental Health, 2001). Methyl parathion was the most commonly observed pesticide. Further, the urinary levels of pesticide metabolites were highest in children aged 13 to 24 months. The extent to which these higher-than-normal levels impact neurodevelopmental status is unknown. In addition to agricultural settings, pesticide exposure to children is also very high in urban settings (Adgate et al., 2001), probably as a result of the heavy use of pesticides in many city dwellings.

Given that the chemical mechanisms of pesticides all have neurological effects and that development of the CNS can be impacted postnatally as well as prenatally, the outcomes of those children who experience low-level exposure to pesticides in their homes postnatally is of concern. Secondary to the identification of those toxins in the environment is the question of the impact of the identified toxins on brain development. For example, the morpholine derivatives of pesticides affect the balance of inhibitory and excitatory thresholds in the CNS (Barbieri & Ferioli, 1994). As noted earlier, other pesticides involve the inhibition of AChE in the CNS (Adgate et al., 2001; Jeyaratnam & Maroni, 1994; Machemer & Pickel, 1994) when OP compounds and carbonates are included. In the case of pyrethroids, the sodium channels that are implicated in potentiation are affected

(He, Liu, & Zhang, 1994), while with OC compounds, the CNS is stimulated (Tordoir & Van Sittert, 1994). With the fromamidines, the effect on the CNS is through changes in the alpha-2 catecholamine receptors. Prenatal exposure to polychlorinated biphenyls (PCBs) is believed to disrupt thyroid function (Roegge & Schantz, 2006); by reducing the level of thyroxine, it is believed that this in turn affects the developmental timeline of the cerebellum. Similar subtle neurodevelopmental and behavioral concerns have been found with prenatal and postnatal exposure (Lai et al., 2002; Ribas-Fito, Sala, Kobevinas, & Sunyer, 2001). Thus, depending on the toxin, there are potentially multiple impacts on the chemical balance of the CNS and resulting neurobehavioral functioning.

Lead

For lead exposure, there is a much larger body of literature than for pesticides (Cory-Slechta, 1994; D. C. Rice, 1993); lead has been described as the most widely studied of pediatric neurotoxicants (Dietrich et al., 2005). While the median blood lead concentration has decreased considerably over the past 20 years, children of diverse cultural and linguistic backgrounds and children living in poverty continue to evidence blood lead levels well above the median (Dilworth-Bart & Moore, 2006; Gump et al., 2007); because culturally and linguistically diverse children are more likely to live in poverty, their risk for exposure to potentially harmful environmental toxins is much higher than for white children (Schell, 1997). Lead exposure can result from a variety of environmental sources; the greatest source of lead poisoning in children is through ingestion of dust and chips from surfaces with lead paint that are deteriorating or from drinking water that is carried through lead pipes in some urban areas with high levels of poverty. Thus, although the overall numbers for toxic blood lead levels (10 μg/dL; CDC, 1991) has decreased, this decrease has disproportionately favored whites and the nonpoor as opposed to culturally and linguistically diverse groups (Dilworth-Bart & Moore, 2006).

At low levels, minimal effects have been noted among preschool children with more equivocal results as children approach school age (for review, see Phelps, 1999). Blood lead levels as low as 10 μg/dl are believed to be associated with lower performance on general measures of intelligence (Bellinger, Stiles, & Needleman, 1992) as well as problems with auditory processing, reaction time, and motor stability (Després et al., 2005; Dietrich, Succop, Berger, & Keith, 1992). Based on existing evidence, there is a causal relationship between lead exposure and impairment at specific levels of exposure (Canfield, Gendle, & Cory-Slechta, 2004). Results of meta-analyses (Needleman & Gatsonis, 1990; Pocock, Smith, & Baghurst, 1994; J. Schwartz, 1994; J. H. G. Williams & Ross, 2007) consistently indicate possible loss of cognitive functioning as a result of lead exposure in infancy with estimates of an effect size of about 0.25 IQ points per 1 μg/dL increase in blood level (J. Schwartz, 1994). As a result, although the CDC and the World Health Organization (WHO) have designated that a blood concentration greater than or equal to10 μg/dL is considered a concern, there is no threshold level of lead exposure that is considered safe. In fact, various researchers have called for reassessment of the 10 μg/dL level (Lanphear et al., 2005). This is based, in part, on recent evidence that academic skills can be adversely affected with lead exposure below the 10 μg/dL level (Lanphear, Dietrich, Auinger, & Cox, 2000).

Peak lead levels generally occur between 18 and 30 months of age in the United States (Chen, Dietrich, Ware, Radcliffe, & Rogan, 2005). At extremely high levels, lead can cause deafness, blindness, coma, convulsions, and death. Signs of lead poisoning (e.g., sluggishness, headache, stomachache, irritability, poor appetite) often can be mistaken for other problems, including the flu (Lidsky et al., 2007). At lower levels, it is believed that the effects of lead exposure tend to be diffuse, affecting general brain development (J. H. G. Williams & Ross, 2007). It has been argued that, at high levels, lead toxicity interferes with the production and transmission of the neurotransmitters involved in establishing synaptic connections and deletions, thus affecting whole brain functioning (Cooper, Suszkiw, & Manalis, 1984; Petit, 1986). In particular, it has been demonstrated that lead affects dopamine function (Brockel & Cory-Shlechta, 1999; Canfield, Kreher, Cornwell, & Henderson, 2003). Some research suggests a cerebellar effect of lead (Bhattacharya, Shukla, Dietrich, & Bornschein, 2006) resulting in problems with gait and postural balance or sway.

Others have investigated the effect of lead exposure on the brain development and organization specific to language function (Yuan et al., 2006). Yuan and colleagues, using functional magnetic resonance imaging (fMRI) in young adults, found that higher mean childhood blood levels were associated with decreased activation of left frontal and left middle temporal regions (i.e., corresponding generally with Broca's and Wernicke's areas). At the same time, higher childhood blood lead levels were associated with increased right middle temporal lobe activation, suggesting a possible compensatory mechanism by the analogous right hemisphere for Wernicke's area. Yuan et al. concluded that this finding supported the contention that the childhood lead exposure has long-term effects for brain organization and the functional system associated with language. Postnatal exposure to lead was significantly correlated with impairments identified in school-age children and beyond, regardless of prenatal exposure.

Mercury

Research related to other toxins (e.g., the various forms of mercury) and their effects on children is much more limited (D. C. Rice, 1996) but recently has received more attention in relation to autism and autistic spectrum disorders. In conjunction with autism spectrum disorders, the predominant concern has been with the presence of thimerisol, which is approximately 50% mercury by weight and breaks down to ethylmercury and thiosalicylate. Ethylmercury is not the same as methylmercury; thimerisol appears to be removed from the blood and body more rapidly than methylmercury. As a result of the concerns for potential effects of thimerisol, the Food and Drug Administration has worked with vaccine manufacturers to reduce or eliminate thimerisol from vaccines. Several cases of acute mercury poisoning from thimerisol-containing products were found in the medical literature, with total doses of thimerisol ranging from approximately 3 mg/kg to several hundred mg/kg (Axton, 1972; Matheson, Clarkson, & Gelfand, 1980; Pfab, Muckter, Roider, & T., 1996; Rohyans, Walson, Wood, & MacDonald, 1994). In 2001, the Institute of Medicine convened a committee (the Immunization Safety Review Committee) to review issues related to the use of thimerisol in immunizations. The first review completed by this committee focused on a potential link between autism and the combined mumps, measles, and rubella vaccine. The second review focused on a potential relationship between thimerisol use in vaccines and neurodevelopmental disorders (Institute of Medicine, 2001). These investigations were in response to the hypothesis that autism is a form of mercury poisoning (S. Bernard, Enayati, Redwood, Roger, & Binstock, 2001). In its initial report, the committee concluded that there was insufficient evidence to establish or negate a causal relationship between thimerisol exposure from childhood vaccines and the neurodevelopmental disorders of autism, attention deficit hyperactivity disorder (ADHD), and speech or language delay. Because the committee concluded that arguments suggesting that exposure to thimerisol-containing vaccines could be associated with neurodevelopmental disorders was plausible, additional efforts to remove thimerisol from vaccines were initiated. The final report further examined the relation between vaccines and their causal relation to autism, incorporating additional epidemiological evidence. The committee concluded that the evidence favored a rejection of a causal relationship between thimerisol-containing vaccines and autism. The report further stated that the evidence in favor of use of vaccinations far outweighs the speculations. Additional studies have examined the relation between thimerisol-containing vaccines and autism spectrum disorders; these studies have found no consistent association between vaccines with thimerisol and neurodevelopmental outcomes (Ball, Ball, & Pratt, 2001; K. M. Madsen et al., 2003; Stehr-Green, Tull, Stellfeld, Mortenson, & Simpson, 2003; Verstraeten et al., 2003).

Exposure to mercury can come from many sources other than vaccinations (Després et al., 2005; McKeown-Eyssen, Ruedy, & Neims, 1983); in particular, exposure may occur prenatally through maternal ingestion of contaminated foods or through ingestion by the child directly, through household accidents, or occupational exposure (Lidsky et al., 2007). Blood levels of mercury should not exceed 3.6 μg/dl while urine levels should not exceed 15 μg/dL. Symptoms of mercury poisoning may be seen when mercury levels exceed 20 μg/dL in blood and 60 μg/dl in urine. One study examining toxic levels in the hair of children with autism found that children with autism in Kuwait had higher in-hair concentrations of mercury, as well as of uranium and lead, than a control group, but no explanation for the levels of mercury was identified (Fido & Al-Saad, 2005). Exposure may be direct or through fetal transfer (Yoshida, 2002) with some indications that the fetal brain accumulates mercury at higher levels than that of the brain of the mother (Feng et al., 2004). Inorganic mercury affects multiple systems through its actions on neurotransmitters including the aminergic and cholinergic systems (J. W. Allen, Mutkus, & Aschner, 2001; Castoldi, Candura, Costa, Manzo, & Costa, 1996; Hare, Rezazadeh, Cooper, Minnema, & Michaelson, 1990; Moretto et al., 2004). Methlymercury is absorbed more easily and is more toxic than inorganic mercury (Verity & Sarafian, 2000).

Arsenic, Aluminum, Manganese, and Other Metals

In addition to lead and mercury, a number of other metals are being investigated, including arsenic (As), cadmium, manganese, and aluminum (Al). Arsenic and its compounds are found in pesticides, herbicides, insecticides, and alloys. One mechanism for arsenic exposure is through contamination of groundwater. Arsenic contamination of groundwater has been found in Bangladesh (Meharg, 2005), Thailand, and China but also in parts of Michigan, Wisconsin, Minnesota, and the Dakotas (Knobeloch, Zierold, & Anderson, 2006). The standard for safe levels of arsenic in drinking water is 10 parts per billion, although skin cancer has been associated with even lower levels (Knobeloch et al., 2006). Arsenic effects occur through its interference in the adenotriphosphate (ATP) production and synthesis. Lead hydrogen arsenate is one of the more common insecticides with indications of brain damage to agricultural workers. More recently, monosodium methyl arsenate (MSMA), which is less toxic, has replaced arsenate in most agricultural settings. Arsenic in the form of chromated copper arsentate (Tannalith) was also used in the treating of various timbers, but this also has been discontinued. The risk at this time is with the disposal of timber treated this way in the past as even the ash can be poisonous (Knobeloch et al., 2006). Historically, arsenic or some variant has been included in articles of bronze, in various medications, and for cosmetic purposes.

Since arsenic is rapidly cleared from the blood, blood arsenic levels may not be very useful in diagnosis; in the urine (measured in a 24-hour collection following 48 hours without eating seafood), levels may exceed 50 μg/dl in people with arsenic poisoning. Arsenic may be detected in the hair and nails for months following exposure. The majority of studies examining arsenic effects have focused on cancer risk. Relatively fewer studies have examined neurotoxicity, and even fewer have examined neurotoxicity in children. A case study was published about a girl who was exposed to an arsenic-based pesticide, copper acetoarsenite. She evidenced multiple clinical signs of arsenic poisoning, including bands in her fingers and toenails, encephalopathy, seizures, and demyelinating polyneuropathy (Brouwer et al., 1992). In another study, with adults and exposure through drinking water, a strong association between arsenic concentration and abnormalities on electromyelograph were found (Hindmarsh et al., 1977).

Less is known about aluminum, cadmium, and manganese. Manganese is a trace element that occurs in nature and that, in appropriate levels, is needed for healthy development (Erickson, Syversen, Aschner, & Aschner, 2005). Common sources of organic manganese include pesticides. Exposure to cadmium is through secondhand smoke, foods, and contaminated water (Agency for Toxic Substances and Disease Registry [ATSDR], 1999; Järup, Berglund, Elinder, Nordberg, & Vahter, 1998). It is unknown if exposure to cadmium alone is related to neurodevelopmental effects in humans, but delays have been found with mice (ATSDR, 1999).

Carbon Monoxide

Another environmental toxin, carbon monoxide poisoning, is a leading cause of death in the United States. When not fatal, the evaluation of severity of intoxification and the long-term effects is difficult and variable (Thom & Kelm, 1989). At acute levels, the most common effects are manifest neurologically or in the form of cardiac injury. Neurological dysfunction as a result of carbon monoxide exposure is most likely to occur in young children and the elderly. The true incidence of carbon monoxide poisoning is unknown; it is estimated that up to one-third of all nonlethal cases may not be diagnosed as such (Dolan, 1985). Sources of carbon monoxide in the environment vary, but the most common source is that of smoke inhalation; most commonly, carbon monoxide poisoning occurs during winter months with fires, heating systems that burn fuels, and exhaust from motor vehicles (Varon, Marik, Fromm, & Gueler, 1999). Another source of carbon monoxide is cigarette smoke (A. Ernst & Zibrak, 1998). The mechanism of action that potentially results in neurological dysfunction derives from the propensity of the inhaled carbon monoxide to bind to hemoglobin, resulting in carboxyhemoglobin. Because the affinity of the carbon monoxide is about 200 times that of oxygen (Rodkey, O'Neal, Colilson, & Uddin, 1974), the availability of oxygen in the bloodstream is drastically compromised. Research indicates that 10% to 14% of severely poisoned individuals evidence some degree of brain damage (Thom et al., 1995).

COURSE AND PROGNOSIS

Course and prognosis varies depending on a variety of factors, including the teratogen, age and duration of exposure, and so on. A summary of effects by teratogens is provided in Table 13.1.

Table 13.1 Environmental Toxins and Domains Affected

Toxin/Teratogen	Domains Affected
PCBs	Auditory Executive functioning Attention problems Psychomotor abilities
Trichloroethylene (TCE), toluene, common solvents	Auditory Difficulty with multitasking Visual system (color blindness)
Organophosphates (OPs)	Visual system (blurred vision) Decreased gestational period Motor tremors Somatosensory Visual-motor, constructional ability Attentional problems, hyperactivity, impulsivity Autistic-type behaviors
Lead	Lower general ability Auditory/linguistic deficits Visual system and scotopic vision deficits Constructional praxis/visual-motor/spatial deficits Working memory deficits Sequencing problems Attention and behavior regulation problems Externalizing behaviors Executive functioning deficits Motor functions: posture, balance, gait problems
Methylmercury (MeHg)	Auditory system impaired Visual system impaired Motor tremors Somatosensory deficits Externalizing behaviors
Arsenic (As)	Verbal ability lower Long-term memory deficits Reading and spelling problems Visual-motor/constructional abilities affected Externalizing behaviors
Cadmium	Externalizing behaviors
Manganese	Emotional issues Motor impairments Movement disorders (including tremor, dystonia and rigidity) Memory deficits
Aluminum	Externalizing behaviors
Carbon Monoxide	Aphasia Apraxia Gait disturbance

Pesticide Exposure

Along the U.S.–Mexico border, pesticide use continues to be associated with major congenital malformations (Garcia et al., 2001). More subtle neurodevelopmental effects may be present but currently are not being identified or monitored in a systematic fashion. In a study of prenatal exposure, maternal exposure to OPs during the pregnancy was found to be associated with shortened gestational duration, particularly with higher levels of exposure at later points in the pregnancy (Eskenazi et al., 2004). The study did not include follow-up data on the status of the neonates. Infant/childhood exposure to neurotoxins has been associated with cognitive delays as well as with neurological diseases (Claudio et al., 2000). There are also some indications of increased incidence of autism spectrum disorders associated with higher levels of OPs in the environment, but no mechanism for this increase was identified (E. M. Roberts et al., 2007).

Colosio et al. (2003) found that acute poisoning with OPs resulted in short-term impairment of neurobehavioral performance but not long-term neurobehavioral impairment. There are some indications that effects of exposure to heavy metals may be transitory, but the more extensive literature suggests more long-term effects. In some instances, for example, effects may be observed both short term and long term. For less intense exposure and chronic exposure to OPs, effects on neurobehavioral and emotional status are equivocal. With children at varying age levels exposed to low levels of neurotoxins continuously, it is conceivable that there may be cumulative effects, particularly on those functional systems that are still developing postnatally (Colosio et al., 2003). Rogan and Gladen (1991) and Gladen and Rogan (1991) investigated the effects of OCs in large groups of children based on transplacental exposure and exposure through breast milk. Results indicated that that while PCB exposure was associated with mild motor delays (Ribas-Fito et al., 2001; W. J. Rogan & Gladen, 1991), DDT and dichlorodiphenyldichloroethylene (DDE) exposure were not associated with delays up to age 2 or age 5 (Gladen & Rogan, 1991; W. J. Rogan & Gladen, 1991). In a study that compared the performance of Yaqui preschool children from a homogeneous agricultural community (with pesticide exposure) to a group of children in the foothills who had no pesticide exposure, the exposed children demonstrated deficits in stamina, eye-hand coordination, visual-motor integration (i.e., drawing), and memory (Guillette, Meza, Aquilar, Soto, & Garcia, 1998). Longer follow-up data for effects of pesticide exposure are not available.

Lead Exposure

Lead has been found to cause lifelong learning problems in children, particularly when exposure occurs prenatally; effects of lead on functional domains based on existing research are summarized in Table 13.1. Inverse relations have been found between prenatal maternal blood lead concentrations and developmental status at 4 years of age (Wasserman et al., 2003). Long-term effects of lead on attention and constructional praxis also have been identified (Ris, Dietrich, Succop, Berger, & Bornschein, 2004). For exposure after the prenatal period, effects may be more subtle, depending on the duration and level of exposure. Investigations of 60-month blood level in 174 children indicated that higher blood lead levels were associated with impaired rule learning, spatial span, and planning (Froehlich et al., 2007). These effects were more pronounced (i.e., a demonstrated interaction effect) for boys as compared to girls. Ris et al. (2006) also concluded that boys were at increased risk for effects of lead exposure on attention and visual-motor/constructional praxis. Results further indicated an interaction effect of blood lead levels with socioeconomic status and cognition/learning abilities. Coscia, Ris, Succop, & Dietrich (2003) used growth curve analyses to examine cognitive effects for 196 children, ages 6 to 15 years, with lead exposure. At age 15, higher lead levels were associated with lower verbal comprehension scores over time and greater decline in vocabulary development. Similar negative trajectories were not evidenced for perceptual areas (Coscia et al., 2003). Notably, effects of blood lead levels on cognition appear to be moderated by high blood folate levels (Solon et al., 2008).

Language, cognition, and educational functioning are not the only domains affected by lead exposure. Notably, research indicates that lead exposure also is associated with greater absenteeism, lower graduation rates, and delinquency (Dietrich, Ris, Succop, Berger, & Bornschein, 2001). In a follow-up study of 780 children with high blood lead levels at 12 to 33 months of age, blood lead levels at age 5 were not significantly correlated with behavior problems; however, at age 7, blood lead levels were related directly to externalizing and school problems (Chen, Cai, Dietrich, Radcliffe, & Rogan, 2007). Children with elevated lead levels are more inattentive, hyperactive, aggressive, disorganized, and less able to follow directions; elevated bone lead levels are associated with elevated risk for delinquency and aggression as well (M. Marlowe, Bliss, & Schneider, 1994; Needleman, 2002; J. H. G. Williams & Ross, 2007). Among children with emotional disturbance, hair lead levels were associated with aggression, withdrawal, distractibility, and social problems (M. Marlowe, Errera, Ballowe, & Jacobs, 1983). Some of the domains affected by lead exposure include poor attention, executive function, working memory, and language delays as well as delays in motor development (Bellinger, Leviton, Waternaux, Needleman, & Rabinowitz, 1987; Bellinger, Leviton, Waternaux, Needleman, & Rabinowitz, 1988; Bellinger et al., 1992; Wigg, Vimpani, McMichael, & Baghurst, 1988).

Given that some focal deficits may emerge at differing ages, it is imperative that longitudinal data be examined across functional domains. For example, in one study, cognitive ability at age 10 best correlated with blood lead levels at 2 years of age (Bellinger et al., 1992) and tooth lead levels (Hansen, Trillingsgaard, Beese, Lyngbye, & Grandjean, 1989). In another study, executive function set shifting was best correlated with concurrent blood lead levels (Stiles & Bellinger, 1993), as was processing speed (Hansen et al., 1989). Long term, low levels of lead have been associated with fine motor deficits that become evident only at school age (Dietrich, Berger, & Succop, 1993). Specific to PCB (and mercury) exposure and 7-year-old children, identified deficits included verbal naming, reaction time, and long-term memory (Grandjean et al., 2001).

Mercury Exposure

Indications from research are that domains affected by mercury poisoning (see Table 13.1) include the auditory system, the visual system, the motor system (e.g., the presence of tremors), and impairments in the somatosensory system, including parasthesias and decreased sensitivity to vibration (D. Campbell, Gonzales, & Sullivan, 1992; P. W. Davidson et al., 2000). Some studies have indicated that, in boys, abnormal muscle tone and deep tendon reflexes (Cordier et al., 2002), as well as poor leg coordination and impaired visual-spatial skills (McKeown-Eyssen et al., 1983) and impaired fine motor skills (G. J. Myers et al., 2003), have been associated with higher maternal mercury concentrations. Others have found impaired performance in children at age 7 but noted confounding factors, such as nutrition, that could have accounted for some or all of the differences (Grandjean et al., 2001); still others believe that prenatal exposure to methylmercury affects the development of the cerebellum, with specific concerns for the interaction of PCBs and methylmercury, both of which can occur in fish and seafood (Roegge & Schantz, 2006). Still others have found that high levels of mercury are associated with higher levels of aggression among children identified with emotional disturbance (M. Marlowe et al., 1983). Prenatal methylmercury exposure has been found to be associated with multifocal and permanent effects (Debes, Budtz-Jorgensen, Weihe, White, & Grandjean, 2006). Alternatively, the results of the Seychelles Child Development Study, with over 700 children, does not support a consistent pattern of association between child outcomes and prenatal exposure to methylmercury from maternal consumption of fish (P. W. Davidson et al., 2006).

Effects of Arsenic and Other Metals

Arsenic, cadmium, and aluminum levels all have been found to be positively related with behavior problems (e.g., disruptive or externalizing behaviors) in children identified as emotionally disturbed (M. Marlowe et al., 1983; M. Marlowe, Stellern, Moon, & Errera, 1985). Another study focused on the effects of exposure to arsenic and lead on the neuropsychological development of Mexican children (Calderón et al., 2001). Theirs was a cross-sectional study with actual concentrations of arsenic (from urinalysis) and blood lead levels for an exposed group and a reference group. Unlike many other studies, Calderón et al. included a height for age index (HAI) as an indicator of malnutrition and body mass. Results indicated that impaired verbal abilities and long-term memory were associated with increased levels of arsenic; lower scores on attentional and sequential tasks were associated with higher levels of lead; and the HAI was positively correlated with Full Scale IQ and visual-perceptual abilities. They concluded that environmental exposure to lead and arsenic have differential effects on CNS function beyond those associated with poverty and malnutrition.

Over the short term, impaired attention and memory deficits were found to be associated with arsenic exposure, but these effects dissipated over time (Potasová & Biro, 1994). In a study of 69 children in Wyoming, increases in arsenic levels, as well as the interaction of arsenic and lead, were found to be associated with decreased reading and spelling achievement (Moon, Marlowe, Stellern, & Errera, 1985). Long-term exposure to arsenic has been associated with impaired psychomotor abilities, speed of recall, long-term memory, and visual-perceptual deficits (Knobeloch et al., 2006). Prolonged exposure to high levels of manganese has been associated with emotional disturbance and motor problems, with some concern that children may be more susceptible to the effects (manganism) than adults (Agency for Toxic Substances and Disease Registry, 2001). Similarly, increases in aluminum, as well as the interaction of aluminum with lead, were found to be associated with impaired visual-motor performance (Moon et al., 1985).

Carbon Monoxide Effects

Neuropsychological sequelae to carbon monoxide may appear immediately or up to 240 days following the exposure (A. Ernst & Zibrak, 1998). These sequelae include aphasia, apraxia, and gait disturbance as well as personality changes. Neurological assessments reveal evidence of abnormalities in association with moderate to severe poisoning; abnormalities included hypodensity of the basal ganglia or other gray matter (Choi, 1983; Ginsberg, 1995; Min, 1986; Zagami, Lethlean, & Mellick, 1993).

EVIDENCE-BASED INTERVENTIONS

The extent to which there is an evidence/research base to support interventions for exposure to environmental toxins and associated deficits is provided in Table 13.2. One intervention specific to exposure to heavy metals is chelation therapy, a medical intervention used to speed the process by which the body rids itself of specific minerals or metals (e.g., lead, mercury, iron). In the chelation process, a chelating agent (e.g., calcium disodium edetate, dimercaprol, penicillamine) specific to the metal involved is given orally, intramuscularly, or intravenously (Kwiatkowski, 2008). The chelating agent encircles and binds to the metal in the body's tissues, facilitating its release from the tissue to the bloodstream, to be excreted through the kidneys and urine. This process can be lengthy and painful; it has been found to be effective in reducing lead, mercury, and arsenic levels, but not for cadmium. The process is not without risks, and even when the levels of the target substance are decreased with chelation, the levels may rebound as a result of concentrations in bone or teeth that gradually are released back into the circulatory system. As a result, chelation therapy may have to be done more than once, even when exposure is not ongoing (Kwiatkowski, 2008). The benefits of chelation for the reduction of the metals are not disputed, and effectively lowering levels may abate further damage (Counter, Ortega, Shannon, & Buchanan, 2003).

At the same time, even with attempts to remove lead, for example, results of changes in cognitive, behavioral, or neuropsychological functioning are equivocal. For example, in the Treatment of Lead-Exposed Children Study across three states (Dietrich et al., 2004), at age 7, one-half of the children with lead levels between 20 to 44 μg/dl received chelation therapy (succimer therapy) while the other half received placebo. Chelation

Table 13.2 Evidence-Based Status for Interventions Associated with Toxic Exposure

Interventions	Target	Status
Chelation therapy	Lead, calcium, iron, mercury levels in blood	Positive practice (Aydinok et al., 2007; Giardina & Grady, 2001; Olivieri et al., 1995; W. Rogan et al., 2001)
Chelation therapy	Cognitive deficits	Ineffective (Dietrich et al., 2004; Haynes et al., 2003; W. Rogan et al., 2001)
Chelation therapy	Motor: gait and posture	Inconclusive (Bhattacharya, Shukla, Auyang, Dietrich, & Bornschein, 2007)
Chelation therapy	Mercury and autism	Inconclusive/adverse effects (Baxter & Krenzelok, 2008; L. Curtis & Patel, 2008)
Nutrition, including breast feeding	General development and CNS function	Promising practice (Haynes et al., 2003; Lai et al., 2002; Ribas-Fito et al., 2001)
Hyperbaric (100%) oxygen therapy	Correcting oxygenation levels (e.g., those compromised due to carbon monoxide)	Promising practice (R. A. M. Myers, Snyder, & Emhoff, 1995; Thom & Kelm, 1989; Thom et al., 1995)

therapy was effective in lowering average blood lead levels for approximately 6 months but resulted in no change in cognitive, behavioral, or neuromotor functioning (Dietrich et al., 2004). Similar studies with the same chelation agent and blood lead levels also found no change in cognitive functioning (Haynes et al., 2003; W. Rogan et al., 2001). In contrast, in a randomized control study of 161 children who had high lead levels, the group that received the chelation therapy (succimer therapy) to lower lead levels demonstrated significant improvement in gait and postural balance (Bhattacharya et al., 2007). The extent to which these positive effects would be sustained long term remains to be determined. Similarly, positive effects of lowering iron levels with chelation therapy in beta-thalassemia (using deferiprone) have been found (Giardina & Grady, 2001; Olivieri et al., 1995; W. Rogan et al., 2001); no information on the extent to which iron chelation affects neurodevelopment was provided. Although some have suggested that chelation might be effective as a treatment for autism, there is no scientific evidence to support the use of chelation therapy as a cure for autism.

For exposure to carbon monoxide, treatment with 100% oxygen is indicated; treatment with hyperbaric oxygen is indicated when the individual evidences unconsciousness or altered neurological or cardiac function due to exposure (Thom & Kelm, 1989; Weaver et al., 2002). Results consistently demonstrate reduced risk of delayed neuropsychological sequelae for up to 12 months (Weaver et al., 2002).

CASE STUDY: DEMETRIC—LEAD EXPOSURE

The next report is from a hospital-based clinic. Identifying information, such as child and family name, teacher or physician name, and school information, has been altered or fictionalized to protect confidentiality.

Reason for Referral

Demetric is an 8-year 11-month-old African American boy referred for reevaluation by his pediatrician, who is following Demetric for a history of early lead exposure, specific language impairment, learning disability, and attentional difficulties.

Background Information

Home

Demetric resides with his mother and stepbrother. Demetric's father is deceased; he died in 1996 as a result of lung cancer. His father was a carpenter who had completed 2 years of college. Demetric's mother is 29 years of age, has a 2-year college education, and works as a nursing assistant. His brother is 13 years old and is entering the eighth grade in the fall. Demetric is an A/B student who is reported to be in good health. Maternal family medical history is significant for lupus, sickle cell anemia, and heart disease. Paternal family history is not known.

Developmental and Medical History

Review of Demetric's developmental and medical history indicates that he is the product of an 8-month pregnancy, 30-hour labor, and vaginal delivery, weighing 5 pounds 3 ounces at birth. His mother indicates that she experienced a single "blackout" spell during her eighth month of pregnancy and was sent to the hospital, where she stayed for

5 days. Demetric exhibited no apparent problems after delivery and went home from the hospital with his mother on schedule. At his 6-month checkup, however, initial lead screening revealed an elevated concentration in his blood (37 μg/dl). The lead concentration in Ms. Young's blood was also assessed and found to be abnormally high as well. The level of lead in Demetric's blood was monitored periodically by the Health Department from 9 months (46 μg/dl) until a normal level was obtained at 29 months (5.7 μg/dl). Demetric attained his early developmental motor milestones within normal limits, with walking occurring at 12 months of age. In contrast, developmental language milestones were delayed significantly. Demetric's language skills primarily consisted of "babbling" until age 3. Demetric's mother was concerned about his "speech" when he turned 2 years old and was not saying words like other children his age. As a result, at 2 years of age, he was evaluated by a speech and language pathologist, who diagnosed a severe expressive and receptive language delay; he began receiving group language therapy shortly thereafter. Subsequently, Demetric was evaluated by an occupational therapist, who recommended that Demetric participate in an occupational/speech therapy group two times a week for 90-minute sessions to address delays in the areas of gross motor, personal/social, and speech/language skills. Demetric was reevaluated by the speech and language pathologist at age 3 and exhibited a severe receptive language delay and a moderate to severe expressive language delay. Subsequent evaluations at age 4 revealed similar findings. Demetric finally began speaking in complete sentences at age 5. Aside from the usual childhood illnesses and the elevated lead levels, Demetric's past medical history was not significant, and currently he is in good health.

Educational History

Review of educational history indicates that Demetric was enrolled in a prekindergarten program in a private daycare at the age of 4. After 2 weeks, the teacher requested that Demetric's mother remove him from the program because he was not talking and not participating; he also had left class and wandered around outside by himself. Demetric's mother removed him from the program and decided to have him stay at home so she could work with him. Demetric's grandmother also spent time working with Demetric. At age 5, Demetric attended kindergarten. During that year, he was assessed again by a speech/language therapist and was found to have articulation problems in conjunction with a severe expressive and receptive language disorder. As part of Demetric's special education Individualized Education Plan (IEP), it was recommended that Demetric receive 1.5 hours of speech/language therapy per week. Significant improvement was noted; however, Demetric was also experiencing academic difficulty and a short attention span in the classroom. As a result, he repeated kindergarten the following year at the same school. He continued receiving speech/language therapy for 1.5 hours each week.

At age 6, Demetric was referred for a psychoeducational evaluation by his teacher because his language problems substantially limited his ability to be successful in the regular classroom. Based on that evaluation, Demetric's cognitive abilities were in the average range as measured by the Leiter International Performance Scale, a nonverbal (NV) measure of intelligence (NVIQ = 95). His visual-motor skills were in the average range; in contrast, Demetric's receptive vocabulary was considerably lower, supporting his history of significant language difficulties. At that time, Demetric's mathematics abilities were below average; however, his reading comprehension was in the average range, and his word identification skills were above average. Adaptive behavior was generally below average, particularly in daily living skills areas. Based on the results of this evaluation, consideration for special education classroom services was recommended.

Demetric was then referred for a neuropsychological evaluation. At that time, he demonstrated average nonverbal intellectual ability as measured by the Test of Nonverbal Intelligence, Second Edition (TONI-2 = 95). Demetric exhibited relative strengths (average performance) in areas of visual-spatial perception, visual-motor integration/construction, and immediate/working memory for visual/nonverbal material. These strengths were contrasted by relative weaknesses (generally deficient to borderline) in auditory processing, expressive and receptive language, auditory/verbal immediate/working memory, and fine motor tapping speed of the right hand. Academically, Demetric demonstrated significant strengths (average to above average) in basic word identification and spelling contrasted by relative weaknesses (borderline to low average) in numerical reasoning/calculation and reading comprehension. Behaviorally, Demetric was displaying significant levels of inattention and impulsivity. His pattern of neuropsychological test performance was felt to be consistent with a diagnosis of specific language impairment (receptive and expressive type), central auditory processing disorder, learning disability in reading comprehension and mathematics, in conjunction with hyperlexia (elevated word recognition). It was recommended that Demetric be placed in a self-contained special education classroom for children with specific language impairment. If this setting was not available, it was recommended that Demetric receive individual and group language therapy in conjunction with learning disability resource classroom services. Home-based language therapy also was recommended to help generalize the results of language therapy. Behavioral management was recommended as part of Demetric's IEP to help him stay on task and complete his assignments. It also was recommended that Demetric receive a formal central auditory processing evaluation and an occupational therapy evaluation.

As a result of these evaluations, during first and second grade, Demetric received special education resource services in a classroom for children with autism under the category of "Specific Learning Disability" (SLD). Within this placement, Demetric received instruction in receptive and expressive language skills, reading comprehension, mathematical calculation, and mathematical reasoning. He also received individual language therapy for 30 minutes a session, three times a week. Review of a school report form recently completed by Demetric's teachers indicated that Demetric "has good spelling and reading skills, although his written work is often difficult to understand and he often has trouble relating experiences." Demetric is scheduled to attend the third grade this fall. He will continue to receive individual language therapy 1.5 hours a week, and he will also have 10 hours/week of special education resource time in the autism class via the SLD program.

Assessment Procedures

Clinical interview (parent)

Behavioral observations

Leiter International Performance Scale—Revised (Leiter-R)

Test of Nonverbal Intelligence, Third Edition (TONI-3)

Neuropsychological Assessment (NEPSY)/Neuropsychological Assessment, Second Edition (NEPSY-2; selected subtests)

Clinical Evaluation of Language Fundamentals, Fourth Edition (CELF-IV; selected subtests)

Peabody Picture Vocabulary Test, Fourth Edition (PPVT-IV)

Wepman Test of Auditory Discrimination
Detroit Tests of Learning Ability, Third Edition (DTLA-3)
Boston Naming Test (BNT)
Wechsler Intelligence Scale for Children, Fourth Edition (WISC-IV; selected subtests)
Test of Visual Perceptual Skills (TVPS; selected subtests)
Kaufman Assessment Battery for Children, Second Edition (KABC-2; selected subtests)
Beery Developmental Test of Visual Motor Integration, Fifth Edition (DTVMI-V)
Rey Osterreith Complex Figure Test
Clock Face Drawing Test
Finger Test Tapping (manual) Test
Children's Memory Scale (CMS)
Wide Range Achievement Test, Fourth Edition (WRAT-4)
Gray Oral Reading Test, Fourth Edition (GORT-4)
Test of Written Language, Third Edition (TOWL-3)
Woodcock Johnson Tests of Achievement, Third Edition (WJ III; selected subtests)
Behavior Assessment System for Children, Second Edition (BASC-2; Parent and Teacher Rating Scales)
Vineland Adaptive Behavior Scale, Interview Edition (VABS)
DSM-IV ADHD Checklist (Parent and Teacher)

Behavioral Observations

Demetric presented himself for testing as a neatly groomed youngster who was in no apparent physical distress. Demetric separated appropriately from his mother and accompanied the examiner to the testing room willingly. Demetric was oriented and related appropriately toward this examiner with good social eye contact noted. In response to direct questions, as well as when conversation was spontaneous, Demetric's use of language was dysfluent; he often told stories to the examiner that were incoherent. Throughout this one-to-one testing session, which consisted of two sessions separated by a lunch break, Demetric demonstrated an age-appropriate span of attention. Lateral dominance is firmly established in the right hand and foot. Vision was not formally screened; however, Demetric's mother reported that this has been evaluated in the past and reported as within normal limits. Hearing was formally assessed by the audiology service and was reported to be within normal limits.

Assessment Results and Interpretation

To assess cognitive ability, Demetric was administered the Leiter International Performance Scale-Revised (Leiter-R) and the Test of Nonverbal Intelligence, Third Edition (TONI-3) in an attempt to control for his history of language disorder as well as to allow for comparison with previous evaluations. The Leiter-R is a nonverbal measure of intelligence that assesses reasoning ability through various tasks such as Figure Ground, Design Analogies, Form Completion, Sequential Order, Repeated Patterns, and Paper Folding. The TONI-3 is another measure of nonverbal ability/reasoning. Using these two nonverbal measures (i.e., when language had been controlled for as a potential confound), Demetric was found to be functioning in the low-average to average range of nonverbal ability/reasoning (see Table 13.3). These scores are consistent with his previous evaluation.

In order to assess higher-order executive functions, Demetric was administered the Tower subtest of the Neuropsychological Assessment (NEPSY). On this task, he was required to move three colored balls to target positions on three pegs in a prescribed number of moves. In addition, there were rules and time constraints that increase task difficulty and necessitate planning/forethought. Demetric scored within the borderline range on this task, suggesting that he has poor planning/sequencing reasoning skills.

Assessment of linguistic functioning was conducted in order to evaluate expressive and receptive language development. Analysis of Demetric's performance indicates that, at the present time, his expressive and receptive language development continue to be significantly below nonverbal intellectual expectancy. Most of his receptive language skills, including receptive vocabulary development, sentence imitation, the ability to follow verbal directions, and understanding sentence structure, have improved since his last evaluation; however, Demetric continues to exhibit a significant deficit in auditory discrimination. Comparison of Demetric's expressive language standard scores would indicate little improvement, if any, since his last evaluation. Specifically, confrontational naming of pictures remains in the borderline range; Demetric's rapid naming skills have declined to the borderline range. His ability to define words is still deficient, and his ability to formulate sentences, which requires linguistic planning, is in the borderline range. The latter score represents some improvement since his last evaluation. Clearly, although Demetric has made some progress with continuation of therapy, his language skills are still very low, and they are not commensurate with his nonverbal ability.

In order to assess visual spatial perception/discrimination ability without a motor component, Demetric was administered the Visual Discrimination subtest of the Test of Visual Perceptual Skills (TVPS), the Gestalt Closure subtest of the Kaufman Assessment Battery for Children, Second Edition (KABC-2), and the Arrows subtest of the NEPSY-2. Analysis of Demetric's performance indicates that his current visual-perceptual functioning is variable, ranging from deficient to well above average. He continues to demonstrate average to above-average visual discrimination and closure skills; however, Demetric experienced significant difficulty on a task requiring scanning/tracking and judging spatial orientation.

Constructional praxis, as measured by the Developmental Test of Visual Motor Integration, Fifth Edition (DTVMI-V), the Rey Complex Figure (RCF) copying task, and a clock face drawing with the requested time of 10:20, is found to be in the low-average range. In contrast, Demetric scored in the average range on Block Design from the WISC-IV. Qualitative analysis of Demetric's performance indicated that he had difficulty with motor planning and organization, as exhibited by number spacing problems while drawing the clock face and his poorly integrated Rey. Finally, it should be noted that Demetric had difficulty telling time to the minute. Fine motor finger oscillation as measured by a manual finger tapper is found to be within normal age-level expectancy bilaterally; however, Demetric continues to exhibit a relative depression in right hand functioning.

In order to assess learning and memory, Demetric was administered the Children's Memory Scale (CMS). Analysis of his performance on the subtests comprising the Attention/Concentration Index and the Picture Locations subtest (supplemental) indicates that Demetric is exhibiting attention/verbal working memory skills that are generally in the borderline to low-average range. Further, it should be noted that Demetric's poor performance on the Numbers subtest was due to an inability to comprehend the task demands

Table 13.3 Psychometric Summary for Demetric

	Standard Scores	
	Evaluation 1	Evaluation 2
Leiter International Performance Scale – Revised (Leiter-R)	95	84
Test of Nonverbal Intelligence, Third Edition (TONI-3)	95	102
Neuropsychological Assessment, Second Edition (NEPSY-2)		
Tower Task (from NEPSY)		70
Phonological Processing		85
Verbal Fluency	85	70
Arrows		60
Peabody Picture Vocabulary Test, Fourth Edition (PPVT-IV)	58	75
Boston Naming Test (BNT)	77	74
Clinical Evaluation of Language Fundamentals, Fourth Edition (CELF-IV)		
Formulated Sentences	65	75
Sentence Structure	65	85
Concepts and Directions	65	75
Detroit Tests of Learning Ability, Third Edition (DTLA-3)		
Sentence Imitation	75	80
Wepman Auditory Discrimination	54	51
Wechsler Intelligence Scale for Children, Fourth Edition (WISC-IV)		
Vocabulary	55	60
Block Design	90	100
Test of Visual-Perceptual Skills	95	125
Visual Discrimination		
Kaufman Assessment Battery for Children, Second Edition (KABC-2)		
Gestalt Closure	105	100
Developmental Test of Visual-Motor Integration, Fifth Edition (DTVMI-V)		
Visual Motor Integration	97	80
Rey Complex Figure Test (copy)		84
Clock Face Drawing		
Form	96	89
Time (3:00)		58
Time (10:20)		53
Finger Tapping		
Right (dominant) Hand	73	89
Left (nondominant) Hand	80	103
	Evaluation 2	
Children's Memory Scale (CMS)	**Scaled Score**	**Standard Score**
Attention/Concentration Index		78
Numbers	4	
Sequences	5	
Picture Locations	13	
General Memory Index		63

Table 13.3 (*Continued*)

	Evaluation 2	
	Scaled Scores	Standard Scores
Stories	6	
Word Pairs	5	
Visual Immediate Index		72
Dot Locations	8	
Faces	3	
Family Pictures	10	
Verbal Delayed Index		78
Stories	6	
Word Pairs	7	
Visual Delayed Index		73
Dot Locations	10	
Faces	1	
Family Pictures	10	
Delayed Recognition Index		66
Stories	7	
Word Pairs	2	
Learning Index		78
Word Pairs	6	
Dot Locations	7	
Gray Oral Reading Test, Fourth Edition (GORT-4)		
Fluency		100
Comprehension		70
Wide Range Achievement Test, Fourth Edition (WRAT-4)		
Reading		105
Spelling		106
Arithmetic		83
Test of Written Language, Third Edition (TOWL-3)		
Written Language Quotient		81
Woodcock-Johnson Tests of Achievement, Third Edition (WJ-III)		
Applied Math		65
Behavior Assessment Scale for Children, Second Edition (BASC-2)		
	T-Scores	
	Parent	Teacher
Clinical Scales		
Hyperactivity	63	55
Aggression	44	47
Conduct	49	47
Anxiety	48	62
Depression	46	61
Somatization	39	42
Atypical	50	73
Withdrawal	44	55
Attention	68	62

(continued)

Table 13.3 ***(Continued)***

	T Score	
	Parent	Teacher
Learning Problems	NA	53
Adaptive Scales		
Adaptability	33	43
Social Skills	25	48
Leadership	28	44
Study Skills	NA	50
Vineland Adaptive Behavior Scale		**Standard Score**
Communication Domain		87
Daily Living Skills		68
Socialization		80
Composite		74
	Raw Scores	
DSM-IV ADHD Checklist	Parent	Teacher
Inattention	26/27	10/27
Hyperactivity/Impulsivity	16/27	2/27

of the backward section (Forward standard score = 95, Backward = 60). In contrast, his visual working memory is above average and significantly better than his verbal working memory. This finding is consistent with his history of auditory processing and language problems.

Demetric's General Memory Index (GMI = 63) is significantly below average and well below his measured nonverbal ability; however, more detailed analysis of his performance indicates that he is demonstrating significant variability in his ability to learn and remember. Results indicate that his ability to learn auditory/verbal material is borderline to low average with fairly good delayed recall (30 minutes) of the material he did learn. In contrast, his visual-memory skills are average when he is asked to learn spatial location and is provided with repetition and structure to learn the material (Dot Locations). He also does better with multisensory, experiential learning (remembering scenes of family activities—Family Pictures). He does not demonstrate the same ability, however, on memory for faces; however, this was in part due to difficulty comprehending task directions.

In order to assess word recognition, spelling, and numerical calculation skills, Demetric was administered the Wide Range Achievement Test, Fourth Edition (WRAT-4). Demetric demonstrated average word recognition, average spelling, and low-average calculation skills. As this test measures reading recognition as opposed to reading comprehension, Demetric was also administered the Gray Oral Reading Test, Fourth Edition (GORT-4). On this measure, Demetric was required to read stories aloud and then respond to multiple-choice questions related to the story content. The Passage score assesses both reading speed and accuracy while the Comprehension score assesses understanding of what is read. Demetric's reading speed and accuracy are commensurate with nonverbal intellectual expectancy, suggesting that he has good decoding skills, and consistent with the results of the WRAT-4. In contrast, his comprehension of what he reads is well below average, as would be consistent with his history of specific language impairment.

In order to assess written expression, Demetric was administered the Test of Written Language, Third Edition (TOWL-3). On this instrument, Demetric was required to write a story about a picture. The story was then evaluated for development of a theme, vocabulary usage, punctuation and capitalization style, spelling, and syntax. Demetric's written expression skills are in the borderline to low-average range. Qualitatively, Demetric's story contained numerous spelling errors, a single run-on sentence (lack of punctuation), and a poorly integrated theme/story line.

Demetric also was administered the Applied Problems subtest of the Woodcock-Johnson Tests of Achievement: Third Edition (WJ III). This subtest assesses the child's knowledge of concepts and ability to solve word problems. Demetric scored in the deficient range, again suggesting that he experienced difficulty with comprehension.

Thus, achievement results indicate that Demetric has relative strengths in word recognition (decoding) and spelling (encoding). These are contrasted by relative weaknesses in the areas of math reasoning and reading comprehension; his weaknesses in these areas are consistent with his history of language difficulties.

Adaptive behavior was measured using the Vineland Adaptive Behavior Scale, Interview Edition (VABS), with the mother serving as informant. Results indicate that Demetric's overall adaptive behavior falls within the borderline range. Demetric's communication and socialization skills were rated as low average in contrast to deficient daily living skills.

In order to assess behavioral/emotional functioning, the Behavior Assessment System for Children, Second Edition (BASC-2) was completed by Demetric's mother and teacher. In addition, a behavior rating scale that reflects items related to the diagnostic criteria for Attention-Deficit/Hyperactivity Disorder was also completed. Analysis of the behavior rating scale data appears to indicate that, at the present time, Demetric continues to have attention difficulties at home, in conjunction with difficulty adapting to change in routine and poor social skills. His mother reported that although his attention span has gotten better, he continues to be distracted easily. He gets upset if he loses when playing with children younger than himself, although he plays appropriately with older children. He likes to interact with people face to face; he does not like it if someone comes up to him from behind. Similar behavioral difficulties were not endorsed by Demetric's teacher in the classroom. His teacher's responses indicated that Demetric exhibits social/emotional immaturity, as evidenced by behaviors such as "humming to himself."

Summary and Diagnostic Impressions

In summary, Demetric is an 8-year 11-month-old African American boy with a history of early and significant lead exposure, resulting in specific language impairment, learning disability, and attentional difficulties. This is the second time he has been evaluated by this service. The results of the current neuropsychological evaluation indicate that Demetric continues to function within the average range of intellectual ability when nonverbal IQ assessment is used as the best estimate of his ability. Demetric demonstrates relative strengths in areas of visual-spatial perception, visual construction when motor planning requirements are minimized, visual working memory, and learning and memory for visual-spatial material when repetition and structure are provided. These are contrasted by relative weaknesses in problem-solving/sequential reasoning ability, expressive and receptive language, auditory/verbal working memory and learning, motor planning, and fine motor functioning of the right (dominant) hand. Academically, Demetric demonstrates relative strengths in basic word identification and spelling contrasted by significant weaknesses in math reasoning and reading comprehension consistent with his history of language impairment. Behaviorally, Demetric continues to have attention difficulties at home, in conjunction with difficulty adapting to change in routine and poor social skills. These difficulties were not endorsed by his teacher at school. Taken together, this pattern of neuropsychological test performance continues to be consistent with a diagnosis of specific language impairment (receptive and expressive type), with associated specific learning disability in reading comprehension and mathematical reasoning. Demetric's attention problems reportedly are improving at home, and his teachers did not observe his attention as problematic in the classroom.

Recommendations

- Continued and intensive language therapy is needed.
  - In order for the benefits of the language therapy to generalize and be maintained across settings, the therapy should be implemented across settings.
  - To facilitate this, it is suggested that Demetric's mother participate in a home-based language therapy program developed and monitored by Demetric's speech-language therapist.
  - In this way, Demetric's mother could learn about new techniques for supporting his special needs, and Demetric could learn the importance of using these skills on a consistent basis.
- Given his deficient linguistic and auditory working memory skills, it is recommended that reading/writing instruction emphasize visual and multisensory approaches instead of phonetic approaches. For example, emphasis should be placed on memorizing words commonly used in text, such as the Dolche sight-word list.
- In order to enhance Demetric's learning/retention, new material should be presented in an organized format that is meaningful to him. Instruction should be supplemented with visual aids, demonstrations, and experiential learning, given his strengths in visual learning and memory. Procedural learning also should be emphasized.
- In light of his deficits in receptive language, adults (e.g., teachers, therapists, parents) should keep in mind several general rules when interacting with Demetric:
  - Eye contact should be ensured.
  - A prompt to look at the speaker before directions are presented will be helpful.
  - Instructions and directions should be kept short, simple, and concrete.
  - Requests should be limited to single commands.
  - Complex tasks should be broken down into smaller components or steps, and instructions should be presented several times, orally and in writing.
- Demetric also will benefit from accommodations, including preferential seating, extended time, shortened assignments, and one-on-one assistance (in order to clarify directions, etc.).
- Training in word processing is strongly encouraged. Most word processing programs are equipped with spell check, as well as cut and paste options. Appropriate instruction on how to use these functions effectively will be increasingly valuable as written expression demands increase during Demetric's education.

  Given Demetric's deficits in executive functioning, he may require instruction on how to organize and plan his approach to novel and complex tasks. Direct instruction in basic organizational strategies will assist Demetric in knowing what to do, when to do it, and how to do it.

- He should be guided in the use of checklists and other organizational aids.
- As Demetric approaches middle school, study skills training will be warranted, emphasizing such techniques as the appropriate outlining of lecture notes and how to study for tests.
- He also will benefit from being taught how to take notes using a shorthand (outlining) method.

- A behavior management program also should be implemented as part of Demetric's Individualized Education Plan both at home and within the classroom to provide Demetric with the structure and positive reinforcement he needs to stay on task, listen, and complete his assignments.
- At home and at school, Demetric should be encouraged to participate in chores, engage in independent self-care, and become more capable in areas of daily living. This may require initial assistance and direction, fading adult assistance gradually over time.

Further Discussion of Case Study

Demetric met the classic picture of lead exposure; however, it is necessary to discern, or at least try to discern, the extent to which these deficits are the result of lead poisoning as opposed to socioeconomic status and psychosocial issues. Based on Demetric's family history, there is no indication that he would be at risk for these difficulties other than as a result of lead exposure. Results indicating weaknesses in language skills and auditory working memory were able to inform educational programming, so that Demetric could experience maximal benefit from instruction.

CONCLUDING COMMENTS

The vulnerability of the CNS to environmental toxins, prenatally and postnatally, is well documented and necessitates the consideration of detailed environmental history when children, particularly those living in at-risk areas (e.g., urban poor, agricultural), are referred for neuropsychological evaluation (Hussain, Woolf, Sandel, & Shannon, 2007). With the strong association of toxic exposure effects and poverty, evaluation of possible toxicity may need to be accounted for when assessing children from low socioeconomic status. Although the United States has restricted the use of many environmental toxins, the same is not true in other countries; toxic levels of lead, for example, can be found in refugee children (Bustos & Goldstein, 2008). The extent to which exposure (at what level, for what duration) contributes to specific disorders (e.g., ADHD, learning disabilities, autism spectrum disorders) remains unknown. Although the overall effect of exposure may be small, it has been argued that any decrease in functioning significantly changes the proportion of the affected population that is in the lower ends of the normal distribution (Needleman, 1994). Review of the status of what is known about children's exposure to varied neurotoxins indicates a need for further information related to the identification of developmental benchmarks that may be affected by exposure as well as the monitoring of exposure access over time with multiple methods to yield aggregate exposure models (Cohen Hubal et al., 2000).

As with other insults or injuries to the CNS, it has been suggested that there is a critical period for impairment by neurotoxins (Mendola, Selevan, Gutter, & Rice, 2002; D. C. Rice, 1996); although Rice made this argument specific to lead and PCBs, the same argument would apply to environmental toxins of any kind. Different functional domains of the brain develop at different times and differing rates (Luria, 1980); thus, it would be expected that differential effects would occur as a result of variance in exposure levels over the developmental course. Results of Aldridge et al. (2005) further suggest that depending on the developmental period, even exposure levels generally considered to be nontoxic may have lasting effects on the CNS. Much of the literature specific to PCB and lead effects is equivocal and has been criticized as lacking in systematic, prospective design (Cicchetti, Kaufman, & Sparrow, 2004; Phelps, 1999).

It is important to remember that some of the developmental effects may not be seen immediately following exposure but may unfold over the developmental course (Colborn, 2006). For all neurotoxins, what continues to be questionable is the extent of subtle deficit that may be associated with chronic as well as acute exposure during the developmental process. Disabling effects of environmental toxins on the developing neurological system are associated with considerable controversy and misunderstanding; there is still too little known about the developmental impacts and long-term outcomes in relation to type, duration, intensity, and timing of exposure (Dietrich, 2000). Future research needs to address these methodological concerns; further, there is a need for future research to consider not only all environmental and chemical exposures but social context and genetic influences in developing a neurodevelopmental phenotype for exposure to environmental toxins (Dietrich et al., 2005).

Chapter 14

NEUROTOXINS, PREGNANCY, AND SUBSEQUENT DISORDERS

DEFINITION AND ETIOLOGY

Environmental toxins (see Chapter 13) are not the only teratogens that can have an impact on neurodevelopmental functioning; studies consistently indicate that substance use and use of medications by pregnant women places their unborn children at risk. Regardless of whether the substance is alcohol, opiates, cocaine, or nicotine, the associated deficits in self-regulation, attentional control, overreactivity, and excitability have been noted (Bandstra, Morrow, Anthony, Accornero, & Fried, 2001; Bard, Coles, Platzman, & Lynch, 2000; Molitor, Mayes, & Ward, 2003). These effects likely are associated with neuronal suppression and neuronal cell death (i.e., apoptosis) as a result of exposure; whether effects are cognitive, sensory, or behavioral is believed to be related to the timing and duration of exposure. With increased knowledge of the effects of drugs on the developing fetus, considerable caution also is exercised with regard to the use of medications of any type by pregnant women (Bercovici, 2005). In some cases, however, such as women with epilepsy, bipolar disorder, or schizophrenia, avoidance of medication is not feasible; in other instances, medications may be prescribed to address concerns with the maintenance of the pregnancy (e.g., diethylstilbestrol, thalidomide). Consistently, although to differing degrees, effects of medications taken by the mother on the developing fetus have been identified (Pillard et al., 1993; Titus-Ernstoff et al., 2003), with increased vulnerability perceived as a function of genotype (Meador, Baker, Cohen, Gaily, & Westerveld, 2007).

Recreational Substances: Alcohol

Of the recreational substances, fetal alcohol effects are the most studied and one of the more common known causes of mental retardation (Stratton, Howe, & Battaglia, 1996). Fetal alcohol syndrome (FAS) is estimated to be present in 1.9 to 4.8 per 1,000 live births globally (Abel & Sokol, 1987), with some effects in up to 9.1 per 1,000 live births (Sampson et al., 1997). Although this is the case, many individuals who suffer from prenatal alcohol exposure do not meet the full criteria for FAS yet suffer from many of the negative effects that accompany FAS (Green, 2007). Fetal alcohol exposure can have a variety of negative effects on a child's brain structure that can lead to neuropsychological anomalies; the damage to the brain is believed to vary depending on the specific circumstances surrounding the intake of alcohol with potential discernible effects on the fetus (Green, 2007). It is important to note that alcohol easily crosses the placenta, with the fetus experiencing the same blood alcohol levels as the mother (Stratton et al., 1996; Streissguth, 1997). The range of deficits associated with prenatal alcohol exposure are subsumed under the global heading of fetal alcohol spectrum disorders (FASD). FASD, fetal alcohol syndrome (FAS), fetal alcohol effects (FAE), Partial fetal alcohol syndrome (pFAS), alcohol-related neurodevelopmental disorders (ARND), static encephalopathy alcohol exposure (SEAE), and alcohol-related birth defects (ARBD) are all disorders that occur when a pregnant woman consumes alcohol. Diagnosis of FASD is based on a combination of (1) prenatal or postnatal growth deficiency; (2) facial dysmorphology, including smaller eye openings, smooth philtrum (i.e., underdeveloped groove between the nose and upper lip), and flattened cheekbones; and (3) central nervous system (CNS) dysfunction (Stratton et al., 1996).

The range of characteristics associated with FASD includes low birth weight, small head circumference, failure to thrive, developmental delays in motor and language areas, and poor socialization skills. Many children exposed to alcohol do not exhibit these symptoms to the same degree; hence the adoption of FASD as representing the potential continuum of alcohol-related disorders (Streissguth et al., 2004). ARND is a recently identified category of those children in the FASD spectrum who exhibit only the behavioral and emotional problems without any signs of developmental delay or physical growth deficiencies. ARND and FAE are most likely underdiagnosed due to more subtle deficits. Exposure to alcohol during fetal development disrupts the development of brain cells as well as cell migration and also affects the neural circuitry of the brain. Consequently, an imbalance in electrophysiological and neurochemical functions occurs, causing an inadequate and dysfunctional message transmission within the brain (Ferraro & Zevenbergen, 2001). Initial studies indicated that FAS was associated with dysmorphogenesis of the brain, giving rise to the multiple functional abnormalities associated with the syndrome (Delis, Jones, Mattson, & Riles, 1998; K. L. Jones & Smith, 1973; Roebuck, Mattson, & Riley, 1998).

Neurological Correlates

Fetal alcohol exposure may have a variety of presentations depending on exposure characteristics and vulnerability of the CNS at the time of exposure such that the brain regions and cell populations that are developing at the time will be more susceptible to impact (Kaemingk & Paquette, 1999). Dysmorphogenesis of the brain may present as small brain volume, small basal ganglia, small cerebellum, or a small or absent corpus callosum (Ferraro & Zevenbergen, 2001), with the continuum of potential consequences of fetal alcohol exposure ranging from severe to mild deficits (C. M. Clark, Conry, Conry, Li, & Loock, 2000). Microcephaly is one of the frequent findings associated with fetal alcohol exposure (Kaemingk & Paquette, 1999); there are three possible ways in which ethanol could result in microcephaly (Sampson et al., 1997). Microcephaly in FAS individuals could be the result of ethanol affecting the neural membranes and impairing their growth; alternatively, ethanol may affect the intermediary metabolism that could affect cell proliferation and growth. Finally, microcephaly may be the outcome of alcohol's effects on transmitter function, which could alter development and consequently stunt growth. There is some evidence that fetal alcohol exposure could result in abnormal functioning of the CNS via the effects on brain ion channels (Costa, Savage, & Valenzuela, 2000); however, the majority of these studies have been with rodents or other animals rather than humans. Various studies have indicated that the smaller brain volume is due primarily to differences in the frontal lobe and left-hemisphere volume (Jernigan et al., 2002; Rasmussen, 2005). For example, in a study of 70 pregnant women who were moderate to heavy drinkers between 12 and 42 weeks of gestation, it was found that exposure to ethanol was clearly related to the size of the child's frontal cortex (Rasmussen, 2005). Furthermore, the study found that 23% of the fetuses exposed to alcohol had a frontal cortex that was below the 10th percentile in size, in comparison to the control group, where only 4% experienced below-average-size frontal lobes.

In addition to volumetric differences, there has been investigation of the differential loss of cells in white or gray matter (S. L. Archibald et al., 2001). In a study using magnetic resonance imaging (MRI) of children prenatally exposed to alcohol, it was found that there was a deterioration of both white matter mass and gray matter mass in the cerebrum, but white matter volumes were more impacted than gray matter volumes. A spin-off study conducted by the same group of researchers sought to examine the possibility of gray matter or white matter disproportionately being affected in the cerebellum and/or cerebrum. In agreement with prior findings, a significant reduction of white matter occurred in the cerebrum, in addition to a smaller, nonsignificant, white matter reduction observed in the cerebellum (S. L. Archibald et al., 2001). Thus, in individuals diagnosed with FASD, white matter hypoplasia is more severe than gray matter hypoplasia in the cerebrum; it was further noted that both white and gray matter volumes were reduced in the parietal lobe, with increased volumes of white matter in the occipital lobe (S. L. Archibald et al., 2001). Based on MRI analysis with a group of six children and adolescents with FASD, it was determined that both the lenticular region of the basal ganglia and the caudate were significantly smaller in the participants with FASD (S. N. Mattson, Riley, & Roebuck, 1998) with anticipated effects in the children's ability to shift tasks, inhibition of inappropriate behavior, and spatial memory (S. N. Mattson, Riley, & Schoenfeld, 2001). In a study of 14 participants with FAS, 12 participants with prenatal exposure to alcohol, and 14 control participants, there was a disproportionate reduction of caudate nucleus volume in FAS volunteers in comparison to the exposure and nonexposure groups (S. L. Archibald et al., 2001). This was further supported by a single case study of a child with FAS conducted with positron emission tomography (C. M. Clark, Conry, Li, & Loock, 1993).

Since the 1970s, studies have found significant abnormalities to the cerebellum due to prenatal alcohol exposure for both animal studies (A. Y. Goodlet et al., 2001) and humans (Obrzut & Wacha, 2007). Autopsy studies with FAS participants have found a range of cerebellar abnormalities, including cerebellar dysgenesis, cerebellar heterotopic cell clusters, and agenesis of the cerebellar vermis (C. R. Goodlet, Hannigan, Spear, & Spear, 1999). The most commonly reported anomaly found in autopsy studies is cerebellar hypoplasia; however, hypoplasia does not arise in every FAS individual. Findings in animal studies have demonstrated that neonatal alcohol exposure generates a significant loss of cerebellar Purkinje cells (A. Y. Goodlet et al., 2001). With regard to the corpus callosum, there is not only increased likelihood of agenesis of the corpus callosum, but autopsy studies also have found abnormalities of the anterior commissure ranging from agenesis to underdevelopment. MRI studies have also had equivocal results. In a study of 9 individuals with FAS, MRI found partial agenesis in 3 out of 9 individuals, hypoplasia in one case, and midline abnormalities in another case (S. N. Mattson, Riley, & Roebuck, 1998).

Illicit Drug Use

Cocaine and Amphetamine Abuse

Consistent with the findings that prenatal alcohol exposure can result in long-term adverse effects on brain development, there is evidence that illicit drug exposure also impacts on brain function and development in the fetus. Of the illicit drugs, cocaine is the most extensively studied. Despite initial beliefs that there would be significant findings, most notably, cocaine use is associated with low birth weight and decreased gestational age (R. W. Keller & Snyder-Keller, 2000; Schempf, 2007). Similarly, amphetamine abuse is also associated with prematurity and poor fetal growth (Cox, Posner, Kourtis, & Jamieson, 2008). Cerebral infarctions, reduced head circumference, and increased risk of seizures also have been identified (R. W. Keller & Snyder-Keller, 2000). Results of other studies have not consistently suggested any relation between maternal cocaine use and infant outcome (Richardson & Day, 1991).

Opiates, Marijuana, and Other Drugs

Use of opiates and marijuana also are associated with lower birth weight or shorter gestational age (Schempf, 2007). There are some indications that prenatal opiate exposure is associated with attention problems and impulsivity (Accornero et al., 2007; Suess, Newlin, & Porges, 1997). In contrast, prenatal exposure to marijuana is associated with decreased social engagement and increased fearfulness as well as problems with inattention and impulsivity (Faden & Graubard, 2000). In another study, there was a nonlinear relationship between marijuana use and child intelligence such that heavy use during the first trimester was associated with lower verbal reasoning, but heavy use during the second trimester was associated with lower composite scores as well as deficits in short-term memory and quantitative scores. Heavy use in the third semester was associated with lower quantitative scores (Goldschmidt, Richardson, Willford, & Day, 2008). Methodological problems with these and other studies (e.g., not controlling for psychosocial, nutritional, environmental factors) make interpretation of these findings difficult (Schempf, 2007).

Polydrug Exposure

Often children who were exposed to one drug were exposed to multiple drugs. Polydrug exposure is associated with either increased or decreased reactivity and arousal (Lewis & Weiss, 2003) as well as increased irritability, hyperactivity, increased startle reactions, and problems with being consoled (Higley & Morin, 2004; Lester et al., 2002; S. J. Weiss & Wilson, 2006). As noted earlier, the extent to which these effects are related primarily to the polydrug use, as opposed to psychosocial and environmental factors, including access to prenatal care and nutritional status, is unknown (Schempf, 2007).

Fetal Anticonvulsant Syndromes

Consistently, although to differing degrees, effects of medications taken by the mother on the developing fetus are being identified; however, results are equivocal (Adab, Tudur, Vinten, Williamson, & Winterbottom, 2004). In general, polytherapy exposure and exposure to antiepileptics is associated with poorer outcomes (Adab, Tudur et al., 2004; P. Crawford, 2002). The mechanisms by which maternal medications can impact the developing fetus are believed to occur due to either effects on neurotransmitters prenatally (and associated changes in neural organization) or effects of withdrawal at the time of birth (Bercovici, 2005). The effects of maternal medications are believed to differentially impact the developing child. Onc factor that mediates the effects of medication is that of timing. During the very early stages of the pregnancy, there is the greatest risk of major changes due to the rapid cell division, differentiation, and migration (Gilstrap & Little, 1998). There is still continued risk beyond the embryonic period, with more minor abnormalities or physiological defects. Risk does not end at birth; most drugs can be detected in breast milk, but at low concentrations (Arnon, Schechtman, & Ornaoy, 2000).

Of particular interest are those medications used in the control of epilepsy, given that 6.1 per 1,000 pregnancies occur in women with epilepsy (Fairgrieve et al., 2000). Prenatal exposure to antiepileptics is associated with increased risk of neurodevelopmental effects (Atkinson, Brice-Bennett, & D'Souza, 2007; Kulkarni, Zaheeruddin, Shenoy, & Vani, 2006; Moore et al., 2000) with an incidence of 6% to 9% (Kaneko et al., 1999). The possible effects include prematurity, low birth weight, increased fetal and neonatal death rates, congenital malformations, developmental delay, and behavioral/ cognitive defects (Meador et al., 2006). Neural tube defects, cardiac malformation, and orofacial defects are the more common anatomic abnormalities (Meador et al., 2006). Exposure to antiepileptic drugs continues through lactation, although to a lesser degree. Combined with the potential benefits, the potential risks lead to considerable controversy over the practice of breastfeeding by mothers on these medications (Pennell et al., 2007). Common characteristics of fetal anticonvulsant syndromes include congenital malformation, distinct facial features, myopia, joint laxity, and other minor anomalies (J. Dean et al., 2007). Animal studies consistently indicate the potential for multiple teratogenic effects of anticonvulsant drugs (Meador, 2002b).

While most of the research has been retrospective, the establishment of various pregnancy registries and follow-up procedures have added to a growing prospective knowledge base. Exposure effects have been identified for various medications; however, in general, the continued use of phenytoin (Dilantin) and lamotrogine (Lamictal) is less often associated with major birth defects (J. Dean et al., 2002; Eberhard-Gran, Eskild, & Opjordsmoen, 2006). Of the antiepileptic drugs, sodium valproate (Depakote) often is prescribed due to its broad anticonvulsant action as well as its less sedative and behavioral side effects as compared to other antiepileptic drugs (Carrion et al., 2007). For example, of 414 children exposed to lamotrogine alone and 182 exposed to lamotrogine and some other antiepileptic other than valproate, major birth defects occurred in 2.9% and 2.7% respectively (Cunningham, Tennis, & International Lamotrigine Pregnancy Registry Scientific Advisory Committee, 2005). In contrast, for the 88 children who were exposed to lamotrogine and valproate, the incidence of major birth defects increased to 12.5% (Cunningham et al., 2005). Notably, a majority of major malformations are identified within the first five days after birth, particularly with valproate exposure (Meador et al., 2006; Wyszynski et al., 2005). Carbamazepine (Tegretol) is another antiepileptic medication. In utero exposure to carbamazepine monotherapy was not associated with decreased cognitive function (Wide, Henning, Tomson, & Winbladh, 2002).

Fetal Valproate Syndrome

The risks associated with in utero exposure to valproate (Wide, Winbladh, & Källén, 2004) led to the identification of fetal valproate syndrome (FVS) as a potential result when pregnant women are taking sodium valproate. Sodium valproate is a widely used medication for the treatment of epilepsy that first was approved for use in 1978; it also is increasingly used for managing bipolar and other mood disorders. Sodium valproate or valproic acid acts either by inhibiting gamma-aminobutyric acid (GABA) metabolism or by a direct effect on mitochondria, thereby impairing cellular energy metabolism (J. K. Brown, 1988); it binds to plasma proteins and may displace other drugs if used in combination with other antiepileptics, giving rise to toxicity. The first adverse report on the developing fetus was published in 1980 (Dalens, Raynaud, & Gaulme, 1980); since then, considerable case studies and clinical research have been conducted to examine the potential teratogenic effects of valproic acid. It is estimated that there is six to seven times greater likelihood of malformations in infants of mothers who took sodium valproate (Kulkarni et al., 2006). Various factors contribute to the likelihood of neurodevelopmental effects of valproic acid, including the number of drugs that are coadministered, drug dosage, differences in metabolism (both infant and mother), and the gestational age of the fetus at exposure, length of exposure, and hereditary susceptibility (Alsdorf & Wyszynski, 2005; H. Malm et al., 2002). It is known that valproic acid crosses the placenta and is present in a higher concentration in the fetus than in the mother (Clayton Smith & Donnai, 1995; Jager-Roman et al., 1986). Based on available research, valproate above 800 to 1,000 mg/day increases the risk of congenital malformations and FVS, in excess of the risks with other antiepileptics (Meador et al., 2009; Perruca, 2005; Tomson & Battino, 2005; Wyszynski et al., 2005). At the same time, however, it is acknowledged that valproate requires fewer dose adjustments and is more effective in seizure control than other antiepileptics (Vajda et al., 2006).

FVS is characterized by distinctive facial appearance as well as other minor and major anomalies; it has been suggested, however, that the extent to which dysmorphic features are solely the result of exposure to antiepileptics is inconclusive (J. Dean et al., 2002; Kini et al., 2006). Some of the more frequent major congenital malformations are neural tube defects, congenital heart defects, oral clefts, genital abnormalities, and limb defects. Approximately 10% of babies are small for gestational age; a low Apgar score and withdrawal symptoms during the neonatal period are common (Clayton Smith & Donnai, 1995; Thisted & Ebbeson, 1993). The most frequent of withdrawal symptoms are irritability, jitteriness, hypotonia, and seizures, which typically occur between 12 and 48 hours of life; these tend to be dose related (Clayton Smith & Donnai, 1995; Thisted & Ebbeson, 1993). Prenatal diagnosis tends to be focused on the detection of neural tube defects as these are frequent major malformations (Alsdorf & Wyszynski, 2005; Yerby, 2003). Neural tube defects have been estimated to occur at around 10 to 20 times the normal incidence with prenatal exposure to valproate; this appears to be specifically related to valproate therapy rather than to other anticonvulsants (Alsdorf & Wyszynski, 2005; Clayton Smith & Donnai, 1995). Neural tube defects are more likely to present as spina bifida than as anencephaly, and there is predisposition for very low lumbar or sacral defects, suggesting that there is increased likelihood of valproate affecting primarily the lowest closure site of the neural tube (Van Allen, Kalousek, & Chernoff, 1993). The likelihood of neural tube defects is associated with the use of medications during the first trimester, low serum folate concentration, and low level of maternal education (Kaaja, Kaaja, & Hiilesmaa, 2003); there is also increased risk of neural tube deficits if there is a family history of such defects (J. Dean et al., 2007). Other less frequent abnormalities include hernia, supernumerary nipple, postaxial polydactyly, bifid ribs, and preaxial defect of feet (Christianson, Cheslar, & Kromber, 1994). Postnatal growth appears to be normal, and general health is good. In some cases, the malformations are consistent with Baller-Gerold syndrome, suggesting that changes in the biochemical environment may precipitate the Baller-Gerold phenotype (Santos de Oliveira, Lejeunie, Arnaud, & Renier, 2005).

Mood Stabilizers

Depression can affect 10% to 16% of pregnant women (Laine, Heikkinen, Ekblad, & Kero, 2003); bipolar disorder is estimated to affect 0.5% to 1.5% of individuals with a typical age of onset at late adolescence or early adulthood (Yonkers et al., 2004). Further, it is during the childbearing years that women are at greatest risk for depression; this increases the likelihood that a woman taking antidepressants will become pregnant (J. L. Morrison, Riggs, & Rurak, 2005). Management of bipolar disorder in women of childbearing age presents many challenges due to the potential for complications and adverse effects of continued medication during the pregnancy weighed against potential risks of not providing medical intervention; notably, valproate and carbamazepine are now also used frequently in the treatment of bipolar disorder. Use of mood stabilizers, including lithium, has been associated with poor neonatal adaptation (Eberhard-Gran, Eskild, & Opjordsmoen, 2005). In particular, lithium may increase the rate of congenital heart defects (Arnon et al., 2000) or goiter and hypothyroidism (Frassetto et al., 2002). Although results are equivocal, significantly lower Apgar scores, longer hospital stays, and high rates of neuromuscular problems have been associated with higher lithium levels at birth (Newport et al., 2005).

Management of depression with tricyclic antidepressants and selective serotonin reuptake inhibitors (SSRIs) historically has been judged to be less teratogenic (Arnon et al., 2000). There are no indications, for example, that SSRI exposure in utero is associated with major congenital malformations (Kulin, Pastuszak, & Koren, 1998; Kulin, Pastuszak, Sage et al., 1998), although there are some indications of minor anomalies (Chambers, Johnson, Dick, Felix, & Jones, 1996). SSRIs affect the serotonin levels, potentially impacting on sleep cycles, circadian rhythms, and the hypothalamic-pituitary-adrenal axis (J. L. Morrison et al., 2005); low birth weight and prematurity are common among infants exposed prenatally to SSRIs (G. Simon, Cunningham, & Davis, 2002). To the extent that some research findings indicate effects, it is not clear if effects are from withdrawal or toxicity (Knoppert, Nimkar, Principi, & Yuen, 2006). Behaviors associated with neonatal withdrawal include irritability, poor feeding, respiratory distress, seizures, and jitteriness (Haddad, 2001; A. Lee, Inch, & Finnigan, 2000). These symptoms can emerge as early as 72 hours postpartum with varying duration. Animal studies indicate that chronic neonatal exposure to specific SSRIs alters serotonin synthetic enzymes as well as serotonin transport expression and that these changes continue into adulthood (Maciag et al., 2006; J. L. Morrison et al., 2005). Mean levels of platelet serotonin (5-HT) in newborns exposed to SSRIs in utero was found to be substantially lower as compared to newborns not exposed; 5-HT levels increased and were found to be at near-adult levels by 1 month of age (G. M. Anderson, Czarkowski, Ravski, & Epperson, 2004). Overall, results of studies investigating the effects of SSRIs are equivocal (Chambers et al., 1996; Koren, 2001; Vorhees et al., 1994). In general, there are no major structural abnormalities; however, there are some subtle motor deficits, behavioral issues, and minor anomalies associated with maternal use of fluoxetine (Prozac), for example, during pregnancy (Casper et al., 2003; Chambers et al., 1996; Zeskind & Stephens, 2004).

Anxiolytics

Benzodiazepines are among the most frequently prescribed medications for anxiety disorders; the mechanism of action for benzodiazepines is via the gamma-amino butyric receptor A (GABA A), an inhibitory receptor (Bercovici, 2005). It has been suggested that 2% of pregnant women may be taking benzodiazepines (Koren, 2001). Benzodiazepines during first trimester are associated with orofacial clefts as well as difficulties with neonatal adaptation (Eberhard-Gran et al., 2005). Sufficient evidence exists to suggest a phenotype for benzodiazepine syndrome (Gilstrap & Little, 1998; Iqbal, Sobhan, & Ryals, 2002; Laegreid, Olegard, Walstrom, & Conradi, 1992) similar to FASD. Characteristics include facial dysmorphism (slanted eyes and epicanthal folds), hypotonia, delayed motor development, microcephaly, varying degrees of mental retardation, and convulsions. Potential neonatal withdrawal similar to that evidenced with SSRIs has been noted as well (Gilstrap & Little, 1998; Iqbal et al., 2002). More research on the effects of benzodiazepine use on the developing fetus is needed (G. M. Anderson, 2004).

COURSE AND PROGNOSIS: FASD AND ILLICIT DRUGS

FASD

Outcomes associated with FASD include effects on general cognitive ability and difficulties with learning and memory and visual-spatial function (S. N. Mattson, Riley, Gramling, Delis, & Jones, 1998); one of the hallmarks of FASD is a deficit in attention (S. N. Mattson, Calarco, & Lang, 2006; Riley & McGee, 2005). Behaviorally, children exposed to alcohol prenatally may exhibit hyperactivity, increased anxiety, and decreased self-regulation. Variability in expression of FASD is related to a number of risk factors, including blood alcohol levels, the pattern of exposure, timing of exposure, genetic vulnerability, and interaction with nutritional variables as well as synergistic reactions with other drugs (Delis et al., 1998; S. N. Mattson et al., 1998).

Infants prenatally exposed to alcohol demonstrated decreased arousal and slower habituation to stimuli within a few days postpartum (Ferraro & Zevenbergen, 2001). Infants exposed in utero also demonstrated unusual reflexive responses and slower information processing compared to infants that had no in utero exposure to alcohol (Jacobson, 1998). At 8 weeks of age, prenatal drug exposure and preterm status were related to dysregulation (Bard et al., 2000). Over time, fetal alcohol exposure is characterized by neuropsychological impairments that include deficits in declarative learning, cognitive flexibility, processing speed, memory, attention, visual-spatial abilities, lower IQ scores, hyperactivity, impulsivity, problem solving, and learning problems (Caine, Delis, Goodman, Mattson, & Riley, 1999; Carmichael, Feldman, Streissguth, & Gonzalez, 1992; Green, 2007; Kodituwakku, Handmaker, Cutler, Weathersby, & Handmaker, 1995; S. N. Mattson, Goodman, Caine, Delis, & Riley, 1999; S. N. Mattson, Riley, Gramling et al., 1998; Rasmussen, 2005).

Facial characteristics associated with FASD become less distinctive over time; however, adolescents and adults with FASD continue to be shorter and to have slightly smaller heads as compared to controls (Streissguth et al., 1991). For example, there is a higher likelihood of conduct problems among children with prenatal alcohol exposure (D'Onofrio et al., 2007). For the 61 adolescents and adults in the Streissguth et al. (1991) study, there was significant variability in cognitive ability. Academically, math deficits were prominent; behaviorally, deficits in social judgment and problem solving as well as increased distractibility were evident. Problems associated with FASD tend to intensify as children move into adulthood. These can include mental health problems, troubles with the law, and the inability to live independently.

Related to the decreased volume of the frontal lobes, there is evidence of executive function deficits associated with FASD. Using the Wisconsin Card Sorting Test (WCST), children with FASD made more perseverative responses and were less accurate at the categories they achieved than controls who did not have exposure to alcohol; however, the performance of the children with FASD was consistent with their overall cognitive ability (Cutler, Handmaker, Handmaker, Kodituwakku, & Weathersby, 1995). Similarly, using the Delis-Kaplan Executive Function Scale (D-KEFS), in comparison to the control group, the children exposed to alcohol exhibited discrepancies on measures of cognitive flexibility, planning ability, selective inhibition, concept formation, and reasoning (Caine et al., 1999; S. N. Mattson et al., 1999). More recent research has continued to demonstrate that children with FASD perform lower on executive function tasks than do control groups (Obrzut & Wacha, 2007). Children with FASD tend to use the same problem-solving approaches or responses, even after they know they are incorrect from past responses, which also demonstrates a malfunction in executive skills (Obrzut & Wacha, 2007). Regardless of whether the substance is alcohol, opiates, cocaine, or nicotine, deficits in executive function, including self-regulation, attentional control, overreactivity, and excitability, have been noted (Bandstra et al., 2001; Bard et al., 2000; Molitor et al., 2003). By age 12, it is estimated that 90% of individuals with FASD have mental health problems and 50% experience difficulties in school and trouble with the law (Streissguth, Barr, Kogan, & Bookstein, 1996). Further, polysubstance use tends to be associated with inattention and impulsivity (D'Onofrio et al., 2007). Characteristics associated with various substances are summarized in Table 14.1.

Of the many deficiencies associated with FAS, short-term and long-term memory often are impacted in a negative way by prenatal exposure to alcohol (Streissguth, 1997). Using a variety of measures including the Wechsler Memory Scale, the Seashore Rhythm Test, the Peabody Picture Vocabulary Test (PPVT), and a stepping-stone maze with 7 individuals with FAS, it was determined that participants performed below the (same sex, same age) control group on all of the assessments, consistent with impairment to memory due to prenatal alcohol exposure (Streissguth et al., 1991). Although research concerning working memory is sparse, there are indications that working memory also may be impacted by fetal exposure to alcohol. For example, children exposed to alcohol have been found to perform below average on the digit span task (H. M. Barr, Sampson, & Streissguth, 1990; Jacobson, 1998). In adulthood, fetal exposure to alcohol has been associated with impaired performance on the consonant trigrams test (Rasmussen, 2005).

Potentially related to frontal lobes or hippocampal effects of exposure, in a study of 15 Native American children with FAS or FAE, researchers used the Memory for Objects task and found that the children with hippocampal damage performed significantly lower on both immediate and delayed recall for object locations (Kaemingk & Paquette, 1999).

Table 14.1 Deficits Associated with Use of Specific Recreational Substances During Pregnancy

Alcohol	Processing speed Attention Emotional regulation Conduct problems/externalizing behaviors Motor deficits
Cocaine	Sustained attention Distractibility High reactivity High impulsivity Poor emotional regulation
Marijuana	Use in first trimester: lower verbal reasoning; second trimester: general ability, short-term memory, quantitative skills; third trimester: quantitative skills Behavioral problems (inattention, fearfulness, poor socialization)

On a test of object recall, however, the children could remember the object in question but could not recall spatial information regarding the object needed to accomplish the requirement necessary to fulfill the task (Nadel & Uecker, 1998). Thus, the research suggests that prenatal alcohol exposure can have effects on memory that are likely to be evidenced from childhood to adulthood.

Illicit Drugs

Some studies indicate that prenatal exposure to cocaine is associated with difficulty with emotional regulation, higher levels of arousal, increased reactivity, and problems with sustained attention and distractibility (Accornero et al., 2007; Bandstra et al., 2001; Bard et al., 2000; Coles, Bard, Platzman, & Lynch, 1999; R. W. Keller & Snyder-Keller, 2000; Molitor et al., 2003; S. J. Weiss, St. Jonn-Seed, & Harris-Muchell, 2007). Although there are some indications of initial behavioral irritability and high levels of reactivity, these behaviors are less noticeable one month after birth (R. W. Keller & Snyder-Keller, 2000). Alternatively, preschoolers exposed to cocaine were more likely to exhibit impulsivity (i.e., increased commission errors) while preschoolers exposed to marijuana were more likely to exhibit attentional problems (i.e., increased omission errors) in a large sample of children (Noland et al., 2005). Preschoolers exposed to cocaine in utero were more likely to have mild receptive language delays (B. A. Lewis et al., 2004) and to score lower on the mental development index (L. T. Singer et al., 2002). At 7 years of age, it was found that mean scores of children exposed to cocaine in utero evidenced lower cognitive ability, depressed visual-motor abilities, and depressed motor skills (Arendt et al., 2004). In one study, it was found that cocaine-exposed children were 2.8 times more likely to be identified with a learning disability by age 7 as compared to a control group (Morrow et al., 2006). Results, however, are equivocal, with other studies failing to find differences (L. T. Singer et al., 2004). Also through at least age 7, there are some indications of cocaine-associated deficits in attention (Accornero et al., 2007). A major problem with determining effects of prenatal exposure, with any of the illicit drugs are the difficulties with parceling out environmental and psychosocial factors associated with maternal drug use (Schempf, 2007). Further, most of the studies do not examine effects through adolescence or adulthood. It has been suggested that the greatest risk associated with maternal substance use is that of poverty, neglect, and maltreatment as well as chaotic home environments and potential foster care placement (Hans, 1999). In general, children with in utero exposure to alcohol and illicit drugs tend to be at risk for learning disabilities, attentional problems, and impulsive behaviors; however, the extent to which this is due to the exposure or ongoing maternal drug use and related environmental factors is unknown (Pulsifer, Butz, O'Reilly Foran, & Belcher, 2008; Schempf, 2007).

CASE STUDY: CALEB—FETAL ALCOHOL SYNDROME

The next report is from a hospital-based clinic. Identifying information, such as child and family name, teacher or physician name, and school information, has been altered or fictionalized to protect confidentiality.

Reason for Referral

Caleb is a 7-year-old first grader who is being initially evaluated by the pediatric neuropsychology service at the request of his maternal aunt/adoptive mother who is requesting an assessment of cognitive functioning due to a history of fetal alcohol exposure throughout the pregnancy. As a result, neuropsychological evaluation was undertaken in order to assess higher cortical functioning and make appropriate recommendations regarding school placement and the need for supportive therapies.

Assessment Procedures

Clinical interview

Behavioral observations

Wechsler Intelligence Scale for Children, Fourth Edition (WISC-IV)

Behavioral Rating Inventory of Executive Functioning (BRIEF)

Neuropsychological Assessment (NEPSY)/Neuropsychological Assessment, Second Edition (NEPSY-2; selected subtests)

Kaufman Assessment Battery for Children, Second Edition (KABC-2; selected subtests)

Expressive One Word Picture Vocabulary Test (EOWPVT)

Developmental Test of Visual Motor Integration, Fifth Edition (DTVMI-V)

Children's Memory Scale (CMS)

Peabody Picture Vocabulary Test, Fourth Edition (PPVT-IV)

Boston Naming Test (BNT)

Clock Face Drawing Test

Clinical Evaluation of Language Fundamentals, Fourth Edition (CELF-IV; selected subtests)

Finger Tapping Test

Behavior Assessment System for Children, Second Edition (BASC-2)

DSM-IV ADHD Checklist

Gray Oral Reading Test, Fourth Edition (GORT-4)

Wechsler Individual Achievement Test, Second Edition (WIAT-II)

Background Information

Caleb resides with his maternal aunt/adoptive mother and her three children. According to his maternal aunt, Caleb has an older half brother, Paul (different father), who is 20 years of age, dropped out of school, and obtained a general equivalency diploma (GED). Paul has been living with the maternal grandmother; he was previously diagnosed with Attention-Deficit/Hyperactivity Disorder (ADHD) and bipolar disorder. No information about Caleb's father was available. Caleb's biological mother is 42 years of age; she quit school in the ninth grade and has not obtained a GED. She has a history of alcohol and substance abuse since the age of 12 or 13 years old; she has been diagnosed with antisocial personality disorder. There is a strong maternal family history of alcohol and drug abuse. Further, there are two uncles with histories of academic difficulty, one of whom has a son who is also experiencing academic difficulty.

Review of developmental and medical history with, his maternal aunt indicates that Caleb is the product of a 36-week pregnancy complicated by alcohol and substance abuse throughout. Delivery was by emergency cesarean section due to premature separation of the placenta with excessive bleeding. Caleb was reported to weigh 2,420 gm (<10th percentile) with a head circumference of 30 cm (10th percentile). Caleb went home with his mother to live in the home of the maternal grandmother. Exact developmental motor and language milestones were not available; however at the age of 2 years 8 months, Caleb was placed in the custody of the state child protection agency due to neglect and substance abuse in the home. According to Ms. Daniels, at that time, Caleb was not talking and was acting out behaviorally. He was placed in foster care but returned to the mother at age 4 years after she completed treatment for alcoholism. Later that year, Caleb was placed back in foster care. At 4 years 10 months, Caleb came to live with Ms. Daniels, where he has remained to the present. Aside from the usual childhood illnesses, Caleb's past medical history is significant for allergy to milk and eggs. There is no known history of seizures or head injury although Caleb did suffer a broken arm at age 2.

Since coming to live with Ms. Daniels, Caleb has exhibited significant conduct problems at home and at school. Caleb is described as inattentive, easily distractible, and impulsive, and he has difficulty maintaining appropriate social boundaries and with stealing. He is easily upset and has frequent anger outbursts. Due to the history of behavioral acting out, Caleb originally was evaluated by a psychologist, who referred the family to a child advocacy center where Caleb subsequently began therapy.

At age 5 years 10 months, Caleb had an initial psychological evaluation. At that time, Caleb was found to be functioning in the low-average to average range of intellectual ability as measured by the General Ability Index of the Wechsler Intelligence Scale for Children, Fourth Edition (GAI = 94). It should be noted that this result was felt to be an underestimate of intellectual potential due to Caleb's short attention span and variable compliance. Analysis of the Index scores revealed average verbal reasoning (Verbal Comprehension Index = 106) and auditory working memory (WMI = 97) contrasted by low-average nonverbal reasoning (Perceptual Reasoning Index = 84) and borderline to low-average processing speed (Processing Speed Index = 80). Academic assessment with the Wechsler Individual Achievement Test, Second Edition (WIAT-II) indicated that Caleb was performing in the high-average to superior range in the areas of word recognition, spelling, and mathematical reasoning with average mathematical calculation skills. Parent and teacher behavior rating scales were significant for inattention, hyperactivity, oppositional behavior, aggression, and poor social skills. Based on these results, Caleb was diagnosed with ADHD, combined type, and oppositional defiant disorder.

At age 6, Caleb began seeing a child psychiatrist who started him on Depakote to manage mood swings and aggression; however, after approximately one month, Caleb was switched to dexmethylphenidate hydrochloride (Focalin) in order to improve attention span. Shortly thereafter, risperidone (Risperdal) was added. Due to little improvement in attention, the Focalin was switched to dextroamphetamine mixed salts (Adderall XR). In addition, Caleb began seeing a behavior therapist. Caleb has continued on these medications; however, the Adderall XR was changed to regular Adderall and is now administered in a twice-a-day dosing pattern.

That same year, Caleb was evaluated by the FAS Interdisciplinary Evaluation Team at a private hospital. Based on the results of the evaluation, the team believed that Caleb did not meet formal diagnostic criteria for fetal alcohol syndrome because he only met three of the four criteria. Specifically, prenatal exposure to alcohol was confirmed based on the history. There was evidence for growth retardation at birth (birth weight = 2,420 gm; <10th percentile, head circumference at birth = 30 cm; < 10th percentile), and Caleb exhibited a significant degree of alcohol-related dysmorphic features (posterior rotation of the ears, anteverted nares, smooth philtrum, thin vermillion border of the upper lip, and clinodactyly of the fifth fingers). Previous psychological evaluation, however, did not suggest evidence of neurodevelopmental deficits. Further, Caleb was administered the

Differential Ability Scales (DAS), on which he obtained a General Conceptual Ability standard score of 106, which was in the average range. His Verbal Cluster score was in the high average to superior range (Scaled Score [SS] = 121), with average Nonverbal Reasoning (SS = 95) and Spatial (SS = 97) Cluster scores. Adaptive functioning using the Vineland Adaptive Behavior Scales, Second Edition, with Ms. Daniels serving as the informant was found to be average (Composite Score = 94), and Caleb's performance on academic screening with the WIAT-2 was above average to superior (Word Reading = 132; Spelling = 132; Numerical Operations = 111). Finally, behavior rating scales completed by Ms. Daniels and Caleb's teacher were significant for short attention span, aggression, and rule-breaking behavior.

Review of educational history indicates that Caleb began attending the prekindergarten class at church. According to Ms. Daniels, "Caleb bit, hit, and kicked" other classmates on the very first day, and this aggressive behavior continued throughout the remainder of the school year. Caleb began attending kindergarten within the local public school system. Prior to the beginning of school, Ms. Daniels met with the assistant principal to secure a "firm teacher" for Caleb; however, on the second day, she was notified that Caleb was "totally out of control." His poor frustration tolerance, poor anger control, and aggressive behavior continued; as a result, the classroom aide was forced to spend an excessive amount of time each day managing Caleb. In April of that year, a special education staffing was held, and Caleb was found eligible for services under the "Other Health Impaired" category secondary to a diagnosis of ADHD and fetal alcohol exposure. Following the meeting, Caleb began receiving resource classroom services for reading and mathematics, support instruction in the regular classroom, occupational therapy as a related service, and special transportation. In addition, a behavioral intervention plan was developed. This year, Caleb is attending first grade with continuation of his special education Individualized Education Plan. Since he reads well, Caleb is working on improving written expression and mathematics with his resource teacher.

Behavioral Observations

Caleb presented himself for testing as a very verbal, neatly groomed youngster of short stature with blond hair and blue eyes. He was casually dressed in a red sweater, jeans, and sneakers. He separated without difficulty from Ms. Daniels and accompanied the examiners to the testing room without difficulty. Caleb was oriented, demonstrated good social eye contact, was very animated, and appeared very comfortable engaging in conversation with the examiners. In response to direct questions, as well as when conversation was spontaneous, Caleb's use of language was fluent and prosodic with excellent vocabulary development noted. Caleb began the evaluation off medication; however, after approximately 30 minutes, he began to exhibit difficulty sustaining attention, became more impulsive, and his activity level increased markedly to the point that he was in and out of his chair, leaning over the testing table, and at times was under the table. As a result, a break was taken in order to allow Caleb to take his medication. Even with medication, Caleb continued to exhibit difficulty sustaining attention, and he became silly and at times verbally inappropriate toward the end of the morning session. During the afternoon session following a second dose of medication during the lunch break, Caleb's attention span, activity level, and ability to filter his verbalizations was somewhat improved. He typically approached tasks enthusiastically and put forth good effort when confronted with more challenging tasks; however, on occasion, Caleb would attempt to bargain with the examiner to avoid a task or receive a break sooner ("no one's looking so we don't have to do this work"). Lateral dominance is firmly established in the right hand for paper-and-pencil manipulation. Vision with corrective lenses for nearsightedness appeared to be functioning normally. Hearing was screened and was reported as normal.

Assessment Results

The results of neuropsychological evaluation indicate that Caleb currently is functioning within the average to high-average range of intellectual ability as measured by the General Ability Index of the Wechsler Intelligence Scale for Children, Fourth Edition (WISC-IV; see Table 14.2). Analysis of the Index scores reveals that Caleb continues to exhibit a significant strength on subtests measuring verbal conceptual ability (above average) contrasted by a significant weakness in his information processing speed (borderline). Additional assessment indicates that while Caleb demonstrated average sequential reasoning/problem solving capability on the Tower subtest of the Neuropsychological Assessment (NEPSY), Ms. Daniels endorsed significant executive functioning deficits in planning/organizational ability, working memory, and behavioral regulation on the Behavior Rating Inventory of Executive Functioning (BRIEF). Consistent with Caleb's performance on the WISC-IV, he demonstrated above-average to superior expressive and receptive language skills. Visual-spatial perception and visual-motor integration/construction were found to be in the average range; however, motor planning deficits were very much in evidence. Further, fine motor tapping speed is found to be in the average range bilaterally, with a relative weakness in right (dominant) hand tapping speed noted as measured by the Finger Tapping Test.

Analysis of Caleb's performance on the Children's Memory Scale indicates that, at the present time, he is exhibiting average ability to hold material in immediate/working memory. When asked to learn and remember (30 minutes later) newly presented material, Caleb demonstrated average ability to learn and recall auditory/verbal material such as stories that were read to him and a list of rote word pairs presented over three learning trials. Within the visual domain, Caleb demonstrated superior ability to learn and recall the spatial location of an array of dots (where) contrasted by a significant deficit in his ability to recall a series of pictured human faces (what). Academically, Caleb continues to demonstrate superior word recognition, oral reading fluency, and reading comprehension. Caleb exhibited average to above-average numerical reasoning and calculation skills, and low-average to average written expression skills, which is significantly below expectation based upon his verbal conceptual abilities. Further, it should be noted that to obtain his score on the written expression subtest, Caleb wrote the letters of the alphabet and three words for things that are round (e.g., circle, head, eye). He did not always copy sentences correctly or combine two sentences to make one good sentence. In addition, his handwriting is very poor, and he reversed some letters.

Adaptive functioning is deficient per Ms. Daniels's report. Behaviorally, analysis of rating scales completed by Ms. Daniels and Caleb's teacher indicates that, at the present time, both raters continue to endorse significant concern with regard to short attention span, hyperactivity, aggression, conduct problems, depressed mood, and poor social skills both at home and at school, even with the benefit of medication.

Summary and Diagnostic Impressions

Caleb is a 7-year-old boy with a history of fetal alcohol exposure and behavioral difficulties. Taken together, this pattern of neuropsychological test performance is consistent with a continued diagnosis of attention deficit hyperactivity disorder, combined type, and oppositional

Table 14.2 Psychometric Summary for Caleb

	Scaled Score	Standard Score
Wechsler Intelligence Scale for Children, Fourth Edition (WISC-IV)		
Full Scale IQ		103
General Ability Index		115
Verbal Comprehension Index		119
Similarities	14	
Vocabulary	14	
Comprehension	12	
Perceptual Reasoning Index		106
Block Design	10	
Picture Concepts	11	
Matrix Reasoning	12	
Working Memory Index		99
Digit Span	9	
Letter-Number-Sequencing	11	
Processing Speed Index		75
Coding	6	
Symbol Search	5	
Neuropsychological Assessment, Second Edition (NEPSY-2)		
Tower Task (NEPSY)		105
Comprehension of Instructions		100
Phonological Processing		110
Word Generation—Semantic		90
Word Generation—First Letter		130
Arrows		110
Peabody Picture Vocabulary Test, Fourth Edition (PPVT-IV)		123
Boston Naming Test (BNT)		109
Clinical Evaluation of Language Fundamentals, Fourth Edition (CELF-IV)		
Formulated Sentences		115
Kaufman Assessment Battery for Children, Second Edition (KABC-2)		
Gestalt Closure		105
Developmental Test of Visual-Motor Integration, Fifth Edition (DTVMI-V)		
Clock Face Drawing Test		96
Form		96
Time (9:30)		102
Time (10:20)		81
Finger Tapping Test (Taps per 10 seconds)		
Right (dominant) Hand		103
Left (nondominant) Hand		113

(continued)

Table 14.2 *(Continued)*

	Scaled Score	Standard Score
Children's Memory Scale (CMS)		
Attention/Concentration Index		94
Numbers	8	
Sequences	10	
Picture Locations	9	
General Memory Index		90
Verbal Immediate Index		97
Stories	10	
Word Pairs	9	
Visual Immediate Index		94
Dot Locations	15	
Faces	3	
Verbal Delayed Index		100
Stories	12	
Word Pairs	8	
Visual Delayed Index		82
Dot Locations	13	
Faces	1	
Delayed Recognition Index		106
Stories	13	
Word Pairs	9	
Learning Index		112
Word Pairs	10	
Dot Locations	12	
Gray Oral Reading Test, Fourth Edition (GORT-4)		
Fluency		125
Comprehension		130
Wechsler Individual Achievement Test, Second Edition-II (WIAT-II)		
Word Reading		132
Pseudoword Decoding		126
Written Expression		93
Spelling		111
Mathematical Reasoning		112
Numerical Operations		103
Behavior Rating Inventory of Executive Functioning (BRIEF)		**T-Score (Parent)**
Behavioral Regulation Index		73
Inhibit		80
Shift		63
Emotional Control		64
Metacognitive Index		75
Initiate		71
Working Memory		73
Plan/Organize		74
Organization of Materials		72
Monitor		73

Table 14.2 ***(Continued)***

	T-Scores	
	Parent	Teacher
Behavior Assessment System for Children, Second Edition (BASC-2)		
Clinical Scales		
Hyperactivity	88	89
Aggression	87	99
Conduct	108	85
Anxiety	50	39
Depression	67	64
Somatization	56	54
Atypicality	65	82
Withdrawal	49	64
Attention	76	69
Learning Problems	NA	58
Adaptive Scales		
Adaptability	30	38
Social Skills	34	35
Leadership	38	40
Study Skills	NA	36
DSM-IV ADHD Checklist	**Raw Score**	
Inattention	24/27	26/27
Hyperactivity/Impulsivity	27/27	27/27

Note. NA = Not applicable.

defiant disorder in conjunction with significant executive functioning deficits, learning disability in the area of written expression, developmental coordination disorder, poor adaptive functioning, and social skill deficits. Further, it is now evident that Caleb meets the neurodevelopmental deficit criteria necessary for a formal diagnosis of fetal alcohol syndrome.

Recommendations

It is recommended that Caleb continue to receive special education resource and inclusion services designed for children with learning disabilities and emotional/behavior disorder under the eligibility category of "Other Health Impaired." Resource placement should be utilized for development of written expression, executive functioning skills (planning/organizational skills, behavioral regulation), and social skills. Continuation of occupational therapy as a related service will be necessary to improve fine motor and adaptive functioning. Caleb also will require continuation of his behavior management plan focused on enhancing his attention, listening skills, and task completion while decreasing oppositional acting-out behavior and aggression toward peers and adults. As part of this plan, rules and expectations should be presented simply, clearly, and consistently and reviewed frequently. This plan should place a large emphasis on consistently rewarding Caleb's "good" behavior, such as positive social interactions, working on classwork, and following directions, rather than having a punitive system that primarily calls attention to his mistakes. In other words, he should have a high ratio of positive reinforcement to punishment (ratio = 5:1). Consequences for both appropriate and inappropriate behavior should be enforced on a consistent basis through positive reinforcement and response cost. This could be managed in the form of a contracting system, given Caleb's age and intellect. The behavioral plan should be coordinated with Ms. Daniels to ensure consistency between home and school, including target behaviors, reinforcers, and punishments.

In order to enhance Caleb's learning/retention, new material should be presented in an organized format that is meaningful to him. The material to be learned should be pretaught, broken down into smaller components/steps, and presented in a highly structured format with frequent repetition to facilitate new learning. Instruction should not be supplemented with complex visual aids or demonstrations, given his deficit in visual learning and memory. As Caleb progresses to middle school, he would benefit greatly from being taught how to use mnemonic strategies when learning new material and studying for tests. These include but are not limited to:

- Rehearsal—showing Caleb how to repeat information verbally, to write it, and to look at it a finite number of times.
- Transformation—instructing Caleb in how to convert difficult information into simpler components that can be remembered more easily.
- Elaboration—showing Caleb how to identify key elements of new information and to create relationships or associations with previously learned material.
- Chunking—instructing Caleb in how to group or pair down long strings of digits or different items into more manageable units and thereby facilitating encoding and retention.

When studying for tests or doing multiple homework assignments on the same day, similar subject material should be separated in order to lessen interference.

Accommodations will be necessary to enhance Caleb's ability to succeed in the classroom, including preferential seating away from bulletin boards, doorways, windows, or other students, if necessary, where excessive stimuli might prove distracting. Instruction should be provided in small-group settings, and efforts should be made to redirect his attention. Given his learning disability in written expression and ADHD, a reduction in the amount, but not the difficulty level, of written assignments may assist Caleb in completing classroom tasks and homework in a timely manner. Moreover, whenever possible, he should be given additional time to complete assignments. Tests should be in multiple-choice/matching/short-answer formats instead of an essay format and should be administered individually/orally, with additional time provided when necessary. Caleb also will benefit from the use of graph paper or different color highlighters to maintain place value when doing written calculation, and having an outline of the steps necessary to complete multistep math problems available for reference. Finally, he should be allowed and encouraged to use various compensatory devices, such as a computer with word processing capability. Most word processing programs are equipped with spell checks, cut and paste, and can be adapted for voice dictation if necessary.

As Caleb approaches middle school, study skills training will be warranted, emphasizing such techniques as the appropriate outlining of lecture notes and how to study for tests. He also will benefit from being taught how to take notes on text material and plan written reports using an outlining method. In a related vein, training in word processing is strongly encouraged. Caleb also may require instruction on how to organize and plan his approach to his studies, as executive functioning is an area of weakness for him. In addition, direct instruction in basic organizational strategies will assist Caleb in knowing what to do, when to do it, and how to do it. Specifically, he should be guided in the use of checklists and other organizational aids, such as a daily planner. With help from teachers and parents, he ideally will plan each day of the week, including time after school. Training in active problem solving also may prove helpful. One problem-solving technique involves teaching the student a four-step procedure: (1) identifying the problem, (2) generating ways to solve the problem, (3) selecting the best solution, and (4) checking out the success of the choice. In the beginning, positive reinforcement should be incorporated into each step of this training to facilitate learning and encourage consistent implementation of the techniques.

Caleb and his family will continue to benefit from behavioral therapy to treat his ADHD and behavior disorder, especially since medication management appears to be minimally successful at this point. Finally, Caleb will continue to require psychiatric follow-up for management of his medications.

Further Discussion of Case Study

This case highlights the occurrence of late effects in terms of cognitive and behavioral impairment as a result of prenatal exposure to alcohol. Three of the formal criteria are more readily identified: exposure, growth retardation, and alcohol-related dysmorphic features. Only over time have the neurocognitive deficits emerged; in all likelihood, additional deficits in behavioral regulation and executive function will become more evident as demands change over the course of development. Also since an early age, there were the behavioral issues, particularly attentional problems, disinhibition, and hyperactivity. Repeated evaluations will be needed to ensure that intervention planning and programming are appropriate as deficit areas are identified.

COURSE AND PROGNOSIS: ANTIEPILEPTICS AND FVS

In contrast to FAS, the distinctive facial phenotype of fetal valproate syndrome tends to evolve over time (Dilberti, Farndon, Dennis, & Curry, 1984; Winter, Donnai, Burn, & Tucker, 1987). The facial features seen in FVS include triangular prominence of the forehead and closely set eyes (i.e., trigonocephaly), high forehead with bifrontal narrowing, hypertelorism, epicanthic folds, infraorbital groove, medial deficiency of eyebrows, flat and broad nose, shallow or smooth philtrum, long upper lip with thin borders, thick lower lip, and small downturned mouth (Ardinger et al., 2005; Clayton Smith & Donnai, 1995; Dilberti et al. 1984; Schorry, Oppenheimer, & Saal, 2005). Valproate also is associated with increased likelihood of diagnosis of autism (S. Duncan, 2007; Rasalam et al., 2005; G. Williams & Hersh, 1997; G. Williams et al., 2001). It has been proposed that early exposure results in neuroanatomical abnormalities that underlie autism spectrum disorders (Arndt et al., 2005). In one study, for example, of 260 children with a history of exposure to antiepileptics, 4.6% met criteria for autism spectrum disorder; of the antiepileptics, valproate was the one most commonly associated with this disorder (Rasalam et al., 2005). Animal models for autism support the association of autistic tendencies with valproate exposure, prenatally and postnatally through lactation (G. S. Wagner, Reuhl, Cheh, McRae, & Halladay, 2006).

Exposure to sodium valproate, as well as exposure to other antiepileptics, has been associated with developmental and learning difficulties (Adab, Jacoby, Smith, & Chadwick, 2001; Adab, Kini et al., 2004; Ardinger et al., 2005; Clayton Smith & Donnai, 1995; J. Dean et al., 2002; G. Williams et al., 2001) as well as decreased cognitive ability, particularly verbal abilities (Vinten et al., 2005). The extent to which cognitive and verbal abilities are impacted is mediated by mothers' cognitive level, the number of seizures experienced by the mother during the pregnancy, and the exposure level (Vinten et al., 2005). In a recent study of a total of 69 cases of FVS, 12% of the affected children died in infancy, and 29% of the surviving children had developmental delays/mental retardation (Kozma, 2001). In another study, 15 cases of FVS presented with dysmorphic features; evidence of mild to moderate developmental

Table 14.3 Deficits Associated with Specific Prescribed Medications Taken During Pregnancy

Drug	Deficit
Valproate	Neural tube defects Microcephaly Ocular abnormalities Decreased cognitive ability likely, particularly in verbal areas Hypotonia Cleft lip or palate defects Communication/Language disorder Cardiovascular and genitourinary abnormalities Autism spectrum disorders Developmental delay and learning problems requiring special education Delayed motor development Memory problems Behavior problems in general Difficulties in adaptive areas
Carbamazepine	Neural defects Cardiac abnormality Growth deficiency Learning problems requiring special education Delayed motor development at 12 months
Phenytoin	Delayed motor development at 12 months Increased anterior fontanelle at age 6 to 12 months Microcephaly Craniofacial abnormalities Growth deficiencies Delayed ability to sit without support
Benzodiazepines	Orofacial clefts Adaptation problems Facial dysmorphism (slanted eyes and epicanthal folds) Hypotonia, delayed motor development Microcephaly Varying degrees of mental retardation
Lithium	Adaptation problems
Lamotrigine (Lamictal)	Orofacial clefts Various major birth defects
Selective serotonin reuptake inhibitors	Low birth weight Delayed/subtle motor deficits Hyperactivity, irritability Respiratory problems and seizures postpartum Hypotonia

delay was found in 10 (67%) on follow-up (Ardinger et al., 2005). In a study of 154 children with antiepileptic exposure and 130 control children, the children with exposure demonstrated deficits in attention, memory, fine motor, and auditory attention areas. More recently, research suggests delays in both motor and cognitive development in children under age 3 with prenatal exposure to antiepileptic drugs (Thomas et al., 2008). The deficits in auditory attention were most pronounced among those children exposed to valproate (Kantola-Sorsa, Gaily, Tsoaho, & Korman, 2007). Results of other studies (Viinikainen et al., 2006) further indicate the need for educational support for children with FVS as they progress with school. For example, in a small sample of children born between 1989 and 2000, 62% of those exposed to valproate and 23% of those exposed to carbamazepine required educational support of some type. Exposure to valproate also was associated with increased frequency of behavioral problems (Viinikainen et al., 2006). Characteristics associated with various medications taken during pregnancy are summarized in Table 14.3.

CASE STUDY: KEISHA—FETAL VALPROATE SYNDROME

The next report is from a hospital-based clinic. Identifying information, such as child and family name, teacher or physician name, and school information, has been altered or fictionalized to protect confidentiality.

Reason for Referral

Keisha is a 6-year-old youngster who is being evaluated as part of a National Institute of Health research study examining the possible effects of exposure to antiepileptic drugs in utero. As part of this project, Keisha was administered a battery of cognitive tests in order to assess her cognitive/developmental functioning.

Assessment Procedures

Differential Ability Scales (DAS)
Neuropsychological Assessment (NEPSY)
Expressive One Word Picture Vocabulary Test (EOWPVT)
Beery Developmental Test of Visual Motor Integration (DTVMI)
Children's Memory Scale (CMS)
Grooved Pegboard Test
Wide Range Achievement Test, Third Edition (WRAT-3)
Adaptive Behavior Assessment System (ABAS)
Behavior Assessment System for Children (BASC)

Background Information

Keisha lives with her mother, father, and older sister. Keisha's parents are both high school educated. Maternal IQ was low average to average (Full Scale quotient 89) as measured by the Wechsler Abbreviated Scale of Intelligence. Keisha's sister is healthy and doing well at school. Keisha currently attends first grade at a public school, and reports from her teacher indicate that she is doing well; however, she is receiving extra support in the classroom due to difficulty with spelling.

Review of the developmental and medical history indicates that the pregnancy with Keisha was uneventful in terms of complications with all ultrasounds reported as normal. Preconception folic acid was taken by Keisha's mother until 12 weeks' gestation (approximately). Keisha's mother denies consuming alcohol or smoking during the gestational period. Keisha's mother was prescribed sodium valproate (Depakote) for idiopathic generalized epilepsy. This medication was continued throughout the pregnancy with Keisha at 200 mg four times per day. Keisha's mother remained seizure free throughout her pregnancy. Keisha was born at 41 weeks' gestation by spontaneous vaginal delivery. Apgar scores were 9, 10, and 10 after 1, 5, and 10 minutes respectively. The newborn assessment indicated that Keisha was jaundiced but that everything else was normal. Keisha was reported to have a normal level of consciousness and normal spontaneous motor movements. Satisfactory muscle tone was reported, and reflexes were also reported as normal.

Keisha was assessed previously at age 3 years. At that time, Keisha's head circumference was 48.0 cm, her weight was 14.0 kg, and she was 91 cm in height. Neurological assessment was normal, eye movements were normal, and no tremors were reported; however, she was found to have minor physical abnormalities including overlapping toes on the left foot and a prominent sternum that was slightly asymmetric. In addition, Keisha was found to have mild eczema over her whole body. Keisha's neuropsychological assessment revealed borderline to low-average intellectual functioning as measured by the Differential Ability Scales (General Conceptual Ability standard score = 79) with average nonverbal ability (Nonverbal Composite Standard Score = 99). More detailed assessment of linguistic functioning with the Pre-school Language Scale, Fourth Edition, revealed that Keisha demonstrated average receptive language capability (Auditory Comprehension standard score = 92) contrasted by borderline expressive language (Expressive Language Standard Score = 77). Keisha has not received the services of a speech therapist to date.

Behavioral Observations

Keisha presented as a pleasant, neatly groomed young lady who was in good spirits. She separated from her mother and accompanied the examiner to the testing room without difficulty. She made good social eye contact and related appropriately toward the examiner throughout the testing session, which consisted of a morning session lasting approximately two hours with a 20-minute break. After an hour lunch break, testing resumed for an additional hour and a half with a 15-minute break.

In response to direct questions, as well as when conversation was spontaneous, Keisha's use of language was poor for her age, both expressively and in terms of her comprehension. Keisha's attention span, activity level, and impulsivity within the context of this one-to-one assessment were felt to be age appropriate. Lateral dominance is firmly established in the right hand for paper-and-pencil manipulation. Vision and hearing were not formally screened; however, they appeared to be functioning adequately for the purposes of this evaluation.

Assessment Results

Cognitive and Neuropsychological Functioning

The results of neuropsychological evaluation indicate that Keisha currently is functioning within the borderline to low-average range of intellectual ability as measured by the

Differential Ability Scales with a significant discrepancy noted between her borderline to low-average verbal reasoning skills and her average nonverbal reasoning skills. As a result, it is felt that the Nonverbal Reasoning Cluster score represents her best estimate of intellectual potential. Of further note is the significant variability in performance evident across the subtests comprising the Spatial Cluster. The low score on the Recall of Designs subtest appears to be the result of poor visual immediate/working memory and mild fine motor difficulty. Additional assessment indicates that Keisha demonstrates low-average sequential reasoning/problem-solving capability (see Table 14.4).

Within the linguistic domain, Keisha's receptive language skills are generally in the low-average range. In contrast, her expressive language continues to be more problematic, consistent with prior assessment at age 3. Specifically, Keisha exhibited significant difficulty naming pictures to confrontation and providing definitions for vocabulary words provided by the examiner.

Visual-spatial perception and visual-motor integration/construction were found to be generally in the average range with slightly more difficulty noted when Keisha was asked to construct with paper and pencil. Fine motor dexterity as measured by the Grooved Pegboard Test was found to be in the average range bilaterally.

Keisha's attention span was found to be within the average range for visual information but below average when information was presented auditorally. Analysis of Keisha's performance on the Children's Memory Scale indicates that, at the present time, she is exhibiting borderline to low-average ability to hold verbal material in immediate/working memory. When asked to learn and remember (30 minutes later) newly presented material, Keisha also exhibited borderline to low-average ability to encode and recall auditory/verbal information contrasted by low-average to average ability to learn and recall visual/nonverbal information. Academically, Keisha demonstrated low-average to average word recognition and spelling skills, contrasted by average numerical reasoning and calculation skills.

Social-Emotional and Behavioral Functioning

Behaviorally, analysis of rating scales completed by Keisha's mother and teacher indicates that, at the present time, Keisha's mother endorsed concern with regard to Keisha's leadership and social skills while behaviors consistent with anxiety and depressed mood are apparent in the classroom. Adaptive functioning is within normal limits based on parental and teacher reports.

Summary and Diagnostic Impressions

Taken together, Keisha demonstrates relative strengths in visual perceptual (nonverbal) areas, with relative weaknesses in auditory-linguistic (verbal) areas. This pattern of neuropsychological test performance is consistent with a picture of dysfunction involving the more anterior aspects of the left cerebral hemisphere resulting in deficits of expressive language, working memory, and the ability to encode and retrieve verbal information. These deficits have resulted in a specific language disorder, expressive type, and will place Keisha at risk for development of a learning disability in the areas of reading and written expression as she progresses in elementary school. As a result, it is recommended that Keisha be referred for a more complete language evaluation and therapy in order to remediate her expressive language disorder.

In addition, a referral to the response to intervention or student support team at her school is also recommended so that an intensive (Tier 2) intervention program can be

Table 14.4 Psychometric Summary for Keisha

		Standard Score
Differential Ability Scales (DAS) (School-Age Level)		
General Conceptual Ability		84
Special Nonverbal Composite		78
Verbal Cluster		82
Word Definitions		78
Similarities		78
Nonverbal Reasoning Cluster		84
Matrices		100
Sequential & Quantitative Reasoning		103
Spatial Cluster		68
Recall of Designs		49
Pattern Construction		95
Neuropsychological Assessment (NEPSY)		
Tower Task		85
Comprehension of Instructions		90
Phonological Processing		85
Verbal Fluency		105
Sentence Repetition		85
Arrows		100
Visual Attention		105
Expressive One Word Picture Vocabulary Test (EOWVT)		68
Developmental Test of Visual-Motor Integration (DTVMI)		87
Children's Memory Scale (CMS)	**Scaled Score**	**Standard Score**
Attention/Concentration Index		75
Numbers	6	
Sequences	6	
Verbal Immediate Index		72
Stories	6	
Word Pairs	5	
Visual Immediate Index		88
Dot Locations	7	
Faces	9	
Verbal Delayed Index		66
Stories	6	
Word Pairs	3	
Visual Delayed Index		97
Dot Locations	10	
Faces	9	
Delayed Recognition Index		75
Stories	7	
Word Pairs	5	
Learning Index		72
Word Pairs	6	
Dot Locations	6	
Wide Range Achievement Test, Third Edition (WRAT-3)		
Reading		91
Spelling		89
Arithmetic		99

(continued)

Table 14.4 *(Continued)*

Behavior Assessment System for Children	T-Scores	
	Parent	Teacher
Clinical Scales		
Hyperactivity	53	43
Aggression	40	48
Conduct	42	43
Anxiety	35	64
Depression	45	65
Somatization	44	46
Atypicality	41	46
Withdrawal	49	62
Attention	55	38
Adaptive Scales		
Adaptability	38	50
Social Skills	36	48
Leadership	32	47
Study Skills	NA	36
Adaptive Behavior Assessment System	**Standard Scores**	
Conceptual	98	102
Social	98	104
Practical	102	89
General Composite	101	94

developed to monitor and remediate Keisha's relative deficiencies in reading and written expression. Keisha's parents are strongly encouraged to become involved in this process. They should feel comfortable that adequate steps are being taken to ensure that:

- The chosen interventions involve the use of research-based methodologies.
- Appropriate assessment tools are being used to monitor Keisha's progress over the 8- to 12-week intervention period.
- The instructor is properly trained in the implementation of the interventions.

If the interventions prove to be ineffective in significantly improving Keisha's language arts abilities, a referral for special education learning disability services under the eligibility category of "Specific Learning Disability" should be initiated.

Given her pattern of strengths and weaknesses, it is recommended that academic instruction in reading/writing instruction emphasize phonetic and multisensory approaches. In order to enhance Keisha's learning/retention, new material should be presented in an organized format that is meaningful to her. The material to be learned should be pretaught, broken down into smaller components/steps, and presented in a highly structured format with frequent repetition to facilitate new learning. Instruction should be supplemented with visual aids, demonstrations, and experiential/procedural learning whenever possible. When studying for tests or doing multiple homework assignments on the same day, similar subject material should be separated in order to lessen interference. Finally, Keisha should be provided with periodic review of previously learned material in order to enhance long-term retention.

Accommodations will be necessary to enhance Keisha's ability to succeed in the classroom, including preferential seating; a reduction in the amount, but not the difficulty level, of assignments; and additional time to complete written assignments. Tests should be in multiple-choice/matching/short-answer formats and administered individually/orally, with additional time provided when necessary. As Keisha progresses through school, she also may require various compensatory devices, such as textbooks on tape/reading pen and a computer with word processing capability. Most word processing programs are equipped with spell checks and cut and paste, and can be adapted for voice dictation if necessary.

Further Discussion of Case Study

Keisha's profile and performance most closely resemble that of a child with specific language impairment (see Chapter 4); the major difference is that the assumption is an etiology that was complicated by maternal valproate. Further, some physical and motor anomalies have been evident since her initial evaluation. Based on the auditory-linguistic differences, Keisha is at risk for significant difficulties in academic areas, with possible identification of learning disabilities as she progresses through school. Although not problematic at this time, monitoring in other areas (fine motor and visual-motor integration) also may be warranted.

EVIDENCE-BASED INTERVENTIONS

Few evidence-based interventions have been investigated with children exposed to substances, legal or illicit, during pregnancy (see Table 14.5). As with other disorders, and regardless of the substance, early intervention is critical not only for the child affected by exposure. For recreational substances, intervention also can help decrease the risk for later-born children. One such program, the Birth to 3 Program, has been shown to have some positive effects with high-risk mothers in at least two studies (C. C. Ernst, Grant, & Streissguth, 1999; Grant, Ernst, & Streissguth, 1999). This program uses paraprofessionals to work with the mother and child, linking them with community services, and providing at-home visitations and training. Results have indicated that there are fewer affected children, reduced foster care placement, and reduced dependence on welfare as a result of the early intervention efforts (C. C. Ernst et al., 1999). For infants with fetal valproate syndrome, identification of possible ocular sequelae and neurodevelopmental sequelae

Table 14.5 Evidence-Based Status for Interventions Related to Toxic Exposure in Utero

Interventions	Target	Status
Folate/folic acid supplements during pregnancy	Decrease risk of neural tube deficits associated with valproate	Supported in general but equivocal as protection against teratogenic effects of antiepileptics (Yerby, 2003)
Birth to 3 Program	Decrease alcohol and drug effects on child outcome	Emerging: potential support from initial studies (C. C. Ernst et al., 1999) but needs replication

are important as well, in order to provide appropriate early intervention (Carrim, McKay, Sidiki, & Lavy, 2007).

Few interventions used for reading, written expression, or math skills have been studied specifically with children with FVS or FAS, but there are some indications that the evidence-based interventions identified in earlier chapters (e.g., cover-copy-compare) may have some benefit (Gryiec, Grandy, & McLaughlin, 2004). The use of computer software to decrease the reliance on handwriting and motor skills also may facilitate school progress. Children with FVS or FAS also may benefit from progress monitoring, tutoring, and other programs used for children with learning disabilities. For those lower-functioning children, particular attention may be needed in the area of functional living skills.

CONCLUDING COMMENTS

Clearly, there are some situations (e.g., recreational substance use) in which the mother can and should take those efforts necessary to ensure a healthy child. Unfortunately, some of the effects of substances may occur prior to the mother's awareness that she is pregnant; in other cases, the mother may not be aware of the extent to which substance use can affect the unborn child. Good prenatal care and education to ensure appropriate knowledge and supplemental vitamins, particularly folic acid, appear to be standard practices. Combined with the public information programs, there may be a decrease in the incidence of fetal alcohol syndrome and other syndromes directly the result of maternal substance use or abuse. Alternatively, there are medications that expectant mothers need to continue taking during the pregnancy; which these are and the minimal dose level need to be determined on an individual basis so that risk is minimized for both mother and child. At the same time, parents and professionals working with these families need to be aware of the potential risks and the need for early identification and intervention services.

Extensive education and training for the parents, health care professionals, and teachers who work with children who are affected by maternal medications or substances are essential and need to be focused not on blame but on positive steps to maximize positive child outcome. Given increased likelihood of developmental issues, including autism, it is important that children born to mothers taking sodium valproate, and likely other antiepileptics, be screened in order to initiate early intervention efforts and maximize outcomes. Early intervention also is warranted to decrease potential effects of demographic, environmental, and psychosocial factors that are associated with maternal substance use. Future studies need to investigate further the impact of in utero exposure not only to recreational substances but to prescribed medications that cannot be discontinued. This research needs to investigate not only immediately obvious effects but more long-term and subtle effects across neuropsychological domains (Meador et al., 2007, 2009).

Chapter 15

CHROMOSOMAL ANOMALIES

Although there are genetic components to most neurodevelopmental disorders, specific disorders have confirmed single-gene etiology and transmission that is autosomal or sex linked. These include a number of different disorders, particularly those usually associated with mental retardation; however, this chapter cannot cover all of these disorders. Down syndrome, fragile X, Williams syndrome, and Angelman and Prader-Willi syndromes are covered here. For many of these disorders, assessment with traditional standardized measures has significant limitations; alternative methods are being explored but are not commonly used (Kogan et al., 2009). In addition to the disorders generally associated with mental retardation, three additional disorders that involve the sex chromosome (Turner syndrome, Klinefelter syndrome, Noonan syndrome) also are discussed briefly.

AUTOSOMAL ABNORMALITIES: DOWN SYNDROME

Definition

All autosomal (non–sex linked) disorders affect the central nervous system and typically result in multiple physical abnormalities. The three most common of the autosomal abnormalities include Down (trisomy 21), Edwards (trisomy 18), and Patau (trisomy 13) syndromes. Most infants with Edwards or Patau die before reaching 1 year of age; children with Down syndrome, however, have a much better prognosis. John Langdon Down, an English physician, published the first accurate description of a person with Down syndrome in 1866 (Batshaw, Pellegrino, & Roizen, 2007; Cody & Kamphaus, 1999). Characteristics of the syndrome had been recognized previously, but Down described the condition as a distinct and separate entity. Physical characteristics include microcephaly (small head), hypotonia (low muscle tone), slanted eyes with an epicanthal fold on the inner corner of each eye, flattened nose, and enlarged tongue. Down syndrome accounts for approximately one-third of all children with mental retardation (MR); cognitive ability varies with most in the mild to moderate MR range (Batshaw et al., 2007; Cody & Kamphaus, 1999).

Incidence

The estimated incidence of Down syndrome is 1 in 700 to 1,000, or 13.65 per 10,000 live births. It is generally agreed that the occurrence of Down syndrome is related to maternal age (Ypsilanti & Grouios, 2008); it occurs across all racial/ethnic groups and levels of income. When the trisomy is of maternal origin, it is believed to occur in the first or second meiotic stage (Garchet-Beaudron et al., 2008; Jyothy et al., 2001; F. Muller, Reviffé, Taillandier, Oury, & Mornet, 2000).

Etiology

Three genetic variations can cause Down syndrome (Patterson & Lott, 2008). Approximately 92% of the time, Down syndrome is caused by the presence of an extra chromosome 21 in all cells of the individual (nondisjunction). When this occurs, and there are three copies of chromosome 21 present in all cells of the individual, it is called trisomy 21. In contrast, approximately 2% to 4% of cases of Down syndrome are due to mosaic trisomy 21. In mosaic trisomy, the extra chromosome 21 is present in some but not all of the individual's cells. With mosaic trisomy 21, the individual typically has 46 chromosomes in some cells but has 47 chromosomes (including an extra chromosome 21) in others. The range of physical and cognitive problems may vary, depending on the proportion of cells that carry the additional chromosome 21 in the mosaic trisomy. Finally, approximately 3% to 4% of individuals with Down syndrome have cells containing 46 chromosomes but still have the features associated with the syndrome due to translocation. With translocation trisomy 21, genetic material from one chromosome 21 gets stuck or translocated onto another chromosome, either prior to or at conception. Individuals with translocation to chromosome 21 have two normal chromosome 21s but also have additional chromosome 21 material on the translocated chromosome. This translocation results in some of the indicators of Down syndrome but not all (Dreux et al., 2008).

Diagnostic procedures are available for prenatal diagnosis of Down syndrome and are recommended by physicians usually based on maternal age or family history. These include chorionic villus sampling (CVS), amniocentesis and percutaneous umbilical blood sampling (PUBS). These procedures involve a small risk of miscarriage, but are about 98% to 99% accurate in the detection of Down syndrome. Amniocentesis usually is performed between 15 and 22 weeks of gestation, CVS between 9 and 14 weeks, and PUBS after 18 weeks. Risk factors for Down syndrome include advanced maternal age, parental balanced translocation, parents with chromosomal disorders, and a previous child with Down syndrome or other chromosomal disorder (M. A. Davidson, 2008). Because the risk of Down syndrome increases with mother's age, testing is encouraged in women over age 35. There is no evidence of toxins, drugs, vitamin deficiencies, or viruses that increase the risk of Down syndrome (M. A. Davidson, 2008).

Neurological Correlates

Few studies have investigated the neurological correlates of Down syndrome; imaging studies do not suggest any major structural differences in children with Down syndrome (Smigielska-Kuzia & Sobaniec, 2007). There is some evidence of reduction of frontal and parietal gray matter volumes; when stereotypies and other autism-related behaviors are present, there is also evidence of hyperplasia of white matter in the cerebellum and brain stem (J. C. Carter, Capone, Kaufmann, 2008; Lubec & Engidawork, 2002). Some research also has found evidence of hippocampal dysfunction (Nadel, 2003; Pennington, Moon, Edgin, Stedron, & Nadel, 2003) and reduced size of both the hippocampal formation and the corpus callosum relative to total brain volume (Teipel & Hampel, 2006). Based on regional cerebral blood flow, perfusion abnormalities (hypoperfusion) are most evident in the fronto-parieto-temporal region and occurred more frequently in the right hemisphere than in the left (Aydin, Kabakus, Balci, & Ayar, 2007). In another study, it was found that the hypoperfusion was associated with the presence of epilepsy and other coexisting conditions as well as greater cognitive deficits (Altiay et al., 2006).

In middle-age adults with Down syndrome, imaging indicated higher glucose metabolic rate and decreased gray matter in the hippocampal and parahippocampal region, the thalamus, the caudate, and the frontal lobe, consistent with what is seen in those at-risk for dementia (Haier, Head, & Lott, 2008). Down syndrome is associated with a risk for epilepsy with focal onset (Persad, Thompson, & Percy, 2002; Pueschel, Louis, & McKnight, 1991). A general decline in functioning in adulthood is associated with degeneration of the hippocampal and cerebellar regions (Pennington et al., 2003). Another neurological characteristic of Down syndrome is a tendency for premature aging and dementia—Alzheimer's type (M. A. Davidson, 2008; Teipel & Hampel, 2006).

Course and Prognosis

Medical problems frequently are associated with Down syndrome (Roizen, 2002). For example, 30% to 50% of the individuals with Down syndrome have heart defects, many of which are correctable with surgery (M. A. Davidson, 2008). In addition, 8% to 12% of individuals with Down syndrome have gastrointestinal tract abnormalities that are correctable by surgery. Children with Down syndrome have a higher incidence of infection, respiratory, vision and hearing problems as well as thyroid and other medical conditions, including Type I diabetes, leukemia, and immune system defects. Celiac disease is evident in 5% to 15% of individuals with Down syndrome and results in multiple gastric problems (M. A. Davidson, 2008). Life expectancy for individuals with Down syndrome is increasing; with this increased life span come problems in orthopedic areas (Mik, Gholve, Scher, Widmann, & Green, 2008) as well as increased risk of dementia (Haier et al., 2008). Dementia–Alzheimer's type is clearly associated with Down syndrome. This is related to the amyloid precursor protein gene, located on chromosome 21, and is believed to be overexpressed in trisomy 21. Additionally, mitochondrial dysfunction may provide a link between Down syndrome and Alzheimer's type dementia (Roizen & Patterson, 2003).

Neurocognitive Correlates

Individuals with Down syndrome range in intellectual ability from moderate retardation to the normal range (Saenz, 1999). Areas of functioning often affected in conjunction with Down syndrome are summarized in Table 15.1. In addition to overall global ability, motor skills and language skills tend to be impaired in individuals with Down syndrome (Laws, Byrne, & Buckley, 2000; Silverman, 2007). Linguistic abilities of children with Down syndrome have been studied extensively (Ypsilanti & Grouios, 2008). For individuals with Down syndrome, left ear advantage on dichotic listening tasks is found frequently (Bunn, Welsh, Simon, Howarth, & Elliott, 2003; T. N. Welsh, Elliott, & Simon, 2003) and was associated with greater errors on imitation tasks, further supporting a connection between language and motor skills (Bunn, Roy, & Elliott, 2007). Laterality of speech/language function tends to be atypical (Heath et al., 2005; Shoji, Koizumi, & Ozaki, 2009). In the speech/language area, expressive language skills tend to be more impaired than receptive language skills (Abbeduto et al., 2001; Abbeduto, Warren, & Conners, 2007; Silverman, 2007) with considerable difficulty with syntax (Abbeduto et al., 2003; Silverman, 2007) and speech production (J. E. Roberts, Price, & Malkin, 2007). Receptive vocabulary level for individuals with Down syndrome emerges as a relative strength, often comparable to typically developing children matched for nonverbal cognitive skills (Laws & Bishop, 2003). The disparity between expressive and receptive areas is marked and evident prior to the use of verbal language, with infant use of gestures expressively in Down syndrome delayed as well (J. F. Miller, Leddy, Miolo, & Sedey, 1995). In addition, deviations in phrasing, rate, placement of sentence stress, and voice

Table 15.1 Neuropsychological Deficits Associated with Down Syndrome

Global Domain/Specific Deficits	Phenotype
Cognition	Mental retardation common but range includes average ability
Auditory-linguistic/Language function	Delays in canonical babbling that is precursor to language development Impaired language, particularly expressive language Deviations in phrasing, rate, placement of sentence stress, voice quality (prosody) occur Difficulty with semantics at vocabulary and conceptual level Syntactical deficits with delayed progression from phrases to sentences Oral apraxia, due in part to structural differences in facial musculature and structure Stuttering common
Learning and memory	Impaired verbal memory
Visual perception/Constructional praxis	Visual-spatial and visual-motor skills tend to be relative strengths
Attention/Concentration	Difficulty with sustained and selective attention
Processing speed	Increased latency in movement
Motor function	Imitation of motor patterns impaired
Achievement/Academic skills	Sight vocabulary a relative strength Decoding of novel words and reading comprehension relative weaknesses

quality (prosody) occur (Stoel-Gammon, 1997); dysfluency or stuttering is also common (Van Borsel & Tetnowski, 2007). Processing speed for verbal information appears to be slowed by laterality differences in expressive and receptive language areas (Heath, Grierson, Binsted, & Elliott, 2007). Across adaptive areas, communication emerges as the more significant weakness relative to daily living skills and socialization skills (E. M. Dykens, Hodapp, & Evans, 2006).

Related to language ability, even when cognitive ability is considered, children with Down syndrome demonstrate deficits in verbal working memory (Silverman, 2007) and verbal short-term memory (Jarrold, Purser, & Brock, 2006). Verbal short-term memory and functional ability of the phonological loop also are believed to account for difficulty in expressive language development in Down syndrome (Jarrold et al., 2006). Deficits in verbal short-term memory and both verbal and spatial long-term memory have been noted and are believed to be related to hippocampal dysfunction (Pennington et al., 2003). Other than long-term recall, visual-spatial processes appear to be relatively spared (Pinter, Eliez, Schmitt, Capone, & Reiss, 2001). Motor difficulties and increased latency in response to verbal cues has been found (T. N. Welsh & Elliott, 2001). Depending on the individual, strengths may be evidenced in visual memory, visual-motor integration, or visual imitation (Fidler, 2005).

Educational Implications

Early intervention during the first three years of life is critical (Abbeduto et al., 2007). Children with Down syndrome typically are delayed in certain areas of development, particularly language areas; the focus of early intervention is not to eliminate problems but to optimize (maximize) the child's possible development. Intervention should come from multiple perspectives to address speech and language, motor development, social skills, self-help skills, and academic skills. Children with Down syndrome tend to learn to read predominantly through sight-word/whole-word approaches, but there is evidence to suggest that they can benefit from phonological awareness training (Goetz et al., 2008). In contrast to children with autism, children with Down syndrome evidence relative strengths in joint attention as well as gestural communication (Franco & Wishart, 1995). Some children will be able to function in general education classrooms, in general education classrooms with aides, or may need special education services. Sight vocabulary is a relative strength; decoding of novel words and reading comprehension are relative weaknesses (Cupples & Iacono, 2002). More teens and adults with Down syndrome are graduating from high school and going on to postsecondary settings; others will need more structured, vocational settings after age 21.

Emotional/Behavioral Functioning

Historically, it was suggested that about 10% to 12% of individuals with Down syndrome also met criteria for autism spectrum disorder (Kent, Evans, Paul, & Sharp, 1999). This may reflect some of the shared language and communication deficits as well as some behavioral components. Behavioral concerns associated with Down syndrome include temper tantrums or misbehavior that result from poor language skills and poor coping skills for dealing with frustration (Jahromi, Gulsrod, & Kasari, 2008). There is some evidence that children with Down syndrome will rely on social behaviors as a means to avoid cognitively challenging tasks and exhibit deficits in means-end (instrumental) thinking (Fidler, 2006). In addition, there is a lack of attention to basic concerns for safety (e.g., these children tend to be overly friendly to strangers, easily victimized), issues with sexuality and making appropriate choices (e.g., birth control, safe sex). Individuals with Down syndrome often are described as stubborn and may exhibit behaviors associated with anxiety, depression, and withdrawal as they increase in age (E. M. Dykens & Kasari, 1997), as well as compulsions (Evans & Gray, 2000).

As they get older, many individuals with Down syndrome are active participants in educational, vocational, social, and recreational arenas. Some are able to find employment and live independently; others will need more structured work and living situations. Transitional planning and preparation is important regardless of ability level. With increased life expectancy among adults with Down syndrome, cognitive declines are being noted. There is evidence that by age 60, a majority of individuals with Down syndrome will present with symptoms of Alzheimer's type dementia (Roizen & Patterson, 2003).

Evidence-Based Interventions

The primary area of focus for treatment parallels the primary neurocognitive deficits: language and communication. It is important for early intervention to be in place, with some indications that even a few months' delay in onset of stimulation can result in poorer development of gross and fine motor, language, and social skills (Saenz, 1999). In conjunction with a focus on communication, management of otitis media and any associated hearing loss is important enough to warrant routine screening (Saenz, 1999).

For other areas of concern, and as part of early intervention, addressing the motor, balance, and gait problems of individuals with Down syndrome may be appropriate. A number of interventions using treadmills and other motor apparatus have been employed to increase ambulation difficulties in individuals with Down syndrome (J. Wu, Ulrich,

Looper, Tiernan, & Angulo-Barroso, 2008). Specific recommendations during early childhood that have been offered for improving speech development include vocal stimulation (Warren, Fey, & Yoder, 2007), increasing the level of speechlike babbling, and facilitating reciprocal interaction (Rondal, Elbouz, Ylieff, & Docquier, 2003). Early on, parents can be trained to respond to any and all speech production; as speech progresses, parents can be trained to respond to only specific productions for target words; there is consistent evidence that maternal responsivity is critical in the development of language, cognition, and social-emotional development among children with developmental delays as seen in Down syndrome (Warren & Brady, 2007). A combination of phonological awareness training has been used successfully with children with Down syndrome (Goetz et al., 2008) to address early literacy, but this has not demonstrated an effect on speech production (E. J. Kennedy & Flynn, 2003). Although short-term memory is believed to account for much of the variance in speech and language development, no specific interventions have been found to be effective in this area for children with Down syndrome.

One program, the Learn at Play Program (LAPP) was specifically developed for children with Down syndrome and their parents (Iarocci, Virji-Babul, & Reebye, 2006). Theoretically driven from a systems perspective, LAPP focuses on the development of interpersonal skills and social competence in early childhood. Positive results were found with the program (Iarocci et al., 2006); however, replication of these results is needed. Consistent with treatment approaches used when mental retardation is present, behavioral approaches, including positive behavior support, may be appropriate for use with individuals with Down syndrome (Feeley & Jones, 2006; R. J. Morris & Morris, 1998). As with other disorders, some alternative methods have been used with children with Down syndrome. Dietary supplements, including antioxidants and folinic acid, have been suggested; however, randomized clinical trials did not yield any evidence to support the use of such nutritional supplements (Ellis et al., 2008). With increased occurrence of scoliosis, hip instability, patellar instability, and other foot problems identified, early screening for orthopedic problems is recommended so that surgery can be avoided (Mik et al., 2008). Another program, the Responsivity Education/Prelinguistic Milieu Teaching (RE/PMT) was developed and tested with a mixed group of children with developmental delays. Thus far, the results of this program have been equivocal (M. Fey et al., 2006; Warren et al., 2008). Evidence-based interventions with children with Down syndrome are summarized in Table 15.2.

In addition to interventions, specific accommodations or modifications may be appropriate for children with Down syndrome. For example, it has been recommended that it may be beneficial to capitalize on strengths in visual modalities, increasing the intensity, frequency of exposure, and duration of exposure to new vocabulary and incorporating familiar context to increase comprehension (Fidler, Philofsky, & Hepburn, 2007).

FRAGILE X

Definition

Fragile X is the most common chromosomal disorder that causes mental retardation after Down syndrome (Cornish, Levitas, & Sudhalter, 2007; Fryns et al., 2000). Fragile X was first identified by geneticist Herbert Lubs, who observed the chromosomal defect responsible for the syndrome in 1969. Fragile X is an X-linked disorder that is the result of a defect in the distal end of the X chromosome at the location of the fragile mental

Table 15.2 Evidence-Based Status for Interventions for Children with Down Syndrome

Interventions	Target	Status
Vocal stimulation, articulation exercises, reinforcement	Early intervention for speech production	Emerging (Rondal et al., 2003; Warren & Yoder, 1997)
Sign language or other alternative visual communication strategy	Fostering communication	Emerging (J. F. Miller et al., 1995; E. M. Roberts et al., 2007; Rondal et al., 2003)
Behavioral approaches	Reciprocal interactions in communicative contexts	Emerging (Rondal et al., 2003)
Treadmill interventions	Motor accuracy and gait	Promising (Angulo-Barroso, Wu, & Ulrich, 2008; J. Wu et al., 2008)
Behavioral approaches (reinforcement, shaping, positive behavioral support)	Aggression, noncompliance, defiance, other challenging behaviors	Inconclusive (Feeley & Jones, 2006)
Behavioral approaches (chaining, use of contingencies)	Means-end thinking, problem solving	Emerging (Fidler, 2006)
Responsive teaching	Cognitive, language, and social domains	Inconclusive (Mahoney, Perales, Wiggers, & Herman, 2006)
Responsive Education/Prelinguistic Milieu Teaching (RE/PMT)	Nonverbal requesting	Inconclusive (M. E. Fey, 2006; Warren et al., 2008; Yoder & Warren, 2002)
Learn at Play Program (LAPP)	Social competence	Inconclusive for birth to 3 years old (Iarocci et al., 2006)
Structured, phonics-based reading intervention	Reading skills	Promising practice (Goetz et al., 2008)
Structured, phonics-based reading intervention	Speech production	Inconclusive (Goetz et al., 2008)
Verbal rehearsal strategies	Short-term memory	Ineffective (Jarrold, Baddeley, & Hewes, 2000)
Errorless compliance training	Noncompliance and other behavior problems	Promising practice (A. S. Davis, 2008)
Nutritional supplements	Cognitive ability, appearance	Ineffective (Roizen, 2005; Salman, 2002)
Piracetam (Nootropil)	Cognitive ability	Ineffective, adverse effects (Lobaugh et al., 2001)

retardation 1 (*FMR1*) gene (Verkerk et al., 1991). This is the location of the information needed for production of the fragile X mental retardation protein (FMRP) that is needed by the body's cells to develop and function normally; with fragile X, the end or some portion of the end is attached only by a thin membrane or may be broken off. The extent to which the production and usability of this protein is affected contributes to the severity of presentation of fragile X (Cornish et al., 2007). Because it is X-linked, it primarily affects males; however, fragile X syndrome does not behave in the typical manner of an X-linked trait. Nearly 20 percent of fragile X males are silent carriers with a permutation or alleles with 55 to 200 repeats; they are unaffected by the syndrome but can pass the fragile X chromosome to their female offspring. Further, about one-third of female fragile X carriers, who would be expected to be asymptomatic, exhibit some symptoms of the disorder. Neurological correlates include decreased size of the posterior vermis of the cerebellum and differences in functioning via functional magnetic resonance imaging (fMRI) of the caudate nucleus and the hippocampus (Cornish et al., 2007).

Incidence

The incidence of fragile X is difficult to discern as it may be misidentified as mental retardation or learning disability. Across studies, it has been estimated that approximately 1 in 3,500 to 8,900 males is affected by the full mutation of the *FMR1* gene, while 1 in 1,000 males has the premutation form of the *FMR1* gene. Further, it was estimated that 1 in 250 to 500 females in the general population has the permutation, and 1 in 4,000 females is affected by the full mutation (D. C. Crawford, Acuña, & Sherman, 2001; Finucane, McConkie-Rosell, & Cronister, 2002).

Course and Prognosis

Individuals with the full mutation tend to be of small stature with a large head. Facial features include a long and narrow face, ear anomalies (e.g., large, pointed), large jaw (prognathism), high arched palate, and a prominent forehead (Hatton et al., 2009; Lachiewicz, Dawson, & Spiridigliozzi, 2000). Additional physical characteristics include large testicles (macroorchidism), double jointedness, and hypotonia. Initial signs of fragile X may be subtle, such as delayed attainment of developmental milestones (Maes, Fryns, Ghesquiére, & Borghgraef, 2000); diagnosis is most likely to occur at 8 years of age (Centers for Disease Control, 2002; Kau, Reider, Payne, Meyer, & Freund, 2000). Notably, research suggests a significant negative correlation between age and IQ, and between age and adaptive behavior for children with Fragile X (Fisch et al., 2007).

Neurocognitive Correlates

Mental retardation is common; a decline in cognitive ability may occur in middle childhood (Lachiewicz et al., 2000). Additionally, assessment is more difficult as a result of the low language abilities and may be best accomplished with nonverbal measures (Hooper, Hatton, Baranek, Roberts, & Bailey, 2000). A summary of the functional domains often affected with fragile X is provided in Table 15.3. Individuals with fragile X syndrome evidence moderate to severe delays in communication skills, particularly in expressive language; they also evidence deficits in repetitive speech and tangential language and poor speech intelligibility in conversation (Belser & Sudhalter, 2001; J. E. Roberts, Mirrett, & Burchinal, 2001). These deficits in language areas continue across the life span, with difficulties in grammar, vocabulary, pragmatics, and speech development reported in adolescents and adults with fragile X syndrome (Abbeduto et al., 2003). Notably, there is some

Table 15.3 Neuropsychological Deficits Associated with Fragile X

Global Domain/Specific Deficits	Phenotype
Cognition	Mental retardation common; decline in cognitive ability occurs in middle childhood
Auditory-linguistic/Language function	Expressive language typically more affected than receptive Difficulties in perseverative speech, but vocabulary acquisition relative strength Language comprehension a relative weakness Relative weaknesses in gesturing, reciprocity, and symbolic communication Dysfluency frequent
Motor function	Fine motor problems frequent
Learning and memory	Memory for meaningful information is strength, but memory for abstract information impaired Relative strength in verbal short-term memory
Visual-perception/Constructional praxis	Visual-perceptual processing intact Visual-motor coordination may be impaired
Attention/Concentration	Selective attention intact; attentional control and inhibition impaired High co-occurrence of Attention-Deficit/Hyperactivity Disorder (ADHD)
Executive function	Impairment evident
Processing speed	Impairment in processing speed dependent on cognitive impairment and specific permutation
Achievement/Academic skills	Difficulties in arithmetic Reading proficiency may or may not be impaired
Emotional/Behavioral functioning	High frequency of autistic symptoms and ADHD Common psychiatric problems include social phobia, depression, obsessive-compulsive disorder, panic disorder, and mood dysregulation

indication that cognitive ability declines with age as a function of the increased demands for higher-order, abstract reasoning (Fisch et al., 1999, 2007). The apparent decline is believed to reflect the slower gains made by children with fragile X such that they fall farther and farther behind (Fisch et al., 2002). Alternatively, frontostriatal connections are implicated as a result of the higher-order/executive function and attentional deficits (Gothelf, Furfaro, Penniman, Glover, & Reiss, 2005). For younger children, receptive language emerges as a relative strength, but this is not evident in older children with fragile X (J. E. Roberts et al., 2001).

Educational Implications

The most noticeable and consistent effect of fragile X is on intelligence (Cornish et al., 2007). More than 80% of males with fragile X have an IQ of 75 or less. The effect of fragile X on intelligence is more variable in females. Some females have mental impairment, some have learning disabilities, and some have a normal IQ. Research suggests that some individuals with learning disability/specific language impairment may have a less severe form of fragile X (Cornish et al., 2007). Speech/language difficulties are common and include echolalia, perseveration or repetitive speech, poor language content, and cluttering (dropping of letters or syllables when speaking). Language comprehension is a relative weakness (Philofsky, Hepburn, Hayes, Hagerman, & Rogers, 2004; J. Price, Roberts, Vandergrift, & Martin, 2007; J. E. Roberts et al., 2001) but expressive language typically is more affected than receptive language (J. E. Roberts et al., 2001). Notably, vocabulary acquisition is a relative strength (Cornish et al., 2007) while comprehension is a relative weakness (J. Price et al., 2007). Verbal aspects are not the only areas of language that are affected; individuals with fragile X also evidence relative weaknesses in gesturing, reciprocity, and symbolic communication (J. E. Roberts et al., 2001).

Despite verbal deficits, a relative strength in verbal short-term memory has been found (Freund, Peebles, Aylward, & Reiss, 1995). Further, memory for meaningful information is a relative strength while memory for abstract information is impaired (Cornish et al., 2007). In at least one study, group differences were not observed in processing speed specific to fragile X; processing speed was compromised in association with cognitive impairment (Hooper et al., 2008) as well as in conjunction with specific chromosomal permutations (J. Grigsby et al., 2008). Similarly, fine motor abilities may be compromised in those children with fragile X who are lower functioning or have co-occurring autism spectrum disorder (Zingerevich et al., 2009).Visual-perceptual processing is usually intact (Cornish et al., 2007); however, visual-motor coordination may be impaired (Freund et al., 1995). Attentional control and inhibition are impaired (Cornish et al., 2007), as are other components of executive function (Gothelf et al., 2005; J. Grigsby et al., 2008; Hooper et al., 2008). Poor sensory skills and mathematical ability (J. E. Roberts et al., 2005) sometimes are found in conjunction with relatively strong reading skills (Hodapp & Fidler, 1999). Motor skills also are affected with toe walking frequent. In addition, stuttering is a common occurrence (Van Borsel & Tetnowski, 2007). Affected females tend to have particular difficulty with mathematics (see Chapter 3).

Social-Emotional/Psychological Implications

Two-thirds of children with fragile X evidence maladaptive behavior (Fisch et al., 2008). Individuals with fragile X may exhibit hyperactivity, self-abusive behavior, and self-isolation as well as other autistic symptoms. Fragile X is one of a very few disorders where there is a certainty of autistic features (Cornish et al., 2007); approximately 90% of individuals with fragile X also have autistic-like features or autism. It is estimated that 15% to 25% of children with fragile X syndrome are diagnosed with autism (D. B. J. Bailey et al., 2004; Lathe, 2009) and 5.5% of males with autism test positive for fragile X syndrome (Hagerman, 2002). This is likely predicated by the fact that the diagnosis of autism spectrum disorder includes the presence of language deficits (see Chapter 5). In addition to language deficits, social approach deficits are also frequent in children with fragile X (J. E. Roberts, Weisenfeld, Hatton, Heath, & Kaufmann, 2007). Consistent with the relative frequency of autistic-like tendencies, hypersensitivity and hyperarousal are recognized as prominent behavioral features. Children with fragile X also tend to demonstrate low levels of initiation of interaction, gaze avoidance, and failure to engage in joint attention; these then lead to social problems. In addition to autism or autistic-like behaviors, children with fragile X also demonstrate problems with attention and hyperactivity, often leading to a diagnosis of ADHD (see Chapter 6), particularly for affected boys (Cornish, Munir, & Wilding, 2001). Common psychiatric problems include social phobia, depression, obsessive-compulsive disorder, panic disorder, and mood dysregulation (Tsiouris & Brown, 2004). For girls with fragile X, there is increased co-occurrence of anxiety disorder or avoidant personality disorder (Freund et al., 1995).

Medical Implications

As with Down syndrome, many health problems are associated with fragile X (Hagerman, 2002). Early on, this includes ear infections (otitis media) that may affect hearing and contribute to the speech and language problems evidenced by these children. Strabismus and other vision problems also may be present. Dental problems frequently occur as well and may further exacerbate speech problems. Heart problems, including mitral valve prolapse, are associated with fragile X, and occasional seizures can occur (Cornish et al., 2007). Children with fragile X are also at increased risk of seizure disorder (Sabaratnam, Venkatesha Murphy, Wijeratne, Buckingham, & Payne, 2003).

Evidence-Based Intervention

Early intervention is critical (Cornish et al., 2007; Hatton et al., 2000; Mirrett, Roberts, & Price, 2003), with identification of comorbid conditions, particularly ADHD and autism. For children who exhibit comorbid conditions, one avenue for identifying potential interventions is to examine the evidence-based practices for the target behavior as demonstrated with the comorbid condition (see Chapters 5 and 6), keeping in mind that no studies have examined the use of these methods with comorbid fragile X populations. Similarly, when considering medication as a treatment alternative, there have been few studies on the use of drugs in children with fragile X (Cornish et al., 2007). Medication classes often used to address some of the behavioral issues associated with fragile X include stimulants, selective serotonin reuptake inhibitors (SSRIs), and alpha-2 agonists, including fenobam (Berry-Kravis et al., 2009; Berry-Kravis & Potanos, 2004), as well as lithium (Berry-Kravis et al., 2008).

A multidisciplinary approach to treatment that includes medical management, educational accommodations, speech-language and occupational therapy, as well as therapy to address social emotional and behavioral challenges would constitute best practice (Friefeld et al., 1993; Schwarte, 2008). Standard treatment includes special education, speech and language services, and behavioral programs to address behavioral concerns. Because of the variability of language profiles among children with fragile X, it is important to match the treatment to the specific profile presented (Fidler et al., 2007). Teaching strategies for school-age children with fragile X include ensuring that the teacher has an awareness of the child's learning style and incorporates simultaneous processing activities (Harris-Schmidt, 2003). This may include the use of whole-word methods for reading and spelling; increased use of visual cues, including pictures, sign language, logos, and words; use of concrete, high-interest examples and materials; and modeling and imitation for both behavioral and communication goals. Genetic counseling will benefit families of affected persons. Other treatment is symptomatic and supportive based on individual needs. A summary of evidence-based practices with children with fragile X is provided in Table 15.4.

WILLIAMS SYNDROME

Definition

Williams syndrome or Williams-Beuren syndrome was identified initially by cardiologists, who noted that a group of patients had not only the same cardiac problems but also similar facial features and mental retardation (Mervis & Morris, 2007). Williams

Table 15.4 Evidence-Based Status for Interventions for Fragile X Syndrome

Interventions	Target	Status
Medications: stimulants such as methylphenidate (Concerta, Ritalin)	Attention span, inhibition, hyperactivity	Emerging, some adverse effects (Hagerman & Hagerman, 2002; Torrioli et al., 2008)
Medications: clonidine (Catapres)	Hyperactivity	Emerging (Hagerman & Hagerman, 2002)
Medications: tricyclic antidepressants	Hyperactivity	Inconclusive (Hagerman & Hagerman, 2002)
Medications: SSRIs	Aggression, hyperactivity, depression, and self-injurious behaviors	Emerging (Hagerman & Hagerman, 2002)
Medications: L-acetylcarnitine	Attention problems	Emerging (Torrioli et al., 2008)
Medications: fenobam	Attention problems, impulsivity	Emerging with adults (Berry-Kravis et al., 2009)
Medications: lithium (Lithobid)	Behavior problems	Emerging (Berry-Kravis et al., 2008)
Behavioral approaches	Sleep problems	Emerging (Weiskop, Richdale, & Matthews, 2005)

syndrome is easily identifiable due to the characteristic facial features, which include at least nine of the following:

- Epicanthal folds
- Periorbital fullness
- Broad brow
- Bitemporal narrowing
- Short upturned nose
- Lacy iris pattern
- Strabismus (crossed eyes)
- Full or bulbous nasal tip
- Full cheeks
- Full prominent lips
- Wide mouth
- Small jaw
- Small teeth
- Dental malocclusion (poor bite)
- Prominent earlobes (C. A. Morris, 2006)

Children with Williams syndrome tend to appear younger than their age, in part due to their short stature and facial features. Notably, they tend to stare at human faces, and it has been suggested that this behavior is unique to Williams syndrome (Mervis & Morris, 2007).

Incidence/Prevalence

Williams syndrome is estimated to occur in 1 of 20,000 to 25,000 live births (Sarpal et al., 2008). Williams syndrome occurs equally as often in males and females, although the medical complications are more common in males. The syndrome occurs across ethnic groups; as with gender, the occurrence of medical complications may vary across ethnic groups (Sarpal et al., 2008).

Etiology

It is now known that Williams syndrome is a microdeletion of chromosome 7q11.23 (Ewart et al., 1993; Sarpal et al., 2008); the deleted portion contains about 25 genes; thus, Williams syndrome constitutes a contiguous gene deletion syndrome, potentially affecting multiple systems (Hillier et al., 2003). In addition, the size of the deletion can vary. Due to these differences, the resulting phenotype is variable. The facial dysmorphology is attributed to the elastin gene haploinsufficiency that is connected to 7q11.23 (Ewart et al., 1993). Other genes also are being investigated (Sarpal et al., 2008).

Neurological Correlates

Using magnetic resonance imaging (MRI), it was found that individuals with Williams syndrome had significantly reduced intracranial volume as compared to controls (Reiss et al., 2000; Sampaio et al., 2008). Compared to age-matched peers, individuals with Williams syndrome evidence increased gyrification in the right parietal and right occipital lobes as well as the left frontal region, based on MRI (J. E. Schmitt, Eliez, Bellugi, Galaburda, & Reiss, 2002). In addition, fMRI yielded reduced activation in the parietal lobe of individuals with Williams syndrome (Meyer-Lindenberg et al., 2004). Other studies also have found reduced gray matter in areas related to visual-spatial processing, including the occipitoparietal sulcus/vertical area of the intraparietal sulcus (Eckert et al., 2005; Meyer-Lindenberg, Mervis, & Berman, 2006; Reiss et al., 2004) as well as the left parieto-occipital region (Boddaert et al., 2005). Reduced volume also was noted in the brain stem (Reiss et al., 2000). As such, individuals with Williams syndrome tend to have a greater ratio of frontal to posterior tissue (Reiss et al., 2000). The central sulcus has also been implicated, particularly the dorsal end bilaterally (Jackowski & Schultz, 2005). In contrast, there appears to be relative sparing of the cerebellar and superior temporal gyrus volumes (Reiss et al., 2000). The typical left-greater-than-right asymmetry of the superior temporal gyrus was not present; finally, the usual correlation between overall cognitive ability and the volume of the superior temporal gyrus was not found in individuals with Williams syndrome, suggesting a disruption in this area of the brain that is likely related to the linguistic difficulties exhibited (Sampaio et al., 2008).

Despite reduced intracranial volume and reductions in both white and gray matter, MRI revealed that the right-hemisphere perisylvian cortex and inferior temporal zone were thicker in individuals with Williams syndrome as compared to controls (P. M. Thompson et al., 2005). Surface complexity also was found to be increased and correlated with the gyrification differences in the temporoparietal region based on Steinmetz criteria (P. M. Thompson et al., 2005). In response to faze and gaze processing tasks, individuals with Williams syndrome evidenced increases in right fusiform gyrus as well as several frontal and temporal regions; regions activated by the control group were bilateral fusiform gyri, occipital, and temporal lobes (Mobbs et al., 2004). Further, relative to controls, the group with Williams syndrome demonstrated more activation in the right inferior, superior, and medial frontal gyri; in the anterior cingulate; and in subcortical regions, including the superior thalamus and caudate. These findings were interpreted to suggest relative sparing of the frontal and temporal regions and impairment of the occipital (visual) regions consistent with visual-spatial deficits and difficulties with gaze and face processing (Mobbs et al., 2004).

Using fMRI, it also was found that children with William syndrome exhibited significantly reduced activity in the striatum and the dorsolateral prefrontal and dorsal anterior cingulate cortices when performing a go-no go task as compared to a control group (Mobbs et al., 2007). This supports the hypothesis that frontostriatal circuits are not engaged to the same extent in individuals with Williams syndrome and accounts for the deficits in response inhibition that are evident (Mobbs et al., 2007). Positron emission tomography and fMRI of 12 children with Williams syndrome indicated reduction in resting blood flow and absent differential response to visual stimuli in the anterior hippocampal formation (Meyer-Lindenberg et al., 2005). No differences in size of the hippocampus were found, but subtle differences in shape were present. It was concluded that these differences may contribute to the deficits in spatial navigation and long-term memory associated with Williams syndrome (Meyer-Lindenberg et al., 2005).

Research further suggests some differences in the corpus callosum in individuals with Williams syndrome (Tomaiuolo et al., 2002). In particular, it was found that the corpus callosum of individuals with Williams syndrome tended to be more convex and smaller as compared to controls. The volumetric difference was most notable in the splenium and caudal sections; these differences may further underlie some of the deficits associated with Williams syndrome (Tomaiuolo et al., 2002). Finally, volumetric differences have been noted in the relative size of the cerebellum relative to the cerebrum in adults and children with Williams syndrome (W. Jones et al., 2002).

Course and Prognosis

Multiple medical issues are associated with Williams syndrome (Mervis & Morris, 2007). These include difficulty with feeding and lack of coordination of the suck and swallow process, part of which may be due to hypotonia. Inguinal hernias occur in about 40% of children with Williams syndrome; this is treated surgically. Williams syndrome is associated with high serum calcium levels, which can cause irritability and constipation; the syndrome also is associated with gastroesophageal reflex and colic. Problems with feeding and gastrointestinal issues may account for the slow pattern of growth over the first 4 years as well as the increased incidence of failure to thrive among infants and toddlers with Williams syndrome (C. A. Morris, 2006). These problems continue into childhood and adulthood with frequent complaints of abdominal pain. Because of the potential for endocrine problems, including hypothyroidism, monitoring of growth is recommended (Mervis & Morris, 2007). Profiles of children with Williams syndrome are somewhat similar to those with fragile X, with similar long-term trajectories (Fisch et al., 2008).

Vision problems, either hyperopia (farsightedness) or strabismus (crossed eyes), are common but do not account for the significant visual-motor problems (Mervis & Morris, 2007). There are some indications of higher than expected rates of sensorineural hearing loss in school-age children with Williams syndrome, possibly progressive (Marler, Effenbein, Ryals, Urban, & Netzloff, 2005). Williams syndrome can co-occur with Arnold Chiari malformation of the cerebellum, which further complicates the presentation of the disorder. Cardiovascular disease occurs frequently and accounts for the relatively lower life expectancy of individuals with Williams syndrome (Sadler et al., 2001).

Taken together, the health, visual, and motor problems associated with Williams syndrome may explain why children with this disorder evidence oral language prior to gestural language (Mervis et al., 2000). Children with Williams syndrome also have deficits in nonverbal joint attention (E. Laing et al., 2002). Articulation is not an issue with children with Williams syndrome (Meyerson & Frank, 1987). Although spoken language precedes nonverbal communication, and verbal abilities generally are far better developed than spatial abilities (Bellugi, Lichtenberger, Jones, Lai, & St. George, 2000), children with Williams syndrome do evidence language delays relative to typically developing children (Gordon, 2006; E. Laing & Jarrold, 2007).

Adults with Williams syndrome evidence a high frequency of problems across multiple organ systems, compromising health and overall functioning (Cherniske et al., 2004). These problems include mild to moderately high frequency sensory neural hearing loss, cardiovascular problems and hypertension, diabetes, gastrointestinal difficulties, subclinical hypothyroidism, and decreased bone density. As a result, there is increased likelihood that adults with Williams syndrome will be living in group homes or other supported living environments rather than independent living situations. There is also some indication of premature or accelerated aging that may complicate progression in adulthood (Cherniske et al., 2004).

Neurocognitive Correlates

Although some individuals with Williams syndrome do have average intelligence, most individuals have mild to moderate mental retardation (Howlin, Davies, & Udwin, 1998; Mervis & Morris, 2007; Tassabehji et al., 1999). There is a general pattern of verbal abilities stronger than visual-spatial abilities (Bellugi, Lichtenberger, Mills, Galaburda, & Korenberg, 1999; Braden & Obrzut, 2002; Mervis et al., 2000). Frequently impaired domains include visual-spatial construction (praxis), motor skills, abstract relational vocabulary, and math skills. In contrast, verbal short-term memory, language ability, and concrete vocabulary as well as reading skills tend to be relative strengths (Gothelf et al., 2005; Mervis & Morris, 2007). As such, it has been suggested that with Williams syndrome, any composite intelligence score is misleading, given the typical pattern of strengths and weaknesses associated with the syndrome (Stinton, Farran, & Courbois, 2008). Within language areas, children with Williams syndrome frequently evidence strengths in language areas, particularly concrete vocabulary; abstract relational vocabulary is more likely to be a relative weakness (Mervis & Morris, 2007; Mervis, Robinson, Rowe, Becerra, & Klein-Tasman, 2004). Comprehension problems emerge early in life despite relatively even development of receptive and expressive language (Mervis & Klein-Tasman, 2000). Deficits in language areas, include word-finding difficulty and pragmatic deficits similar to those with autism spectrum disorder (Bellugi et al., 2000, 2007; Philofsky, Fidler, & Hepburn, 2007; Udwin & Yule, 1991). Similarly, Williams syndrome is associated with a disconnect between language and face processing (Bellugi et al., 1999).

Individuals with Williams syndrome have difficulty with mental rotation tasks (Farran, Jarrold, & Gathercole, 2001; Vicari, Bellucci, & Carlesimo, 2006). These difficulties are not ameliorated when salience of the stimulus is increased (Stinton et al., 2008) but may relate to their difficulties in visual-spatial areas. In early childhood, the presence of hypotonicity can contribute to delayed motor milestones; however, over time, the child may become hypertonic in lower limbs with increased deep tendon reflexes and tightening of the Achilles' tendon. Both hypotonicity and hypertonicity affect motor functions. As a result, motor performance and dexterity are delayed (S.-W. Tsai, Wu, Liou, & Shu, 2008).

Table 15.5 Neuropsychological Functioning Associated with Williams Syndrome

Global Domain/Specific Deficits	Phenotype
Cognition	Mental retardation common; general pattern of verbal abilities stronger than visual-spatial abilities
Auditory-linguistic/Language function	Strengths in language areas, particularly concrete vocabulary; abstract relational vocabulary a relative weakness Relative even development of receptive and expressive language Comprehension problems Word-finding difficulty Pragmatic deficits similar to those with autism spectrum disorder
Learning and memory	Relative strength in verbal short-term memory
Visual perception/Constructional praxis	Visual-spatial and constructional abilities significantly impaired
Motor function	Motor performance and dexterity delayed
Achievement/Academic skills	Reading skills better developed than math skills
Emotional/Behavioral functioning	High co-occurrence of ADHD (Mervis & Morris, 2007) and Autism High rate of behavioral problems, poor social relationships, anxiety, obsessions, and communication problems

Educational Implications

Consistent with higher verbal ability and lower nonverbal ability, reading skills are better developed than math skills (Mervis & Morris, 2007). As suggested by the deficit areas in Table 15.5, children with Williams syndrome evidence significant academic and behavioral problems. In a study of 20 individuals with Williams syndrome, academic achievement in the area of reading was highly variable (Lew, Smith, & Tager-Flusberg, 2003). Notably, the level of reading was correlated not with verbal ability (vocabulary) but with nonverbal ability (matrices). Further, although expected relations were found between phonological awareness and reading level, rapid naming was not significantly related to reading in this sample (Lew et al., 2003).

Psychological Implications

In general, children and adults with Williams syndrome tend to be highly social (Bellugi et al., 1999). There is a higher than expected incidence of ADHD and anxiety among individuals with Williams syndrome (Mervis & Morris, 2007). There is also a high comorbidity of autism spectrum disorders among children with Williams syndrome (Klein-Tasman, Mervis, Lord, & Philips, 2007). Even when not diagnosed, there is a high rate of behavioral problems, poor social relationships, anxiety, obsessions, and communication problems associated with Williams syndrome (M. Davies, Udwin, & Howlin, 1998; Einfeld, Tonge, & Rees, 2001).

Evidence-Based Intervention

The available research on the use of cognitive-behavioral approaches with individuals who have mental retardation is limited; there is even less available research when there is

Table 15.6 Evidence-Based Status for Interventions for Williams Syndrome

Intervention	Target	Status
Cognitive-behavioral therapy	Obsessive, compulsive behavior	Emerging (Klein-Tasman & Albano, 2007)
Behavioral approaches	Food refusal	Emerging (O'Reilly & Lancioni, 2001)
Desensitization training	Hypersensitivity to sound	Emerging (Myerson & Frank, 1987)

a specific etiology to the mental retardation, such as Williams syndrome (Klein-Tasman & Albano, 2007). Based on case study results, and targeting areas of social skills, obsessions, and compulsions, Klein-Tasman and Albano concluded that cognitive-behavioral approaches may hold promise for some individuals with Williams syndrome. A summary of available research is presented in Table 15.6.

ANGELMAN SYNDROME

Definition

Angelman syndrome was initially described by Harry Angelman and came to be known as happy puppet syndrome or puppet children syndrome based on his initial descriptions (Angelman, 1965). Angelman syndrome is characterized by severe developmental delay, speech impairment, ataxia with a puppetlike gait, and frequent laughing, smiling, and excitability (C. A. Williams & Driscoll, 2007). Physical characteristics include somewhat flattened head; protruding tongue, with widely spaced teeth; and pronounced occipital groove (Buntinx et al., 1995; R. J. Morris & Morris, 1998). Additionally, hypopigmentation (light skin, blue eyes, light hair color) occurs in about 70% of cases. Behaviorally, Angelman syndrome is associated with jerky movements and a puppetlike gait as well as bouts of laughter, believed to be due to defects in the brain stem. Children with Angelman smile frequently, often as a precursor to seeking adult attention (Oliver et al., 2007). Most children with Angelman syndrome are functionally mute. Further, they may have vision problems, with optic pallor or atrophy frequently noted (R. J. Morris & Morris, 1998).

Incidence

Angelman syndrome is estimated to occur in 1 in 12,000 to 16,000 live births (C. A. Williams, 2005). It occurs worldwide, but incidence may be underestimated due to the diagnostic challenge the syndrome presents to neurologists and other medical personnel. Consensus criteria have been developed (C. A. Williams & Driscoll, 2007); these criteria rely predominantly on genetic testing and observed features.

Etiology

The gene involved has been identified as 15q11–q13; this is the area of the gene that is subject to imprinting and encompasses a cluster of gamma-aminobutyric acid (GABA) receptor subunit genes (Guerrini, Carrozzo, Rinaldi, & Bonanni, 2003). With Angelman, it is thought that there is a flaw in the genomic imprinting. It is believed to be maternally transmitted but can occur through several possible mechanisms. The most frequent mechanism is the deletion form associated with maternal transmission, accounting for about 70% of those with Angelman and associated with the most severe phenotype (C. A. Williams, 2005). An additional 25% are due to mutation of the ubiquinine-protein ligase (UBE3A) gene (Kishino, Lalande, & Wagstaff, 1997). In other cases, the mechanism may be paternal uniparental disomy or inheritance of two copies of the paternal gene and no maternal contribution. It is believed that the manifestation of Angelman varies as a result of the conflict between the alleles donated by the mother (with deletion of the maternally imprinted region) and father (Oliver et al., 2007). In some cases, mutations of the MECP2 gene (the gene mutation in Rett syndrome) also may be present. Severity of manifestation of deficits associated with Angelman syndrome appears to be reflective of the genotype or mechanism of occurrence (Sahoo et al., 2006). In particular, children with larger, class I deletions are at greater risk of comorbid autism, decreased cognitive functioning, and poorer expressive language skills; children with larger deletions are also more likely to require multiple medications to control seizures (Sahoo et al., 2006).

Neurological Correlates

The brain in Angelman syndrome is structurally normal; there are reports of individuals having cerebellar hypoplasia, unilateral temporal lobe hypoplasia, and vermian cyst (Laan, van Haeringen, & Brouwer, 1999). Neuroimaging studies suggest cortical atrophy, microencephaly, and ventricular dilation; these differences are presumed to be related to expression of UBE3A in areas of the neocortex, hippocampus, striatum, and Purkinje cells of the cerebellum (Dindot, Antalffy, Bhattacharjee, & Beaudet, 2007). Additionally, there are some indications of thinning of the corpus callosum and decreased myelination. Based on histological studies, there may be decreased dendritic arborization, decreased GABA in the cerebellum, and increased glutamate in the frontal and occipital regions. Research with MRI and computed tomography indicate mild cortical atrophy, cortical anomalies, or generalized ventricular enlargement or some combination (C. A. Williams, 2005; C. A. Williams & Frias, 1982). Craniofacial abnormalities are likely the result of decreased brain growth. The language disturbance is believed to be due to misrouting of long projection axons during prenatal development.

Angelman syndrome is associated with diffusely abnormal electroencephalogram (EEG), with high-amplitude spike and slow waves at 2 to 3 cycles per second, sometimes more prominent anteriorly, persistent rhythmic 4 to 6 cycles per second spikes not associated with drowsiness, or spikes mixed with 3 to 4 cycles per second components mainly posteriorly and facilitated by, or only seen with, eye closure (Boyd, Harden, & Patton, 1988; Clayton Smith, 2001). These patterns often lead to genetic testing and ultimately to the diagnosis (C. A. Williams, 2005). Evidence of transient myoclonic status epilepticus has been reported in up to 50% of individuals with Angelman syndrome (Viani et al., 1995). Abnormalities are most evident in posterior regions (Paprocka et al., 2007). It is estimated that 90% of individuals with Angelman syndrome will develop a seizure disorder in infancy or early childhood of variable severity (Valente et al., 2006); notably, Angelman syndrome accounts for up to 6% of those with epilepsy (Guerrini et al., 2003). In Angelman syndrome with epilepsy, there is characteristic paroxysmal discharge in the occipital region and diffuse high-voltage slow wave on EEG (Kumada et al., 2005).

Course and Prognosis

The behaviors and delays associated with Angelman syndrome usually are not evident at birth, with most children having a normal prenatal and birth history and no major birth defects. Nonspecific features may include microcephaly, developmental delay, or motor ataxia/hypotonia similar to cerebral palsy, making early diagnosis difficult (C. A. Williams, 2005). Although there may be some genetic overlap with Rett syndrome, there is no regression or loss of skills evident with Angelman syndrome. Angelman usually is identified in infancy or early childhood when atypical facial features and behaviors become problematic and more clearly present as a clinical syndrome (R. J. Morris & Morris, 1998; C. A. Williams, 2005). Age of diagnosis is between 3 and 7 years (C. A. Williams et al., 1995), with one study reporting a median age at diagnosis of 3.9 years (Paprocka et al., 2007). Problems with feeding and hypotonia may be the first indicators; developmental delays often are first noted at about 6 months of age. The unique features of Angelman syndrome that facilitate diagnosis often are not evident until after age 1.

Puberty may be delayed but is generally normal. Individuals with Angelman syndrome can have children but this is rare, likely due to restricted access rather than physiological reasons (C. A. Williams & Driscoll, 2007). Young adults are generally in good health aside from seizures; scoliosis develops with increasing age. Because of retardation, independent living is not possible, but most live at home or in group homes. Life expectancy appears to be normal, but it is important to monitor diet and activity level to keep weight down; scoliosis may result in cardiorespiratory complications later in life (Clayton Smith, 2001).

Neurocognitive Correlates

Neurocognitive aspects associated with Angelman are summarized in Table 15.7. Mild to moderate retardation is common; higher-functioning abilities are associated with imprinting defect or unipaternal disomy (Jolleff, Emmerson, Ryan, & McConachie, 2006); lower cognitive ability is associated with full deletion or type I (Lossie et al., 2001). Differences in cognitive ability by molecular class indicate an overlap across subtypes (S. U. Peters, Beaudet, Madduri, & Bacino, 2004). One of the major domains affected is that of communication. Better development of language and communication is associated with Angelman caused by imprinting or unipaternal disomy as opposed to maternal deletion in the areas of comprehension of phrases, spoken language and use of gestures for communication, and oromotor functions (Jolleff et al., 2006). Attentional problems are also frequent and may compromise intervention (Walz & Benson, 2002). Motor dysfunction is noted frequently in individuals with Angelman syndrome, including distal limb spasticity, ataxic-like gait, stiffness in lower limbs, and coactivation during movement (Beckung, Steffenburg, & Kyllerman, 2004). Greater than expected asymmetry of muscle strength was evident. Notably, although evidencing spasticity and decreased muscle

Table 15.7 Neuropsychological Deficits Associated with Angelman Syndrome

Global Domain/Specific Deficits	Phenotype
Cognition	Mild to moderate retardation common
Auditory-linguistic/Language function	Limited to no speech development
Attention	Short attention span
Emotional/Behavioral functioning	Socialization is a strength Affect not always appropriate; aggression and noncompliance may be present Smiles and laughter frequent in response to any social interaction High frequency of co-occurring autism and ADHD

strength, abnormalities usually are not sufficient to warrant a diagnosis of cerebral palsy (Beckung et al., 2004).

Educational Implications

Most individuals with Angelman syndrome function in the severe to profound range of mental retardation (R. J. Morris & Morris, 1998). Educational programs are best designed to develop and improve adaptive skills and increase independence to the extent possible. Because oral language does not develop, sign language or other nonverbal means of communication may be needed. Physical therapy may be appropriate to increase ambulation (C. A. Williams & Driscoll, 2007). Of adaptive skills, children with Angelman syndrome tend to exhibit strengths in socialization areas and deficits in motor skills (S. U. Peters, Goddard-Finegold, Beaudet, & Madduir, 2004).

Emotional/Behavioral Concerns

The most notable behavior is the excessive and inappropriate laughter as well as a generally happy demeanor. In particular, smiles and laughter were noted to occur frequently in response to any social interaction (Horsler & Oliver, 2006).

Research suggests that children with Angelman respond to social cues from adults and gain positive attention in response to smiles (Oliver et al., 2007). Thus, these behaviors may be being positively reinforced despite their inappropriateness to a given situation. Based on case study review and parent report, children with Angelman syndrome also exhibit inattention, hyperactivity, eating and sleeping problems, aggressive behavior, defiance, noncompliance, and tantrums. Further, they have a tendency to mouth objects and engage in repetitive and stereotypic behavior, such as hand flapping (Summers, Allison, Lynch, & Sandler, 1995). In a study examining problem behaviors in children with Angelman syndrome, caregiver/parent reports indicated that the behaviors of greatest concern were the lack of speech, overactivity, eating problems, and sleep problems (D. J. Clarke & Marston, 2000). Notably, 68% of the children were reported to have a fascination with water while only 57% were reported to have inappropriate bursts of laughter (D. J. Clarke & Marston, 2000).

Related to some of the shared behaviors with autism and findings of four individuals with Angelman syndrome who met full criteria for autism, it has been suggested that Angelman syndrome be considered as a possible etiology when the combination of autism, epilepsy, and mental retardation are present (Steffenburg, Gillberg, Steffenburg, & Kyllerman, 1996). The co-occurrence of Angelman and autism is most likely to be present with type I deletions; these children also are likely to have lower functioning levels (Sahoo et al., 2006). In one study of children with Angelman, 42% met criteria for autism (S. U. Peters, Beaudet et al., 2004). One significant behavioral difference identified was that relative to individuals with autism, children with Angelman exhibit more flexibility in their behavioral approach to task (Didden et al., 2008). In addition, socialization is a strength, while motor skills and communication are relative weaknesses (S. U. Peters, Beaudet et al., 2004). When both Angelman and autism were evident, the children demonstrated lower levels of language, communication, and socialization as compared to children who only had Angelman syndrome (Peters, Beaudet et al., 2004).

Evidence-Based Intervention

There is no cure for Angelman syndrome, so treatment must address the individual manifestation. Some specific practices are listed in Table 15.8. Seizure control may or may not

Table 15.8 Evidence-Based Status for Interventions for Angelman Syndrome

Interventions	Target	Status
Picture Communication System (PECS)	Communication	Unknown (R. J. Morris & Morris, 1998)
Behavioral approaches	General compliance	Promising practice (R. J. Morris & Morris, 1998)
Medications: vigabatrin (Sabril) and tiagabine (Gabitril)	Seizure control	Adverse effects (C. A. Williams & Driscoll, 2007)
Medical: surgical reimplant of salivary ducts or use of scopolamine patches	Excessive drooling due to tongue protrusion	Ineffective (C. A. Williams & Driscoll, 2007)

be maintained with or without medication (see Chapter 10); the use of anticonvulsants that increase brain GABA levels (e.g., vigabatrin [Sabril] and tiagabine [Gabitril) are not recommended for individuals with Angelman syndrome (C. A. Williams & Driscoll, 2007). Medical complications need to be addressed as they occur. Occupational therapy/physical therapy may be indicated depending on the effects on the motor system. If motor problems are severe, braces or surgery may be indicated. It is important to monitor children with Angelman syndrome for seizures, vision problems, and reflux. As they enter adolescence, it is important to encourage activity to avoid obesity (C. A. Williams & Driscoll, 2007).

As with other developmental disorders, early intervention, including stimulation and enrichment while establishing functional communication, is important. Morris and Morris stressed the importance of focusing on those skills that the person with Angelman syndrome is likely to be able to develop rather than, for example, focusing on speech, which is not likely to be achieved. Behavioral approaches (e.g., positive reinforcement, shaping) have been found to be effective in teaching self-help skills, social skills, sign language, and prevocational skills (R. J. Morris & Morris, 1998). For communication, the Picture Exchange Communication System (PECS) or a similar system has been recommended; no specific studies with Angelman syndrome were identified. Individualization and flexibility is important in meeting the needs of these children in school.

PRADER-WILLI SYNDROME

Definition

Prader-Willi syndrome (PWS) was first described in 1956 and later identified in 1981 (Reddy & Pfeiffer, 2007). It is a rare chromosomal disorder and, like Angelman syndrome, is associated with a missing segment from chromosome 15, but with PWS, the transmission is from the father. Prader-Willi syndrome is characterized by hypotonia, hypogonadism, cognitive impairment, and clinical obesity. Early on, there is low or diminished fetal activity that results in the identification of the disorder. In infancy, there is usually poor muscle tone (hypotonia) and underdeveloped sex organs (hypogonadism) as well as feeding problems (Reddy & Pfeiffer, 2007). Children with PWS tend to have a narrow palatal arch, characteristic craniofacial features (e.g., almond-shaped eyes, downturned mouth), fair complexion, and small hands.

Prevalence

The estimated prevalence is 1 out of 10,000 to 20,000 births (E. M. Dykens & Kasari, 1997). All persons with PWS share the same characteristics and traits regardless of sex, race or culture.

Etiology

Prenatally, DNA testing usually is initiated due to a lack of movement as reported by the mother. In most cases, PWS is the result of a loss of multiple genes on chromosome 15 on the paternal component of section 11–13 on the long arm of the chromosome (J. L. Miller, Couch et al., 2007). In a very few cases (about 5%), what is inherited is an imprinting defect rather than a deletion from the father. The imprinting does not allow the expression of the genes, but there is a 50% chance of passing the syndrome to offspring as a result of the defect. There is some indication that those having type I deletions present with more severe problems (Samaco, Nagarajan, Braunschweig, & La Salle, 2004).

Neurological Correlates

PWS symptoms are caused by a dysfunction of the hypothalamus in the brain, which regulates hunger and many other systems in the body. Individuals with PWS feel hungry most (if not all) of the time and yet can eat only about half the calories of an average person (E. M. Dykens & Cassidy, 1999). The mechanism of this problem in appetite regulation is less clear. Imaging studies of individuals with PWS revealed multiple morphometric abnormalities including ventriculomegaly, decreased volume of brain tissue in the parietal occipital lobe, sylvian fissure polymicrogyria, and incomplete insular closure (J. L. Miller, Couch et al., 2007). A case study of a female infant with PWS using MRI indicated evidence of a diffusely abnormal cerebral gyral folding pattern such that cortical malformation from an early point in development is likely associated with PWS (Yoshi, Krishnamoorthy, & Grant, 2002).

With diffusion tensor imaging, results indicated that trace was significantly higher for the individuals with PWS in left frontal white matter as well as the left dorsomedial thalamus (Yamada, Matsuzawa, Uchiyama, Kwee, & Nakada, 2006). In contrast, fractional anisotropy was reduced in the internal capsule bilaterally, the right frontal white matter, and the splenium of the corpus callosum (Yamada et al., 2006). White matter lesions in individuals with PWS also have been noted using MRI but were not evident with sibling controls (J. L. Miller et al., 2006). In other studies, individuals with PWS demonstrated greater blood oxygen level-dependent activation in the ventromedial prefrontal cortex in response to food stimuli as compared to controls, even after an oral glucose load. Functional MRI in response to pictures of food offered some insight into the lack of appetite regulation (J. L. Miller, James et al., 2007). These findings support the role of the frontal cortex in modulating the response to food in general and to the increased reward value of food for individuals with PWS (J. L. Miller, James et al., 2007). Further, with regard to problematic and challenging behaviors (e.g., temper outbursts), imaging results suggest abnormalities in the frontal regions, particularly on attention-switching tasks (Woodcock, Oliver, & Humphreys, 2008). Other regions and structures of the brain have been implicated as well. A case study of a 3-year-old male with PWS revealed right cerebellar hypoplasia (Titomanlio et al., 2006).

Course and Prognosis

The manifestation of Prader-Willi is complex and affects all areas of functioning: physiological, cognitive, educational, and behavioral. In early childhood, some of the manifestations include hypotonia and a poor sucking reflex (Medved & Percy, 2001). This may result in early presentation as failure to thrive due to feeding difficulties. Infants with PWS tend to have small hands and feet; males have undescended testes and small genitalia. Although there may be initial feeding problems, as the infant grows, there is a significant increase in eating, with an insatiable appetite, or hyperphagia (Medved & Percy, 2001). As toddlers, children with PWS evidence developmental delays. Physical characteristics, including stunted height and straight ulnar borders, have been noted. Research indicates that children with PWS are at risk for epilepsy with febrile seizures occurring frequently in childhood (Kumada et al., 2005). Finally, they have limited sex hormone production, which, combined with their uncontrollable eating, leads to obesity and often to diabetes in adolescence (Van Lieshout, De Meyer, Curfs, Koot, & Fryns, 1998). A related concern is that they have decreased tendency (a higher threshold) for vomiting in response to toxicity, placing them at risk for food poisoning (Medved & Percy, 2001). Vision problems, including myopia and strabismus, are common. Related to body mass index and other factors, scoliosis occurs in about one-third of children with PWS (de Lind van Wijngaarden et al., 2009).

Notably, one area of concern with PWS more than many other disorders is the effect on the family system (Hodapp & Fidler, 1999). In particular, behaviors related to overeating, skin picking, hypoactivity, and compulsions often lead to high levels of stress in parents. Because of the additional needs of the child with PWS, these families often have to do without amenities or forgo activities more so than with children with other developmental disorders (Hodapp & Fidler, 1999). Across studies, parents of children with PWS are more likely to experience marital conflict and divorce as compared to parents of children with fragile X or Williams syndrome (Van Lieshout et al., 1998); this is believed to be due to the increased need for monitoring (Medved & Percy, 2001). Adult outcomes vary depending on the individual with PWS. In one study of adult outcomes, only 10% had a certificate of completion of secondary education, 15.7% were employed in sheltered workshop settings, and about 33% attended some form of adult training or care during the day (Waters, Clarke, & Corbett, 1990).

Neurocognitive Correlates

A summary of neurocognitive correlates is provided in Table 15.9. Individuals with PWS present with mild to significantly impaired intellectual ability as well as language difficulties (E. M. Dykens, Hodapp, & Finucane, 2000; Medved & Percy, 2001; State, Dykens, Rosner, Andres, & King, 1999). Overall ability may be associated with genetic alteration responsible with higher IQ associated with uniparental disomy (Roof et al., 2000). Simultaneous processing may emerge as a relative strength in comparison to sequential processing (E. M. Dykens, Hodapp, Walsh, & Nash, 1992).

Speech also is affected with hypernasal resonance and high pitch, in conjunction with speech motor deficits (Akefeldt, Akefeldt, & Gillberg, 1997; B. A. Lewis, Freebairn, Heeger, & Casidy, 2002; Van Borsel & Tetnowski, 2007). Dysfluency is present in about 34% of individuals with PWS (Kleppe, Katayama, Shipley, & Foushee, 1990). As with other disorders in this chapter, expressive language is more impaired than receptive language; language is more impaired than visual-spatial processing

Table 15.9 Neuropsychological Deficits Associated with Prader-Willi Syndrome

Global Domain/Specific Deficits	Phenotype
Cognition	Mental retardation common, often in mild range; some may be in borderline range, others in moderate range Simultaneous processing may emerge as stronger than sequential processing
Auditory-linguistic/Language function	Auditory linguistic processing more delayed than visual processing Expressive language more impaired than receptive language Hypernasal quality to speech Dysfluency in about 34% of individuals with PWS
Learning and memory	Short-term memory deficient but long-term memory strong Immediate memory most impaired when stimuli required sequencing
Motor function	Developmental motor milestones delayed Relative weakness in fine motor ability and strength
Visual-perception/Constructional praxis	May emerge as a strength, with jigsaw puzzles a preferred activity
Attention/Concentration	Difficulties with attention switching
Executive function	Difficulties with impulse control, perseveration Deficits in executive functioning noted
Perceptual/Sensory Perception	Sensory perception appears to be intact
Achievement/Academic skills	Learning difficulties or learning disabilities common Reading may emerge as relative strength; more difficulty with math
Emotional/Behavioral functioning	Hyperphagia/compulsive eating Obsessive compulsive, behaviors such as ordering and grouping of objects; repetitive, rigid, and routinized behavior Skin picking Excessive verbalization, chattering Temper outburst, emotional lability, irritability Co-occurring psychosis, bipolar or other psychiatric disorder

(Curfs, Hoondert, Van Lieshout, & Fryns, 1995). Within language areas, expressive language tends to be more impaired than receptive language. Developmental motor milestones also are delayed with relative weakness in fine motor ability and strength (E. M. Dykens & Cassidy, 1999).

In contrast to language and motor areas, visual-spatial skills emerge as a strength, with jigsaw puzzles a preferred activity (Medved & Percy, 2001). In regard to memory and learning, short-term memory is deficient, but long-term memory is strong (E. M. Dykens & Cassidy, 1999). Notably, immediate memory was most impaired when stimuli required sequencing (Jauregi et al., 2007). Deficits in attention switching (Woodcock et al., 2008) as well as executive function have been noted as well (Jauregi et al., 2007). In particular, children with PWS often demonstrate difficulties with impulse control and perseveration (A. J. Martin et al., 1998). Of the neurocognitive domains, somatosensory function is generally intact (E. M. Dykens & Cassidy, 1999).

Educational Implications

As expected, learning difficulties or learning disabilities are common (E. M. Dykens & Cassidy, 1999). Despite language difficulties, reading may emerge as a relative strength; many individuals with PWS exhibit more difficulty with math, but this is not always the case (F. A. Conners, Rosenquist, Atwell, & Klinger, 2000).

Emotional/Behavioral Implications

Although children with PWS are generally likable in early years, as they mature, they present with more troublesome behaviors, including verbal aggressiveness, self-assaultive behavior, and rage (Greenswag & Alexander, 1988). Behavioral issues emerge early in childhood and initially center around food-related problems. This manifests as hyperphagia/compulsive eating (E. M. Dykens & Kasari, 1997; Medved & Percy, 2001). These problems gradually evolve beyond food-related situations, presenting as poor coping skills and conduct problems (Akefeldt & Gillberg, 1999). Specific behaviors have included temper outbursts, emotional lability, stealing, and impulsivity (Curfs et al., 1995; E. M. Dykens & Kasari, 1997; Medved & Percy, 2001). Some children with PWS may be secretive and manipulative; the majority will resort to temper tantrums (Medved & Percy, 2001). Additional problem behaviors include excessive verbalization and chattering (E. M. Dykens & Kasari, 1997; Greenswag & Alexander, 1988). In more severe cases, there is co-occurring psychosis, bipolar, or other psychiatric disorder (Descheemaeker et al., 2002).

While there are a preponderance of externalizing problems in early childhood, by adolescence, there is a high co-occurrence of internalizing disorders. Depression (E. M. Dykens & Cassidy, 1999; Van Lieshout et al., 1998), psychosis (Verhoeven et al., 1998), and obsessive-compulsive disorder (Medved & Percy, 2001; State, Dykens, Rosner, Martin, & King, 1999). Individuals with PWS exhibit a range of deficits in social behavior, including social withdrawal (Jauregi et al., 2007). Associated with the obsessive-compulsive behaviors, individuals with PWS frequently engage in skin picking, particularly on the head and front of the legs (E. M. Dykens & Kasari, 1997; Symons, Butler, Sanders, Feurer, & Thompson, 1999). Obsessions and repetitive compulsivelike behaviors are manifest as central distinguishing features of PWS (Curfs et al., 1995; E. M. Dykens & Kasari, 1997; Wigren & Hansen, 2003). It has been suggested that individuals with PWS exhibit a wide range of psychopathology, including problems with conduct/externalizing behaviors, anxiety, and attention problems (Reddy & Pfeiffer, 2007).

Evidence-Based Intervention

Treatment approaches and foci vary across the life span (see Table 15.10). In infancy, interventions may be needed to address basic physiological needs. For example, gavage feeding or other mechanism may be appropriate to alleviate the poor sucking response. Once the infant is identified as having PWS, additional assessments to rule out or identify associated problems may be needed. This may include screening by a pediatric ophthalmologist for myopia and strabismus as well as evaluation and consideration of surgical treatments for cryptorchidism. As the child develops, various hormone therapies may be considered for height and muscle increase and to encourage secondary sexual characteristics. Across the life span, there is a need for vigilant monitoring of daily food and firm limit setting. Moderate physical activity and regular physician visits to monitor health concerns will be necessary as well (Medved & Percy, 2001). Environmental and behavioral interventions have been most effective in weight management.

Table 15.10 Evidence-Based Status for Interventions for Prader-Willi Syndrome

Intervention	Target	Status
Medications: donepezil (Aricept), galantamine (Razadyne)	Cognitive ability, memory	Emerging (Spiridigliozzi et al., 2007)
Medications: risperidone (Risperdal)	Problem behaviors (temper tantrums, noncompliance)	Emerging (Medved & Percy, 2001)
Medications: SSRIs	Aggression, hyperactivity, depression, and self-injurious behaviors	Emerging (Medved & Percy, 2001)
Growth hormone	Scoliosis	Emerging (de Lind van Wijngaarden et al., 2009)

General considerations in adolescence include transition planning with options for continued residence with parents or a group home with other individuals who have PWS. Regardless of setting or age, individuals with PWS will need a structured environment with monitoring of eating behavior and weight balance to prevent morbid obesity. Because of the tendency for obsessive-compulsive behavior, it is suggested that schedules be very predictable and repetitive; change in the environment can precipitate behavioral problems (Medved & Percy, 2001). Coping skills and social skills present as problematic deficits for individuals with PWS, but no studies of interventions for these specific skills with individuals with PWS were identified. There is some research to suggest that serotonin reuptake inhibitors or other medications, such as risperidone, may have indirect and positive effects on weight management by decreasing other problem behaviors (Medved & Percy, 2001).

Educational Interventions

As with their home environment (or work environment), students with PWS need constant monitoring to restrict their eating behaviors. This means that even restroom behavior needs to be monitored to ensure that they are not eating soap or other objects that may have been left there by other children. Lunch and snack time will have to be monitored carefully.

Emotional/Behavioral Interventions

Children with PWS frequently engage in temper tantrums and other aggressive or noncompliant behavior, usually associated with either food or difficulty with shifting of attention (Akefeldt & Gillberg, 1999). Throughout activities, parents, teachers, and other professional staff need to be attentive to the potential for children with PWS to bully (to gain food objects from others) as well as to be bullied. Although not physically coordinated or athletic, children with PWS need to be engaged in physical activity at their level on a regular basis (Medved & Percy, 2001). With the increased family stress associated with PWS, support in the form of education, support groups, or caregiver assistance may be appropriate (Medved & Percy, 2001; van den Borne et al., 1999). Some form of mental health support for siblings of a child with PWS also may be appropriate, but no specific research is available in this area.

CASE STUDY: GEORGE—ANGELMAN SYNDROME

The next report is from a hospital-based clinic. Identifying information, such as child and family name, teacher or physician name, and school information, has been altered or fictionalized to protect confidentiality.

Reason for Referral

George is 10 years 3 months of age. He was referred for comprehensive evaluation as part of his participation in an ongoing, collaborative study of the natural history of Angelman syndrome (AS) and in a neuroimaging study in children with AS. George's diagnosis of AS has been confirmed by the results of genetic testing, which revealed the typical deletion associated with AS.

Assessment Procedures

Parent interview
Behavioral observations
Bayley Scales of Infant Development, Third Edition (BSID-III)
Vineland Adaptive Behavior Scales, Second Edition (VABS-2)
Preschool Language Scale, Fourth Edition (PLS-4)
Aberrant Behavior Checklist (ABC)
Autism Diagnostic Observation Schedule (ADOS), Module 1

Background Information

George was born to a 19-year-old mother and a 20-year-old father. He was born at 34 weeks via vacuum extraction and weighed 4 pounds 13 ounces. He had respiratory syncytial virus twice during the first year of life and was hospitalized both times. He had a history of difficulties with feeding, had reflux, and was given propulsid (Cisapride) as well as ranitidine hydrochloride (Zantac). George had surgery to correct strabismus in 2003 (age 5) and had ear tubes placed in 2004 (age 6). George also has a history of difficulties with sleep but now sleeps through the night six of seven nights per week. He began having seizures at age 17 months, but since being taken into foster care in 2004, his seizures are well controlled. He was taken into foster care secondary to parental mental illness and substance abuse. Results of a recent brain MRI (done at age 10) revealed that he has a prominent cerebrospinal space dorsal and inferior to the cerebellum, and the corpus callosum has a minor dysmorphic appearance.

In terms of George's developmental milestones, he sat alone at 15 months, pulled to stand at 18 months, and began walking independently at 6 years of age. He smiled responsively at 9 months of age and started to gesture/point at 18 months of age but has never used single words. He started to follow commands without gestures at 24 months of age. He started to finger-feed at 16 months of age. Behaviorally, he has a history of temper tantrums and aggressive behaviors (pinching and scratching), though these behaviors have lessened with intensive behavioral therapy. He has a long history of receiving physical therapy, occupational therapy, and speech therapy services both in and out of school. He currently is served within a life skills classroom with some inclusion.

Behavioral Observations

George is a 10-year 3-month-old boy who acknowledged the examiner by smiling, using good eye gaze, and waving to her in greeting. He did not exhibit any difficulties with making the transition from the waiting room to the evaluation room. During the evaluation of his cognitive skills, George was easily engaged and smiled at his foster father throughout the evaluation. When items were more difficult for him, he would throw test objects and exhibited more sensory issues (i.e. by "tasting" some test objects). In spite of these behaviors, he was at least able to attempt all items that were presented to him. Thus, these results are judged to be an accurate reflection of his overall abilities.

Although George did not use any words, he did vocalize using vowel sounds (but not vowel/consonant combinations). He used a range of nonverbal gestures (pointing, nodding his head) and demonstrated a range of facial expressions. There were no indications of problems with vision or with hearing.

Assessment

As part of the standard battery in place for this study of children with AS (because they are largely nonverbal), George was given the Bayley Scales of Infant Development, Third Edition (BSID-III). His performance on the cognitive scale was most like that of a child around the age of 13 months. George was able to uncover hidden objects, suspend a ring from a string, and remove a small food object from a bottle. Results are provided in Table 15.11.

George's overall language abilities also were assessed using the BSID-III. His receptive language skills were most like those of a child about the age of 9 months. George was able to respond to his name, discriminate sounds, and understood what "no" means. His expressive language skills were slightly lower, falling at the 7-month-old level. This pattern is not uncommon among children with AS. George was able to use gestures, participate in play routines, gain the attention of others, and vocalize using vowel sounds.

George's motor skills also were assessed using the BSID-III. His fine motor skills were most like those of a child about 8 months of age. He was able to bring objects to midline and could transfer objects from hand to hand. His gross motor skills were more advanced by comparison and fell at the 14-month-old level. George can walk alone, throw a ball, and squat without support.

George's foster father, Mr. Fine, provided information regarding George's adaptive behavior. Using the Vineland Adaptive Behavior Scales, Second Edition (VABS-2), George's adaptive behavior composite is 43, which falls within the moderate deficits range of the low adaptive level. This is slightly higher as compared to his overall cognitive abilities as assessed on the BSID-III. Mr. Fine reported moderate deficits for George in the area of communication and noted that his abilities fell between the 8-month-old level (for his expressive language skills) and the 13-month-old level (for his receptive language skills). His self-help skills fell within the moderate deficits range and clustered between the 7-month-old level (for his domestic skills) and the 1-year 6-month-old level (for his community skills). His socialization skills also fell within the moderate deficits range of the low adaptive level and fell between the 9-month-old level (for his interpersonal relationship skills) and the 13-month-old level (for his play/leisure skills).

Mr. Fine provided information about George's behavior by completing the Aberrant Behavior Checklist (ABC)—Community Version. The ABC—Community Version is a behavior rating scale that assesses a range of maladaptive behaviors in children,

Table 15.11 Psychometric Summary for George

Bayley Scales of Infant Development, Third Edition (BSID-III)		**Age Equivalent**
Cognitive Scale Developmental Age		13 months
Language Scale: Receptive Communication		9 months
Language Scale: Expressive Communication		7 months
Motor Scale: Fine Motor		8 months
Motor Scale: Gross Motor		14 months
Preschool Language Scale, Fourth Edition (PLS-4)		
Auditory Comprehension		8 months
Expressive Communication		7 months
Total Language		7 months
Vineland Adaptive Behavior Scales, Second Edition (VABS-2)		
	Standard Score	
Communication	43	
Receptive		2 years, 6 months
Expressive		1 year, 1 month
Daily Living Skills	43	
Personal		1 year, 1 month
Domestic		7 months
Community		1 year, 6 months
Socialization	47	
Interpersonal Relationships		9 months
Play/Leisure		1 year, 1 month
Coping Skills		10 months
Composite	43	
Aberrant Behavior Checklist	**Raw Score**	**Mean for Age**
Irritability	15	10.33
Lethargy/Withdrawal	14	5.65
Stereotypy	9	4.15
Hyperactivity	29	13.18
Inappropriate Speech	0	1.18

adolescents, and adults with mild to profound mental retardation. The community version of the scale is designed for use with children who are not residing in institutional settings. The rating scale consists of five factors:

1. Irritability
2. Lethargy/Withdrawal
3. Stereotypy
4. Hyperactivity/Noncompliance
5. Inappropriate speech

George's scores on the ABC reflected significant elevations in the areas of irritability, lethargy/withdrawal, stereotypy, and hyperactivity at this time. This is significant as these scores were normed on patients with genetic disorders and mental retardation.

Because many children with Angelman Syndrome also demonstrate some characteristics of autism, George was also given the Autism Diagnostic Observation Schedule (ADOS), Module 1. The ADOS is a semistructured, standardized assessment of communication, social interaction, and play for use with individuals with possible autism spectrum disorders. Both the reliability and validity of the ADOS demonstrate its utility in distinguishing between those children who have cognitive and language delays only as opposed to those who have autism spectrum disorders. The evaluation consists of a series of activities that permit observation of behaviors specific to autism spectrum disorders, given a person's age and developmental level. Although the ADOS consists of four modules, an individual is given only one module, which is selected based on his or her developmental level and overall expressive language ability. George was given Module 1, which is designed for young children who have no speech and a maximum of simple phrases. It consists of 10 activities with 29 accompanying ratings. The activities focus on the playful use of toys and other materials that are salient to children with developmental ages of less than 3.

During the administration of the ADOS, George did not use any recognizable words, but when he vocalized, all of his vocalizations were socially directed. He did use the examiner's hand as a tool to make requests. He also, however, made requests by reaching to objects with coordinated eye gaze. He used eye gaze very well to modulate social interactions, demonstrated a range of facial expressions, exhibited shared enjoyment in interactions, and demonstrated play skills that were appropriate as compared to his developmental level.

Mr. Fine also completed the Behavior and Sensory Interests questionnaire, which assesses more details related to behaviors that are not uncommon in children with autism and a variety of other genetic syndromes. George has repetitive hand and finger movements, taps objects in a repetitive manner, throws objects, and is quite obsessed with plastic. He has some unusual sensory interests as well (looking at things out of the corner of his eyes, licking objects as a way of exploration, and smelling objects). Some aggressive behaviors (e.g., occasional hitting and biting) were noted for George as well.

Summary and Diagnostic Impressions

George is a 10-year 3-month-old boy who was evaluated as part of a study of children with Angelman syndrome. His diagnosis of Angelman syndrome has been confirmed by the results of genetic testing. The results of this evaluation reveal that George's cognitive/developmental skills are most like that of a child around the age of 13 months. His receptive language skills fell at the 9-month level and, as is consistent with children with AS, are significantly better developed as compared to his expressive language skills, which fell at the 7-month-old level. His fine motor skills fell at the 8-month level and are not as well developed as his gross motor skills, which fell at the 14-month-old level. Mr. Fine provided information regarding George's adaptive behavior. His overall adaptive behavior is slightly higher than his cognitive skills and falls within the moderate deficits range of the low adaptive level. Based on his overall cognitive/developmental skills as well as his adaptive behavior at home, George does meet criteria for a child with severe mental retardation (*DSM-IV* 318.0).

Recommendations

It is very important to note that despite his cognitive and language delays, George has developed good socialization skills. His level of play is at least consistent with and, in some cases, exceeds expectations, given his developmental level. Specifically, George showed/shared toys with his father and the examiner. He also shows a range of facial expressions, exhibits shared enjoyment in interactions with others, and has many methods of making requests for desired objects (e.g. he gestures, vocalizes). When making requests for desired objects, he coordinates his use of eye contact with a vocalization.

It is not uncommon for some older, higher-functioning children with Angelman syndrome to exhibit compulsions and rituals. This clearly seems to be the case for George at this time. If his "fixations" (e.g., with plastic) and his sensory issues begin to impact his ability to learn and focus in school, additional behavioral and possibly pharmacological treatments may be indicated for him.

In the meantime, we recommend that George continue in his intensive school program (to include extended-year services). He also should continue to receive occupational therapy, speech therapy, and physical therapy school support services to address his needs in all areas. To insure his progress across all domains, it will be important that George's foster parents, his therapists, his physicians, and his teachers maintain close contact with one another. They should reinforce similar goals, and any changes in his behavior should be noted by all involved in his care.

Further Discussion of Case Study

As can be seen in this case study of George, the most important information gained from the assessment is not the diagnosis of Angelman syndrome—that is based on genetic testing. It also probably was not necessary to do a comprehensive neuropsychological examination to determine that George met criteria for severe mental retardation. What is gained, however, from the comprehensive assessment is awareness of George's strengths (socialization), which can be built on in planning his intervention, particularly in language and communication areas. Similarly, understanding of Angelman syndrome provides some suggestions of what behavioral issues to anticipate (rituals, compulsions), and can inform proactive interventions in this regard. As noted in the recommendations, because of the complexities associated with Angelman syndrome, maximizing George's outcome will require collaboration of parents, teachers, medical personnel, and related services personnel, in and out of the school setting.

SEX CHROMOSOME DISORDERS

In addition to the chromosomal disorders discussed already, all of which result in some level of cognitive impairment, there is another group of congenital disorders, all of which involve sex chromosome anomalies. These include Turner syndrome, XXX syndrome, Noonan syndrome, Klinefelter syndrome, and XYY.

Turner Syndrome

Definition, Incidence, and Etiology

Turner syndrome is caused by the loss or abnormality of genetic material from one of the sex chromosomes at the pseudoautosomal region; in effect, individuals with Turner syndrome are missing all or part of one of their sex chromosomes (Davenport, Hooper, & Zeger, 2007; Wodrich & Tarbox, 2008). Approximately half of the girls with Turner syndrome have only one X chromosome (45, X); others with Turner syndrome have a mosaic pattern such that some of their cells are missing an X chromosome (45, X) while other cells have a different chromosomal composition (Sävendahl & Davenport, 2000). In another third, the individuals have two X chromosomes, but part of one X is missing; an X chromosome may be fragmented, have portions deleted, or have other structural problems, such as the ring X formation. The more severe manifestation is a complete loss of an X chromosome or a ring X, while the least severe is a mosaic karyotype involving a normal 46XX cell line.

Turner syndrome is the most widely known and examined of the chromosomal abnormalities in females, but it is often underdiagnosed (Davenport et al., 2007). Diagnosis can be made via karyotype testing of cells in the amniotic fluid before birth and on cells in the blood after birth. It may be diagnosed at any age but most likely during adolescence at the onset of puberty and gonadal development failure. It is estimated that Turner syndrome affects 1 in 1,900 to 2,500 female live births, or about 1.5 million women worldwide. The most marked characteristics of Turner syndrome are short stature and ovarian/gonadal failure; however, three physical systems are affected—skeletal, reproductive, and lymphatic—with myriad symptoms and conditions as a result (Davenport et al., 2007).

Neurological Correlates

Based on existing research, a number of structural differences have been identified (Davenport et al., 2007). These include reduced volume of the parietal lobes bilaterally and reduced volume of the right hippocampus. These reductions are contrasted by increased volume of the right superior temporal gyrus and left amygdala gray matter. Functional imaging studies indicate reduced activation of parietal regions at rest, with abnormal engagement of parietal and prefrontal areas during more challenging tasks as well as decreased activation in the dorsolateral prefrontal cortex, caudate, and inferior parietal lobes during visual-spatial working memory tasks. Based on these differences, it was concluded that Turner syndrome is associated with deficient engagement of frontoparietal circuits (Cutter, Daly, Robertson, & Chitnis, 2006; Davenport et al., 2007).

Course and Prognosis

During infancy, cardiac abnormality, poor sleeping, and poor feeding may be evident (Davenport et al., 2007). Feeding problems may be caused by structural problems, including a high palate or small jaw, and underdeveloped chewing skills. Toddlers may refuse solid food or have problems digesting food; input from dieticians and speech therapists may be needed. Appearance of those with Turner syndrome may include short neck, high arched palate, low-set and prominent ears, low hairline, webbed neck, hands and feet that are swollen or puffy at birth, and soft nails that turn upward. Children with Turner syndrome may develop or evidence strabismus (crossed eyes); this occurs in about one-third of such children. Stature is generally below average, with a slowed rate of growth (Davenport et al., 2007).

Puberty and reproductive function are implicated specifically with most girls not beginning puberty at a normal age and most women losing their ovarian function at an early age. As a result, women with Turner syndrome cannot become pregnant naturally. Further, because these women do not get adequate estrogen, they are at increased risk for osteoporosis and related complications (Davenport et al., 2007). The cardiovascular system is also affected, with frequent structural problems of the heart or major blood vessels (P. Chang et al., 2000; Davenport et al., 2007). Overall, high blood pressure affects about 40% of adults with Turner syndrome. In addition to the reproductive problems and cardiovascular complications, females with Turner syndrome are at higher than normal risk for kidney problems (P. Chang et al., 2000).

Neurocognitive effects of Turner syndrome have been investigated (Davenport et al., 2007; J. Rovet, 2004); these are summarized in Table 15.12. The incidence of mental retardation in Turner syndrome is about the same as in the general population and is more likely to occur if the individual has the small ring X chromosome (C. Turner, Dennis, Skuse, & Jacobs, 2000). In general, girls and women with Turner syndrome most often have verbal IQ scores similar to the general population. In contrast, Performance IQ (PIQ) tends to be somewhat lower due to the difficulties in tasks that require visual-spatial processing. The consistency of the verbal/nonverbal difference has been attributed to disruption of visual-spatial processing abilities and involvement of the frontoparietal region with additional deficits in executive function (Lasker, Mazzocco, & Zee, 2007). Girls with Turner syndrome also evidence related difficulties in visual attention, visual-motor, and fine motor coordination domains; dysfluency (stuttering) also may be present (Van Borsel & Tetnowski, 2007). In addition, deficits in short-term memory, nonverbal processing speed, and reaction time may be affected by decreased estrogen levels but may be alleviated by hormone replacement therapy (Ross et al., 2004). Other specific deficits include problems with visual and working memory; these appear to continue across the life span. Deficits persist in visual-perceptual areas, visual-motor integration, affect recognition, visual memory, attention, and executive function (Ross et al., 2004). One theory regarding this imbalance within the brain is that females with Turner syndrome have a diffuse right-hemisphere dysfunction (i.e., nonverbal learning disability).

Table 15.12 Neurocognitive Correlates of Turner Syndrome

Global Domain/ Specific Deficit Area	Phenotype
Cognition	Cognitive impairment with Turner syndrome as frequent as in general population
Auditory-linguistic/Language function	Language skills tend to be spared Stuttering or dysfluency common
Learning and memory	Visual/spatial memory more likely to be impaired than auditory/verbal memory
Motor function	Visual-motor integration likely to be impaired; reaction time longer than expected; clumsiness frequent
Visual perception/Constructional praxis	Deficits in visual-spatial and visual-perceptual areas evident
Attention/Concentration	Attention problems occur frequently
Executive function	Deficits evident in executive function
Achievement/Academic skills	Severe learning problems, especially in math, may be present Reading and spelling less likely to be affected
Emotional/ Behavioral	Deficits in social skills, affect recognition occur frequently

Turner syndrome does not affect intelligence but can cause problems similar to those associated with nonverbal learning disabilities (NVLDs). The difficulties in visual-spatial domains are believed to be related to white matter anomalies as well as gray matter alterations (S. J. Hart, Davenport, Hooper, & Belger, 2006; Holzapfel, Barnea-Goraly, Eckert, Kesler, & Reiss, 2006). Turner syndrome sometimes is associated with severe learning difficulties and dysmorphism. In particular, the reduced volume in the parietal lobes is associated with visual-spatial difficulties and arithmetic difficulties. Other commonly observed weaknesses include difficulty imagining objects in relation to each other (difficulty driving and poor sense of direction) and trouble appreciating subtle social cues, such as facial expression. Persons with Turner syndrome also may evidence clumsiness, psychomotor problems, and poor dexterity (Davenport et al., 2007). Due to the potential for subtle deficits, it has been recommended that every child with Turner syndrome should be provided with an educational evaluation so that any problems can be identified early (Davenport et al., 2007). It is recommended that the comprehensive assessment should include measures of intelligence, achievement (mathematics and reading), nonverbal (visual-perceptual skills), memory, and personality domains at minimum. In particular, girls with Turner syndrome have been found to perform an average of 2 years behind grade level on mathematics achievement tests (M. M. Murphy & Mazzocco, 2008; T. J. Simon et al., 2008). This is believed to reflect the parietal dysfunction. Within the math area, problems tend to be more related to the conceptual/factual area than to the actual computational area. In contrast, spelling and reading skills appear to remain intact (M. M. Murphy & Mazzocco, 2008).

Overall, research has shown that girls with Turner syndrome have fewer psychiatric disorders than girls in the general population (Davenport et al., 2007). When problems are present, ADHD-related behaviors are not uncommon; anxiety, depression, and social withdrawal also may occur (H. F. Russell et al., 2006). Personality studies indicate a tendency toward high extroversion and low neuroticism (Boman, Hanson, Hijelmquist, & Möller, 2006). In addition, personality characteristics associated with Turner syndrome include high stress tolerance, unassertiveness, overcompliance and a lack of emotional maturity. Girls with Turner syndrome have some of the negative symptoms, such as a lack of emotional reactivity and poor relationships with peers, that may be related to their difficulties with internalizing disorders and social withdrawal (Davenport et al., 2007). Alternatively, the social problems may be related to difficulties with affective expression and affective recognition as in nonverbal learning disability (McCauley, Kay, Ito, & Treder, 1987).

Evidence-Based Interventions

Early identification and intervention are key to preventing and addressing some of the potential problems associated with Turner syndrome (see Table 15.13). Many medical approaches are used to address some of the associated problems. Surgical interventions may be necessary as a result of cardiac and renal abnormalities, strabismus, and inner ear defects (M. P. Powell & Schulte, 1999). For feeding/gastrointestinal problems, elimination of gluten has been effective for some but not all girls with Turner syndrome. Specific accommodations can be made for small stature (e.g., blocks for bicycle or car pedals), and in some cases, the introduction of human growth hormone (hGH) in early childhood may increase height (M. P. Powell & Schulte, 1999).

Parents need to be aware of their child's needs and be advocates for their child at school. Teachers need to be aware of and address the learning needs of the student with Turner syndrome as well. An Individualized Education Plan to address deficits and concerns

Table 15.13 Evidence-Based Interventions for Turner Syndrome

Intervention	Target	Status
Gluten-free diet	Gastrointestinal problems, feeding issues	Inconclusive (Gillett et al., 2000)
Estrogen replacement therapy	Secondary sexual development	Promising practice (Davenport, 2008)
Human growth hormone (hGH)	Increase stature	Promising practice (Denson, 2008)
Androgen therapy	Advance linear bone growth	Promising practice (Davenport, 2008)

in educational areas (e.g., math, handwriting) may be appropriate. Counseling at various points in development may be appropriate to ensure that the girl with Turner syndrome understands her disorder and its impact long term; as needed, counseling to address issues of self-esteem, affective expression and reception, and social skills may be appropriate for some individuals. Finally, as the child ages, she will need to become an advocate for herself.

Klinefelter Syndrome

Definition, Incidence, and Etiology

Another sex chromosome anomaly, Klinefelter syndrome, affects males rather than females. This syndrome was first identified by Klinefelter et al. in 1942 based on males demonstrating testicular failure, breast enlargement, and inability to produce sperm (Cody & Hynd, 1999). The genetic karyotype of Klinefelter syndrome was determined to be 47, XXY, with a mosaic of 47, XXY/46, XY (Ross et al., 2004). Although it is always associated with an extra X chromosome in some or all genes, variants exist with 48, XXYY and 48, XXXY, and 49, XXXXY. Regardless of karyotype, the same genetic and endocrine features are in place, but with the more severe karyotype, there is greater likelihood of severe cognitive deficits. The Klinefelter phenotype includes childhood onset of testicular failure, tall stature, disproportionately long legs, elevated levels of gonadotropins, and breast development (gynecomastia) as well as behavioral and cognitive features (Ross, Stefanatos, & Roeltgen, 2007; Ross et al., 2008; Visootsak & Graham, 2006). Additional physical characteristics include decreased facial, pubic, and body hair; hypertelorism (widely spaced eyes); increased likelihood of left-hand dominance; and increased risk for obesity. The primary physical manifestations emerge during puberty, so this is when Klinefelter syndrome is most likely to be identified and diagnosed. Klinefelter syndrome is the most common sex-linked genetic disorder. It occurs in about 1 per 426 to 1,000 males (0.1 to 0.2% of population) and accounts for 3.1% of infertile males. It is equally distributed across socioeconomic status and racial/ethnic groups (Ross et al., 2007).

The manifestation of testicular failure and the inability to produce sperm relate to the levels of endogenous testosterone. It is believed to be evident initially in the absence of the typical burst of testosterone during the last trimester of pregnancy, followed by continued lower than normal levels of testosterone during infancy and early childhood and throughout adulthood. Because testosterone levels are affected, androgen levels also are affected. Brain development may be altered by androgen deficiency, but this has not been a focus for diagnosis or research (Ross et al., 2007, 2008).

Klinefelter syndrome is a common cause of developmental delay (Khalifa & Struthers, 2002), but deficits tend to be in discrete areas rather than diffuse (Cody & Hynd, 1999). Cognitive ability tends to be within normal limits or to follow normal distribution. In children, verbal ability (Verbal Comprehension) tends to be lower than nonverbal abilities (Perceptual Reasoning), but this is not the case in adulthood. Neurocognitive implications include motor dysfunction as a prominent feature; in addition, executive function often is impaired (Geschwind, Boone, Miller, & Swerdloff, 2000). There is a tendency for decreased strength, impaired fine motor coordination and upper limb coordination, decreased motor speed, decreased dexterity, and decreased muscle tone (hypotonia). As a result, motor milestones may be delayed; the child may evidence hypoactivity (decreased activity levels) or atypical movement patterns. In language areas, results from dichotic listening suggest that boys with Klinefelter syndrome tend to be right-hemisphere dominant for language. Further, 70% to 80% of boys with Klinefelter syndrome have deficits in language development and language-based learning. Language problems may appear initially as delays in early expressive language and speech development, with later deficits evident in word retrieval, expressive grammar, and development of narrative discourse. Receptive language areas of phonemic awareness, verbal processing, and understanding of morphology and grammar also may be affected (Cody & Hynd, 1999; Ross et al., 2008).

Consistent with language dysfunction (see Chapter 4), educational implications include a tendency for boys with Klinefelter syndrome to evidence reading difficulty as well as speech language delays (Ross et al., 2007). It is estimated that 50% to 75% of boys with Klinefelter syndrome will exhibit specific reading disability at some point in development; it is also estimated that about 60% to 80% will need special education services. By age 7, boys with Klinefelter syndrome may have severe problems with spelling but not arithmetic; however, by age 10, problems in math areas also emerge. The result is a pattern of generalized learning difficulties by middle school (Ross et al., 2008; J. Rovet, Netley, Keenan, Bailey, & Stewart, 1996). Despite these difficulties, most boys with Klinefelter syndrome do graduate from high school; few go on to higher education (Ross et al., 2007).

There are also psychological effects of Klinefelter syndrome (Ross et al., 2007). By age 12, issues with tall stature, skinny frame, and a lack of secondary sex characteristics increase the risk for teasing and ridicule by peers (e.g., in association with changing for physical education). Boys may exhibit shyness and social anxiety or be described as having a quiet, unassertive personality, diminished self-esteem, and generalized anxiety. With adolescence, there may be increased social isolation and decreased sexual interest (Ross et al., 2007).

Evidence-Based Interventions

Medical interventions include testosterone/androgen replacement prior to puberty, but no studies demonstrate this empirically; there is also no indication that addition of testosterone results in increased aggression or cognitive profile (Ross et al., 2007, 2008). Counseling and supportive services to help with coping skills have been recommended (Ross et al., 2007). It is important that teachers be aware of potential issues with teasing and take appropriate actions to squelch this behavior.

Noonan Syndrome

Noonan syndrome is another chromosomal anomaly with variable expression (Tramboo et al., 2002). It was originally believed that Noonan syndrome was the male counterpart to Turner syndrome; however, it is now known that they are very different disorders with different mechanisms of occurrence (Allanson, 2007). Noonan syndrome actually affects both males and females. The incidence of Noonan syndrome is estimated at 1 in 1,000 to 2,500 children worldwide. It is one of the most common genetic syndromes associated with congenital heart disease.

Etiology

Family studies consistently have suggested that Noonan syndrome is genetically transmitted with autosomal dominant transmission but variable expression. The gene implicated in Noonan syndrome has been mapped to the long arm of chromosome 12 and specifically the chromosomal region 12q24 (Tramboo et al., 2002). In families with multiple family members affected, Noonan syndrome maps to chromosome 12q24.1. In one study, it was determined that about half of the participants had a mutation of the PTPN11 gene at that location. This gene is responsible for encoding protein tyrosine phosphatase SHP-2 (Tartaglia et al., 2001) and is part of several intracellular pathways that are involved in embryonic development and formation of cardiac valves. In addition to PTPN11, SOS1, the human deltex gene (DLT 3 1), or KRAS genes also have been implicated (Medved & Percy, 2001; Tramboo et al., 2002). Duplication of this same region (12q24) that involves PTPN11 can result in Noonan syndrome as well.

Course and Prognosis

In addition to the heart malformations, the principal features include short stature, chest indentation, impaired blood clotting, and characteristic facial features (Teeter, 1999). In particular, individuals with Noonan syndrome tend to have large heads with triangular faces, broad forehead, a short neck with a low hairline, and curly hair. Hypertelorism (wide-set eyes) occurs in about 95% of individuals with Noonan syndrome; in some cases, proptosis (bulging eyes) is also evident. Vision may be affected with refractive errors, strabismus, or nystagmus present. Ears tend to be low set and rotated backward with a thick outer rim. In males, cryptorchidism (failure of testicles to descend) occurs in almost all cases (Teeter, 1999). Eating problems, including failure to thrive, are not uncommon. Although these problems may be evident to some extent in all individuals with Noonan syndrome, the range and severity of features varies greatly, and the syndrome is not always identified at an early age (Teeter, 1999). Some individuals may have co-occurring Van Willebrand or Arnold Chiari malformation. About one-third of individuals with Noonan syndrome have impaired cognitive ability to the extent of being identified with mental retardation (Teeter, 1999). For those individuals with Noonan syndrome who do not evidence mental retardation, visual-spatial abilities tend to be better developed than verbal abilities (D. A. Lee, Portnoy, Hill, Gillberg, & Patton, 2005; Troyer & Joschko, 1997). Others may evidence milder developmental delays, speech and language difficulties, learning disabilities, poor coordination and clumsiness, poor attention, and impaired motor abilities (Troyer & Joschko, 1997). Speech problems may be related to micrognathia (small lower jaw), high arched palate, and poor tongue control. In contrast to deficit areas, memory may be intact (Troyer & Joschko, 1997). No consistent emotional problems have emerged as yet in conjunction with Noonan syndrome (D. A. Lee et al., 2005). Consistent with impaired attention, it has been suggested that there is a need to consider the co-occurrence of ADHD in children with Noonan syndrome (Horiguchi & Takeshita, 2003).

Evidence-Based Interventions

A multidisciplinary intervention approach is recommended for individuals with Noonan syndrome that is tailored to the specific needs of the individual and incorporates medical follow-up, psychoeducational interventions, vocational training, and parental support (Teeter, 1999). Growth hormone has been considered as one means of addressing some of the issues associated with Noonan syndrome (Noordam, van der Burgt, Sengers, Delemarre-van de Waal, & Otten, 2001).

CASE STUDY: WALTER—NOONAN SYNDROME

Reason for Referral

Walter is a 6-year-old kindergarten student who is being followed by his pediatrician for a history of Noonan syndrome (autosomal dominant; PTPN11 gene located on chromosome 12q24 with associated dysmorphic features (short stature, widely spaced down-slanting eyes) and congenital heart defect (supravalvular pulmonary stenosis), which required surgical repair. In addition, Walter has exhibited a history of developmental delay, short attention span, and hyperactivity. It should be noted that approximately 25% to 30% of individuals with Noonan syndrome have learning problems. As a result, Walter's pediatrician requested neuropsychological evaluation in order to assess higher cortical functioning and make appropriate recommendations regarding school placement and the need for supportive therapies.

Background Information

Walter resides with his parents, Phil and Trish, and his two older brothers. Pat is 11 years of age and an A student in the fifth grade. According to the mother, Pat has a history of ADHD for which he has taken methylphenidate (Concerta) in the past. Tim is 9 years of age and an A student in the third grade. Both siblings are reported to be in good health. The father is 43 years of age, a college graduate with a degree in agriculture, who is currently employed as a store manager. The mother is 42 years of age, a college graduate with a degree in nursing, who is currently employed as a registered nurse and working toward a master's degree. Both parents are reported to be in good health.

Review of Walter's developmental and medical history indicates that he is the product of a 37-week-gestation pregnancy complicated by chylothorax diagnosed by routine sonogram three days prior to delivery. The delivery was vaginal, and Walter was reported to weigh 5 pounds 11 ounces at birth. Due to the chylothorax, Walter was intubated, and a bilateral thoracentesis was performed. Walter was subsequently transferred to the neonatal intensive care unit, where he remained for approximately 28 days. He was discharged with a nasogastral tube for feeding and a referral to the Babies Can't Wait program. His mother was unable to recall Walter's exact developmental, motor, and language milestones; however, she felt that all of these were delayed. Toilet training was fully accomplished prior to 3 years of age without significant difficulty. In addition to Walter's neonatal history, at approximately 12 months of age, he was diagnosed with pulmonary aortic stenosis by his pediatric cardiologist. At 1 year 10 months, Walter was evaluated by a pediatric geneticist, who diagnosed Walter with Noonan's syndrome. At 4 years 1 month, Walter underwent surgical repair for supravalvular pulmonic stenosis.

According to his mother, Walter has always been "busy"; however, his attention span did not become problematic until he began attending preschool. His mother went on to report that Walter always has experienced difficulty falling asleep at night. As a result, he likes to be rocked by his father until he falls asleep in the den. Walter wakes up almost every night about 1:00 to 2:00 a.m. and spends the rest of the night sleeping with his parents. Walter is very restless off and on during sleep. More recently, his mother reports that Walter has been experiencing headaches in which he typically wakes up at night or in the early morning complaining of headache with associated vomiting. Walter enjoys a good appetite, and there is no history for seizure disorder or significant head injury.

Review of Walter's academic history indicates that at 2 years of age, he began attending a nursery program at Toddler Tech. In addition, he also was cared for during the day by his maternal grandparents. At 3 years of age, Walter attended the 3-K program at Toddler Tech. His mother reported that on occasion he would "get in trouble." At 4 years of age, it was decided to have Walter remain in the 3-year preschool program due to the heart surgery. At 5, Walter attended the 4–K program at Toddler Tech. This was the first year that he was actually asked to perform readiness skill activities. According to his mother, Walter got in trouble frequently, requiring "time out." The infractions typically included not following directions, not completing work, and behaving like the "class clown." Review of a school report form completed by Walter's 4–K teacher indicates that she characterized Walter as

> very easygoing and laid back. He is a happy child. Walter's attention span wanders often. At the table, he will put his hands on the other children, not to hurt them but to pick at them. He likes to be a clown and will make faces and/or hand gestures to make children laugh. He also makes noises when he is working, resting, sitting, etc. Whenever he is corrected about any behavior, he smiles or laughs about it.

She went on to estimate that Walter's readiness skill development was below average for grade placement.

At present, Walter is attending a kindergarten program at his local elementary school. According to his mother, Walter has experienced behavioral difficulty right from the start, which has resulted in a disciplinary referral and a half day of in-school suspension. Walter's infractions include constantly playing, making noises, and not following directions. Review of a similar school report form completed by Walter's current teacher indicates that she characterizes Walter as

> outgoing, active, social, loves to be a clown and make others laugh. All the children like him. He is always happy. He is never rude to me or my paraprofessional. Walter just has trouble being still and paying attention to group instruction. He is not disrespectful to others. He is easily distracted from his work.

Walter's teacher again estimated that he is performing at a below average level for grade placement in readiness skill development.

Assessment Measures

Clinical interview
Developmental history
Differential Ability Scales, Second Edition (DAS-II), Early Years Level
Neuropsychological Assessment (NEPSY)/Neuropsychological Assessment, Second Edition (NEPSY-2)
Peabody Picture Vocabulary Test, Fourth Edition (PPVT-IV)

Expressive One Word Picture Vocabulary Test (EOWVT)
Kaufman Assessment Battery for Children, Second Edition (KABC-2)
Beery Developmental Test of Visual-Motor Integration, Fifth Edition (DTVMI-V)
Finger Tapping test
Children's Memory Scale (CMS)
Wide Range Achievement Test, Fourth Edition (WRAT-4)
Bracken Basic Concept Scale (Expressive)—Revised (BBCS-R)
Adaptive Behavior Assessment System, Second Edition (ABAS-2)
Behavior Assessment System for Children, Second Edition (BASC-2; Parent and Teacher Rating Scales)
DSM-IV ADHD Checklist (Parent and Teacher Scales)

General Observations and Impressions

Walter presented himself for testing as a somewhat immature youngster with blond hair and blue eyes who was casually dressed in a maroon T-shirt, plaid shorts, and sneakers. He exhibited difficulty separating from his mother and, as a result, she accompanied Walter and the examiners to the testing room. Even with his mother present, Walter initially was hesitant to begin testing. As a result, his mother phoned her husband in order to get Walter to cooperate. Following the phone call, Walter's level of cooperation improved dramatically and testing proceeded. Throughout the evaluation, which consisted of two sessions separated by a lunch break, Walter exhibited good social eye contact, a broad range of affect, and readily initiated conversation with the examiners. Walter's language usage was fluent and prosodic with word-finding difficulty noted. Walter's attention span was felt to be extremely short, necessitating frequent verbal redirection from the examiners along with providing Walter with periodic breaks. In addition, Walter was observed to be very restless, in and out of his seat, and he often would respond impulsively on verbal as well as visual-motor tasks. Lateral dominance is firmly established in the right hand for paper-and-pencil manipulation. His mother reported that Walter's vision and hearing were screened by the health department and reported to be normal.

Test Interpretation

The results of neuropsychological evaluation indicate that Walter currently is functioning within the low-average to average range of intellectual ability as measured by the Differential Ability Scales—Second Edition (DAS-II). Analysis of the various Cluster scores reveals that Walter exhibited average verbal conceptual and nonverbal reasoning ability contrasted by borderline visual-spatial/constructional ability. In contrast, review of Walter's performance on the subtests comprising the Spatial Cluster indicates that Walter's low score was due to his poor performance on a paper-and-pencil copying task. His constructional ability was found to be low average when fine motor requirements were minimized. Additional assessment indicates that Walter demonstrated borderline to low-average sequential reasoning and problem solving capability on the Tower subtest of the Neuropsychological Assessment (NEPSY). Test results are summarized in Table 15.14.

Walter's language skills are generally in the low-average to average range. Specifically, Walter exhibited average vocabulary development, low-average to average phonological

Table 15.14 Psychometric Summary for Walter

		Standard Score
Differential Ability Scales, Second Edition (DAS-II), Early Years Level		
General Conceptual Ability		83
Special Non-verbal Composite		80
Verbal Cluster		96
Verbal Comprehension		105
Naming Vocabulary		89
Non-verbal Reasoning Cluster		90
Picture Similarities		91
Matrices		95
Spatial Cluster		75
Pattern Construction		87
Copying		69
Neuropsychological Assessment, Second Edition (NEPSY-2)		
Tower (NEPSY)		80
Phonological Processing		90
Sentence Repetition		90
Comprehension of Instructions		80
Word Generation		80
Arrows		95
Peabody Picture Vocabulary Test, Fourth Edition (PPVT-IV)		91
Expressive One Word Picture Vocabulary Test (EOWVT)		92
Kaufman Assessment Battery for Children, Second Edition (KABC-2)		
Gestalt Closure		105
Developmental Test of Visual-Motor Integration, Fifth Edition (DTVMI-V)		
Visual Motor Integration		60
	Taps /10 sec.	
Finger Tapping		
Right (dominant) Hand	16.0	60
Left (nondominant) Hand	15.3	65
Children's Memory Scale (CMS)		
Attention/Concentration Index		
Numbers		65
Sequences		70
Picture Locations (supplemental)		80
Verbal Immediate Index		
Stories		105
Visual Immediate Index		
Dot Locations		80
Verbal Delayed Index		
Stories		90
Visual Delayed Index		
Dot Locations		100
Delayed Recognition		
Stories		105

(continued)

Table 15.14 *(Continued)*

	Standard Score		
Wide Range Achievement Test, Fourth Edition (WRAT-4)			
Reading		84	
Spelling		69	
Arithmetic		67	
Bracken Basic Concept Scale (Expressive), Revised (BBCS-R)			
School Readiness Composite		71	
Adaptive Behavior Assessment System, Second Edition (ABAS-2)			
General Adaptive Composite		75	
Behavior Assessment System for Children, Second Edition (BASC-2)			
		T-Score	
Clinical Scales	Parent	Teacher	Teacher
Hyperactivity	74	76	75
Aggression	84	60	58
Anxiety	42	47	44
Depression	58	44	49
Somatization	58	42	74
Atypical	66	46	70
Withdrawal	45	38	43
Attention	69	67	66
Adaptive Scales			
Adaptability	39	59	65
Social Skills	39	54	55
Activities of Daily Living	31	NA	NA
Functional Communication	36	57	44
DSM-IV ADHD Checklist		**Raw Score**	
Inattention	27/27	10/27	18/27
Hyperactivity/Impulsivity	23/27	26/27	16/27

processing and sentence imitation skills, and borderline to low-average rapid verbal naming ability when asked to provide items belonging to a specific category. Walter's performance on measures of verbal comprehension was highly variable with more difficulty noted when he was confronted with multipart directions. Visual-spatial perception is found to be well within the average range; however, Walter's performance on visual-motor/constructional tasks was deficient and consistent with his performance on the DAS–II. Fine motor tapping speed is found to be bilaterally depressed as measured by the Finger Tapping test.

Analysis of Walter's performance on the Children's Memory Scale (CMS) indicates that, at the present time, he is exhibiting deficient to borderline ability to hold material in immediate auditory working memory contrasted by borderline to low-average visual working memory. When asked to learn and remember (30 minutes later) newly presented material, Walter demonstrated average ability to recall stories that were read to him as well as average ability to recall the spatial location of an array of dots presented over three structured learning trials once he mastered the placements. It should be noted that due to poor task comprehension, Walter was unable to perform in a valid manner on the Word Pairs and Faces subtests.

Academically, assessment of Walter's readiness skill development indicates that he currently is underachieving as compared with his performance on the Verbal Cluster of the DAS-II, which is felt to be a best estimate of his potential to learn. Specifically, Walter demonstrated a firm grasp of color and shape recognition, and he could write his first but not his last name successfully. In contrast, Walter's letter recognition and sound symbol relationship skills are not automatic, and he has not developed a beginning sight word vocabulary. Walter is able to count to 14 with one-to-one correspondence; however, his single-digit number recognition is not automatic, he had difficulty showing a requested amount with his fingers, and he was unable to perform word problems involving addition or subtraction, such as "3 pennies spend 1." Finally, Walter's handwriting was quite poor and labored. Adaptive functioning is found to be in the borderline range per his mother's report. Behaviorally, analysis of rating scales completed by Walter's mother and his K-4 and K-5 teachers indicates that Walter is exhibiting significant difficulty focusing and sustaining his attention; he is hyperactive and emotionally immature both at home and in the classroom. In addition, his mother endorsed a significant concern with regard to verbal aggression in the home.

Summary and Diagnostic Impressions

Taken together, this pattern of neuropsychological test performance is consistent with a diagnosis of ADHD, combined type, in conjunction with executive dysfunction (poor problem solving, difficulty with rapid word retrieval and holding information in immediate working memory, and poor behavioral regulation) and developmental coordination disorder, which together are placing Walter at significant risk for development of a learning disability as he progresses through elementary school. These findings are consistent with Walter's diagnosis of Noonan syndrome in that approximately 25% to 30% of children with this disorder develop learning disabilities.

Recommendations

As a result, it is recommended that Walter be considered for resource/inclusion special education services designed for children with learning difficulties under the eligibility category of "Other Health Impaired." Special education services should be utilized for development of academic readiness skills as well as basic reading, language arts, and mathematics skills.

In addition, Walter will require support services within the regular education setting, including the development and implementation of a behavioral plan focused on enhancing his attention span, listening skills, task completion, and social skills as part of his Individualized Educational Plan. As part of this plan, rules and expectations should be presented simply, clearly, and consistently and reviewed frequently. This plan should place a large emphasis on consistently rewarding Walter's "good" behavior, such as positive social interactions, working on classwork, and following directions, rather than having a punitive system that primarily calls attention to his mistakes. Consequences for both appropriate and inappropriate behavior should be enforced on a consistent basis through positive reinforcement and response cost. At the same time, it is recommended that he have a high ratio of positive reinforcement (gaining points, tokens, etc.) to punishment (losing points, etc.), as would be consistent with positive behavioral support. The behavioral plan should be coordinated with the parents to ensure consistency between home and school, including target behaviors, reinforcers, and punishments.

Given Walter's pattern of strengths and weaknesses, it is recommended that academic instruction in reading/writing instruction emphasize multisensory approaches along with continued training in phonetic word attack skills. In order to enhance Walter's learning/retention, new material should be presented in an organized format that is meaningful to him. The material to be learned should be pretaught, broken down into smaller components/steps, and presented in a highly structured format with frequent repetition to facilitate new learning. Instruction should be supplemented with visual aids, demonstrations, and experiential/procedural learning whenever possible. When studying for tests or doing multiple homework assignments on the same day, similar subject material should be separated in order to reduce interference. Finally, Walter should be provided with periodic review of previously learned material in order to enhance long-term retention.

In light of his inattention, impulsivity, and executive deficits, there are several general rules teachers, therapists, and parents should keep in mind while interacting with Walter.

- Eye contact should be ensured.
- A prompt to look at the speaker before directions are presented will be helpful.
- Instructions and directions should be kept short, simple, and concrete.
- Requests should be limited to single commands, and instructions should be presented several times.
- Training in active problem solving also may prove helpful. One problem-solving technique involves teaching the student a four-step procedure:
  1. Identifying the problem
  2. Generating ways to solve the problem
  3. Selecting the best solution
  4. Checking out the success of the choice

In the beginning, positive reinforcement should be incorporated into each step of this training to facilitate learning and encourage consistent implementation of the techniques.

Walter should undergo occupational therapy evaluation in order to determine if he would benefit from therapy at school focused on minimizing the impact of his fine motor difficulty in the classroom.

Accommodations will be necessary to enhance Walter's ability to succeed in the classroom, including preferential seating away from bulletin boards, doorways, windows, or other students, if necessary, where excessive stimuli might prove distracting. Instruction should be provided in small-group settings whenever possible, and efforts should be made to redirect his attention. Given his ADHD, a reduction in the amount, but not the difficulty level, of assignments may assist Walter in completing classroom tasks and homework in a timely manner. Moreover, whenever possible, he should be given additional time to complete assignments. Tests should be in multiple-choice/matching/short-answer formats instead of an essay format and should be administered individually/orally, with additional time provided when necessary. Walter also will benefit from the use of graph paper or different color highlighter pens to maintain place value when doing written calculation, having an outline of the steps necessary to complete multistep math problems available for reference, and the use of computer programs to solidify basic math facts. Finally, as Walter progresses through school, he should be allowed and encouraged to use various compensatory devices, such as textbooks on tape/reading pen, a calculator to check written calculation, and a computer with word processing capability if necessary.

In addition to the above-mentioned behavior modification program, Walter also may benefit from family therapy designed to assist the parents in developing a similar program for use with Walter in the home. If therapy, classroom accommodations, and a behavioral plan prove ineffective at managing Walter's symptoms of inattention, overactivity, and impulsivity, consultation with his pediatrician regarding a trial of medication management should be considered. Finally, a referral to a child neurologist in order to further evaluate and manage Walter's headaches is strongly recommended.

Further Discussion of Case Study

The diagnosis of Noonan syndrome with Walter should alert the clinician of areas to be concerned with as part of the assessment process. As with George, Walter is evidencing many early signs of potential later problems; identification and appropriate early intervention can address these issues and increase the likelihood of a more positive academic outcome. In addition, the evaluation indicated co-occurring ADHD, which likely is exacerbating his learning difficulties. Finally, although not specifically an issue at Walter's age, school personnel will need to be aware of, and sensitive to, the likelihood that Walter may be the victim of bullying or teasing, ultimately with the potential for psychosocial issues to emerge in adolescence.

CONCLUDING COMMENTS

This chapter has reviewed what is known about specific chromosomal abnormalities and presented two case studies. Notably, across these disorders, there is consistency in the research, indicating that early intervention is critical to the later outcome for children with these disorders; further, at the root of much of the educational and behavioral difficulties are deficits in communication status. Across disorders, deficits in expressive language may result in an underestimate of overall ability; moreover, individuals with these disorders vary in terms of functioning level. Specific components of neuropsychological assessment may be useful in differentiating strengths and weaknesses as well as in differentiating between chromosomal disorders (Kogan et al., 2009). Comprehensive and regular evaluation to monitor changes in function over time and as contextual demands change is needed. Finally, consideration of quality of life issues and transition are particularly important with these disorders. At the same time, however, there is little research establishing an evidence base for interventions for children with these disorders.

Chapter 16

NEUROCUTANEOUS DISORDERS

Neurocutaneous disorders are those that involve the nervous system and the skin. Of the neurocutaneous syndromes, three syndromes account for the majority of the referrals to pediatric neurology clinics (Zaroff & Isaacs, 2005): neurofibromatosis, tuberous sclerosis, and Sturge-Weber syndrome. These will be the focus of this chapter, but there are many others as well.

NEUROFIBROMATOSIS

Definition and Etiology

Neurofibromatosis (NF) is classified as a neurocutaneous disorder due to the presenting evidence of patches of hyperpigmentation of the skin (e.g., birthmarks or stigmata). There are two types of neurofibromatosis: Type 1 (NF1), or von Recklinghausen, and Type 2 (NF2). NF1 is one of the most common human single-gene disorders; it affects at least 1 million persons worldwide (A. H. Crawford & Schorry, 2006; Yohay, 2006). The incidence of NF1 is 1 per 2,500–3,000 live births with autosomal dominant transmission (Hersh, 2008). NF1 is caused by mutations of the NF1 gene at chromosome 17q11.2 (Tang et al., 2004). NF2 is also autosomal dominant. Each type is characterized as a multisystem disorder that primarily involves the skin and nervous system. Some features of NF1 are present at birth; others are age-related abnormalities of tissue proliferation and present over the course of development. In general, neurofibromatosis presents as tumors of the central and peripheral nervous system, café-au-lait spots, lesions of the viscera and vascular system, and facial and skull deformities (Hersh, 2008). The café-au-lait spots are most numerous on the trunk; they are usually evident at birth with other signs evident by age 1 (Hersh, 2008; Nilsson & Bradford, 1999). Notably, the presence of more cutaneous stigmata is associated with less central nervous system complications (Nilsson & Bradford, 1999). Children with NF1 exhibit abnormalities in astrocyte growth regulation and are prone to the development of brain tumors or astrocytomas (Dasgupta & Gutmann, 2005). Tumors are most evident on cranial nerve II (optic) and cranial nerve VIII (cochlear); they also may be on the spinal cord. In about 45% to 50% of cases, there are clinical signs of neuropathology (Chalhub, 1976; Hersh, 2008). The level of neuropathology varies with cognitive level. With low IQ, there is a high incidence of cortical and subcortical anomalies including polymicrogyria, pachygyria, heterotopias, and disordered cortical layering (Nilsson & Bradford, 1999). In contrast, with normal IQ, there is a high incidence of heterotopias and abnormal layering. NF2 also is characterized by the development of multiple nervous system tumors, ocular abnormalities, and skin tumors but usually is considered a disease of adults (Ruggieri et al., 2005). Although initial signs and/or symptoms may be evident in childhood, they may go unrecognized. As a result, the majority of neurofibromatosis research with children is specific to NF1.

Genetically, the NF1 gene is involved in cell differentiation, regulation of cell growth, and cell interactions; deletions on chromosome 17 appear to be responsible for NF1 (Nilsson & Bradford, 1999; V. C. Williams et al., 2009), with about 50% of cases familial in nature. The NF1 gene and its protein product, neurofibromin, have been identified (Bonneau, Lenherr, Pena, Hart, & Scheffzek, 2009; Cawthon et al., 1990); any mutation of this gene may affect cell growth during critical developmental periods from conception to puberty and beyond. As with other disorders, the manner of transmission (paternal or maternal) is of importance as well (Lazaro et al., 1996). There also are individual differences that have been identified at the cell level. In contrast to the association of NF1 with chromosome 17, NF2 is associated with 22q (Guttmann et al., 1997).

Neurological Correlates

Few studies have examined the structural or morphological correlates of NF1. Examination of gray and white matter volume in children with NF1 often indicates that they have larger volumes with T2-weighted hyperintensities, macrocephaly, and optic gliomas as compared to matched relatives (Billingsley, Schrimsher, Jackson, Slopis, & Moore, 2002; Greenwood et al., 2005). The greatest difference in white matter volume was in the frontal lobes while the greatest difference in gray matter volume was in the temporal, parietal, and occipital regions. Although IQ was significantly related to gray matter volume in the control group, the same was not true of the children with NF1 (Greenwood et al., 2005). A previous study indicated that volume of gray matter, as well as corpus callosum size, was related to academic achievement (B. Moore, 2000).

Visual-spatial impairment and neuroanatomical abnormalities are considered hallmark features of NF1 (Billingsley et al., 2004; Billingsley, Slopis, Swank, Jackson, & Moore, 2003). Neuroimaging studies have investigated the neural network of visual-spatial processing in NF1 (Clements-Stephens, Rimrodt, Gaur, & Cutting, 2008). Results with normative samples indicate a right-hemisphere network of activation including inferior parietal lobe, dorsolateral prefrontal cortex, and extrastriate regions. In contrast, individuals with NF1 tended to activate left-hemisphere regions, possibly as a result of an inefficient right-hemisphere network. Notably, the NF1 group evidenced decreased activation of the primary visual cortex (Clements-Stephens et al., 2008). Further, individuals with NF1 who showed expected gyral patterns in the right hemisphere performed worse across language measures than those showing an extra (i.e., anomalous) gyrus. In particular, a doubling of Heschl's gyrus in the left and right hemispheres was significantly associated with performance on several neuropsychological measures (Billingsley, Slopis et al., 2003). Also based on magnetic resonance imaging (MRI) study, the left planum temporale in boys with NF1 was significantly smaller in both surface area and gray matter volume as compared to that in girls with NF1 and controls. Boys with NF1 also showed greater symmetry between the left and right hemispheres in this region compared with girls with NF1 and controls. As has been found with the dyslexia research (see Chapter 2), decreased leftward asymmetry of the planum was associated with poorer reading and math achievement in children with NF1 (Billingsley et al., 2002). Differential use of inferior and dorsolateral prefrontal cortical areas relative to NF1 was revealed during phonologic (rhyme) tasks, with increased signal change in the right superior temporal gyrus noted (Billingsley, Jackson et al., 2003). Also using functional MRI (fMRI), individuals with NF1 demonstrated less neuronal hemodynamic activity in occipital and parietal cortices as compared with controls. Further, the NF1 group relied more on areas of the posterior cortex relative to lateral and inferior frontal regions during visual-spatial analysis (Billingsley et al., 2004).

Course and Prognosis

Course and prognosis varies depending on type of NF as well as what triggers the diagnosis and when; in effect, the presentation, course, and prognosis are highly idiographic, necessitating comprehensive evaluation (Nilsson & Bradford, 1999; V. C. Williams et al., 2009). Children with NF2 often first come to medical attention because of ocular, subtle skin, or neurological problems (Ruggieri et al., 2005). Over time, they present with more classic symptoms of neurofibromatosis due to tumors. The clinical course is highly variable, depending on tumor, early surgical intervention, surgical outcome after tumor resection, and any complications (Ruggieri et al., 2005). For individuals with NF1, initial identification may arise as a result of infantile spasms (Ruggieri et al., 2009); over time, there is increased risk of cognitive and learning difficulties. Cognitive deficits are the most common complication in children with NF1, with academic achievement negatively affected (Hyman, Shores, & North, 2006).

Although neurofibromatosis is associated with marked clinical variability, most individuals do well in terms of growth and development (Hersh, 2008). With NF1, health-related quality of life was found to be significantly different in areas of motor, cognitive, and social functioning (Graf, Landolt, Mori, & Boltshauser, 2006). Further, when compared to a normative sample, children and adolescents with neurofibromatosis also demonstrated a reduction of positive and negative emotions. In effect, illness-related variables had a negative impact on the emotional domain of quality of life while positive family relationships positively affected both quality of life and psychological adjustment (Graf et al., 2006). There is some indication of possible manifestation as nonverbal learning disability in conjunction with neurofibromatosis (Cutting, Clements, Lightman, Yerby-Hammack, & Denckla, 2004). Others also have found unusually high proportions of maladaptive behavior associated with neurofibromatosis (Fisch et al., 2008; Nilsson & Bradford, 1999).

Medical Implications

In addition to hearing problems and possible visual problems, research suggests a high frequency of orthopedic complications in children with NF1. Based on a database of 588 children, the incidence of spinal deformity in children with NF1 was found to be 21%; other orthopedic problems occurred in 1% to 25%, depending on the orthopedic problem (A. H. Crawford & Schorry, 2006). As noted earlier, there is an increased risk for the development of astrocytomas with neurofibromatosis, and this may warrant medical intervention.

Neurocognitive Correlates

Cognitive deficits in NF1 have been documented in both the verbal and the visual perceptual and spatial domains (Billingsley et al., 2002; Cutting et al., 2002). The severity of NF1 was associated with the degree of cognitive deficits (Krab, Aarsen et al., 2008). Most commonly, children with NF1 evidence difficulties in language, motor, visual-motor, and visual-spatial deficits (Cutting et al., 2004). The cognitive function of adults with NF1 tends to be compromised in regard to visual-spatial and attention abilities, as would be expected from child research (Pavol et al., 2006). Discriminant function with two measures of visual-spatial skills and one measure of receptive vocabulary were found to account for 45% of the variance between the groups. Based on analyses and findings, it was suggested that while there may be sparing of basic cognitive functions, individuals with NF1 will have greater impairment on tests that use multiple cognitive skills (Pavol et al., 2006). In other studies, nearly all children with NF1 showed visual-perceptual and executive dysfunctions (Descheemaeker, Ghesquière, Symons, Fryns, & Legius, 2005; Schrimsher, Billingsley, Slopis, & Moore, 2003). Attentional deficits also have been found in conjunction with NF1 (Coudé, Mignot, Lyonnet, & Munnich, 2007; Philip & Turk, 2006). For example, in a study of 310 individuals with NF1 and a contrast group of 242 individuals, the occurrence of grade retention (53% and 25% respectively) and the presence of inattentive symptoms (67% and 14% respectively) differed significantly by group; further, grade retention was strongly associated with the degree of inattentive symptoms (Coudé et al., 2007). No specific problems with processing speed (i.e., slower cognitive tempo) have been associated with NF1 consistently (Rowbotham, Pit-ten Cate, Sonuga-Barke, & Huijbreqts, 2009; Zöller, Rembeck, & Bäckman, 1997); stuttering is a frequent problem, however (Van Borsel & Tetnowski, 2007). Both short- and long-term memory emerge as relative strengths for individuals with neurofibromatosis (Hyman, Shores, & North, 2005). Functioning across domains in association with neurofibromatosis is provided in Table 16.1.

Educational Implications

There is a lack of consensus in the literature regarding the frequency of general and specific learning disabilities (Hyman et al., 2006). In a recent study, 75% of the children with NF1 performed more than 1 standard deviation below grade-level peers in at least one academic area (Krab, Aarsen et al., 2008). In addition, children with NF1 have significantly increased risk for retention in grade, placement in special education, and/or were receiving remedial teaching for learning, behavior, speech, or motor problems (Coudé, Mignot, Lyonnet, & Munnich, 2006; Cutting et al., 2004; Krab, Aarsen et al., 2008). In a sample of children with NF1, 20 children (67%) demonstrated deficits in

Table 16.1 Neuropsychological Deficits Associated with Neurofibromatosis

Global Domain/Specific Deficits	Phenotype
Cognition	Likely to be impaired; degree of impairment related to NF1 severity
Auditory-linguistic/Language function	Deficits in language areas common Stuttering common
Learning and Memory	Memory usually a relative strength
Visual perception/Constructional praxis	Visual-motor and visual-spatial deficits common
Attention/Concentration	Deficits in attention common
Processing speed	Processing speed appears to be spared
Motor function	Deficits in motor areas common; motor production may be slowed
Achievement/Academic skills	Achievement tends to be below expectancy Special education frequent
Emotional/Behavioral functioning	Comorbidity with ADHD frequent Problems with peer relations Poor self-concept in specific domains

one or more reading subskills; the majority (75%) met criteria for phonological dyslexia (Watt, Shores, & North, 2008). In a study of 81 children with NF1 and 49 comparison children, problems with academic achievement were present in 52% of children with NF1; however, only 20% of the children with NF1 were diagnosed with a specific learning disability (Gutmann, 1999; Hyman et al., 2006). Of the children with NF1, only males with NF1 were at significant risk for identification as having a learning disability, usually associated with Verbal IQ (verbal abilities) significantly lower than Performance IQ (nonverbal abilities). Further, there was significant comorbidity of literacy-based learning disabilities and Attention-Deficit/Hyperactivity Disorder (ADHD; Hyman et al., 2006). Another study found that as many as 40% of children with NF1 evidenced a learning disability and 65% evidenced impairment in at least one academic area (Gutmann, 1999). Similarly, of 48 children with NF1 in South Africa, the most consistent disability related to the child's level of cognitive functioning. School problems (i.e., learning and behavioral problems) were reported in 70% of school-age children (Ramanjam et al., 2006). In a smaller study of 17 children with NF1, nearly 50% of the children evidenced learning disabilities, particularly in literacy skills. Arithmetic learning disability was rare (Descheemaeker et al., 2005). Notably, even those children with NF1 who were not identified as needing special education often evidenced neuropsychological deficits, with only 10% not displaying any school-related problems (Krab, Aarsen et al., 2008).

Emotional/Behavioral Implications

Children with neurofibromatosis are at increased risk (1 in 6) of presenting with emotional and/or behavioral problems (Fisch et al., 2007; Noll, Reiter-Purtill, Moore et al., 2007). When 58 children with neurofibromatosis, ages 7 to 15, were compared with classroom peers of the same race/gender and age, results indicated that teachers perceived children with neurofibromatosis as more prosocial (Noll, Reiter-Purtill, Moore et al., 2007); however, both teachers and peers viewed children with NF1 as displaying less leadership skills and as being more socially sensitive and isolated (i.e., often left out, trouble making friends); parents also reported lower social functioning. Overall, the children with neurofibromatosis had fewer friendships and were less well liked by peers (B. Barton & North, 2004; Noll, Reiter-Purtill, Moore et al., 2007). Neurological involvement was significantly related to psychosocial problems (Noll, Reiter-Purtill, Moore et al., 2007). Alternatively, in a sample of 75 children and adolescents with neurofibromatosis, the majority reported positive global self-concept, with some exceptions on specific domains (B. Barton & North, 2007). One of these exceptions related to their self-concept in relation to physical and athletic abilities; adolescents also reported significantly lower self-concept for mathematics.

Of 64 children with NF1, there was a higher than expected occurrence of reported difficulties associated with peer relations, hyperactivity, emotional symptoms, and sleep problems, particularly parasomnias (H. Johnson, Wiggs, Stores, & Huson, 2005). Notably, poorer social outcomes than their unaffected siblings, and significantly poorer social skills in comparison with normative data was associated with the presence of ADHD (B. Barton & North, 2004). Given deficits in attentional abilities, it is not surprising that approximately 50% of children with NF1 meet diagnostic criteria for ADHD (Cutting et al., 2004; Mautner, Kluwe, Thakker, & Leark, 2002; Philip & Turk, 2006). Moreover, using the Test of Variables of Attention (TOVA), it was found that children with both NF1 and ADHD evidenced significantly poorer attention than those with only NF1, only ADHD, or a control group. In addition, the comorbid group evidenced more inattention problems on parent rating scales (Mautner et al., 2002). As such, assessment of children with NF1 should include screening for attentional and behavioral difficulties associated with ADHD.

In contrast, regardless of the presence of comorbid difficulties of low achievement or ADHD, children with neurofibromatosis reported somewhat higher academic self-perceptions relative to objective criteria; this may serve as an adaptive or protective mechanism (B. Barton & North, 2007). In addition, there has been some consideration of an association between NF1 and autism (P. G. Williams & Hersh, 1998). In chart review of 74 children with NF1, it was found that in 73%, there was evidence of one or more developmental disorders, including specific language impairment, intellectual deficits, learning disability, motor problems, and/or ADHD; of these cases, 4% met criteria for a diagnosis of autistic disorder. The authors concluded that the rate of occurrence of autistic disorder in the sample was sufficient to warrant adding it as a potential co-occurring disorder (P. G. Williams & Hersh, 1998).

Evidence-Based Interventions

Because of the multifaceted and idiographic presentation of NF, it has been suggested that intervention planning should be both multidisciplinary and forward thinking (Nilsson & Bradford, 1999). In effect, it is important to anticipate problems and take efforts to address potential problems in advance rather than wait for them to develop. One of the components with NF, as with other disorders, is ensuring that the parent(s) and the child have a clear understanding of the disorder, what to look for to ensure appropriate medical intervention, and what to be aware of in terms of educational needs. At the school level, it is important for teachers to be aware of the child's disorder and the potential for the social issues and bullying to occur. Although research indicates needs across academic, behavioral, and social domains, there is minimal to no available research specific to what works for children with NF (see Table 16.2). One study examined the possible benefits to cognitive ability of simvastatin (Zocor), but this was not found to have any effect (Krab, de Goede-Bolder et al., 2008). An additional study examined the effects of stimulant medication in addressing the attentional problems of children with NF1 and co-occurring ADHD with positive effects (Mautner et al., 2002).

Table 16.2 Evidence-Based Interventions for Neurofibromatosis

Intervention	Target/Goal	Level of Support
Stimulant medication	Inattention	Emerging (Mautner et al., 2002)
Simvastatin (Zocor)	Cognitive deficits	No effect (Krab, de Goede-Bolder et al., 2008)
Cochlear implant, brain stem implant	Hearing loss in NF2	Emerging (Colletti, 2007; Lim et al., 2007; Vincent, Pasanisi, Guida, DiTrapani, & Sanna, 2008)

CASE STUDY: GINO—NEUROFIBROMATOSIS TYPE 1

The next report is from a hospital-based clinic. Identifying information, such as child and family name, teacher or physician name, and school information, has been altered or fictionalized to protect confidentiality.

Reason for Referral

Gino is a ninth grader who is being reevaluated at the request of his parents. Gino has a history of neurofibromatosis Type 1 and associated learning difficulties. As a result, neuropsychological evaluation was undertaken in order to monitor higher cortical functioning and make appropriate recommendations regarding school placement and the need for supportive therapies.

Assessment Procedures

Wechsler Intelligence Scale for Children, Fourth Edition (WISC-IV)
Peabody Picture Vocabulary Test, Fourth Edition (PPVT-IV)
Boston Naming Test (BNT)
Wisconsin Card Sorting Test (WCST)
Dichotic Listening Test
Kaufman Assessment Battery for Children, Second Edition (KABC-2; selected subtests)
Delis-Kaplan Executive Function Scales (D-KEFS; selected subtests)
Clinical Evaluation of Language Fundamentals, Fourth Edition (CELF-IV; selected subtests)
Beery Developmental Test of Visual-Motor Integration (DTVMI-V)
Rey Complex Figure Test (RCFT)
Finger Tapping Test
Children's Memory Scales (CMS)
Gray Oral Reading Test, Fourth Edition (GORT-4)
Wechsler Individual Achievement Test, Second Edition (WIAT-II)
Study Skills Questionnaire
DSM-IV ADHD Checklist (Parent and Teacher Scales)
Adaptive Behavior Assessment System, Second Edition (ABAS-2; Parent Scale)
Behavior Assessment System for Children, Second Edition (BASC-2; Parent and Teacher Rating Scales)
Behavior Rating Inventory of Executive Functioning (BRIEF; Parent Scale)

Background Information

Gino resides with his parents and his two sisters. Anna is 18 years old and a graduating senior at a private high school. She will be attending college in the fall. Kathy is 10 years old and an A student who is attending private school as well. Gino's father is a college graduate who operates his family's business. Gino's mother is also a college graduate and full-time homemaker. Both of Gino's parents are in good health. According to Gino's mother, the paternal family history is significant for bipolar disorder in the grandmother and a male cousin. The maternal family history is significant for narcolepsy in an uncle and depression in an aunt. Finally, Anna has a history of ADHD, inattentive type.

Review of Gino's developmental and medical history with his mother indicates that Gino is the product of a full-term pregnancy complicated by frequent illness, and vaginal delivery, weighing 7 pounds 1 ounce at birth. During delivery, Gino's arm "got stuck," but otherwise, Gino did well as a newborn and went home from the hospital with his mother on schedule. Developmental motor milestones were obtained within normal limits, with sitting up occurring at 7 months of age and walking at 14 months of age. Developmental language milestones also were attained within normal limits, with first words coming at 13 months of age; however, his mother noted that Gino's motor and language development seemed slower than that of his sisters. Toilet training was fully accomplished at 3 years of age. Aside from the usual childhood illnesses, Gino's past medical history is significant for frequent crying, difficulty gaining weight, and frequent diarrhea during the first year of life, which improved after beginning a soy formula for feeding. In addition, Gino fell off a counter at 4 months of age. He was taken to his pediatrician, who indicated that he was "fine"; however, the doctor noticed hyperpigmented, or café-au-lait, spots on his back (see Figure 16.1). Gino subsequently was referred to a pediatric geneticist, who diagnosed Gino with neurofibromatosis Type 1. At age 11, Gino underwent scoliosis surgery (midthoracic). At present, Gino is characterized as a picky eater, who is "tired all the time" and "not interested in anything." He "hates school," and it is "difficult to wake him up and get him to school on time." She goes on to report that Gino's mood seems to elevate on weekends and holidays.

Review of educational history indicates that Gino attended a Mother's Day Out program at church from 2 to 4 years of age three days a week from 9 a.m. to 1 p.m. His mother reported that he was off by himself frequently in the preschool program. At the age of 4, Gino began a half-day 4–K program at a private school. Gino was immature, had difficulty with readiness skills, and his teacher recommended retention. The next year, when Gino was 5, he repeated 4–K with a different teacher. Some attention span problems were noticed, but his academic skills were reported as adequate for kindergarten. At the age of 6, Gino attended half-day kindergarten. Gino's mother reported that he did "OK," but the teacher recommended testing prior to first grade.

Gino was tutored during the summer, and in August he underwent psychological evaluation by a psychologist in private practice. At that time (age 7 years 4 months), Gino's intellectual functioning was reported to be in the low-average range as measured by the Wechsler Intelligence Scale for Children, Third Edition (WISC-III; Full Scale [FS] IQ = 86, Verbal IQ = 82, Performance IQ = 93). His academic achievement was much lower, particularly in spelling and arithmetic (Wide Range Achievement Test,

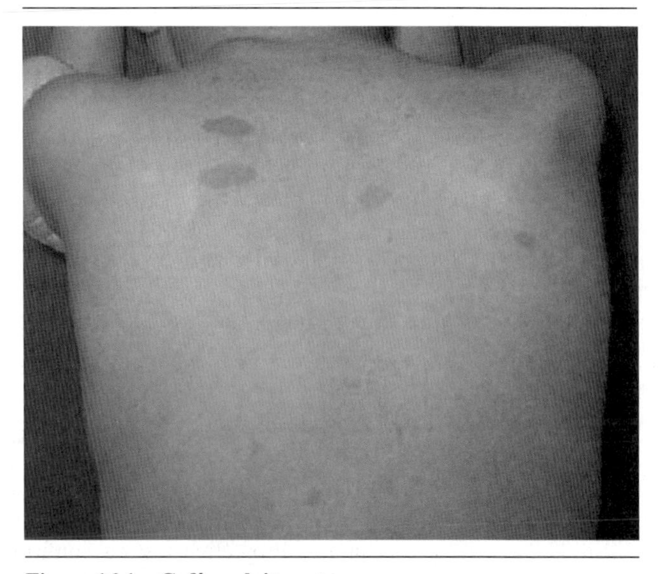

Figure 16.1 Café-au-lait spots.

Third Edition [WRAT-3] Reading = 78, Spelling = 58, Arithmetic = 56). Gino was reported to have problems with attention and concentration during testing, but no serious concerns were noted on the Achenbach Child Behavior Checklist. Self-report measures indicated significant symptoms of anxiety.

In first grade, Gino had difficulties in reading and spelling and continued to exhibit attention span problems. As a result, tutoring was reinstituted. Gino also was given a medication trial with methylphenidate (Ritalin) during April and May of that school year, which negatively affected his mood. As a result, this was discontinued at the beginning of the summer. Gino was evaluated at the Sylvan Learning Center in May of first grade. At that time, his reading was reported to be on an early first-grade level. Gino was reevaluated by the same private psychologist that June. Gino was noted to have a short attention span during testing. His academic achievement as measured by the Wechsler Individual Achievement Test was in the low-average range in most areas, including reading (decoding and comprehension) and mathematics (reasoning and calculation). His spelling skills were borderline; however, his listening comprehension skills were higher, in the average range. Gino scored in the borderline range on the Gray Oral Reading Test, suggesting poor reading skills (rate, accuracy, and comprehension).

For second and third grades, Gino began attending a different private school that had a program for children with learning disabilities. He was mainstreamed for science, physical education, art, and music. Gino continued to experience academic difficulties in reading, spelling, and with memorizing math facts. His self-esteem continued to suffer due to frustration with schoolwork and difficulty making and keeping friends. As a result, Gino was initially evaluated by this service at 10 years of age. The results of neuropsychological evaluation indicated that Gino was functioning within the average range of intellectual ability as measured by the WISC-III (FS IQ = 97; Verbal IQ = 92; Performance IQ = 104). Additional assessment revealed that Gino demonstrated relative strengths in the areas of sequential reasoning/problem solving; most areas of receptive and expressive language; visual-spatial perception and construction; fine motor functioning; visual learning and memory, including visual working memory; and verbal memory for organized, meaningful material. These strengths were contrasted by relative weaknesses in auditory discrimination/processing, word finding/retrieval, motor planning, auditory working memory, and ability to learn rote verbal material. Academically, Gino exhibited relative strengths in reading decoding and reading comprehension contrasted by relative weaknesses in math calculation/reasoning and spelling. Behaviorally, Gino was rated as having clinically significant symptoms of depression. In contrast, his attention span appeared to have improved significantly compared with what was reported previously. Taken together, this pattern of neuropsychological test performance was felt to be consistent with a diagnosis of learning disability in the area of mathematics (dyscalculia), consistent with the known cognitive and behavioral correlates of neurofibromatosis Type 1. While Gino demonstrated significant improvement in his reading skills, he continued to exhibit a dysfluent reading style. In addition, Gino was experiencing depressed mood that appeared to be secondary to his academic difficulties and neurological condition. Based on the results of that evaluation, special education support services were recommended along with classroom accommodations and counseling.

Gino was enrolled in public school for fourth grade. In order to determine if he would qualify for special education services, he underwent additional psychological evaluation by the school psychologist assigned to his school. The results of academic assessment with the Woodcock-Johnson Test of Achievement confirmed the math disability along with poor writing mechanics. Projective testing confirmed poor self-concept, feelings of inadequacy, and social isolation. Following this evaluation, Gino began receiving special education learning disability resource services under the "Other Health Impaired" category in order to improve mathematical calculation and written expression. These services also were provided throughout the fifth grade. It should be noted that during the summer between fourth and fifth grades, Gino also participated in the PACE program at Partners in Achievement. His mother indicated that significant improvement was not evident on completion of this program.

For sixth grade, the parents elected to place Gino in the learning disorders program at another private school in the area. In addition, the parents initiated private tutoring sessions for Gino directed at improving language arts. Gino's mother felt that this was a "wasted year" for Gino. Academic reassessment at the end of the school year with the Wechsler Individual Achievement Test, Second Edition (WIAT-II) and the Gray Oral Reading Test—Revised (GORT-2) revealed significant weaknesses in mathematical calculation, oral reading fluency, and reading comprehension. Based on these results, it was decided that Gino would repeat the sixth grade at another private school that offered academic support services. Gino earned final grades of B in science and Cs in all other academic subjects. Gino went on to attend the seventh grade at the same school, where he again earned final grades of Bs and Cs. It should be noted that Gino received tutoring in math during this time as well. In addition, his pediatrician began medication trials with various stimulant medications in January of Gino's second year in sixth grade. Ultimately, Gino was maintained on methylphenidate (Concerta); 18 mg in the morning, which continued throughout the seventh grade. Finally, Gino also underwent an auditory processing evaluation in September of eighth grade. Results of that evaluation were reported to be consistent with normal hearing acuity, normal language development, and a mild central auditory processing disorder.

At present, Gino is completing the ninth grade, where he earned first-semester grades of Bs and Cs. Review of a school report form completed by Gino's academic support teacher indicates that she characterizes Gino as "very reserved and resistant to efforts to correct his errors when he is being tutored." She went on to report that Gino is "very guarded and is hard to reach at times. He can be quite stubborn."

Behavioral Observations and Impressions

Gino presented himself for testing as a reserved, neatly groomed young man with brown hair and hazel eyes who was casually dressed in a blue-and-white striped polo shirt, khaki shorts, and sneakers. He separated appropriately from his mother and accompanied the examiners to the testing room without difficulty. Gino was oriented; however, his eye contact was intermittent, his affect was restricted, and he spoke only when spoken to. This gradually improved as the evaluation progressed, and Gino always exhibited good manners. In response to direct questions, Gino's use of language was fluent and prosodic with good comprehension noted. Throughout the evaluation, which consisted of two sessions separated by a lunch break, Gino's attention span and impulsivity were felt to be age appropriate; however, he was very fidgety in his chair. When confronted with difficult test items, Gino typically responded in a reflective manner; however, he did not like it when additional queries were given by the examiner. Lateral dominance is firmly established in the right hand and foot. Vision was not formally screened; however, Gino's mother reported that Gino recently was evaluated by a pediatric ophthalmologist, and his vision was normal. Hearing was last assessed as part of the auditory processing disorder (APD) evaluation in eighth grade and reported to be within normal limits bilaterally.

Test Results and Interpretation

The results of neuropsychological evaluation indicate that Gino continues to function within the average range of intellectual ability as measured by the General Ability Index of the Wechsler Intelligence Scale for Children, Fourth Edition with fairly good consolidation noted between his verbal comprehension and nonverbal reasoning abilities. Further analysis of the index scores reveals average performance on subtests measuring immediate auditory working memory, which represents a significant improvement from prior assessment by this service (see Table 16.3). This result is contrasted by a significant decline on subtests measuring information processing and motor speed. Additional assessment indicates that Gino continues to demonstrate average higher-order problem-solving capability, although his mother reports difficulty with initiation and working memory on the Behavior Rating Inventory of Executive Functioning (BRIEF).

Expressive and receptive language development continues to be in the average range, with mild difficulty noted on a measure of rapid verbal naming. Further, language appears to be lateralized in the left cerebral hemisphere as evidenced by a strong right ear advantage on a dichotic listening test for consonant-vowel syllables. Visual-spatial perception and visual-motor/constructional skills continue to be in the average range as well; however, motor planning weaknesses are still evident (Rey Complex Figure). Fine motor tapping speed as measured by the Finger Tapping test is above average bilaterally.

Assessment of Gino's ability to learn and remember new material indicates that at the present time he is demonstrating variability in his ability to hold and manipulate material in immediate working memory, which appears to be due to poor attention regulation. Gino continues to exhibit better ability to learn and recall (30 minutes later) visual as opposed to auditory material; however, his performance across both domains has declined significantly as compared with that obtained on prior assessment (average to above average). Academically, Gino is now demonstrating significant deficits as compared with intellectual expectancy in the areas of word recognition, oral reading fluency, reading comprehension, and written expression along with continued difficulty with numerical reasoning skills. In contrast, he is exhibiting significant improvement in the area of numerical calculation, which is now well within the average range (see Table 16.3).

Review of a study skills questionnaire completed by Gino indicates that he endorsed difficulty "getting started" with homework and that he typically spends one hour a night doing homework. He also endorsed poor time management and test prep skills, he does not use an assignment book, his study area is full of distractions, he has a poor understanding and use of mnemonic strategies, and he has difficulty identifying main ideas during classroom lectures and while reading assigned text material.

Behaviorally, analysis of rating scales completed by Gino's mother and the academic support teacher indicates that both raters endorsed clinically significant symptoms associated with depressed mood, inattention, social emotional immaturity/withdrawal, and difficulty adapting to change. Further, Gino indicated that he "hates school, has no friends, and has nothing to look forward to each day."

Summary and Recommendations

Gino is a 16-year-old ninth grader with a history of neurofibromatosis Type 1 and co-occurring ADHD; he has a history of continued learning difficulties despite average intellectual ability and a variety of support services. Taken together, this pattern of neuropsychological test performance is consistent with a continued diagnosis of learning

Table 16.3 Psychometric Summary for Gino

	Scaled Scores	Standard Scores
Wechsler Intelligence Scale for Children, Fourth Edition (WISC-IV)		
Full Scale IQ		92
General Ability Index		101
Verbal Comprehension Index		104
Similarities	12	
Vocabulary	11	
Comprehension	10	
Perceptual Reasoning Index		96
Block Design	9	
Picture Concepts	9	
Matrix Reasoning	10	
Working Memory Index		91
Digit Span	9	
Letter-Number Sequencing	8	
Processing Speed Index		78
Coding	6	
Symbol Search	6	
Wisconsin Card Sorting Test (WCST)		
Categories Achieved		109
Perseverative Errors		97
Failure to Maintain Set		60
Peabody Picture Vocabulary Test, Fourth Edition (PPVT-IV)		95
Boston Naming Test (BNT)		100
Delis Kaplan Executive Function Scale (D-KEFS)		
Verbal Fluency		85
Clinical Evaluation of Language Fundamentals, Fourth Edition (CELF-IV)		
Formulated Sentences		115
	Number Correct	
Dichotic Listening		
Left Ear	7/30	
Right Ear	17/30	
		Standard Score
Kaufman Assessment Battery for Children, Second Edition (KABC-2)		
Gestalt Closure		105
Developmental Test of Visual-Motor Integration (DTVMI-V)		
Visual Motor Integration		94
Rey Complex Figure (copy)		77
Clock Face Drawing Test		
Form		106
Time (10:20)		106

(continued)

Table 16.3 ***(Continued)***

Finger Tapping Test	**Raw Score**	**Standard Scores**
Right (dominant) Hand	50.3 taps/ 10 seconds	115
Left (nondominant) Hand	46.0 taps/ 10 seconds	115
Children's Memory Scale (CMS)	**Scaled Scores**	
Attention/Concentration Index		82
Numbers	9	
Sequences	5	
Picture Locations (Supplemental)	6	
General Memory Index		83
Verbal Immediate Index		78
Stories	9	
Word Pairs	4	
Visual Immediate Index		88
Dot Locations	9	
Faces	7	
Verbal Delayed Index		85
Stories	8	
Word Pairs	7	
Visual Delayed Index		103
Dot Locations	10	
Faces	11	
Delayed Recognition Index		72
Stories	9	
Word Pairs	2	
Learning Index		78
Word Pairs	4	
Dot Locations	9	
Gray Oral Reading Test, Fourth Edition (GORT-4)		
Fluency		80
Comprehension		85
Wechsler Individual Achievement Test, Second Edition (WIAT-II)		
Word Reading		85
Written Expression		85
Mathematical Reasoning		84
Numerical Operations		96
Behavior Assessment System for Children, Second Edition (BASC-2)		
	T-Scores	
	Parent Rating Scale	Teacher Rating Scale
Clinical Scales		
Hyperactivity	57	64
Aggression	48	57
Conduct	42	56
Anxiety	48	78

(continued)

Table 16.3 *(Continued)*

	T-Scores	
	Parent	**Teacher**
Depression	85	91
Somatization	63	Not Interpretable
Atypical	70	70
Withdrawal	75	78
Attention	78	63
Learning Problems	NA	76
Adaptive Scales		
Adaptability	29	33
Social Skills	25	41
Leadership	27	39
Study Skills	NA	42
Activities of Daily Living	27	NA
Functional Communication	20	36
Behavior Rating Inventory of Executive Functioning (BRIEF-2)		**T-Score (parent)**
Behavioral Regulation Index		59
Inhibit		51
Shift		58
Emotional Control		63
Metacognitive Index		63
Initiate		66
Working Memory		74
Plan/Organize		63
Organization of Materials		52
	Raw Scores	
DSM-IV ADHD Checklist	**Parent**	**Teacher**
Inattention	26/27	22/27
Hyperactivity/Impulsivity	1/27	11/27

Note. NA = Not applicable.

disability in the area of numerical reasoning as well as in the areas of reading fluency, reading comprehension, and written expression. In addition, Gino continues to experience depressed mood, poor self-concept, and poor social skills consistent with a diagnosis of depression.

As a result, it is recommended that Gino complete high school in a setting where he can receive special education support services from a learning disabilities specialist along with classroom accommodations. The support services can be provided as part of the school program or privately through tutoring. In the event that Gino and his parents elect to have Gino attend school within the public setting, these services could be provided under the eligibility category of "Other Health Impaired," due to the fact that his learning disabilities are consistent with the difficulties frequently encountered by students with neurofibromatosis Type 1.

In order to enhance Gino's learning/retention, new material should be presented in an organized format that is meaningful to him. The material to be learned should be pretaught, broken down into smaller components/steps, and presented in a highly structured format with frequent repetition to facilitate new learning. Instruction should be supplemented with visual aids, demonstrations, and experiential/procedural learning. Gino would benefit greatly from being taught how to use mnemonic strategies when learning new material and studying for tests. These include but are not limited to:

- Rehearsal—showing Gino how to repeat information verbally, to write it, and to look at it a finite number of times.
- Transformation—instructing him in how to convert difficult information into simpler components that can be remembered more easily.
- Elaboration—instructing Gino in how to identify key elements of new information and to create relationships or associations with previously learned material
- Chunking—instructing Gino in how to group or pare down long strings of digits or different items into more manageable units and thereby facilitate encoding and retention.
- Imagery—showing him how to visualize and make a "mental picture" of information to be learned.

When studying for tests or doing multiple homework assignments on the same day, similar subject material should be separated in order to lessen interference. Gino should review previously learned material periodically throughout the semester in order to enhance long-term retention. Finally, Gino will need to budget a minimum of two hours each night for the completion of homework and test preparation.

Study skills training will be warranted, emphasizing such techniques as the appropriate outlining of lecture notes and how to study for tests. Gino also will benefit from being taught how to take notes on text material and plan written reports using an outlining method. Gino also will require instruction on how to organize and plan his approach to his studies. Specifically, he should be guided in the use of checklists and other organizational aids, such as a daily planner.

Accommodations will continue to be necessary in order to enhance Gino's ability to succeed in the classroom, including preferential seating and additional time to complete assignments. Tests should be in multiple-choice/matching/short-answer formats instead of essay/short-answer format and should be administered individually, with additional time provided when necessary. Finally, Gino should be allowed and encouraged to use various compensatory strategies, such as a calculator to check written calculations and a computer with word processing capability. Most word processing programs are equipped with spell checks and cut and paste, and can be adapted for voice dictation if necessary. This will be increasingly valuable during Gino's education.

Gino would benefit from psychiatric evaluation to further explore the nature of his chronically depressed mood and determine if medication therapy would be appropriate. Individual therapy to treat his depression also would be helpful. Specifically, therapy should focus on enhancing Gino's self-esteem and improve his coping skills. Finally, the effectiveness of his stimulant medication in addressing attentional problems needs to be monitored over time.

Further Discussion of Case Study

As noted earlier, NF1 is frequently associated with co-occurring academic and social-emotional problems as well as ADHD. In this case, Gino's functioning is being affected at all levels: His learning disabilities and ADHD, in combination with the NF1 stigmata, likely contribute to social difficulties with resulting depression. There is not going to be a single approach to treatment. With combined effects and issues, the treatment must be sufficiently multifaceted to address academic issues, social issues, depression, and attention problems. Often this may necessitate collaboration across disciplines with differing interventions working in concert to yield a more positive outcome.

TUBEROUS SCLEROSIS COMPLEX

Definition and Etiology

Tuberous sclerosis complex was first recognized as a syndrome by Désiré-Magloire Bourneville in 1880; this was followed by a series of reports with similar characteristics (Riccio & Harrison, 1998). Tuberous sclerosis is a neurocutaneous disorder characterized by flesh-colored discrete marks that may resemble acne (adenoma sebaceum) and typically occur in a butterfly distribution in the folds of skin around the nasal area. It was named to reflect the potatolike lesions in the cerebral cortex that result in hard areas of tissues called cortical tubers (Hunt, 2006; Roach, 1992). In addition to the adenoma sebaceum, there may be areas where there is an absence of pigmentation (amelanotic nevus), most often on the trunk and limbs (Chalhub, 1976). Tuberous sclerosis complex involves multiple systems and abnormal growth of a variety of organs, including the skin, kidneys, and central nervous system (Hunt, 2006).

Tuberous sclerosis is an inherited autosomal dominant disorder (Roach, 1992); however, it also may occur as a genetic mutation with no family history. The gene location is believed to be at 9q34 and 11q23 (Connor, 1990). There are also some indications of involvement of chromosome 16 as well as complex genetic interactions (Zaroff, Devinsky, Miles, & Ban, 2004). In its more severe form, tuberous sclerosis complex, mutations are in the tumor suppressor genes, TSC1 (Hamartin) or TSC2 (Tuberin) (Curatolo, D'Argenzio, Cerminara, & Bombardieri, 2008; de Vries et al., 2005; L. A. Devlin, Shepherd, Crawford, & Morrison, 2006). These are proteins that form a cytosolic complex that inhibits the mTOR pathway, thus controlling cell growth and proliferation (Curatolo et al., 2008). Pathologically, abnormalities of neuronal migration, cellular differentiation, and excessive cellular proliferation all contribute to the formation of the different brain lesions associated with tuberous sclerosis.

Prevalence and Incidence

Tuberous sclerosis occurs in about 1 per 12,000 children (de Vries et al., 2005); across age groups, it is estimated to occur in 1 in 14,500 people (Zaroff et al., 2004). Accurate incidence and prevalence is complicated by the variability in severity, extent of symptoms, and the age range at which the syndrome is identified. Furthermore, in individuals of average cognitive ability, diagnosis may not be made until (unless) the child develops a more severe form of the syndrome (Webb & Osborne, 1995; Zaroff et al., 2004).

Neurological Correlates

In a sample of 78 children with tuberous sclerosis, 21 had cerebellar lesions; 9 had right-sided, 10 had left-sided, and 2 had bilateral cerebellar lesions. Children with the lesions were more likely to demonstrate behaviors associated with autism spectrum disorders. Further analysis revealed that children with right-sided cerebellar lesions evidenced higher social isolation as well as greater communicative and developmental impairment as compared to children with left-sided cerebellar lesions (Eluvathingal et al., 2006). In a study of 44 children with tuberous sclerosis, there was no significant relationship between the number and location of tubers and gender, autism, mental retardation or degree of mental retardation, epilepsy, history of infantile spasm, or age at onset of seizures less than 1 year (V. Wong & Khong, 2006). Notably, the presence of cortical tubers in the parietal and occipital lobes was associated with the history of infantile spasm (V. Wong & Khong, 2006).

Course and Prognosis

The lesions are rarely evident before age 2 years; they are increasingly present with age and are easily identified by age 35 (Webb & Osborne, 1995). For these reasons, the consensus panel on tuberous sclerosis recommends that individuals with this disorder undergo regular cognitive and behavioral evaluation, including neuropsychological assessment appropriate for the age and developmental level (de Vries et al., 2005). The average age at initial diagnosis of tuberous sclerosis ranges from 11 to 15 years for those with a comorbid condition (e.g., mental retardation, seizure disorder). Seizure is the most common presenting symptom for tuberous sclerosis, often presenting in the first year of life (Curatolo et al., 2008). Seizure disorder co-occurs in 85 to 95% of those affected by tuberous sclerosis (Curatolo et al., 1991). Electroencephalogram (EEG) may be abnormal with random, high-voltage slow waves and spikes that arise from multiple foci and spread to various cortical areas (Curatolo et al., 2008; J. Jacobs et al., 2008; Leal et al., 2008); over time, the pattern of electrical discharge develops into the more rhythmic activity associated with seizures (J. Jacobs et al., 2008). Seizures initially may manifest as infantile spasms with gradual development into seizures in adolescence and adulthood.; these seizures frequently do not improve with typical antiepileptic drugs (Curatolo et al., 2008). The primary medical complication is epilepsy, but there also is potential for related health problems that affect kidneys, heart, lungs, and bone (Baskin, 2008). The extent of medical involvement is highly variable and may present prior to or precipitate the identification of tuberous sclerosis. Further, there is significant variability in the effects on overall functioning as a result of the tubers; effects often manifest as co-occurring seizure disorder, mental retardation, or learning disability. Some individuals with tuberous sclerosis will exhibit behavioral patterns associated with autism spectrum disorders, schizophrenia, hyperactivity, or aggressive/destructive behavior as well (de Vries et al., 2005).

Neurocognitive Correlates

Children with tuberous sclerosis evidence a wide range of deficits across cognitive, sensory, and motor domains. The heterogeneity of deficits has been attributed to the locations of the tubers within the brain for the individual (de Vries et al., 2005; V. S. Miller & Bigler, 1982; Zaroff et al., 2004). Among those individuals with tuberous sclerosis and average intellectual functioning, suggesting more intact brain function, the pattern of deficits that emerges is related to executive function (de Vries et al., 2005). In particular, these individuals may exhibit problems with multitasking, organizational skills, planning, self-monitoring, and judgment as well as attention problems and memory problems. With regard to memory, deficits are in executive working memory as well as recall; recognition often is spared (Ridler et al., 2007). Memory deficits are believed to be reflective of abnormalities in the distribution of gray and white matter in addition to the lesions or tubers. The anomalous distribution is most evident in the gray matter of the thalamus and basal ganglia components of the frontostriatal circuits (Ridler et al., 2007). Attentional deficits are also frequent with tuberous sclerosis complex (de Vries, Gardiner, & Bolton, 2009). Parents also reported more difficulties in academic areas (de Vries et al., 2005). For those individuals with impaired cognition, neurocognitive function is more likely to resemble that of a child with autism and epilepsy, both of which are likely to co-occur with tuberous sclerosis. As noted earlier, the specific deficits are likely to change over time, requiring monitoring and assessment at regular intervals (de Vries et al., 2005). Neurocognitive and other deficits are summarized in Table 16.4.

Educational Implications

About 50% of individuals with tuberous sclerosis will have intellectual functioning within the normal range (de Vries et al., 2005). For these individuals, there is a high rate of attention problems, although these may not be sufficient to meet criteria for ADHD. Learning problems are frequent among children with tuberous sclerosis even when general cognitive ability is within the normative range (Hunt, 1995; Prather & de Vries, 2004; Zaroff et al., 2004). The cognitive and learning problems evidenced are believed to be a function of co-occurrence with seizure disorder. At the same time, approximately half of the children with tuberous sclerosis have impaired cognitive ability, meeting criteria for mental retardation (Gomez, 1988; Roach, 1992). For those children with tuberous sclerosis and mental retardation, there is a high risk for autism to be present as well (de Vries et al., 2005; Jeste, Sahin, Bolton, Ploubidis, & Humphrey, 2008; Zaroff et al., 2004).

Behavioral/Emotional Implications

There is consistent evidence that tuberous sclerosis is a risk factor for a variety of behavioral issues (de Vries, Hunt, & Bolton, 2007). Co-occurrence of psychiatric problems other than learning problems or mental retardation is about 76% to 83% (I. C. Gillberg, Gillberg, & Ahlsen, 1994; Prather & de Vries, 2004; Smalley, Tanguay, Smith, & Gutierrez, 1992). In one study, approximately 40% of the children with tuberous sclerosis presented with clinically significant behavioral problems, most frequently involving symptoms of autism spectrum disorder, inattention, and hyperactivity (Smalley et al., 1992). Higher seizure frequency, mixed seizure disorder, and low intellectual functioning contributed to the risk for behavior problems (Kopp, Muzykewicz, Staley, Thiele, & Pulsifer, 2008).

Table 16.4 Neuropsychological Deficits Associated with Tuberous Sclerosis

Global Domain/Specific Deficits	Phenotype
Cognition	Mental retardation common, particularly with co-occurring epilepsy
Auditory-linguistic/ Language function	Receptive and expressive language as well as pragmatic communication deficits associated with lower cognitive ability
Learning and Memory	Short- and long-term memory impaired; recognition is spared
Visual perception/ Constructional praxis	No information specific to visual-perceptual skills identified
Attention/Concentration	Deficits in attention common
Processing speed	No information found on processing speed
Motor function	No information found on motor coordination
Achievement/Academic skills	Learning disability; special education placement is frequent
Emotional/Behavioral functioning	Behavioral patterns associated with autistic spectrum disorders, schizophrenia, hyperactivity, anxiety, or aggression Comorbidity with ADHD and autism higher than expected

In another study (Muzykewicz, Newberry, Danforth, Halpern, & Thiele, 2007), of 241 children and adults with tuberous sclerosis complex, more than 25% had a history of mood disorder symptoms, anxiety disorder symptoms, ADHD symptoms, and/or aggressive/disruptive behavior disorder symptoms. Consistent with the Kopp et al. (2008) study, there were significant relationships between symptomatology and seizure history, surgical history, cognitive impairment, and features of autism or pervasive developmental disorder. In addition, emotional and behavioral status were related to neurological manifestations, age, gender, and genetic mutation (Muzykewicz et al., 2007). These results are also consistent with an earlier report of 50 case studies, wherein the most frequent behavior problems associated with tuberous sclerosis included the presence of autism or autistic-like behaviors, hyperactive or impulsive behavior, and aggressive or destructive behavior (Smalley et al., 1992).

The association between autism and tuberous sclerosis is further linked to the occurrence of mental retardation or seizure disorder or both (Riccio & Harrison, 1998). Those children with tuberous sclerosis who had a co-occurring autism spectrum disorder, attention deficit–related symptoms, and speech and language difficulties were more likely to have a history of epilepsy, facial angiofibromata, shagreen patches, and other physical features of the disorder (de Vries et al., 2007). Even those without mental retardation were more likely to have some behavioral issues (e.g., anxiety symptoms, depressed mood, aggressive outbursts). Although the disruptive behaviors and developmental disorders are more pronounced in children, adults with tuberous sclerosis have higher than expected rates of anxiety symptoms and depressed mood (de Vries et al., 2005). Further, among the more able individuals with tuberous sclerosis, the difficulties encountered socially, academically, and in the workplace increase their risk for low self-esteem. Notably, approximately half of the parents in the Kopp et al. (2008) study reported clinically significant parenting stress; the level of stress was associated with specific characteristics of the child, including the presence of current seizures, a history of psychiatric diagnosis, low intelligence, and behavioral problems.

Evidence-Based Interventions

Many of the same interventions used in other disorders may be appropriate for children with tuberous sclerosis. Specific interventions that have been studied with samples of children with tuberous sclerosis are identified in Table 16.5. For example, vigabatrin (Sabril) has proved to be effective against infantile spasms due to tuberous sclerosis (Curatolo, Bombardieri, & Cerminara, 2006). Surgical treatment may be an option for those children with tuberous sclerosis who have refractory epilepsy (Curatolo et al., 2008; Madhavan et al., 2007). Other methods of intervention for epilepsy (see Chapter 10) also have been considered in conjunction with tuberous sclerosis–related epilepsy (Connelly et al., 2006). In addition, citalopram (Celexa) demonstrated efficacy in treating anxiety and depression while risperidone (Risperdal) demonstrated efficacy in treating problematic behaviors (Muzykewicz et al., 2007). With the high co-occurrence of autism, the evidence-based practices discussed in Chapter 5 also may be appropriate.

Academic Interventions

Educational needs will vary depending on the individual. No academic interventions for students with tuberous sclerosis were identified. Interventions appropriate for students with learning disabilities would seem a reasonable starting point.

Table 16.5 Evidence-Based Interventions for Tuberous Sclerosis

Intervention	Target/Goal	Level of Support
Vigabatrin (Sabril)	Infantile spasms	Promising practice (Curatolo et al., 2006)
Surgery, resection of 1 or more tubers	Refractory seizures	Promising practice (Connolly, Hendson, & Steinbok, 2006; Curatolo et al., 2008; Leal et al., 2008)
Citalopram (Celexa)	Anxiety and depression	Emerging (Muzykewicz et al., 2007)
Risperidone (Risperdal)	Problematic (aggressive) behaviors	Emerging (Muzykewicz et al., 2007)

Psychosocial Interventions

Autism is one of the most common problems associated with tuberous sclerosis; as a result, interventions to deal with those autistic-like behaviors present may be needed. These may include structured teaching, behavioral approaches, social skills training, and alternative communication systems (see Chapter 5). Referrals for behavioral intervention and monitoring of parental stress should be included in the medical management of children with tuberous sclerosis (Kopp et al., 2008).

CASE STUDY: HECTOR—TUBEROUS SCLEROSIS

The next report is from a hospital-based clinic. Identifying information, such as child and family name, teacher or physician name, and school information, has been altered or fictionalized to protect confidentiality.

Reason for Referral

Hector is an 11-year-old boy who is being initially evaluated by the pediatric neuropsychology service at the request of his pediatric neurologist, who is following Hector for a history of tuberous sclerosis and infantile spasms that began at 11 months of age and eventually progressed to partial and complex partial seizures. Hector's seizures have remained refractory to medication therapy and vagal nerve stimulator implantation. In addition, Hector underwent stereotactic resection of a subependymal giant cell astrocytoma that was blocking the foramen of Monro. At present, Hector is taking phenytoin (Dilantin) for seizure management; however, he continues to average 8 to 12 seizures per day. Two video EEG monitoring sessions were reported to be significant for interictal spike activity for the right frontal, central, and temporal regions, with ictal discharges coming from the right occipital region (see Figure 16.2). MRI scan of the brain was significant for cortical tubers throughout the brain (see Figure 16.3). As a result, neuropsychological evaluation was undertaken as part of the Phase I Pediatric Epilepsy Surgery Protocol in order to assess higher cortical functioning and make appropriate recommendations regarding school placement and the need for supportive therapies.

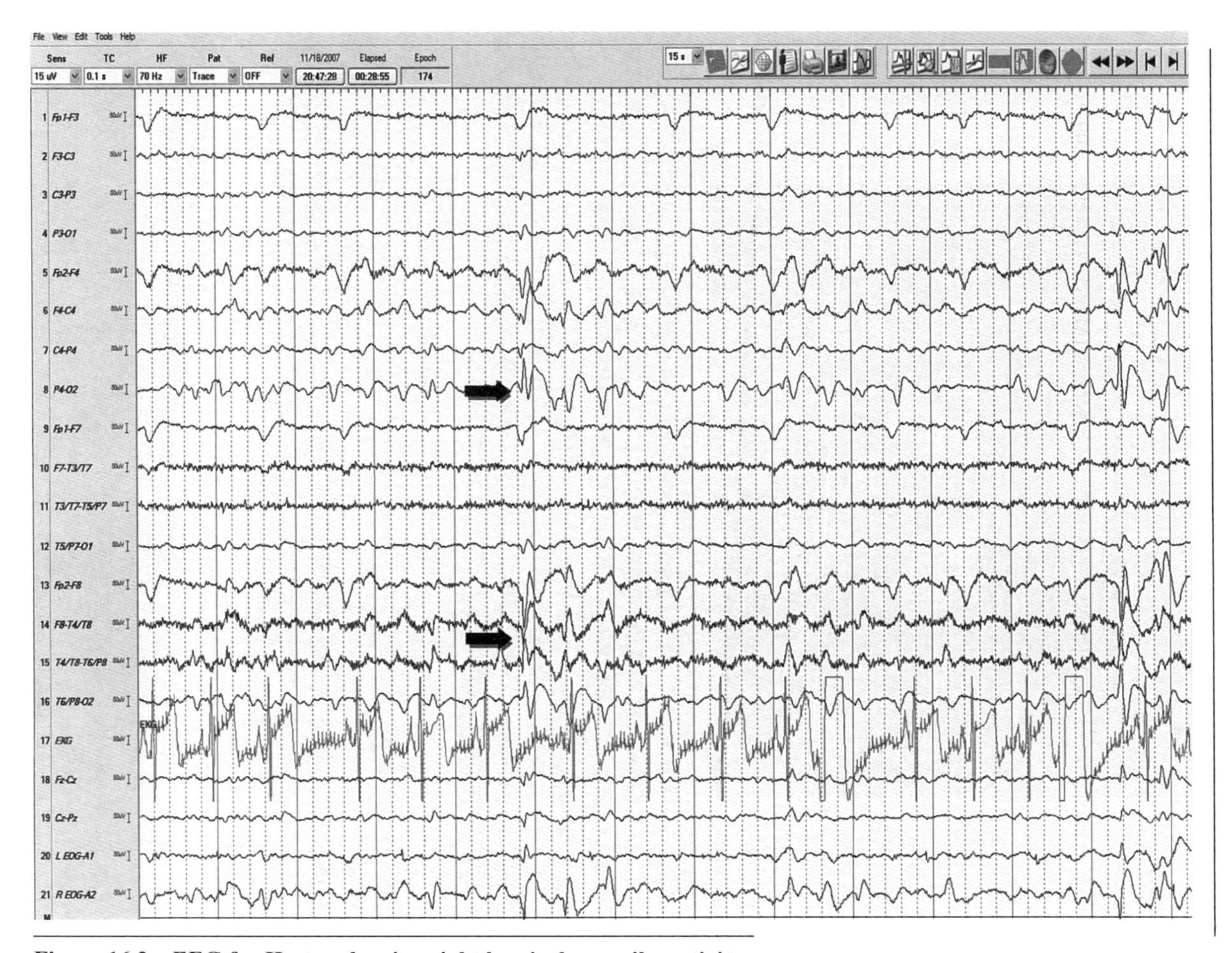

Figure 16.2 EEG for Hector showing right hemisphere spike activity.

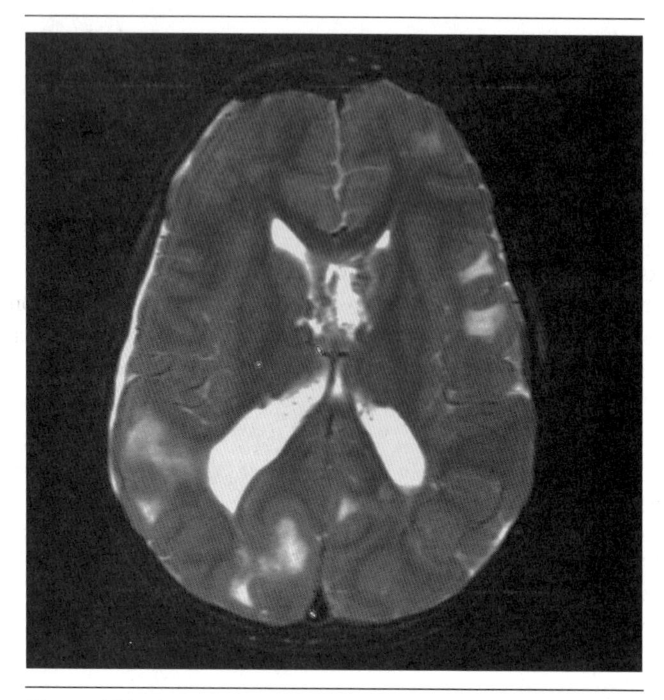

Figure 16.3 MRI for Hector showing the tubers and atrophy associated with tuberous sclerosis.

Assessment Procedures

Clinical interview

Behavioral observations

Wechsler Intelligence Scale for Children, Fourth Edition (WISC-IV)

Peabody Picture Vocabulary Test, Fourth Edition (PPVT-IV)

Boston Naming Test (BNT)

Neuropsychological Assessment (NEPSY)/Neuropsychological Assessment, Second Edition (NEPSY-2; selected subtests)

Delis-Kaplan Executive Function Scales (D-KEFS; selected subtests)

Clinical Evaluation of Language Fundamentals, Fourth Edition (CELF-IV) (selected subtests)

Kaufman Assessment Battery for Children, Second Edition (KABC-2; selected subtests)

Beery Developmental Test of Visual-Motor Integration (DTVMI-V)

Clock Face Drawing Test

Finger Tapping Test

Children's Memory Scales (CMS)

Gray Oral Reading Test, Fourth Edition (GORT-4)

Wide Range Assessment Test, Fourth Edition (WRAT-4)

Test of Written Language, Third Edition (TOWL-3)

DSM-IV ADHD Checklist

Adaptive Behavior Assessment System, Second Edition (ABAS-2)

Behavior Assessment System for Children, Second Edition (BASC-2)

Background Information

Hector resides with his parents and his two older brothers. George is 16 years old, an A student in the 10th grade, and in good health. Manuel is 13 years old and an average student in the eighth grade. He has a history of Attention-Deficit Hyperactivity Disorder (ADHD) and obsessive-compulsive disorder (OCD). Hector's father is 47 years old, a college graduate with a master's degree in mechanical engineering, who is on the faculty at a technical college. He is reported to be in good health. Hector's mother is 44 years of age, a college graduate, who works on a temporary basis. She reports a history of attention span problems and depression. The maternal family medical history is significant for depression and migraine headache in several relatives. The paternal family medical history is significant for a great-aunt with suspected bipolar disorder.

Review of developmental and medical history with his mother indicates that Hector is the product of a normal full-term pregnancy and a planned cesarean delivery, weighing 7 pounds 1 ounce at birth. Hector did well as a newborn and went home from the hospital with his mother on day 3. At that time, a large hypopigmented lesion was noted on Hector's right inner thigh. He began having infantile spasms at 11 months of age and was initially evaluated by his child neurologist. Following EEG and MRI scan of the head, a diagnosis of tuberous sclerosis was made. Developmental motor and language milestones were delayed. Further, Hector has always exhibited fine motor difficulty, which has significantly impacted his self-help skill development. Toilet training was fully accomplished at 3 to 4 years of age; however, Hector still requires some assistance. At present, physical examination is significant for adenoma sebaceum on the face (see Figure 16.4), shagreen patches over the lower back (see Figure 16.5), and multiple ash leaf spots (hypopigmented lesions; see Figure 16.6) consistent with tuberous sclerosis. Hector also exhibits significant separation anxiety from his mother and an excessive preoccupation with bells and traffic lights.

Review of educational history indicates that at 13 months of age, Hector began receiving services from the early intervention program that continued until 3 years of age. At 15 months of age, Hector began attending a developmental center, where he received preschool services along with physical therapy, occupational therapy, and speech/language therapy. He also attended a summer program offered by the center. At 5 years old, Hector began attending a significantly developmentally delayed special education preschool classroom.

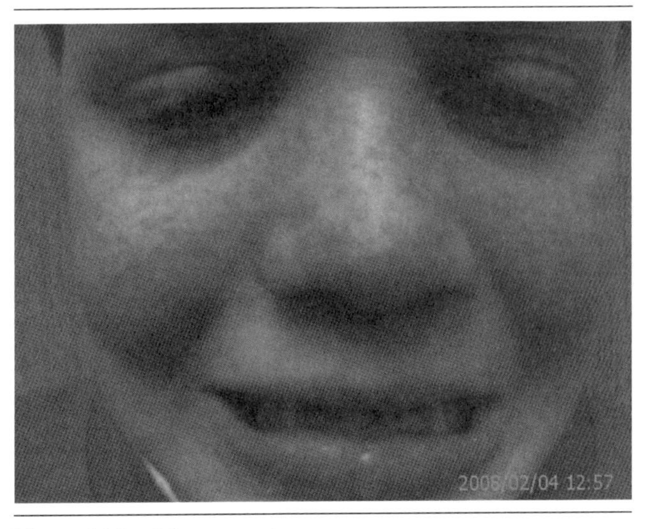

Figure 16.4 Adenoma sebaceum.

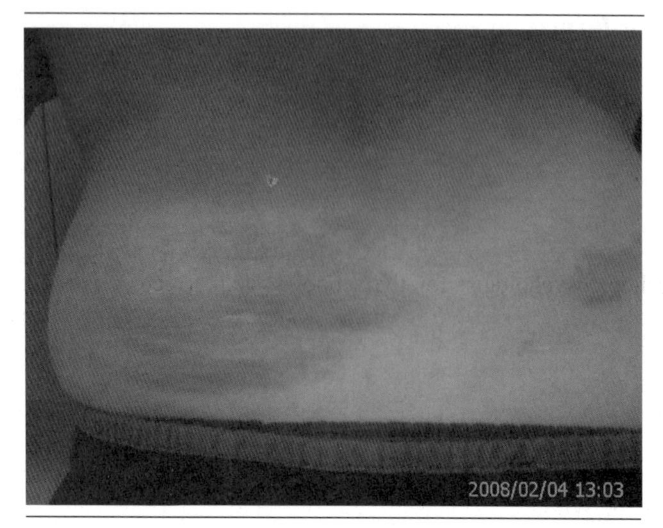

Figure 16.5 Shagreen patches.

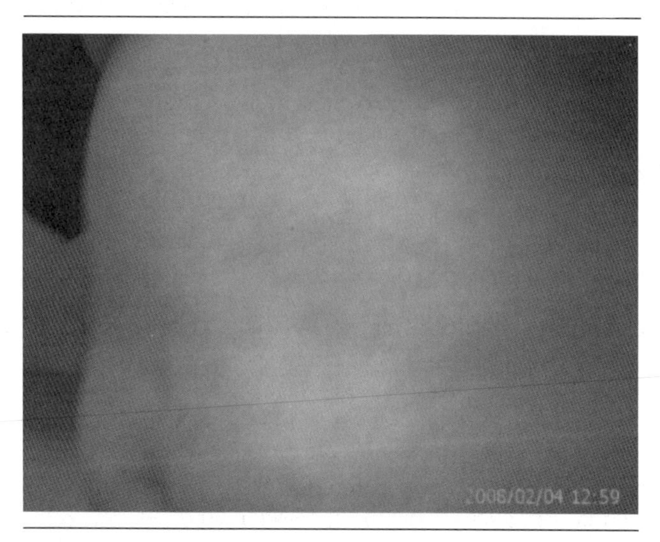

Figure 16.6 Hypopigmentations.

Hector also received occupational therapy and speech/language therapy as related services. At 6 years of age, Hector underwent psychological evaluation by the school psychologist for the school system. At that time, intelligence testing with the Differential Ability Scales (DAS) and the Universal Nonverbal Intelligence Test (UNIT) found Hector to be functioning in the moderate to mild intellectually disabled range with better nonverbal functioning noted. Academic assessment with the Woodcock-Johnson Tests of Achievement indicated that Hector was performing at or above this level of expectancy across all areas assessed.

Hector continued to receive similar special education services until 8 years of age. According to his mother, Hector was placed into a self-contained special education classroom for children with mild intellectual disability under the "Other Health Impaired" category. In addition, he continued to receive occupational therapy and speech/language therapy as related services. At age 9 years 5 months, Hector underwent initial neuropsychological evaluation by a psychologist at a local hospital. At that time, Hector was functioning in the moderate intellectually disabled range as measured by the Reynolds Intellectual Assessment Scales (RIAS); however, his performance on academic assessment with the Woodcock-Johnson Tests of Achievement continued to be above this level of expectancy. Based on these results along with behavior rating scale data, Hector was diagnosed with mild autism, moderate mental retardation, poor coordination, and overanxious disorder.

At 10 years 11 months of age, Hector again underwent psychological reevaluation by the school psychologist for the school system. Hector was attending the fifth grade, and he continued to receive special education classroom and related services. On the Stanford-Binet Intelligence Scale, Fifth Edition, Hector was functioning in the moderate to mild intellectually disabled range; however, his performance on the Comprehensive Test of Nonverbal Intelligence was in the mild intellectually disabled to borderline range. Academic assessment in reading was consistent with nonverbal ability; however, mathematics, written expression, and adaptive functioning were below nonverbal expectancy as measured by the Woodcock-Johnson Tests of Achievement and the Vineland Adaptive Behavior Scales, Second Edition.

At present, Hector is repeating the fifth grade in a self-contained special education classroom for students with mild intellectual disability under the "Multiple Disabilities" category with continuation of occupational therapy and speech/language therapy. Review of a school report form completed by his teacher indicates that he characterizes Hector as a child who "loves to work. He is very easy to get along with and full of excitement. Sometimes if he doesn't get what he wants he might get upset but gets over it quickly. He is a joy to teach."

Behavioral Observations

Hector presented himself for testing as a pleasant, neatly groomed youngster with blond hair and blue eyes who was casually dressed in a red "Cars" shirt, black pants, and Crocs. Hector exhibited significant difficulty separating from his mother. As a result, she walked Hector to the door of the testing room and departed. During the first testing session, which lasted approximately 45 minutes, Hector continued to complain about the work presented and required frequent verbal encouragement from the examiner in order to maintain adequate testing behavior; however, after a snack break, Hector appeared more relaxed and eager to comply with testing demands. It should be noted that Hector's compliance and demeanor steadily improved throughout the day with improved eye contact and socialization noted. In response to direct questions as well as when conversation was spontaneous, Hector's use of language was fluent, prosodic, and concrete in nature with limited vocabulary and poor pragmatics noted. Hector's attention span, activity level, and impulsivity within the context of this one-to-one assessment were felt to be mental age appropriate, and he did experience difficulty with transitions requiring much structure and verbal redirection. Lateral dominance is firmly established in the right hand for paper-and-pencil manipulations. Vision is followed by a local ophthalmologist. According to his mother, Hector wears glasses due to a tuber that is next to the right optic nerve; however, Hector does not like to wear his glasses because they irritate his facial fibromas. Hearing was screened by the school system this year and was reported to be normal. Finally, it should be noted that Hector appeared to experience three very brief seizure episodes during the day. After each episode, he quickly reverted back to baseline; during one instance, he identified the episode as a "seizure."

Test Interpretations

The results of neuropsychological evaluation indicate that Hector currently is functioning within the moderate intellectually disabled range of ability as measured by the Wechsler Intelligence Scale for Children, Fourth Edition (WISC-IV); however, analysis of the various Index scores reveals that Hector is demonstrating a relative strength in his verbal reasoning ability contrasted by moderately deficient performance on the Indexes assessing nonverbal reasoning, auditory working memory, and information processing speed (see Table 16.6). Additional assessment indicates that Hector is exhibiting mildly deficient sequential reasoning/problem-solving capability as measured by the Tower subtest from the Neuropsychological Assessment (NEPSY).

Expressive and receptive language abilities are generally in the mild to moderately deficient range with significant word-finding/confrontational picture naming difficulty evident. Further, language appears to be lateralized in the left cerebral hemisphere as evidenced by a right ear advantage in Hector's ability to repeat consonant vowel syllables presented simultaneously to each ear on a Dichotic Listening Test. Visual-spatial perception and visual-motor integration/construction also were found to be in the mild to moderately deficient range with motor planning difficulty evident. Fine motor tapping speed is found to be depressed in the right (dominant) hand as measured by the Finger Tapping test.

Analysis of Hector's performance on the Children's Memory Scale (CMS) indicates that, consistent with his performance on the WISC-IV, he is exhibiting mildly deficient ability to hold material in immediate/working memory. When asked to learn and remember (30 minutes later) newly presented material, Hector also demonstrated mildly deficient learning and recall capability; however, variable performance was noted within the verbal and visual modalities. Specifically, Hector demonstrated mildly deficient ability to learn and remember organized/meaningful information such as stories that were read to him in contrast to low-average recall of rote verbal material (a list of 14 word pairs) presented over three highly structured learning trials. Within the visual modality, Hector exhibited deficient recall capability when asked to remember pictures of human faces (what) in contrast to borderline to low-average learning and recall of dot locations presented on a page (where).

Academically, Hector continues to demonstrate word recognition/spelling, oral reading fluency, reading comprehension, and numerical reasoning/calculation skills in the mildly deficient range consistent with his verbal conceptual abilities. In contrast, written expression skills are now a relative area of weakness. Adaptive functioning is also within the mildly deficient range. Behaviorally, analysis of rating scales completed by Hector's mother and special education teacher indicates that, at the present time, he continues to exhibit social-emotional immaturity, both at home as well as in the classroom. Hector's mother also endorsed significant concern with regard to inattention and his level of anxiety in the home.

Summary and Recommendations

Taken together, this pattern of neuropsychological test performance is consistent with a diagnosis of pervasive developmental disorder, not otherwise specified, characterized by mild intellectual disability, specific language impairment, developmental coordination disorder, and overanxious disorder of childhood with features of obsessive-compulsive disorder. These deficits are secondary to Hector's history of tuberous sclerosis and seizure disorder.

Table 16.6 · Psychometric Summary for Hector

	Scaled Scores	Standard Scores
Wechsler Intelligence Scale for Children, Fourth Edition (WISC-IV)		
Full Scale IQ		45
Verbal Comprehension Index		63
Similarities	7	
Vocabulary	2	
Comprehension	2	
Perceptual Reasoning Index		49
Block Design	2	
Picture Concepts	1	
Matrix Reasoning	2	
Working Memory Index		54
Digit Span	1	
Letter-Number Sequencing	3	
Processing Speed Index		50
Coding	1	
Symbol Search	1	
Neuropsychological Assessment, Second Edition (NEPSY-2)		
Phonological Processing	1	
Comprehension of Instructions	3	
Arrows	2	
Tower (NEPSY)		65
Peabody Picture Vocabulary Test, Fourth Edition (PPVT-IV)		49
Boston Naming Test (BNT)		<40
Delis-Kaplan Executive Function Scales (D-KEFS)		
Verbal Fluency	2	
Clinical Evaluation of Language Fundamentals, Fourth Edition (CELF-IV)		
Sentence Repetition	1	
Formulated Sentences	1	
	Number Correct	
Dichotic Listening Test		
Left Ear	4/30	
Right Ear	15/30	
		Standard Score
Kaufman Assessment Battery for Children (KABC-2)		
Gestalt Closure		60
Developmental Test of Visual-Motor Integration, Fifth Edition (DTVMI-V)		
Visual Motor Integration		66
Clock Face Drawing Test		
Form		67
Time (9:15)		56

(continued)

Table 16.6 *(Continued)*

Finger Tapping Test	**Raw Score**	**Standard Score**
Right (dominant) Hand	31.0 taps/10 seconds	75
Left (nondominant) Hand	34.0 taps/10 seconds	96
Children's Memory Scale (CMS)	**Scaled Score**	
Attention/Concentration Index		51
Numbers	1	
Sequences	3	
Picture Locations	3	
General Memory Index		50
Verbal Immediate Index		60
Stories	3	
Word Pairs	4	
Visual Immediate Index		60
Dot Locations	6	
Faces	1	
Verbal Delayed Index		69
Stories	2	
Word Pairs	8	
Visual Delayed Index		60
Dot Locations	6	
Faces	1	
Delayed Recognition Index		51
Stories	2	
Word Pairs	2	
Learning Index		66
Word Pairs	4	
Dot Locations	5	
Gray Oral Reading Test, Fourth Edition (GORT-4)		
Fluency		55
Comprehension		65
Test of Written Language, Third Edition (TOWL-3)		
Written Language Quotient		53
Wide Range Achievement Test, Fourth Edition (WRAT-4)		
Reading		60
Arithmetic		55
Spelling		65
Behavior Assessment System for Children, Second Edition (BASC-2)		
	T-Scores	
	Parent	Teacher
Clinical Scales		
Hyperactivity	47	55
Aggression	37	48
Conduct	40	42
Anxiety	64	55
Depression	55	48

(continued)

Table 16.6 *(Continued)*

	T-Scores	
	Parent	**Teacher**
Somatization	53	47
Atypical	65	66
Withdrawal	62	39
Attention	64	49
Learning Problems	NA	58
Adaptive Scales		
Adaptability	39	50
Social Skills	54	65
Leadership	34	59
Study Skills	NA	49
Activities of Daily Living	44	NA
Functional Communication	40	47
Adaptive Behavior Assessment System, Second Edition		**Standard Score**
General Adaptive Composite		61
Communication		80
Community Use		55
Functional Academics		60
Home Living		55
Health and Safety		70
Leisure		65
Self-Care		55
Self-Direction		70
Social		90
	Raw Scores	
DSM-IV ADHD Checklist	**Parent**	**Teacher**
Inattention	7/27	9/27
Hyperactivity/Impulsivity	11/27	10/27

Note. NA = Not applicable.

As a result, it is recommended that Hector continue to receive self-contained special education classroom services with a low pupil-to-teacher ratio designed for children with mild intellectual disability in conjunction with occupational therapy and speech/language therapy as related services. Hector also would benefit from a behavioral plan focused on enhancing his attention regulation, listening skills, task completion, and ability to deal with change/new situations as part of his Individualized Education Plan. As part of this plan, rules and expectations should be simply, clearly, and consistently presented and reviewed frequently. This plan should place a heavy emphasis on consistently rewarding Hector's "good" behavior, such as positive social interactions, working on classwork, and following directions, rather than having a punitive system that primarily calls attention to his mistakes. In other words, he should have a high ratio of positive reinforcement to punishment (ratio = 5:1). Consequences for both appropriate and inappropriate behavior should be enforced on a consistent basis through positive reinforcement and response cost. This could be managed in the form of a token economy, given Hector's age and intellect. The behavioral plan should be coordinated with the parents to ensure consistency between home and school, including target behaviors, reinforcers, and punishments. Further, participation in a social skills training group also may prove beneficial.

Given Hector's pattern of strengths and weaknesses, it is recommended that academic instruction in reading/writing emphasize multisensory approaches. In order to enhance Hector's learning/retention, new material should be presented in a concrete and organized format that is meaningful to him. The material to be learned should be pretaught, broken down into smaller components/steps, and presented in a highly structured format with frequent repetition to facilitate new learning. Instruction should be supplemented with visual aids, demonstrations, and experiential/procedural learning whenever possible. Finally, Hector should be provided with periodic review of previously learned material in order to enhance long-term retention.

In light of his inattention and poor receptive language skills, there are several general rules teachers, therapists, and parents should keep in mind while interacting with Hector:

- Eye contact should be ensured.
- A prompt to look at the speaker before directions are presented will be helpful.
- Instructions and directions should be kept short, simple, and concrete.
- Requests should be limited to single commands, and instructions should be presented several times if necessary.

Accommodations will be necessary to enhance Hector's ability to succeed in the classroom, including preferential seating; a reduction in the amount, but not the difficulty level, of assignments; and additional time to complete assignments. Tests should be in multiple-choice/matching/short-answer formats instead of an essay format and should be administered individually/orally, with additional time provided when necessary. Hector also will benefit from the use of graph paper or different color highlighters to maintain place value when doing written calculation. Finally, as he progresses through school, Hector should be allowed and encouraged to use various compensatory devices, such as textbooks on tape/reading pen, a calculator, and a computer with word processing capability. Most word processing programs are equipped with spell checks, cut and paste, and can be adapted for voice dictation if necessary.

Hector should continue to be followed by his pediatric neurologist for medical management of his tuberous sclerosis and epilepsy. In the event that Hector is found to be a candidate for epilepsy surgery, he should be reevaluated by this service approximately one year from the date of surgery in accordance with the pediatric epilepsy surgery protocol. Finally, once the decision regarding epilepsy surgery is resolved, a psychiatric consultation is recommended for medical management of Hector's anxiety and obsessive-compulsive behaviors along with family counseling to assist the parents in the development of a behavior management program for use in the home.

Further Discussion of Case Study

Hector's profile is fairly typical of a child with tuberous sclerosis, with both epilepsy and components of autism spectrum disorders evident. Like Hector, many children with tuberous sclerosis present with multiple issues, all of which affect the child's long-term outcome. Although there is considerable variability across individuals with tuberous sclerosis, early intervention and frequent monitoring to ensure appropriate intervention planning is needed; comprehensive assessment, such as this one, can help identify those underlying areas (e.g., language, attention, memory) that will present obstacles to learning if parents, teachers, and other professionals are not mindful of the need for multisensory approaches. Similarly, emotional and behavioral issues need to be addressed in order for social, functional, and academic progress to occur. As recommended by the consensus panel (de Vries et al., 2005), even if medical status is maintained, regular reevaluation to ensure appropriate programming over time and development will be needed.

STURGE-WEBER SYNDROME

Definition and Etiology

Sturge-Weber syndrome (SWS; encephalotrigeminal angiomatosis) is a neurocutaneous disorder characterized by a port wine stain (stigmata) on the face, usually with unilateral presence (Welty, 2006). Although the port wine stain results from a vascular disorder (venous dysplasia) rather than a neural disorder (Parsa, 2008), the effects are manifest neurologically. The classical SWS is comprised of a triad of clinical manifestations: specifically, a facial capillary malformation (port wine stain), with a vascular malformation of the eye and/or vascular malformation of the brain (leptomeningeal angioma) (Comi, 2003). Variants with fewer than all three components, however, are not uncommon (Ch'ng & Tan, 2008; Comi, 2003). This neuro-oculo-cutaneous syndrome is believed to be a result of vascular malformations of associated structures during the first trimester (Ch'ng & Tan, 2008). The distribution of stigmata usually follows the divisions of cranial nerve V (Welty, 2006).

According to the most recent view of the pathogenesis of SWS, the signs and symptoms all arise from localized primary venous dysplasia; the venous hypertension then is transmitted to nearby areas via communicating venous passageways and compensatory collateral venous channels (Parsa, 2008). Neurological concerns relate to development of excessive blood vessel growth on the surface of the brain (angiomas). Angiomas typically are located in the occipital region of the brain on the same side as the port wine stain and create abnormal conditions for brain function in the region. In conjunction with the angiomas, weakening or loss of the use of one side of the body (hemiparesis) may develop opposite to the port wine stain (Parsa, 2008). Port wine stains occur in 3 per 1,000 live births. No good data exist for how many people have SWS; however, estimates range from 1 in 20,000 to 50,000 live births (Comi, 2003; Comi, Bellamkonda, Ferenc, Cohen, & Germain-Lee, 2008). Unlike NF and tuberous sclerosis, SWS is a congenital, nonfamilial disorder of unknown incidence and cause (Comi et al., 2008). There is no identified cause or etiology; however, it is believed that the malformation in the blood vessels likely occurs in the first to second month of gestation (Kotagal & Rothner, 1993).

Neurological Correlates

Using imaging, it has been found that microstructural white matter damage extends beyond cortical abnormalities and may contribute to cognitive impairment (Juhász, Batista, Chugani, Muzik, & Chugani, 2007; Juhász, Haacke et al., 2007). Involvement of infratentorial structures is common but may be relatively subtle (M. E. Adams, Aylett, Squier, & Chong, 2009). In some cases, abnormalities of the corticospinal tract may be identified in children with SWS even before severe motor impairment develops (Sivaswamy et al., 2008). Magnetic resonance spectroscopic imaging has been found to be more sensitive than conventional structural MRI for detection of frontal lobe involvement in SWS (Batista et al., 2008). Decreased frontal lobe N-acetyl-aspartate (NAA) is an excellent predictor of motor functions. On computed tomography (CT) scan, there is evidence of intracranial calcification, usually in the occipital and parietal regions, but calcification also may occur in the temporal region. With SWS, structural MRI abnormalities are most common in the posterior brain regions; however, some individuals with SWS evidence abnormal NAA and/or choline lower in the frontal lobe gray matter

(Batista et al., 2008). The calcification is associated with cell atrophy. Research suggests that early, severe unilateral cortical damage in SWS may give rise to increased glucose metabolism in the contralateral visual cortex, probably reflecting functional reorganization (Batista, Juhász, Muzik, Chugani, & Chugani, 2007).

Course and Prognosis

Symptoms depend on the extent and location of the venous dysplasia and frequently include infantile spasms (Barbagallo et al., 2009) and seizures (M. E. Adams et al., 2009). Seizures usually begin within the first years of life and become progressively less manageable. The convulsions usually appear on the opposite side of the body from the port wine stain and vary in severity. Developmental delay of motor and cognitive skills also may occur to varying degrees; mental retardation is common, and neurological symptoms are often progressive (Juhász, Haacke et al., 2007). Based on multivariate regression, hemispheric white matter volume ipsilateral to the angioma is an independent predictor of cognitive ability; no correlation with gray matter volume was identified (Juhász, Lai et al., 2007). Port wine stains that affect the entire V1 distribution predict underlying neurological and/or ocular disorders that require ongoing ophthalmological surveillance and/or neurological management (Ch'ng & Tan, 2008).

With SWS, detrimental metabolic changes occur before 3 years of age coinciding with a sharp increase of developmentally regulated cerebral metabolic demand. Progressive hypometabolism is associated with high seizure frequency in these children; however, metabolic abnormalities may remain limited or even partially recover later in those children with well-controlled seizures. Metabolic recovery accompanied by neurological improvement suggests a window for therapeutic intervention in children with unilateral SWS (Juhász, Haacke et al., 2007). Hypothyroidism is also common (Comi et al., 2008).

Studies suggest that complex molecular interactions contribute to the abnormal development and function of blood vessels in SWS; related to the blood flow, many individuals with SWS have migraine headaches (Kossoff, Balasta, Hatfield, Lehmann, & Comi, 2007). Neurologic deterioration in SWS is likely secondary to impaired blood flow to the brain and is worsened by the presence of seizures (Comi, 2003). For children with SWS and onset of seizures or strokelike events before 6 months of age, the prognosis is worse with a severe early course and persistent neurologic deficits. The course stabilizes after 5 years of age in most cases. In contrast, with late-onset seizures or stroke, there is a more benign course; aspirin use is associated with a stable course, but further studies are needed (Udani, Pujar, Munot, Maheshwari, & Mehta, 2007).

Studies of individuals with SWS focus most often on the medical aspects of this syndrome; considerably less has been studied about the affective and behavioral correlates (Chapieski, Friedman, & Lachar, 2000). What has been found is that children with SWS are more likely to exhibit problems than their siblings across a number of behavioral domains: intellectual/academic, social skills, mood, and compliance. Risk for psychological problems is associated with lower levels of cognitive functioning, seizure disorders, and more frequent seizures. Larger port wine stains were associated with increased mood and social problems, particularly in older children (Chapieski et al., 2000). These problems, combined with limited intelligence and social skills as well as poor aesthetic appearance and seizures, must be addressed in order for individuals with SWS to improve social interactions, obtain gainful employment, and have a better quality of life (Pascual-Castroviejo, Pascual-Pascual, Velazquez-Fragua, & Viaño, 2008).

Neurocognitive Correlates

Epilepsy, hemiparesis, mental retardation, and ocular problems were the most frequent and severe features of children with SWS (Pascual-Castroviejo et al., 2008). Early surgical treatment may control the seizures, but other neurological problems, such as hemiparesis and intellectual deficits, are not affected as positively (Pascual-Castroviejo et al., 2008). In particular, early onset of seizures and poor response to medical treatment, bilateral cerebral involvement, and unilateral severe lesions were predictive of a poor prognosis. A summary of functional concerns is provided in Table 16.7.

Educational and Behavioral Implications

Children with SWS generally have been diagnosed by the time they enter school (Cody & Hynd, 1998). The most frequent reasons for involvement of neuropsychologists or other professionals in the management of SWS include the co-occurrence of mental retardation and behavior problems. The academic problems may be exacerbated by the side effects of many antiepileptic medications (see Chapter 10). No characteristic educational issues were found in the extant literature; however, learning problems with subsequent special education placement are common (Kossoff, Balasta et al., 2007). Behavior problems are common as well and may manifest in conduct problems or problems relating to disinhibition (Cody & Hynd, 1998).

Table 16.7 Neuropsychological Deficits Associated with Sturge-Weber Syndrome

Global Domain/Specific Deficits	Phenotype
Cognition	Developmental delay of motor and cognitive skills may occur to varying degrees; mental retardation common
Auditory-linguistic/Language function	Level of impairment variable
Learning and Memory	Level of impairment variable
Visual perception/Constructional praxis	Level of impairment variable
Attention/Concentration	Attention problems common
Processing speed	With motor difficulties, speed also affected
Motor function	Hemiparesis common
Achievement/Academic skills	Learning disability; special education frequent
Emotional/Behavioral functioning	Behavior problems common

Evidence-Based Interventions

Interventions to address components of learning and behavior problems, medical prevention and compliance, and self-esteem are needed by the child affected by the syndrome. Interventions that have been used with children with SWS are summarized in Table 16.8. It is important to keep in mind that as with other disorders, the progression of the disorder is such that continuous and regular monitoring of progress, medication side effects, and effectiveness of intervention planning is required (Cody & Hynd, 1998).

Medical Management

Sometimes children with SWS are treated with neurosurgery (hemispherectomy) if seizures become intractable. Because of the potential emotional effects, medical intervention to address the adenoma sebaceum, such as dermabrasion, may be indicated

Table 16.8 Evidence-Based Status for Sturge-Weber Syndrome

Interventions	Target	Status
Surgery or laser procedure	Cosmetic removal of port wine stain	Adverse effects (Hennedige, Quaba, & Al-Nakib, 2008; Parsa, 2008)
Triptans (Imitrex, Zomig, Amerge, Maxalt)	Prevention of migraine	Emerging (Kossoff, Balasta et al., 2007)

(Hennedige et al., 2008; Parsa, 2008). Surgeries that eliminate the port wine stains to minimize the cosmetic blemish may reduce collateral venous blood flow passageways. In some instances, this reduction may worsen blood stasis within the brain and potentially exacerbate neurologic symptoms (Parsa, 2008). Laser therapy is one approach for treating port wine stains, but whether it is effective for patients with facial dermatomal port wine stains and SWS is unknown (Hennedige et al., 2008). Based on one study, the portion of cranial nerve V that is affected may be a factor, with unsatisfactory outcomes for those with involvement of the maxillary division of the trigeminal nerve. Additional research specific to those with SWS is needed (Hennedige et al., 2008).

Educational and Psychological Management

No specific studies were found that related to educational or psychological interventions with individuals with SWS. Limited intelligence and social skills, aesthetic appearance, and seizures complicated the integration of children with SWS with their peers. These features must be addressed in order to improve opportunities for positive social interactions, gainful employment, and better quality of life (Pascual-Castroviejo et al., 2008).

CASE STUDY: JULIANA—STURGE-WEBER SYNDROME

The next report is from a hospital-based clinic. Identifying information, such as child and family name, teacher or physician name, and school information, has been altered or fictionalized to protect confidentiality.

Reason for Referral

Juliana is an 8-year 9-month-old third grade student who is being initially evaluated by the pediatric neuropsychology service at the request of her pediatric neurologist, who is following her for a history of Sturge-Weber syndrome (without the classic facial port wine stained nevus), complex partial seizure disorder with secondary generalization, and questionable cognitive decline. At present, Juliana is taking levetiracetam (Keppra) for seizure management along with aspirin. She is allergic to oxcarbazepine (Trileptal), phenytoin (Dilantin), and penicillin. Juliana has not experienced an observed seizure in approximately two months. Neuropsychological evaluation was undertaken in order to assess higher cortical functioning and make appropriate recommendations regarding school placement and the need for supportive therapies.

Assessment Procedures

Clinical interview
Behavioral observations

Wechsler Intelligence Scale for Children, Fourth Edition (WISC-IV)
Peabody Picture Vocabulary Test, Fourth Edition (PPVT-IV)
Boston Naming Test (BNT)
Neuropsychological Assessment (NEPSY)/ Neuropsychological Assessment, Second Edition (NEPSY-2; selected subtests)
Clinical Evaluation of Language Fundamentals, Fourth Edition (CELF-IV; selected subtests)
Kaufman Assessment Battery for Children, Second Edition (KABC-2; selected subtests)
Beery Developmental Test of Visual-Motor Integration, Fifth Edition (DTVMI-V)
Clock Face Drawing Test
Finger Tapping Test
Children's Memory Scales (CMS)
Gray Oral Reading Test, Fourth Edition (GORT-4)
Wechsler Individual Achievement Test, Second Edition (WIAT-II)
Behavior Assessment System for Children, Second Edition (BASC-2; Parent and Teacher Rating Scales)
DSM-IV ADHD Checklist

Background Information

Juliana resides with her mother and her 2-year-old sister, Chablis, who is in good health and developing normally. Juliana's parents were never married, and she had no contact with her father. Juliana's father is reported to be 36 years of age, a high school graduate, who is currently employed as a construction worker. Juliana's mother is 28 years of age, completed the 11th grade and has not earned a general equivalency diploma. She is currently a full-time homemaker. Both parents are reported to be in good health. The family medical history is significant for a paternal aunt who had seizures as a child and sickle cell anemia in a second paternal aunt.

Review of developmental and medical history with Juliana's mother indicates that Juliana is the product of a 39-week pregnancy complicated by elevated blood pressure in the mother during the last trimester that was managed with medication. Delivery was vaginal and without complication. Juliana was reported to weigh 6 pounds 4 ounces at birth. She did well as a newborn and went home from the hospital with her mother on day 2. Juliana's mother was unable to recall Juliana's exact developmental motor and language milestones; however, she felt that Juliana attained these well within normal limits. Toilet training was fully accomplished at approximately 2 years of age without difficulty.

Juliana experienced her initial seizure at 6 years of age; the seizure progressed to status epilepticus and resulted in a hospital admission. Initial MRI of the brain and serial follow-up studies have all been reported to be significant for volume loss involving the right temporal, parietal, and occipital lobes; gyriform calcifications more inferior than superior; and bilateral (R > L) occipital leptomeningeal angiomatosis consistent with a diagnosis of SWS (see Figure 16.7 (MRI)). Serial EEG monitoring has been significant for bilateral posterior and right frontal epileptiform discharges; however, her most recent EEG showed diffuse right frontal discharges that were felt to be a paradoxical false localization from the right posterior region due to the calcifications (see Figure 16.8 (EEG)). Juliana's past medical history is also significant for headaches and Stevens-Johnson syndrome shortly

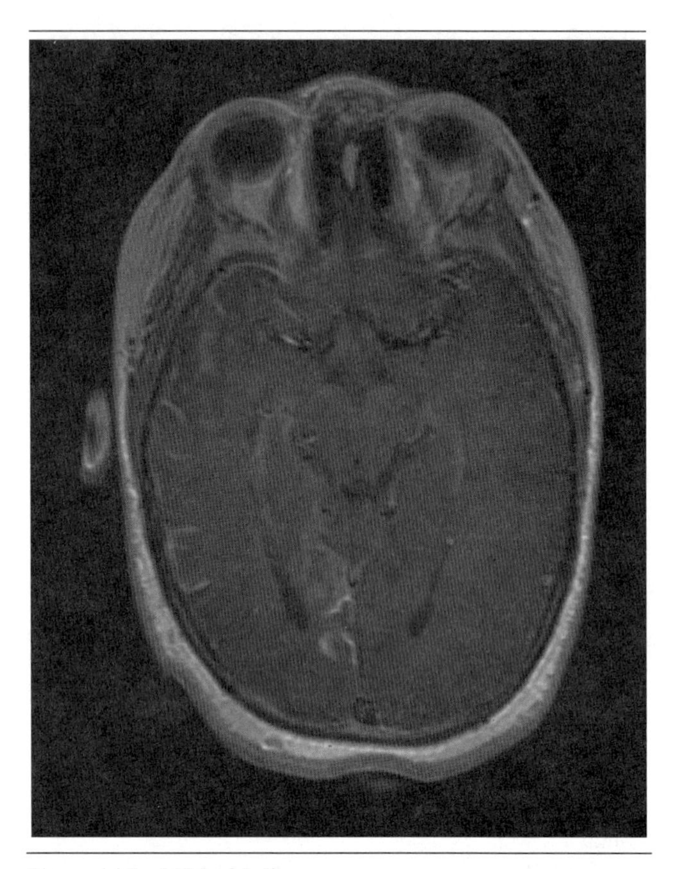

Figure 16.7 MRI of Juliana.

after the initiation of treatment for the seizures with phenytoin (Dilantin) and oxcarbazepine (Trileptal). At present, Juliana enjoys a good appetite and sleeps well. Her mother does not report a history of short attention span or behavioral difficulty in the home.

Review of educational history indicates that Juliana attended Head Start when she was 3 and 4 years of age. According to her mother, Juliana did well in this setting with no significant problems reported. At 5 years of age, Juliana began attending kindergarten within the local school system. Once again, Juliana was reported to do well in this setting. At 6 years of age, Juliana was promoted to first grade, where her mother stated that she made the "all-A honor roll." It was during this school year that Juliana started having seizures. In second grade, Juliana's mother reported that Juliana made the "A/B honor roll" first semester; however, she earned a C in reading second semester.

This year, Juliana is attending third grade, where her mother states that she continues to earn Cs in reading. Further, after experiencing some seizures in October, Juliana's academic performance became highly variable especially in reading (decoding and comprehension). As a result, the student support team at Juliana's school referred her for a psychological screening evaluation by the school psychologist assigned to her school. At that time, Juliana was administered the Kaufman Brief Intelligence Test on which she exhibited a significant verbal-performance discrepancy in favor of her nonverbal reasoning ability (Vocabulary = 60; Matrices = 102). Academic assessment with the Woodcock Johnson Tests of Achievement, Third Edition revealed significant underachievement in the areas of understanding directions and mathematical calculation.

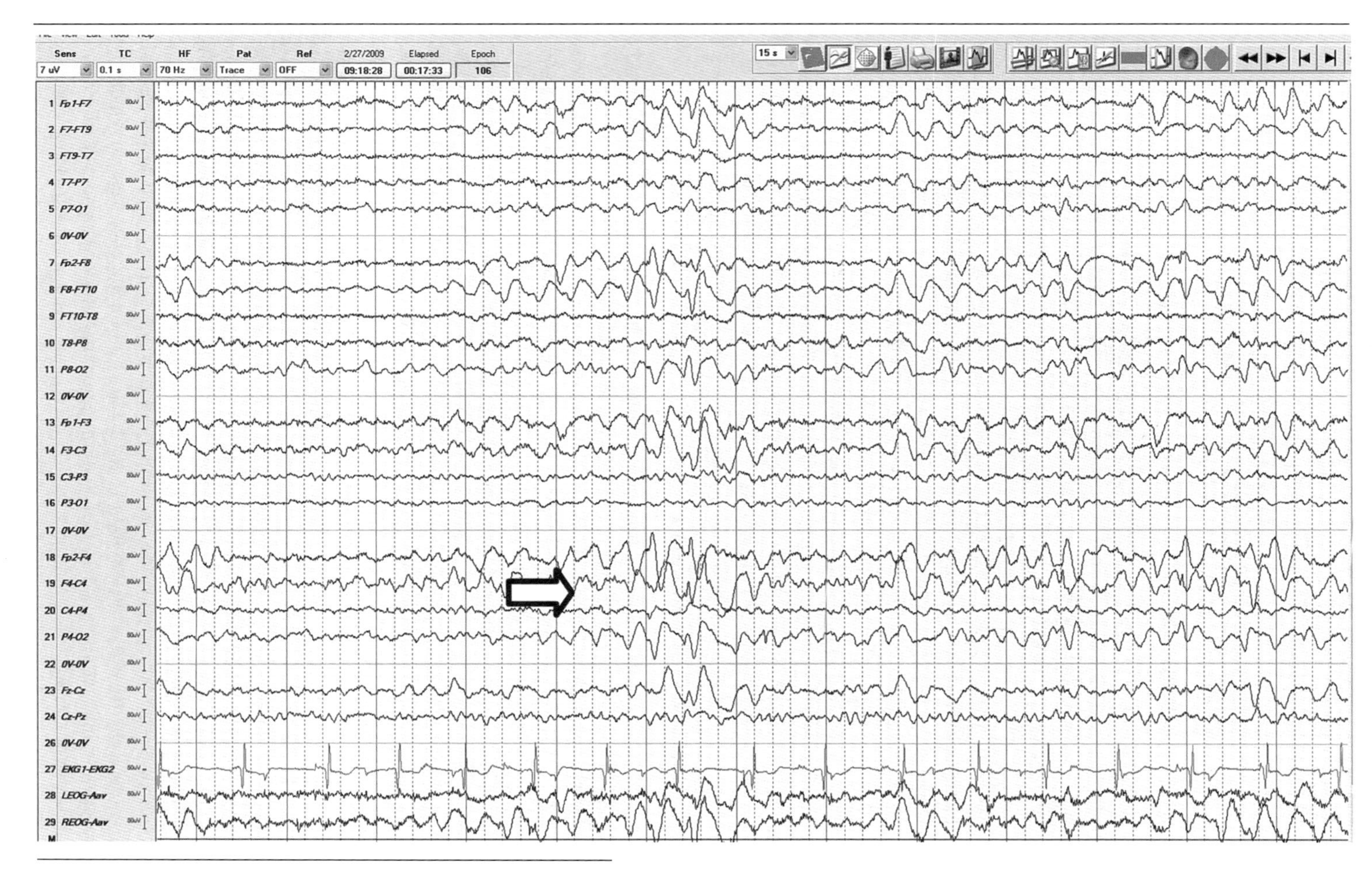

Figure 16.8 Most recent video EEG monitoring of Juliana.

Review of a school report form completed by Juliana's teacher indicates that she characterizes Juliana as "a very quiet soft-spoken student. She has problems with reading fluently and with understanding. Juliana also has problems with various math concepts such as rounding, subtracting, telling time, and counting money." The teacher went on to estimate that Juliana was performing at a failing level in reading and mathematics as compared with her grade level placement.

Behavioral Observations

Juliana presented herself for testing as a pleasant, neatly groomed, overweight young lady who was casually dressed in a yellow top, white skirt, and sneakers. She separated appropriately from her mother and grandmother and accompanied the examiners to the testing room without difficulty. Juliana was oriented, demonstrated good social eye contact, and related appropriately toward the examiners with good manners noted. In response to direct questions as well as when conversation was spontaneous, Juliana's use of language was fluent and prosodic but marked by significant word-finding difficulty. Throughout the evaluation, which consisted of two sessions separated by a lunch break, Juliana's attention span, activity level, and impulsivity within the context of this one-to-one assessment were felt to be age-level appropriate. When confronted with more challenging tasks, Juliana put forth a good effort, and she responded well to praise and encouragement from the examiners. Lateral dominance is firmly established in the right hand for paper-and-pencil manipulation. Vision and hearing were screened by the school system prior to psychological screening evaluation and reported to be within normal limits.

Test Results and Interpretation

The results of neuropsychological evaluation indicate that Juliana is functioning within the deficient to borderline range of intellectual ability as measured by the Full Scale IQ score of the Wechsler Intelligence Scale for Children, Fourth Edition (WISC-IV); however, due to the significant verbal-performance discrepancy in favor of Juliana's average nonverbal reasoning ability, it is recommended that the average Perceptual Reasoning Index score be used to estimate her true intellectual potential. This interpretation is further supported by Juliana's average performance on the Tower Subtest from the Neuropsychological Assessment (NEPSY), which is a measure of sequential reasoning and nonverbal problem solving (see Table 16.9).

Additional assessment indicates that Juliana demonstrated deficient to borderline expressive and receptive language skills with a strength noted on a measure of receptive vocabulary and a significant deficit found on a measure of word-finding/confrontational picture naming. Language appears to be lateralized in the left cerebral hemisphere as evidenced by a right ear advantage in Juliana's ability to report consonant vowel syllables presented simultaneously to each ear on a Dichotic Listening Test; however, it should be noted that Juliana is demonstrating a performance pattern consistent with bilateral ear suppression. Visual-spatial perception and visual-motor integration/construction were found to be in the low-average to average range, consistent with Juliana's performance on the WISC-IV. It should be noted that the deficient score on the Gestalt Closure Subtest from the Kaufman Assessment Battery for Children, Second Edition (KABC-2) resulted from the task requirement to name pictures. Fine motor tapping speed is found to be in the low-average range with a relative depression noted in right-hand performance as measured by the Finger Tapping test.

Analysis of Juliana's performance on the Children's Memory Scale (CMS) indicates that, at the present time, she is exhibiting deficient to borderline ability to hold verbal as well as visual

Table 16.9 Psychometric Summary for Juliana

	Scaled Scores	Standard Scores
Wechsler Intelligence Scale for Children, Fourth Edition (WISC-IV)		
Full Scale IQ		70
Verbal Comprehension Index		63
Similarities	5	
Vocabulary	3	
Comprehension	3	
Perceptual Reasoning Index		90
Block Design	7	
Picture Concepts	11	
Matrix Reasoning	7	
Working Memory Index		83
Digit Span	7	
Letter-Number Sequencing	7	
Processing Speed Index		65
Coding	6	
Symbol Search	1	
Neuropsychological Assessment, Second Edition (NEPSY-2)		
Phonological Processing		90
Comprehension of Instructions		70
Word Generation: Semantic		55
Word Generation: Initial Letter		75
Arrows		90
Tower (NEPSY)		100
Peabody Picture Vocabulary Test, Fourth Edition (PPVT-IV)		72
Boston Naming Test (BNT)		<40
Clinical Evaluation of Language Fundamentals, Fourth Edition (CELF-IV)		
Sentence Repetition		70
Formulated Sentences		75
Dichotic Listening	**Number Correct**	
Left Ear	8/30	
Right Ear	10/30	
		Standard Score
Kaufman Assessment Battery for Children, Second Edition (KABC-2)		
Gestalt Closure		60
Developmental Test of Visual-Motor Integration, Fifth Edition (DTVMI-V)		
Visual Motor Integration		81
Clock Face Drawing Test		
Form		89
Time (10:20)		109
	Raw Score	**Standard Score**
Finger Tapping Test		
Right (dominant) Hand	24.7 taps/10 seconds	81
Left (nondominant) Hand	24.7 taps/10 seconds	87

(continued)

Table 16.9 *(Continued)*

	Scaled Scores	Standard Scores
Children's Memory Scale (CMS)		
Attention/Concentration Index		66
Numbers	3	
Sequences	6	
Picture Locations	1	
General Memory Index		50
Verbal Immediate Index		57
Stories	4	
Word Pairs	2	
Visual Immediate Index		50
Dot Locations	2	
Faces	1	
Verbal Delayed Index		69
Stories	4	
Word Pairs	6	
Visual Delayed Index		57
Dot Locations	5	
Faces	1	
Delayed Recognition Index		63
Stories	6	
Word Pairs	2	
Learning Index		54
Word Pairs	3	
Dot Locations	2	
Gray Oral Reading Test, Fourth Edition (GORT-4)		
Fluency		65
Comprehension		60
Wide Range Achievement Test, Fourth Edition (WRAT-4)		
Word Reading		79
Pseudoword Decoding		83
Written Expression Reading		86
Spelling		91
Mathematical Reasoning		84
Numerical Operations		97

Behavior Assessment System for Children, Second Edition (BASC-2)	T-Scores	
	Parent	Teacher
Clinical Scales		
Hyperactivity	45	42
Aggression	55	43
Conduct	40	42
Anxiety	43	38
Depression	39	45
Somatization	61	66
Atypical	46	56
Withdrawal	35	68
Attention	45	51

(continued)

Table 16.9 *(Continued)*

	T-Scores	
	Parent	**Teacher**
Learning Problems	NA	72
Adaptive Scales		
Adaptability	66	60
Social Skills	69	31
Leadership	64	30
Study Skills	NA	42
Activities of Daily Living	67	NA
Functional Communication	62	42
DSM-IV ADHD Checklist	Raw Scores	
Inattention	7/27	14/27
Hyperactivity/Impulsivity	13/27	0/27

Note. NA = Not applicable for rater.

material in immediate/working memory. When asked to learn and remember (30 minutes later) newly presented material, Juliana experienced significant difficulty processing and encoding the required information into long-term memory. Further, she exhibited significant difficulty with information retrieval as well. Together, these difficulties resulted in deficient to borderline learning and recall performance for both verbal and visual material. Thus, Juliana is experiencing significant difficulty making new memories. Academically, Juliana exhibited average spelling and numerical calculation skills; borderline to low-average word reading/phonetic decoding, reading comprehension, mathematical reasoning, and written expression skills; and deficient oral reading fluency. With the exception of the numerical calculation score, these results are generally consistent with those obtained previously.

Behaviorally, analysis of rating scales completed by Juliana's mother and teacher indicates that, at the present time, Juliana is not exhibiting significant emotional or behavioral difficulty in the home. In contrast, Juliana's teacher endorsed significant concern with regard to social withdrawal and poor social skills in general. In addition, she rated Juliana's functional communication skills as poor along with significant learning problems in the classroom.

Summary and Diagnostic Impressions

Juliana is an 8-year old with a history of seizure disorder believed to be related to the presence of leptomeningeal angiomatosis consistent with Sturge-Weber Syndrome, but without the classic port wine stain. This pattern of neuropsychological test performance is consistent with a picture of dysfunction involving the perisylvian language zone in the left cerebral hemisphere in conjunction with bilateral temporal lobe dysfunction. Taken together, these findings are consistent with a diagnosis of specific language impairment (expressive and receptive type) and learning disability in the area of reading fluency. Further, Juliana's learning and memory deficits will make the acquisition of new learning more difficult and affect her performance across all subject areas.

Recommendations

As a result, it is recommended that Juliana be considered for special education services under the eligibility categories of "Specific Learning Disability/Other Health Impaired," given that her learning difficulties are directly related to her neurological disorder.

Resource placement should be utilized for development of reading skills as well as to support other academic areas that require reading skills as a prerequisite. In addition, language therapy as a related service should be considered. These recommendations are offered with regard to instruction:

- Given Juliana's pattern of strengths and weaknesses, it is recommended that academic instruction in reading/writing instruction emphasize the use of multisensory approaches.
- In order to enhance Juliana's learning/retention, new material should be presented in an organized format that is meaningful to her.
- The material to be learned should be pretaught, broken down into smaller components/steps, and presented in a highly structured format with frequent repetition to facilitate new learning.
- Instruction should be supplemented with visual aids, demonstrations, and experiential/procedural learning whenever possible.
- As Juliana progresses in school, she would benefit greatly from being taught how to use mnemonic strategies when learning new material and studying for tests. These include but are not limited to:
  - Rehearsal—showing Juliana how to repeat information verbally, to write it, and look at it a finite number of times.
  - Transformation—instructing Juliana in how to convert difficult information into simpler components that can be remembered more easily.
  - Elaboration—showing Juliana how to identify key elements of new information and to create relationships or associations with previously learned material.
  - Chunking—instructing Juliana in how to group or pare down long strings of digits or different items into more manageable units and thereby facilitate encoding and retention.
  - Imagery—showing Juliana how to visualize and make a mental picture of information to be learned.
- When studying for tests or doing multiple homework assignments on the same day, similar subject material should be separated in order to lessen interference.
- Finally, Juliana will require periodic review of previously learned material in order to enhance long-term retention.

In light of Juliana's language disorder, teachers, therapists, and parents should keep in mind several general rules while interacting with her:

- Eye contact should be ensured.
- A prompt to look at the speaker before directions are presented will be helpful.
- Instructions and directions should be kept short, simple, and concrete.
- Requests should be limited to single commands, and instructions should be presented several times if necessary.

Accommodations will be necessary to enhance Juliana's ability to succeed in the classroom, including preferential seating, a reduction in the amount, but not the difficulty level, of assignments, and additional time to complete assignments. Tests should be in multiple-choice/matching/short-answer formats instead of an essay format and should be administered individually/orally, with additional time provided when necessary. Finally, Juliana should be allowed and encouraged to use various compensatory devices, such as textbooks on tape/reading pen and a computer with word processing capability. Most word processing programs are equipped with spell checks and cut and paste, and can be adapted for voice dictation if necessary.

Finally, Juliana should continue to be followed by her neurologist for medical management of her epilepsy. If Juliana is found to be a candidate for epilepsy surgery, she should be reevaluated by this service approximately one year from the date of surgery in accordance with the pediatric epilepsy surgery protocol.

Further Discussion of Case Study

Juliana's case is an interesting one in that there is no presentation of a port wine stain, but there is documented presence of Stevens-Johnson syndrome. Stevens-Johnson syndrome is a cutaneous and mucous syndrome that, like SWS, also may take on a red or purplish rash, but is painful and spreads if not treated. Some preexisting disorders increase the risk of Stevens-Johnson syndrome, but not generally SWS (Mayo Clinic Staff, n.d.). The occurrence of this in conjunction with SWS limits some of the analgesic medications and other medications that Juliana can tolerate. For Juliana, the prognosis at this time is of concern, given the difficulty she is experiencing with the formulation of new memories secondary to bilateral temporal lobe involvement. Thus, it is critical that she receive appropriate supports in the classroom. Professionals working with her will have to be vigilant about the potential risk of any further complications, including malformations of blood flow and the development of glaucoma or other ocular difficulties. Frequent monitoring will be needed for Juliana as with all children with SWS (Cody & Hynd, 1998).

CONCLUDING COMMENTS

Neurocutaneous syndromes potentially are associated with cognitive, learning, behavior, and health concerns; even within the syndromes, individual presentation varies significantly. The quality of life and expectation of a full and normal life will be dependent on the characteristics of a given individual. In all three case studies presented here, educational impact is evident. In addition, across these disorders, there is the potential for possible co-occurring problems across domains of psychosocial adjustment, medical issues, and educational issues. Thus, input and combined expertise of a variety of professionals is necessary to comprehensively assess and address the needs of the individual with one of these syndromes (Hunt, 2006). The complexity of issues associated with these disorders demands interdisciplinary collaboration and communication between professionals and contexts (home, school, medical facility) where these children function. Notably, there is a paucity of research on the best approaches to treatment (other than medical) to address the myriad and complex issues associated with these disorders.

Chapter 17

METABOLIC DISORDERS

Any number of metabolic disorders can affect children. Based on frequency and available research, the metabolic disorders that are discussed in this chapter include diabetes mellitus (Type 1), phenylketonuria (PKU), and the mucopolysaccharide disorders. Each is presented separately with concluding comments as appropriate to all.

TYPE 1 DIABETES

Definition

Insulin-dependent diabetes mellitus (also referred to as Type 1 or juvenile onset) is one of the more common disorders in childhood (Bachman & Hsueh, 2008; Strawhacker, 2001). It is classified as an autoimmune disorder that is characterized by insufficient insulin production (P. H. Bennett, 1994; Nattrass & Hale, 1988). The insufficient insulin production can result in excess of unmetabolized glucose (sugars) in the blood and urine, and interferes with the body's ability to use simple sugars. If not identified and treated, diabetes can lead to dangerously high levels of blood glucose due to the inability of the pancreas to produce sufficient insulin (D. W. Foster, 1991). Behavioral symptoms of diabetes may resemble those of someone who has been drinking: confusional state, slurring of speech, and impaired motor coordination. More severe symptoms can include severe dehydration, diabetic coma, and death. Alternatively, if there is too much insulin, the result is hypoglycemia. Hypoglycemia is associated with motor tremor, confusion, weakness, loss of consciousness, and possible seizures. The likelihood of abnormal electroencephalograms (EEGs) is increased with frequency of severe hypoglycemic episodes (D. W. Foster, 1991).

Adult parallels of Type 1 exist and are referred to as Type 2 or late onset, although there is increased incidence of Type 2 in adolescents and children (American Diabetes Association, 2006). Type 2 most typically evidences in mid- to late 40s or early 50s. Another form of diabetes is gestational diabetes. Gestational diabetes occurs in conjunction with pregnancy; the diabetes may remit or may not remit after the child is born (American Diabetes Association, 2006). Of those individuals with diabetes, 5% to 10% are diagnosed with Type 2 diabetes; about 1 in every 400 to 600 people under 20 years of age has Type 2 diabetes (Centers for Disease Control [CDC], 2005).

Incidence

The incidence of Type 1 also is approximately 1 in 400 to 600 school-age children (American Diabetes Association, 2006; Sperling, 1990). The age range for diagnosis of Type 1 diabetes is generally between 10 and 14 years, but it may present earlier or later.

The age-specific incidence increases with age; only about 8% of children under the age of 5 are identified with Type 1 diabetes (Jefferson, Smith, & Baum, 1985). Among all types of diabetes (i.e., Type 1, Type 2, and gestational), Type 1 diabetes is the most prevalent type among youth in the United States; with increased obesity, this statistic is seen as potentially changing in the future with approximately 1 in 6 overweight adolescents evidencing pre-diabetes (American Diabetes Association, 2006). Type 1 is diagnosed across ethnic groups and in both boys and girls. Of note, a greater proportion of non-Hispanic White youth are diagnosed with diabetes under the age of 10, but these ethnic differences are not as pronounced across older age ranges. In contrast, ethnic differences in the older age group are common among youth diagnosed with Type 2 diabetes with Hispanic/Latino and African American groups overrepresented (CDC, 2005; Lawrence et al., 2006). There are some indications that Type 1 diabetes may be more common in Asian families who migrate to the United Kingdom as compared to those who remain in India (Bodansky et al., 1987).

Etiology

Many factors may be associated with Type 1 diabetes including viruses, certain diets, chemicals, and other environmental factors. Genes also are believed to be involved in Type 1 diabetes, with multiple occurrences usually occurring within the family. The genetic link for Type 2 is believed to be stronger but also strongly affected by environmental factors.

Genetic

The genetic base to Type 1 diabetes is such that the risk of a child developing Type 1 diabetes is 1 in 17 when the father has diabetes and 1 in 25 when the mother has diabetes and has the child before the age of 25 (American Diabetes Association, 2006). For some reason, the risk decreases when the mother has diabetes and is over the age of 25 at the time of the child's birth. If both parents have diabetes, the risk increases to 1 in 4 to 1 in 10 that the child will have diabetes. Despite extensive research, a single gene responsible for diabetes has not been identified; rather, up to 19 sections of the human genome may be related to a risk or susceptibility to Type 1 diabetes (Momin et al., 2009).

One section of interest includes genes involved in the development of human leukocyte antigens (HLAs); these proteins help the immune system recognize the body's own cells. Without these proteins, an autoimmune response may occur (Redondo, Fain, & Eisenbarth, 2001). There is also some indication that the specific HLA genes involved in Type 1 diabetes vary by ethnicity/race (Britten, Mijovic, Barnett, & Kelly, 2009; Eike et al., 2009). The genetic link to Type 2 diabetes appears to be stronger than for Type 1 based on twin studies and the frequency among and across racial/ethnic groups. In most cases of Type 2 diabetes, usually more than one gene is involved, and gene combinations may vary across individuals and families (Gloyn & McCarthy, 2001). The genes involved in Type 2 appear to change the way insulin acts on tissues, creating insulin resistance and ultimately increasing the levels of insulin in the bloodstream. Most important, there is a gene by environment interaction such that it is believed that diabetes prevention programs (weight loss and exercise) could decrease the genetic risk of Type 2 diabetes (Ho et al., 2008; Madden, Loeb, & Smith, 2008). The aryl hydrocarbon receptor nuclear translocator (ARNT) gene also appears to be implicated in Type 2 diabetes and may lead to a potential treatment approach in the future (Das, Sharma, Chu, Wang, & Elbein, 2008). Obesity, which is caused by both genetic and environmental factors, increases insulin resistance and the risk of Type 2. Other risk factors for Type 2 diabetes that may involve a genetic component include unhealthy levels of cholesterol and triglycerides (hyperlipidemia), high blood pressure, and a metabolic syndrome. The genetic predisposition is most likely to present in those who eat an unhealthy, high-calorie diet, are overweight, and get little exercise (American Diabetes Association, 2006).

Environmental

There is evidence to suggest that family structure and parental diabetes have adverse effects on the diabetes outcome of children; however, there is no indication that socioeconomic status or disadvantage in and of themselves affect outcome (Baumer, Hunt, & Shield, 1998). In particular, parent perceptions of their children's ability to self-manage may result in poorer glycemic control (Pattison, Moledina, & Barrett, 2006).

Neurological Correlates

No specific structural differences are specifically associated with diabetes, regardless of type. Abnormalities are associated with the occurrence of hypoglycemic convulsions as evidenced by serial EEG recordings (Soltész & Acsádi, 1989). These changes vary depending on the repetitive cycling and frequency of the convulsions.

Course and Prognosis

Course and prognosis with Type 1 diabetes is highly dependent on the level of metabolic control the individual is able to maintain across the life span. If controlled, the risks of medical complications decrease; if not, neurocognitive, educational, psychological, and medical risks increase. As a result of variability in compliance and glycemic control over time, repeated assessment of neurocognitive function is important in ensuring appropriate intervention planning.

Neurocognitive Correlates

Risk factors for neuropsychological impairment differ based on age at onset of disease (later is better), metabolic control of the disorder, and personality factors. The extent to which detrimental effects occur varies, and the majority of individuals do not evidence cognitive decrements. Individuals at risk for cognitive decrements are those with an early age of onset and those with retinopathy or other microvascular complications (Biessels, Kerssen, de Haan, & Kappelle, 2007).

Earlier onset also is associated with deficiencies in children's use of strategies to organize and recall information (Hagen et al., 1990). Duration of disease (time since onset of Type 1 diabetes) also appears to be a factor, with longer duration associated with decreased efficiency on a task that requires attention and speed of processing (Sansbury, Brown, & Meacham, 1997). In effect, longer duration is associated with more negative effects. Further, poor metabolic control is predictive of greater cognitive impairment (C. S. Holmes, Cant, Fox, Lampert, & Greer, 1999; Northam et al., 2001). These findings support the ongoing monitoring of the cognitive functioning of children and adolescents with Type 1, particularly those who are older and have sustained longer duration of the disease, and the implementation of intervention programs aimed at remediating learning problems in these youth (Sansbury et al., 1997). Ethnicity and socioeconomic status (SES) also emerge as factors. In particular, African American children with diabetes, regardless of SES, are at greater risk for cognitive deficits and learning problems than either White children with diabetes or without diabetes (Overstreet, Holmes, Dunlap, & Frentz, 1997).

Another study attempted to control for a number of potential confounds (family factors) by using nondiabetic siblings as the control group (Perantie et al., 2008). Overall, the group with Type 1 diabetes evidenced lower verbal abilities than sibling controls, particularly when there was a history of hyperglycemic episodes, but not hypoglycemic episodes. In contrast, deficits in nonverbal abilities as well as delayed recall were associated with hypoglycemic episodes. This was particularly true if these episodes occurred before the age of 5, suggesting interference in developmental trajectories (Perantie et al., 2008). Children with Type 1 demonstrate lower cognitive ability than controls with some subgroups at greater risk than others. Poorer metabolic control including both recurrent hypoglycemia and severe hyperglycemia, earlier age of disease onset, and longer disease duration have been related to lower IQ scores (C. S. Holmes et al., 1999). Similarly, in a 6-year follow-up study, those children with Type 1 diabetes performed more poorly than a control group on measures of cognition, attention, processing speed, long-term memory, and executive functioning (Northam et al., 2001). Of these neurocognitive domains, attention, processing speed, and executive function were most impaired in children with early onset (i.e., before 4 years of age); in contrast, episodes of severe hypoglycemia were associated with lower Verbal and Full Scale IQ scores (Northam et al., 2001).

The most comprehensive study of neurocognitive effects of Type 1 diabetes was a meta-analysis that included 1393 study participants with Type 1 diabetes and 751 control participants from 19 studies (Gaudieri, Chen, Greer, & Holmes, 2008). In general, children with Type 1 diabetes demonstrated slightly lower overall cognition (Effect Size = –0.13), with small differences compared with control subjects across a broad range of domains. Notably, learning and memory domains were similar for both groups; however, both learning and memory skills were more affected for children with earlier onset. A similar pattern of greater impairment associated with early onset was found for attention/executive function skills (Gaudieri et al., 2008).

For children, frequency of school absences (both as sign of poor control/management of disorder and lack of exposure) are associated with greater impairment. Common neurocognitive deficits occur in memory and fine motor dexterity (J. F. Rovet, 2000). Additionally, there is evidence of disproportionate rates of lower cognitive ability and associated academic skills deficits. During states of low blood sugar, deficits were more pronounced in areas of motor speed, attention, and mental efficiency (Hershey et al., 2005; C. S. Holmes, Hayford, Gonzalez, & Weydert, 1983; Reich et al., 1990; Ryan et al., 1990). Research suggests the ability to problem solve, self-monitor, and utilize working memory are related to higher rates of adherence regardless of age (Bagner, Williams, Geffken, Silverstein, & Storch, 2007). Increased latency or sluggish cognitive tempo (Hagen et al., 1990; C. S. Holmes et al., 1983; Northam et al., 2001; Sansbury et al., 1997) as well as problems with attention (Hagen et al., 1990) have been noted. Further, history of severe hypoglycemia is associated consistently with more neuropsychological impairments, parent reported learning problems, and special education placement (Hannonen, Tupola, Ahonen, & Riikonen, 2003). In particular, metabolic control is associated with memory performance (Hagen et al., 1990; Northam et al., 2001). Specific deficits associated with hypoglycemia included verbal short-term memory and phonological processing (Hannonen et al., 2003). These deficits are summarized in Table 17.1.

It is important to note that some of these deficits may be transient. Although neurocognitive deficits may be identified, there is also evidence of significant improvements in perceptual reasoning, selective attention, divided attention, cognitive flexibility, and

Table 17.1 Neuropsychological Deficits Associated with Diabetes

Global Domain	Phenotype
Cognition	Impaired cognition associated with poor metabolic control
Auditory-linguistic/Language function	Verbal abilities may be impacted by early onset and hyperglycemic episodes
Visual perception/Constructional praxis	Spatial abilities impacted by hypoglycemic episodes
Learning and Memory	Recall of information may be affected by poor metabolic control
Executive function	Complex problem solving, organization, and other aspects of EF compromised
Attention/Concentration	Attentional problems common
Processing speed	Increased latency or sluggish cognitive tempo
Achievement/Academic skills	Academic deficits and placement in special education common
Emotional/Behavioral functioning	Externalizing problems, eating disorders, depression

working memory when metabolic control was established (Knight et al., 2009). Fewer mood-related symptoms were reported (parent, teacher, and self-report), and fewer behavioral problems were noted (parent reports) as well. Thus, children with Type 1 diabetes demonstrated significant improvements across areas of functioning once intervention was in place to improve metabolic control (Knight et al., 2009). This finding suggests that it is important to have some knowledge of the child's level of metabolic control over the previous months (i.e., as indicated by A1c levels) as well as current blood glucose levels when completing evaluations for children with diabetes.

Educational Implications

Lower academic achievement has been found in association with Type 1 diabetes; boys are at greater risk for learning problems than girls (C. S. Holmes, O'Brien, & Greer, 1995). Children with Type 1 diabetes are at risk for high rates of school absenteeism; as such, the interruptions in education, whether due to lack of control, clinic appointments, glucose checks, or other reasons, may result in lower achievement (Ryan, Longstreet, & Morrow, 1985). Academic and behavioral problems also can occur in youth with poor metabolic control. Children in poor control performed significantly worse on reading scores, grade point average, and core total scores (composite of math, reading, and language) than those with good control (McCarthy, Lindgren, Mengeling, Tsalikian, & Engvall, 2003). Findings also indicated that hospitalizations due to poor control negatively affected academic performance. In academic areas, children with Type 1 diabetes are likely to be deficient in both reading and math areas (J. F. Rovet, Ehrlich, & Hoppe, 1988; Ryan et al., 1985), resulting in special education placement due to specific learning disability (J. F. Rovet, Ehrlich, Czuchta, & Akler, 1993). Placement in special education services also is associated with poorer metabolic control and earlier age of onset (C. S. Holmes et al., 1999).

Psychological Implications

In addition to academic issues, children with Type 1 diabetes also are at risk for psychological problems, with 33.3% of adolescents with Type 1 diagnosed with a psychiatric disorder (Kovacs, Goldston, Obrosky, & Bonar, 1997). The comorbidity of diabetes and depression in children and adolescents is a significant problem, affecting children and adolescents with diabetes about two to three times more, respectively, than those without diabetes (Grey, Whittemore, & Tamborlane, 2002). There seems be a higher risk of depression in girls with diabetes than boys (Hood et al., 2006; Lawrence et al., 2006). Possibly as a result of weight gain associated with initiation of insulin treatment, dietary restraints, and potential for insulin underdosing or omission, eating disorders or subthreshold behaviors associated with eating disorders are about twice as common in adolescents with Type 1 diabetes (J. M. Jones, Lawson, Daneman, Olmsted, & Rodin, 2000; Rodin et al., 2002). Even at subthreshold levels, this is a concern because of the effect these behaviors have on metabolic control. Incidence of eating disorder in conjunction with diabetes was correlated with level of family dysfunction (Rodin et al., 2002).

The occurrence of behavior problems is associated with higher-than-normal blood glucose levels as would occur with poor metabolic control (Valdovinos & Weyand, 2006). Further, poor metabolic control (i.e., blood sugar control) in youth with diabetes and depression may be associated with both physiologic and behavioral factors, since depression may make adherence to the diabetes care regimen more difficult; the hypersecretion of cortisol may impair the body's response to insulin (Grey et al., 2002). Many youth with Type 1 diabetes reportedly do not have more behavior problems than their healthy counterparts (Duke et al., 2008; B. J. Leonard, Jang, Savik, Plumbo, & Christensen, 2002); however, those in poor control may have more behavior problems, particularly externalizing problems (B. J. Leonard et al., 2002).

Long-term prognosis depends on lifetime metabolic control. Results of the Diabetes Control and Complication Trial (Diabetes Control and Complication Trial Research Group, 1993) indicated that good metabolic control positively affected the progression of associated complications including retinopathy, nephropathy, and neuropathy. Specifically, lowering blood glucose levels reduced the risk of kidney disease by 50%, eye disease by 76%, and nerve disease by 60%. The group also found that better metabolic control slowed the progression of these diseases by at least 50%. These findings underscore the need for early identification as well as early management of blood glucose concentrations.

Evidence-Based Intervention for Diabetes

The initial goal of treatment with Type 1 diabetes, as well as Type 2 diabetes, is to establish metabolic control (Santiprabhob et al., 2008). This is achieved through dietary control and insulin administered by injection or insulin pump as well as daily exercise (Brink, 1996; Karam, 1996; Nattrass & Hale, 1988). The level of insulin is determined based on blood glucose levels, diet, physical activity, and stress levels; individuals with diabetes need to monitor blood glucose levels throughout the day to avoid hypoglycemic or hyperglycemic episodes that can impair neurocognitive functioning (J. F. Rovet, 2000). The management regimen also includes monitoring of blood sugar levels three to five times per day. Level of care is defined as "intensive" when there is extensive involvement of professionals from varying disciplines, usually in the context of a monthly visit to a diabetes clinic (Wysocki et al., 2006). This is contrasted with "usual care" which is less intensive and requires more self-management skills and parental support. Not surprisingly, research suggests that psychological and behavioral variables moderate the outcomes for adolescents at differing levels of care. In effect, the more intensive involvement may be needed to maintain compliance and metabolic control in adolescents with low self-care autonomy but may not affect outcome for those with high self-care autonomy (Wysocki et al., 2006).

Compliance with monitoring, insulin injection, dietary control, and exercise are critical but not always achieved. For this reason, some research has investigated the use of behavioral and psychosocial procedures to improve compliance with the intent of improving metabolic control in children with Type 1 diabetes (Lasecki, Olympia, Clark, Jenson, & Heathfield, 2008; W. A. Plante & Lobato, 2008). Approaches have included individual and group formats with varying components, small numbers of participants, and varying outcome measures (see Table 17.2). Lasecki et al. explored the use of behavioral consultation and conjoint behavioral consultation; these approaches were found to lead to improved compliance and metabolic control, with particular target behaviors identified for each of the four children in the study. For both conditions, some form of reinforcement was used. Social validity in terms of parent and school nurse feedback was positive (Lasecki et al., 2008). Another study also examined the use of behavioral interventions in diabetes management, with results suggesting that behavioral interventions were moderately effective (mean ES = 0.33) (S. E. Hampson et al., 2000). Across studies, behavioral interventions were found to yield small to medium effects on management in children and adolescents ages 9 to 21 (Rodin, 2001). Additional research needs to be conducted for specific target behaviors (e.g., monitoring blood glucose levels, injecting of insulin when appropriate, eating properly, engaging in exercise). Group approaches, including those focusing on social skills, stress management, and family functioning have been studied, with some

Table 17.2 Evidence-Based Status for Interventions for Diabetes Type 1

Interventions	Target	Status
Regimen of insulin injections, glucose monitoring, dietary control, and daily exercise	Metabolic control	Positive practice (Diabetes Control and Complication Trial Research Group, 1993)
Islet transplant	Metabolic control	Emerging (Hathout, Lakey, & Shapiro, 2003)
Behavioral consultation/Conjoint behavioral consultation	Increasing compliance with prescribed regimen	Emerging (S. E. Hampson et al., 2000; Lasecki et al., 2008)
Behavioral interventions	Metabolic control	Emerging (Rodin, 2001)
Didactic psychoeducational groups	Improve coping and compliance through education	Minimal to no effect (W. A. Plante & Lobato, 2008)
Diabetes skills practice groups	Diabetes self-management	Inconclusive (W. A. Plante & Lobato, 2008)
Psychosocial groups	Family functioning and metabolic control	Inconclusive to no effect (W. A. Plante & Lobato, 2008)
Psychosocial groups	Social skills and metabolic control	Inconclusive to no effect (W. A. Plante & Lobato, 2008)
Psychosocial groups	Stress management and metabolic control	Inconclusive to no effect (W. A. Plante & Lobato, 2008)
Coping skills training	Metabolic control, psychosocial outcome	Emerging (M. Davidson, Boland, & Grey, 1997; Grey, Boland, Davidson, & Tamborlane, 1999)

improvements noted in adherence and overall relationships but minimal changes to metabolic control (W. A. Plante & Lobato, 2008).

One area of support that is vital to diabetes management for children and adolescents is that of the family (Hanson, Henggeler, & Burghen, 1987). Children and adolescents need help and support from their family, specifically parents, to manage and cope with their diabetes. Younger children especially need assistance from the family, as they are not able to perform as many of the diabetes management tasks. Although there is some indication of a tendency to try to shift responsibility to the child in early adolescence, research supports shared responsibility for diabetes self-care through middle adolescence (Helgeson, Reynolds, Siminierio, Escobar, & Becker, 2007). Family relationships and interactions involving diabetes management are especially important during adolescence, when metabolic control tends to worsen; in addition, studies suggest that there is an association between parenting style and metabolic control (Duke et al., 2008; Hanson et al., 1987). Metabolic control in adolescence is affected by the reciprocal relationship among the physiological effects of diabetes, the physiological effects of puberty, and developmental and psychosocial variables.

One area of intervention that often is neglected is ensuring that teachers of children with Type 1 diabetes understand that some of their difficulties may be due to the diabetes and that they can recognize mild hypoglycemic or hyperglycemic episodes (Wodrich & Cunningham, 2008). In particular, it may be helpful if the child's teacher can identify the child's highs and lows, with modifications to scheduling to accommodate the variability. For example, it may be helpful to schedule more challenging tasks at those times of the day when a child's functioning is better (Wodrich & Cunningham, 2008). For those children with fine motor problems that affect their handwriting, it may be appropriate to allow them to respond verbally or provide some alternative format that limits writing requirements; use of a computer to complete writing assignments may be a viable alternative as well (Wodrich & Cunningham, 2008). For children with decreased processing speed, it also may be appropriate to adjust time constraints or decrease the number of items to be completed.

CASE STUDY: SAM—TYPE 1 DIABETES

The next report is from a hospital-based clinic. Identifying information, such as child and family name, teacher or physician name, and school information, has been altered or fictionalized to protect confidentiality.

Reason for Referral

Sam is a 17-year-old Caucasian male who was referred for evaluation by his primary care physician due to concerns regarding increasing problems with memory and mood swings, which appear to be negatively impacting his health care practices and ability to maintain adequate regulation of his blood sugar.

Assessment Procedures

In order to gain historical information about Sam, multiple sources of information were consulted. His father provided comprehensive medical and educational records. Interviews were conducted individually and collaboratively with Sam and his father to gain additional information about Sam's current level of functioning. Direct information from teachers was unavailable as the evaluation was conducted during the summer. Additionally, these assessment measures were utilized during the comprehensive neuropsychological evaluation:

Clinical interview (parent)
Behavioral observations
Wechsler Adult Intelligence Scale, Third Edition (WAIS-III)
Woodcock-Johnson Tests of Achievement, Third Edition (WJ III)
Delis-Kaplan Executive Function System (D-KEFS)
Wechsler Memory Scale, Third Edition (WMS-III)
California Verbal Learning Test, Second Edition (CVLT-II)
Behavior Assessment System for Children, Second Edition (BASC-2; Parent and Self-Report)
Behavior Rating Inventory of Executive Function (BRIEF; Parent Report)

Background Information

Home Environment

Sam lives in a small town with his father, stepmother, and half sister (Ella); Sam's father and stepmother were married when Sam was 4 years old, and both are in good general health. Sam's father is a college graduate and works as a sales professional. His stepmother also completed college and owns an interior design business. Their daughter, Ella, is 10 years old and in good health. She recently completed the fifth grade, is described as a "star student," and is very active in Girl Scouts and a local soccer club.

Sam's father and his biological mother were never married. Sam lived with his mother during his infancy and toddler periods. Following a litigious custody hearing, his father was provided with primary physical and legal custody of Sam when he was 5 years old. Sam's biological mother lives approximately 20 miles away and has only sporadic contact with Sam. She has another son (Joey, 7 years old) who lives with her. According to records and reports from Sam's father, his mother is in good medical health, despite a history of substance abuse and undiagnosed emotional difficulties. She completed high school and works at a local convenience store. Joey is in the second grade and in good health but is reportedly demonstrating elevated levels of hyperactivity and aggression at school; Sam's father reported that he has heard that Joey is being evaluated by the school for possible Attention-Deficit/Hyperactivity Disorder (ADHD). In addition to the aforementioned psychiatric histories, there is also a history of bipolar disorder within the extended family. There are no known medical or learning disorders within the family history.

Medical and Developmental History

Sam's father provided information about Sam's gestational, developmental, and medical history. The pregnancy with Sam was reportedly without complications, and he was born at normal gestational age via normal vertex procedure, weighing 6 pounds 14 ounces. He did not experience any neonatal difficulties and was described as an "easy" baby. Sam achieved language and motor developmental milestones at appropriate ages, with independent walking occurring the day after his first birthday. He began using single words at 9 months of age. Progression of development occurred normally, and Sam was described as a bright and curious child.

Besides the normal childhood illnesses and infrequent ear infections, Sam's medical history was rather uneventful until he reached 12 years of age, at which time he was diagnosed with Type 1 diabetes (diabetes mellitus). Since that time, he has had several episodes of impaired consciousness due to low blood sugar. In fact, when he was 15 years old, he lost consciousness and fell to the floor, hitting his head on a table in the process. Magnetic resonance imaging (MRI) of his brain was reportedly normal, but after this episode he complained of problems with learning new information. Sam has been hospitalized on two other occasions due to poor compliance with his diabetes management. The most recent of these hospitalizations occurred approximately one month prior to the present neuropsychological evaluation. Upon transport to the local pediatric medical center, Sam admitted that he had not checked his blood sugar for approximately two weeks, and he had not been consistent with his insulin injections that were required twice daily following checks of his blood sugar. During this time, Sam had run away from his father's house and was reportedly staying with friends or sleeping in his car.

Educational Background

Sam recently completed 11th grade; he has never been retained nor has he received special education services. For the past two years, he has received 504 accommodations for his "memory loss." Although he has demonstrated a high level academic achievement based on previous evaluation in ninth grade (Wechsler Individual Achievement Test Reading, 148; Mathematics, 133; Language, 135; and Total 146), Sam has difficulty staying organized, completing his work, and turning in his work. He shared that he has difficulty maintaining his motivation and had many missing assignments over the past year because he did not complete them or could not find them to turn in. As a result, his grades often do not reflect his high academic ability. After completing high school, Sam plans on attending a technical school in order to learn to how to be a live sound technician; he shared that he wants to own his own record label.

Psychosocial History

With regard to school behavior, Sam was suspended for breaking the glass in a vending machine by throwing a rock against it in eighth grade. In tenth grade, he was suspended for "mooning" a school bus. He reportedly spent several days in in-school suspension in high school after fighting with another student. Difficulty with noncompliance and aggression are evident to a lesser degree at home. However, additional concerns of hyperactivity, impulsivity, and inattention were noted. Mr. Holiday shared that Sam often talks excessively, has boundless energy, poor judgment, and is easily frustrated. He also is reported to have a low mood and demonstrate withdrawal. Sam has participated in psychotherapy off and on since the eighth grade. He is receiving venlafaxine hydrochloride (Effexor) at the present time, and Mr. Holiday reported that it seems to have a calming effect. Specifically, Sam reported that he is not nearly as irritable and short-tempered with his friends when he is receiving his medication. He stated that he has headaches if he does not take his medication.

With regard to risky behaviors, Sam admitted to illegally taking prescription drugs in the past. His father and stepmother reportedly were concerned about drug use (i.e., huffing), but all drug tests have returned negative. He admitted to a general lack of concern for his health. That is, Sam admitted to piercing several body parts with a safety pin or syringe following use of a topical analgesic he had obtained. Shortly after the completion of 11th grade after he was visiting his mother, he did not return home for nearly two weeks. He has received several speeding tickets over the past 6 months, and he also has been involved in two motor vehicle collisions that were determined to be the result of his carelessness.

With regard to social skills, his stepmother reported that Sam always seeks friendships with younger adolescents. Sam shared that he is dating several girls but is not sexually promiscuous. He previously had a girlfriend who reportedly remains his friend. He admitted to losing friends when he has lied to them in the past. With regard to family relationships, Sam reported that he gets along with his father and stepmother "OK" and shared that they are helping with his medical routine.

Sam is currently employed at a local music store, where he began working approximately two weeks ago. He previously worked at a fast food restaurant, where Sam shared that he got along well with his coworkers. After working there for nearly one year, Sam reported that one day he was feeling overwhelmed and simply walked off the job.

Behavioral Observations

Sam was accompanied by his father to the assessment. He was casually dressed and well groomed. He is appropriate in weight and height for his age. When the psychologist first introduced herself to Sam and his father, he responded appropriately. Rapport was easy to develop and maintain throughout the evaluation. Sam demonstrated adequate effort on all tasks, even on tasks he perceived as difficult (e.g., memory).

Sam's mood was appropriate for the evaluation, and he demonstrated mood-congruent affect. He engaged the psychologist in some spontaneous conversation. He did not appear to have difficulty answering questions or understanding instructions or directions and rarely requested repetition. Sam did not demonstrate any articulation or phonetic errors, substitutions, or dysfluencies. He did not demonstrate difficulty with sustained attention and concentration and exhibited good behavioral inhibition; however, he was somewhat restless, often shaking his leg during the evaluation. With regard to motor skills, Sam ambulated independently without any noticeable difficulty or need for assistance. He used his right hand for writing and drawing and demonstrated a mature tripod pencil grip. Overall, Sam demonstrated adequate rates of attention/concentration, task perseverance, cooperation, and motivation. Therefore, the next test results should be considered a valid estimate of Sam's current neuropsychological functioning.

Assessment

Cognitive and Neuropsychological Functioning

The results of neuropsychological evaluation indicate that Sam currently is functioning within the high-average range of general intellectual ability as measured by the Wechsler Adult Intelligence Scale, Third Edition (WAIS-III), with significant strengths on tasks requiring nonverbal reasoning skills. Relative weaknesses were noted in areas measuring his auditory working memory and cognitive processing speed. Sam's standard scores on the cognitive measure are listed in Table 17.3.

On tasks measuring Sam's executive functioning skills, he generally demonstrated average or better skills (see specific scores in Table 17.3). Specifically, he performed in the average range on tasks measuring his verbal fluency skills and in the average to high-average range on rapid naming tasks that assessed his cognitive inhibition. His nonverbal sequencing, processing speed, and cognitive flexibility fell in the high-average to superior range.

Table 17.3 Psychometric Summary for Sam

	Scaled Score	Standard Score
Wechsler Adult Intelligence Scale, Third Edition (WAIS-III)		
Full Scale IQ		106
General Intellectual Ability		118
Verbal IQ		101
Performance IQ		111
Verbal Comprehension Index		110
Vocabulary	11	
Similarities	11	
Information	14	
Comprehension	11	
Perceptual Reasoning Index		123
Picture Completion	15	
Block Design	12	
Matrix Reasoning	14	
Picture Arrangement	11	
Working Memory Index		86
Arithmetic	7	
Digit Span	8	
Letter-Number Sequencing	8	
Processing Speed Index		88
Digit Symbol-Coding	7	
Symbol Search	9	
Delis-Kaplan Executive Function System (D-KEFS)		
Trail Making Test		
Visual Scanning	11	
Number Sequencing	13	
Letter Sequencing	14	
Number-Letter Sequencing	14	
Motor Speed	12	
Verbal Fluency Test		
Letter Fluency	9	
Category Fluency	10	
Category Switching Total	10	
Color-Word Interference		
Color Naming	11	
Word Reading	12	
Inhibition	12	
Inhibition/Switching	12	
Tower		
Total Achievement Score	10	
Mean First-Move Time	12	
Time-Per-Move Ratio	11	
Move Accuracy Ratio	1	
Rule-Violations-Per-Item Ratio	10	
Behavior Rating Inventory of Executive Function (BRIEF), Parent Form		

(continued)

Table 17.3 *(Continued)*

	T Score	
Clinical Scales		
Inhibit	97	
Shift	58	
Emotional Control	67	
Initiate	76	
Working Memory	85	
Plan/Organize	70	
Organization of Materials	63	
Monitor	68	
Behavioral Regulation Index	78	
Metacognition Index	75	
General Executive Composite	78	
Wechsler Memory Scales, Third Edition (WMS-III)		
	Scaled Score	
Logical Memory		
I Recall	3	
II Recall	5	
Faces		
I Recognition	12	
II Recognition	12	
California Verbal Learning Test, Second Edition (CVLT-II)		
	T Score	
List A Trial 1	45	
List A Trial 5	35	
List A Trials 1–5	41	
List B Free Recall	35	
List A Short-Delay Free Recall	35	
List A Short-Delay Cued Recall	40	
List A Long-Delay Free Recall	35	
List A Long-Delay Cued Recall	45	
Learning Slope	40	
Perseverations	45	
Intrusions	50	
Correct Recognition Hits	40	
False Positives	55	
Woodcock-Johnson Tests of Achievement, Third Edition (WJ III)		
		Standard Score
Letter-Word Identification		127
Reading Fluency		96
Calculation		109
Math Fluency		95
Spelling		97
Writing Fluency		99
Passage Comprehension		116
Applied Problems		112
Writing Samples		91

(continued)

Table 17.3 *(Continued)*

Behavior Assessment System for Children, Second Edition (BASC-2), Self-Report	
	T Score
Clinical Scales	
Attitude to School	42
Attitude to Teachers	39
Sensation Seeking	44
Atypicality	45
Locus of Control	37
Social Stress	40
Anxiety	48
Depression	40
Sense of Inadequacy	44
Somatization	44
Attention Problems	63
Hyperactivity	69
Adaptive Scales	
Relations with Parents	50
Interpersonal Relations	59
Self-Esteem	60
Self-Reliance	33
Composites	
School Problems	39
Internalizing Problems	40
Inattention/Hyperactivity	68
Emotional Symptoms Index	45
Personal Adjustment	51
Behavior Assessment System for Children, Second Edition (BASC-2), Parent Rating Scales (Father)	
	T Score
Clinical Scales	
Hyperactivity	80
Aggression	55
Conduct Problems	99
Anxiety	60
Depression	71
Somatization	65
Atypicality	104
Withdrawal	72
Attention Problems	83
Adaptive Scales	
Adaptability	47
Social Skills	33
Leadership	30
Activities of Daily Living	20
Functional Communication	27
Composites	
Externalizing Problems	81
Internalizing Problems	69
Behavioral Symptoms Index	86
Adaptive Skills	28

Sam also was administered a Tower task that measures an individual's ability to quickly and efficiently solve novel tasks. On this task, Sam had a high-average first-move time, indicating that he initiated problem solving slightly faster than others his age. He also demonstrated an average time-per-move ratio, taking the same amount of time to complete each task as others his age. Overall, Sam completed each task correctly, but not always within the time limit. Although he did not incur any rule violations, his move accuracy fell in the severely impaired range, suggesting inefficient problem solving and haphazard placement of the disks despite arriving at the correct result in the end.

Furthermore, Mr. Holiday completed a questionnaire detailing his perceptions of Sam's executive functioning abilities; his responses were not overly negative or inconsistent, resulting in a valid profile. Based on Mr. Holiday's responses, he has significant difficulties with Sam's ability to inhibit impulsive responses, control his emotions, initiate problem solving or activity, sustain working memory, plan and organize problem-solving approaches, and monitor his behavior. Mr. Holiday has mild concerns with Sam's ability to organize his environment, but he did not note difficulties with Sam's ability to adjust to changes. Based on another questionnaire that was completed by Sam and Mr. Holiday, Sam admitted mild concerns, and Mr. Holiday reported significant concerns, with his ability to regulate his activity level and sustain attention.

Analysis of Sam's performance on the Wechsler Memory Scale, Third Edition (WMS-III; see results in Table 17.3) indicates that, at the present time, he is exhibiting generally average ability to learn and recall visual information. When presented with photographs of faces to remember, he performed in the high-average range after their initial presentation and after a 30-minute delay. He correctly recognized the same number of faces during the immediate and delayed trials, indicating good retention of information he originally learned.

In contrast to Sam's average visual learning and memory skills, however, he exhibited difficulty with learning and remembering complex auditory information. Specifically, when two stories were read to him and he was asked to repeat each story immediately after it was read, Sam performed in the mildly impaired range. When the second story was read to him a second time, he increased his learning very slightly, obtaining a learning slope in the borderline range. Approximately 30 minutes later, he performed in the borderline range when asked to recall each story. Although he did not require a prompt about either of the stories, Sam retained slightly less information after the delay, suggesting that practice and repetition may be necessary to help him encode the information. He also was asked to answer yes/no questions about the stories. Of the five questions he answered incorrectly, he had not previously provided the correct information, suggesting that he had not originally encoded it.

Sam also was asked to learn a list of 16 words. He recalled 6 words of the list after it was read to him the first time, obtaining a score in the average range and suggesting appropriate initial auditory attention. After the list was read to him five times and he had the opportunity to recall the words after each trial, he demonstrated a low-average learning slope, reaching a learning plateau somewhat more quickly than others his age. When presented with a second word list, he recalled only 3 words (borderline range), exhibiting greater than expected vulnerability to proactive interference (i.e., previous learning interferes with new learning). When asked to recall the first list after he was presented with the second list and again after a 20-minute delay, he recalled 8 words each time, which is in the borderline range. Compared to his recall of 10 words during Trial 5, Sam demonstrated an expected amount of retroactive interference (i.e., learning new information interferes with recall of old information). When given semantic cues to help him cluster his answers, Sam recalled more words than he was able to recall during free recall tasks. Furthermore, when given the opportunity to recognize words from the list among distracters, he performed in the low-average range, identifying 14 of the 16 words as part of the original list; he misidentified two nontargets, which is in the average range. An overview of Sam's performance on this test can be found in Table 17.3.

Academic Functioning

The Woodcock-Johnson Tests of Achievement, Third Edition (WJ III) was administered as a measure of academic achievement. Based on his performance, Sam appears to have well-developed reading and math skills, with relative weaknesses in writing. However, his level of academic achievement is generally consistent with his measured intellectual skills. Sam's standard scores on the WJ-III subtests are listed in Table 17.3.

Social-Emotional and Behavioral Functioning

Sam and his father each completed a questionnaire to gain additional information about Sam's emotional and behavioral functioning. There are quite diverse results. That is, Sam denied the presence of any clinically significant concerns. Only mild concerns with attention problems and hyperactivity were noted, in addition to somewhat lower levels of self-reliance. Conversely, his father's responses were excessively negative albeit consistent. However, this level of concern was corroborated by information provided during the clinical interview, and the level of concern noted in the profile should be considered a valid indicator of Mr. Holiday's perception of Sam's current functioning. Generally, Mr. Holiday indicated diffuse dysfunction in the domains of externalizing behaviors (i.e., hyperactivity, conduct problems), internalizing problems (i.e., anxiety, depression, somatization), and other behavioral symptoms (i.e., withdrawal, atypical behaviors, attention problems). Additionally, Mr. Holiday expressed concern with multiple areas of his son's adaptive functioning, including his social skills, leadership abilities, daily living skills, and communication skills. A review of the profiles obtained by Sam and his father can be seen in Table 17.3.

Summary and Diagnostic Impressions

Based on the current neuropsychological evaluation, Sam's general intellectual ability was in the above-average range. His profile was mostly consistent, with select areas of weakness in auditory memory and efficiency of problem solving. He also performed in the low-average or average range in many areas, including processing speed, working memory, and verbal fluency; further, significant concerns were reported with emotional and behavioral functioning.

Due to the moderating effect that poorly managed diabetes can play on an individual's daily functioning, especially with regard to emotional and behavioral regulation, it is difficult to make any definite diagnoses of a mood disorder at the present time. Even if these medical conditions were not interfering with Sam's current presentation, a diagnosis such as bipolar disorder would not be appropriate at this time, as there does not appear to be any history of a manic or a major depressive episode. The behaviors described by Sam and his father appear to be hypomanic in nature. Also, given the presence of bipolar disorder in his family, Sam is more at risk for developing this disorder. Given his history of risky and somewhat reckless behaviors, including use of illicit substances, Sam may cause himself to fall into a manic or depressive episode if illicit substances are used at any time. Use of substances also may cause him to demonstrate memory difficulties and reduced cognitive efficiency. All of these issues should be considered and reevaluated after a time during which Sam demonstrates daily compliance with his medical routine, especially with regard to the monitoring of his blood sugar and consistent use of insulin. After a period during which Sam is medically stable, perhaps six months, reconsideration of diagnostic issues should be completed by a licensed professional (i.e., psychologist, psychiatrist).

Recommendations

Psychological Implications

Consideration of Sam's current psychological functioning is the primary issue at the present time. Stabilization of his mood is important to facilitate not only better emotional coping but also to improve compliance with his medical regimen. As a result, these recommendations are offered:

- Consultation and consideration of Sam's psychiatric medication regimen should be done immediately with an adolescent psychiatrist who can consult with Sam's primary endocrinologist. Although Sam reported that the Effexor seems to regulate his moods somewhat, adding to this or replacing with another medication may help relieve some of the other concerns, including his tendency toward hypomanic periods.
- Because of his significant medical history, Sam may find himself feeling different from other adolescents his age, which may result in emotional difficulties, including depression and anxiety, and externalizing behaviors, such as aggression and conduct problems. Participation in individual psychotherapy with a pediatric psychologist knowledgeable about diabetes is highly recommended.

Educational Implications

Given the impact that Sam's current level of functioning may have on his educational performance, provision of additional accommodations and modifications may be necessary. Although 504 accommodations may be sufficient to provide him the necessary supports, consideration of special education services may be required. Some of the most salient recommendations to benefit Sam's educational performance include:

- Designing the right studying environment is very important. The environment should be structured so as to reduce distracting stimuli. Studying in a public place (i.e., library, bookstore) is not recommended. Turning off the radio and television will be important.
- Make use of visual information as much as possible to compensate for weaknesses in auditory memory. Using encoding strategies, such as mnemonics, chunking, and visual imagery, would be helpful. Repetition and practice, spanned over numerous days, when learning new material would enable Sam to make the most of his memory skills. Massed practice (i.e., cramming) will not be helpful. When learning multiple chunks of information, it is extremely important to present small chunks of information with plenty of time between presentations so as not to reduce his ability to recall old or newly learned information.

- It also would be pertinent not to overwhelm Sam by introducing too much information at once and to provide him with the context of the material before it is presented. When newly presented information is complex and incorporates a variety of modalities, it will be important to reduce the complexity of the information. For instance, when he is learning about a historical event, he should group information according to area. For example, when learning about the Civil War, Sam should group the important battles together, listing the important people and dates associated with each one.
- Sam needs to be encouraged to take time to prepare a task, especially a multistep task, prior to attempting it. It might be helpful to write out the steps before attempting the task or to review an already made list. Brainstorming ideas for a report or other written work also would be helpful. This process will give him time to think through the process of completing such tasks. As he becomes more independent in monitoring his own behavior, his parents can incrementally remove support and increase demands. Sam could have good organizational skills and planning if he is not pressured by time constraints and is encouraged to be accurate in exchange for quickness.

Further Discussion of Case Study

The case of Sam elucidates the often very complex interaction between psychological functioning and diabetes management. Poor management of diabetes can indeed lead to mood fluctuations and aberrant behavior, even mimicking very significant mood disorders such as bipolar disorder; however, children and adolescents may have primary mood, anxiety, or behavior disorders that are further complicated by poor compliance with the medical regimen for diabetes. Compliance issues are especially salient with adolescents, who may be reluctant to adhere to treatment if procedures interfere with social functioning or make them appear "different" from their peers. In general, clinicians should respect these issues and consult with more seasoned colleagues and experts in adolescent endocrinology issues in order to provide a comprehensive and coherent assessment of the individual's functioning.

PHENYLKETONURIA

Definition

Phenylketonuria (PKU) is a genetic error or mutation that affects the individual's ability to break down phenylalanine (Phe) due to the reduced or absent phenylalanine hydroxylase (PAH; Gassió et al., 2008). PAH has been mapped to chromosome 12; PKU is then a genetic disorder. When this gene is defective, a rise in the essential amino acid Phe occurs. The result is a buildup of Phe as well as a decrease in tyrosine, a substance that is normally a by-product of the breakdown of Phe in tissues (Scriver, Kaufman, Eisensmith, & Woo, 2001). Newborn screening programs have been proactive in identifying individuals with PKU; this has resulted in early treatment and prevented mental retardation in a majority of cases (DeRoche & Welsh, 2008). Advances in genetic testing have identified subcategories of individuals who are carriers and who may experience lesser effects, but these individuals generally are not studied to the extent as those presenting with classical PKU.

Infants with PKU appear normal at birth; many have blue eyes and fairer hair and skin than other family members. If untreated, within the first few weeks the infant may begin to show neurologic disturbances, such as epilepsy. By 3 to 6 months, the infant may begin to lose interest in surroundings; by 1 year of age, the infant is developmentally delayed and exhibits other symptoms (Sarkissian, Gámez, & Scriver, 2009). When untreated, PKU can manifest with mental retardation, eczema, seizures, spastic reflexes, and muscle stiffness. In addition, the child may have an awkward gait, motor deficits, behavioral problems, limited to no language abilities, lack of interest in surroundings, self-abusive behaviors (e.g., head banging), and incessant moaning. Childhood autism is often prominent. With classical and untreated PKU, skeletal changes include a small head, small stature, and flat feet; there is a characteristic musky odor to the skin and urine.

Incidence

One of the most common genetic disorders that potentially leads to mental retardation, PKU affects 1 in 10,000 to 20,000 live births (Harding, 2008; Stanbury, Wyndgaarden, & Friedrickson, 1983). PKU affects males and females equally. PKU is fairly common among individuals of European descent with its widespread presence explained by human migration; however, it is very rare among individuals of African descent (Kozák et al., 1997).

Etiology

PKU is an autosomal recessive disorder; a person only gets PKU when he or she inherits two copies of the mutated gene, one from each parent. Many mutations exist in the PAH gene; most children inherit two different mutations, which results in substantial genetic heterogeneity in those with PKU. Each mutation leads to an obstruction in the metabolism of phenylalanine, which is abundant in protein.

Neurological Correlates

Based on MRI of early-treated individuals with PKU, the cerebrum, corpus callosum, hippocampus, intracranial volume, and pons were significantly smaller in those with PKU as compared to a control group (Pfaendner et al., 2005). In contrast, the volume of the lateral ventricles was significantly larger in those individuals with PKU as compared to the control group. Largest differences were found in the pons, hippocampus, cerebrum, and corpus callosum. No significant differences were found for the basal ganglia, cerebellum, and thalamus. Further, no association was found between the volume of specific brain structures and metabolic control (Pfaendner et al., 2005). Untreated PKU is believed to result in decreased myelination and subsequent loss of white matter; research suggests that white matter abnormalities are present even when treatment is initiated early on (P. J. Anderson et al., 2007). White matter pathology is most likely to occur in the posterior periventricular region, frontal region, and subcortical regions. Functioning level of individuals with PKU is associated with white matter abnormalities that may be independent of metabolic control, particularly when white matter pathology extends into the frontal and subcortical regions (P. J. Anderson et al., 2007). At the same time, there is some indication that white matter abnormalities are at least partially reversible if diet is instituted and maintained (Cleary, Walter, Wraith, & Jenkins, 1995).

Course and Prognosis

Historically, PKU was associated with mental retardation, but this is not necessarily the case if treated early and continuously across the life span. Even with early identification, individuals with PKU differed significantly from controls on Full Scale IQ, processing speed, attention, inhibition, and motor control (Moyle, Fox, Arthur, Bynevelt, & Burnett, 2007). Children with untreated PKU often are diagnosed with autism as well as with developmental delay. In most studies, if treatment was delayed initially after the first 3 months of life, the child performed less well than those who were treated earlier. With early treatment, the prognosis is better, and individuals with PKU will demonstrate low average to average cognitive ability (A. Diamond, Prevor, Callender, & Druin, 1997; Scriver et al., 2001; Williamson, Dobson, & Koch, 1977). No direct correlation has been found between allele pattern and cognitive functioning (Ramus et al., 1993). Studies further suggest, however, that noncompliance with dietary restrictions is associated with cognitive decline in school-age children (Waisbren, Schnell, & Levy, 1980). In many neurocognitive domains, early-treated adolescents and adults with PKU function comparably to controls when Phe levels are maintained (Moyle et al., 2007). There are some indications that levels of Phe are related not only to neurocognitive functions but to other nutritional components, such as selenium (Gassió et al., 2008). Similarly, in a study of nine sibling pairs, findings included mental retardation, autistic features, microcephaly, tremor, hypotonia, and diminished reflexes; however, some differences between siblings were noted, suggesting factors beyond genotype that influence the neurologic outcome (Yalaz, Vanli, Yilmaz, Tokatli, & Anlar, 2006).

Neurocognitive Correlates

Motor and executive functions are identified frequently (A. Diamond et al., 1997; M. C. Welsh, Pennington, Ozonoff, Rouse, & McCabe, 1990), including deficits in attention (Gassió et al., 2008). Deficits include children's ability to retain information and use it for problem solving, planning, and sustained attention as well as in the integrative processing skills of reasoning, comprehension, and concept formation (DeRoche & Welsh, 2008). Children and adolescents with PKU demonstrated lower performance on several measures of executive function, including initiation of problem solving, concept formation, and reasoning (VanZutphen et al., 2007). Performance on executive function tasks requiring inhibitory control, cognitive flexibility, and set shifting decreased at higher Phe levels. Phe levels were correlated positively to age and were related inversely to dietary adherence (VanZutphen et al., 2007). Based on meta-analysis, small to moderate effects of PKU emerge on measures of cognitive ability, with moderate to large effect sizes for executive function components of planning and flexibility respectively (DeRoche & Welsh, 2008). Using event-related potentials (ERPs) and a visual go-no-go task, adults with PKU who had been continuously treated from birth manifested subtle impairments in early sensory processing of visually presented information as well as impairments in inhibitory functions (Moyle, Fox, Bynevelt, Arthur, & Burnett, 2006). In addition to executive function deficits, children with PKU have been found to evidence a slower cognitive tempo (Antshel & Waisbren, 2003).

Visual-motor deficits also are prevalent. Even early-treated children tend to have awkward pencil grips and poor handwriting. In particular, fine motor speed is diminished. Copying letters or figures is laborious, and it takes children with PKU longer to complete written or copying tasks. They also have notable difficulties with following of visual demonstrations, diagrams, and models as well as difficulties remembering objects in space. Visualization and abstract concepts that rely on visualization are challenging for them; for example, the number line in math class may be incomprehensible. Working memory and processing speed also may be impacted, with subtle differences noted when diet is not maintained into adulthood (Channon, Goodman, Zlotowitz, Mockler, & Lee, 2007). Neurocognitive functioning associated with PKU is summarized in Table 17.4.

Educational Correlates

When children with PKU have difficulties in school, it is invariably in math and likely is related to their visual-spatial and sequencing difficulties. One study documented a steady decline in math scores in both diet-continued and diet-discontinued children from 6 to 10 years of age (Waisbren et al., 1980). Another study found that mean IQ, reading, and spelling test scores improved between ages 6 and 10 for those children continuing on the diet; however, mean scores on arithmetic, language, and perceptual skills declined at a uniform rate regardless of dietary status for both groups (Fishler, Azen, Friedman, & Koch, 1989). By age 12, achievement scores in math fall again in 90% of the children with PKU. In contrast, decoding skills and spelling are usually strengths for children with PKU. As they become older (usually around fourth grade), difficulties in reading become apparent; this happens when demands for reading comprehension and application of rote skills begin. Even when treated, areas of abstract reasoning, executive function, and attention emerge as weaknesses (A. Diamond et al., 1997; Waisbren, Brown, de Sonneville, & Levy, 1994; M. Welsh & Pennington, 2000). Fourth grade also is when problems in executive functioning and sustained attention interfere with the acquisition of new knowledge and mastery of new skills for all children; with PKU, the deficits in these areas can cause problems in social studies and science classes. Finally, as children progress through the grades, there is increased written work and homework, which can overwhelm children with PKU due to their poor visual-motor skills. Overall, children with PKU present with more school problems than nonaffected peers, probably due to their neurocognitive deficits. The index of dietary control for the last 6 months yielded a close relationship with school performance (Gassió et al., 2005). Even children with PKU who maintain metabolic control are at risk for learning disabilities.

Table 17.4 Neuropsychological Deficits Associated with PKU

Global Domain	Phenotype
Cognition	With early treatment and dietary control, individuals with PKU demonstrate low-average to average cognitive ability
Auditory-linguistic/Language function	With early control, verbal abilities tend to be spared
Visual perception/Constructional praxis	Deficits in visual-perceptual and spatial functioning Also deficits in visual-motor areas, including handwriting
Learning and memory	Subtle deficits may be evident if diet not maintained into adulthood
Executive function	Generalized impairment in executive function
Attention/Concentration	Impaired attentional abilities
Processing speed	Subtle deficits may be evident if diet not maintained into adulthood
Achievement/Academic skills	Difficulties most likely to be in mathematics
Emotional/Behavioral functioning	High rates of self-mutilation, aggression, impulsivity, and psychosis

Psychosocial Correlates

Individuals with untreated PKU are some of the most difficult individuals to manage due to high rates of self-mutilation, aggression, impulsivity, and psychosis (Wacker et al., 1990). Research also suggests a more impulsive cognitive style among children with PKU (D. D. Davis, McIntyre, Murray, & Mims, 1986). With the dietary restrictions, stress in family functioning and relationships has also been explored. Results indicate that lifetime phenylalanine control and child social competence were related to family cohesion and adaptability; family cohesion also was related to cognitive performance (Reber, Kazak, & Himmelberg, 1987). Finally, there are some similarities between the problems exhibited by children with PKU and those with ADHD (Antshel & Waisbren, 2003).

Evidence-Based Intervention

The only cure for this disorder is a liver transplantation; however, this is generally not considered due to the high risk (Harding, 2008). The current recommended treatment for PKU includes a lifetime phenylalanine-restricted diet, a special nutritional formula, and medications. The diet is highly restricted. Individuals with PKU cannot eat any high-protein foods, such as meat, fish, milk, eggs, cheese, soy, most grains, sweets (chocolate) and nuts. Individuals with PKU can eat measured amounts of fruits and vegetables, special low-protein pastas, grains, breads, and cereals. Because they cannot get protein through food sources, the special formula used for individuals with PKU contains all the necessary nutrients (amino acids) in protein except for phenylalanine (MacDonald et al., 2004). Unfortunately, this formula has a distinctive taste and smell. Infants usually accept the formula without difficulties; children find it distasteful; adults deem it unpalatable. To bypass the distasteful component of the formula, some individuals get their formula through tube feedings. In addition to the formula and restrictive diet, individuals with PKU take numerous medications (M. Welsh & Pennington, 2000).

Some controversy has occurred with how long this treatment regimen should be continued (A. Diamond et al., 1997). For example, in the past, it was recommended or permitted to discontinue the diet at 5 to 6 years of age; this was then changed to some allowance to discontinue the diet when blood phenylalanine levels consistently exceeded 15 mg/dl, or at about 8 to 10 years of age. Then it was decided that it would be possible to discontinue the diet when there was no further decline in cognitive or motor functioning; this occurs at a median age of 20 years. Research, however, indicates that if metabolic control is variable throughout childhood, the individual tends to have poorer mental processing skills, slower reaction time, diminished achievement, and lower IQ. Cognitive ability (IQ) is related significantly to the average Phe control between birth and 14 years of age. Further, discontinuation of the restricted diet resulted in diminished IQ in a sizable proportion of children. For children and adults, diet resumption and maintaining metabolic control resulted in improved reaction time and concentration. Notably, the diet regimen is not without risks (Sitta et al., 2009). If overtreated with extreme limitation of protein intake, the result can be Phe depletion, and the child with PKU can experience significant growth retardation, lethargy, and even death.

Over the years, differing products have been developed to try to increase compliance. For example, PKU Express (Vitaflo) was a new low-volume (amino acids 72 g/100 g), low-carbohydrate, Phe-free protein substitute with added vitamins and minerals designed for people with PKU over 8 years of age (MacDonald et al., 2004). Although the product is dense, participants in the 2004 study described the smell and texture as the same as or worse than those of previous protein substitutes. Because of the issues with dietary adherence, there are ongoing efforts to develop viable cell-directed therapies (i.e., cell transplantation and gene therapy) for the treatment of PKU (Harding, 2008). Other new approaches are being explored as well, such as tetrahydrobiopterin (BH4) supplementation; these approaches need to be evaluated with regard to safety, efficacy, and expected outcomes (Burlina & Blau, 2009; Giovannini et al., 2007).

Increasing knowledge among family members and individuals with PKU also has been considered. A study of 71 individuals with PKU participated in a study related to educational resources (Durham-Shearer, Judd, Whelan, & Thomas, 2008). Most respondents were aware of dietary recommendations, although this did not always result in compliance. Education was provided, and there was a significant difference in the extent of change in knowledge score between baseline and 1 month in favor of the intervention group. Unfortunately, improved knowledge was not accompanied by improved compliance (Durham-Shearer et al., 2008). Because of the risks associated with poor dietary control, blood levels and metabolic control need to be monitored. Careful monitoring of neurocognitive status during infancy and school years also is recommended; there is a need to monitor specifically the status of executive function skills during the transition to, and during, adolescence (VanZutphen et al., 2007). Occupational therapy sometimes is recommended for these children due to their motor difficulties. With regard to poor communication and severe behavior problems, behavioral treatment targeting communicative responding and inappropriate behavior were both necessary for maximal control over difficult behavior and resulted in a change in behavior (Wacker et al., 1990). Those interventions with some research support are presented in Table 17.5. Notably, no studies were found that addressed interventions or accommodations for math and visual-perceptual difficulties of children with PKU.

Table 17.5 Evidence-Based Status for Interventions for PKU

Interventions	Target	Status
Regimen of dietary control, protein formula, and medications	Metabolic control	Promising practice (A. Diamond et al., 1997; MacDonald et al., 2004; M. Welsh & Pennington, 2000)
Tetrahydrobiopterin (BH4) supplementation	Metabolic control	Emerging (Burlina & Blau, 2009; Giovannini et al., 2007)
Educational programming	Increasing compliance	Ineffective (Durham-Shearer et al., 2008)
Behavioral approaches	Communication, Inappropriate behavior	Emerging (Wacker et al., 1990)

CASE STUDY: VINNIE—PKU

The next report is from a hospital-based clinic. Identifying information, such as child and family name, teacher or physician name, and school information, has been altered or fictionalized to protect confidentiality.

Reason for Referral

Vinnie is an 8-year-old boy with phenylketonuria (PKU). Due to recent onset of academic difficulty and disruptive behaviors in the classroom, coinciding with rising phenylalanine levels, he was referred for comprehensive evaluation of cognitive functioning by his geneticist.

Assessment Procedures

Review of records
Clinical interview
Behavior Assessment System for Children, Second Edition (BASC-2)
Behavior Rating Inventory of Executive Function (BRIEF)
California Verbal Learning Test—Children's Version (CVLT-C)
Conners' Continuous Performance Test, Second Edition (CCPT-II)
Delis-Kaplan Executive Function System (D-KEFS) selected subtests
Beery Developmental Test of Visual Motor Integration, Fifth Edition (DTVMI-V)
Neuropsychological Assessment, Second Edition (NEPSY-2; selected subtests)
Wechsler Intelligence Scale for Children, Fourth Edition (WISC-IV)
Woodcock-Johnson III Normative Update (WJ III NU), Tests of Academic Achievement

Background Information

Home Environment

Vinnie lives with his mother. He is the product of a full-term pregnancy that was complicated by hospitalization in the second trimester due to maternal fever, headaches, and pain. The pregnancy was otherwise uncomplicated, and there was no reported fetal exposure to alcohol or illicit drugs. Following a vaginal delivery, Vinnie was born weighing 6 pounds 7.5 oz. His neonatal course was characterized as smooth, and he was discharged from the hospital two days after his birth. Vinnie was diagnosed with PKU via newborn screening.

Motor Development

Vinnie acquired early gross motor milestones at typical times. He first sat unsupported around 6 months of age, crawled around 7 months of age, and took his first steps around 11 months of age. No subsequent concerns were reported for gross motor coordination, and Vinnie is skilled at a number of athletic activities. Toilet training was accomplished during the daytime around 3.5 years of age; he continues to have occasional bedwetting accidents. Vinnie had difficulty acquiring fine motor skills. He prefers the use of his right hand for most activities, and his handwriting is characterized as messy. He continues to need assistance when fastening clothes and is not yet able to tie shoelaces. Vinnie has never received occupational or physical therapy.

Language Development

Although Vinnie's mother could not recall the approximate ages when Vinnie acquired early language milestones, she reported that his early language development was typical (i.e., first words by 12 months of age and use of phrases by 24 months of age). No subsequent concerns were reported for problems with articulation or language pragmatics. Vinnie has never received speech/language therapy.

Activities of Daily Living/Adaptive Behavior

Vinnie requires assistance when completing some activities of daily living, including dressing or drying off after a bath. He is responsible for several household chores (i.e., cleaning his room, vacuuming, washing dishes), and he completes these tasks with reminders and assistance. No concerns were reported for sleep or appetite disturbance. Vinnie typically gets 9 to 10 hours of sleep per night. There are no reported problems with sleep onset, maintenance, or habitual, loud snoring. According to Vinnie's mother, he has a healthy appetite and responsibly complies with dietary restrictions associated with PKU.

Medical History

Medical history is positive for PKU that has reportedly been well controlled with dietary interventions. Phenylalanine (Phe) levels have generally ranged from 2.3 to 4.7 mg/dL (therapeutic goal = 3–6 mg/dL) in the past. He has been prescribed Phenex-1; he was then prescribed Phenex-2 (100g/day). Recently, Phe levels have been elevated (6.7 mg/dL in March, 11 mg/dL in May, and 16 mg/dL in June). His Phenex-2 was increased to 130 g/day. He is being followed by the genetics team to monitor his Phe levels frequently. Recent neurological evaluation was within normal limits.

Medical history is otherwise negative for major illness or injury, including seizures, traumatic brain injury, or hospitalizations. Vinnie has sustained minor injuries following minor accidents, including one requiring stitches on his forehead. No loss of consciousness or other sequelae were reported. Vinnie had several ear infections during infancy, and a set of pressure-equalization tubes were placed when he was 12 months of age. There is no history of asthma or allergies. Results of a vision and hearing screen conducted as part of his annual pediatric visit were within normal limits.

Educational History

Vinnie completed the kindergarten and first grade in a regular education classroom. Vinnie's mother reported that he made satisfactory progress acquiring early academic skills, and no concerns were reported by his teachers regarding inattention or disruptive behaviors in the classroom. There were no reported difficulties with the reading acquisition process. Vinnie was described as a B/C student. He has never been referred for psychoeducational assessment or received special education services. During the second grade, Vinnie evidenced increasing academic difficulties, and his teacher reported concern about inattention, "off-task" behaviors, and disruptive classroom behaviors. Retention in the second grade was considered; however, Vinnie was promoted to the third grade.

Currently, Vinnie is enrolled in the third grade, where he is served in a regular classroom. According to his teacher, Vinnie is performing on grade level in areas of basic reading skills, reading comprehension, arithmetic facts and concepts, and oral comprehension. In contrast, he demonstrates mild difficulty with reading fluency, written expression, and writing speed and efficiency. He also demonstrates mild difficulty retaining skills following school breaks. His teacher did not report any current concerns with disruptive behavior problems or social difficulties in the classroom.

Psychosocial History

There is no reported history of psychological diagnosis or intervention or traumatic exposure. Vinnie's mother expressed no concerns about his social relatedness; he makes and keeps friends with ease. Significant disruptive behavior problems were denied (i.e., 0 of 8 *Diagnostic and Statistical Manual of Mental Disorders*, Fourth Edition [*DSM*-IV] criteria for oppositional defiant disorder) as were significant symptoms of inattention, hyperactivity, and impulsivity (i.e., 2 of 9 *DSM-IV* criteria for inattention and 1 of 9 *DSM-IV* criteria for hyperactivity/impulsivity associated with attention deficit hyperactivity disorder). No concerns were reported for depression, anxiety, vocal or motor tics, or perceptual disturbance. Maternal family history is positive for depression; paternal family history is positive for ADHD.

Behavioral Observations

Vinnie was accompanied to this evaluation by his parents. He presented as a casually dressed, friendly child who was small in stature for his age. He willingly separated from his parents, accompanied the examiner to the testing room, and readily established rapport. During the structured evaluation, Vinnie evidenced adequate ability to focus and sustain his attention. Although he was mildly restless, frequently rubbing his eyes, playing with his fingers, or swinging his legs, his level of motor activity did not interfere with his performance during this evaluation. He was an eager conversational partner, frequently introducing and shifting topics with ease. In general, Vinnie was very cooperative, completed all tasks that were presented to him, and seemed to put forth his best effort. Thus, the results presented are deemed a valid and accurate estimate of his current level of cognitive functioning.

Assessment Results

Three types of scores describe Vinnie's performance on measures of cognitive functioning. The first type of score is called a standard score. Standard scores compare a child's performance with typical children his or her age. An average standard score is 100, with an average range of 90 to 110. The second type of score is a percentile (%ile). An average percentile score is 50, and the average range for percentile scores falls between 25 and 75. The third type of score is called a T-score, which has an average of 50 and an average range of 43 to 57.

Intellectual Functioning

Scores obtained on the Wechsler Intelligence Scale for Children, Fourth Edition (WISC-IV) during this evaluation placed Vinnie's current intellectual functioning in the low-average range (see Table 17.6). The range of Vinnie's cognitive abilities was captured by the composite scores. Regarding his language-related skills, his word knowledge, verbal reasoning, fund of verbal information, and knowledge of social conventions were in the low-average range (Verbal Comprehension Index Standard Score = 85). It should be noted that his performance in this domain ranged from borderline to average, and Vinnie demonstrated particular difficulty with verbal concept formation. When required to solve problems using nonverbal/abstract reasoning or constructional praxis, Vinnie's performance was in the average range (Perceptual Reasoning Index Standard Score = 96). On those subtests that required a sturdy working memory, or ability to "hold" information in mind for the purpose of multistep problem solving, Vinnie demonstrated average auditory working memory (Working Memory Index Standard Score = 94). Finally, psychomotor speed was mildly impaired (Processing Speed Index Standard Score = 75).

Table 17.6 Psychometric Summary for Vinnie

	Scaled Score	Standard Score
Wechsler Intelligence Scale for Children, Fourth Edition (WISC-IV)		
Full Scale IQ		84
Verbal Comprehension Index		85
Similarities	5	
Vocabulary	10	
Comprehension	7	
Information	9	
Perceptual Reasoning Index		96
Block Design	8	
Picture Concepts	9	
Matrix Reasoning	11	
Picture Completion	8	
Working Memory Index		94
Digit Span	8	
Letter-Number Sequencing	10	
Processing Speed Index		75
Coding	4	
Symbol Search	7	
Delis-Kaplan Executive Function System (D-KEFS)		
Trail Making Test		
Visual Scanning	12	
Number Sequencing	12	
Letter Sequencing	4	
Number-Letter Sequencing	9	
Motor Speed	10	
Verbal Fluency Test		
Letter Fluency	9	
Category Fluency	10	
Category Switching Total Correct	10	
Category Switching Total Accuracy	11	
Neuropsychological Assessment, Second Edition (NEPSY-2)		
Animal Sorting Total Correct Sorts	12	
Animal Sorting Combined Score	11	
Comprehension of Instructions Total Phonological	6	
Processing Total	9	
Speeded Naming—Time	7	
Speeded Naming Combined Score	5	
Memory for Faces Total Score	10	
Memory for Faces—Delayed	9	
Memory for Faces vs. Delayed Contrast	9	
Developmental Test of Visual-Motor Integration, Fifth Edition (DTVMI-V)		
Visual Motor Integration		97
Visual-Perception		98
Motor Coordination		98

(continued)

Table 17.6 *(Continued)*

California Verbal Learning Test—Children's Version (CVLT-C)	**T-Score**
List A Trial 1	45
List A Trial 5	35
List A Trials 1–5	39
List B Free Recall	50
List A Short-Delay Free Recall	45
List A Short-Delay Cued Recall	30
List A Long-Delay Free Recall	40
List A Long-Delay Cued Recall	30
Learning Slope	40
Correct Recognition Hits	45
False Positives	45
Behavior Rating Inventory of Executive (BRIEF), Parent Form	
Clinical Scales	
Inhibit	37
Shift	40
Emotional Control	47
Initiate	35
Working Memory	45
Plan/Organize	39
Organization of Materials	58
Monitor	44
Indices	
Behavioral Regulation Index	50
Metacognition Index	42
General Executive Composite	41
Behavior Rating Inventory of Executive (BRIEF), Teacher Form	
Clinical Scales	
Inhibit	46
Shift	42
Emotional Control	43
Initiate	44
Working Memory	45
Plan/Organize	42
Organization of Materials	42
Monitor	43
Indices	
Behavioral Regulation Index	43
Metacognition Index	43
General Executive Composite	42
Woodcock-Johnson Tests of Achievement, Third Edition (WJ III)	**Standard Score**
Letter-Word Identification	95
Reading Fluency	91
Calculation	89
Math Fluency	88
Spelling	101
Writing Fluency	84
Passage Comprehension	101
Applied Problems	93
Writing Samples	96

(continued)

Table 17.6 *(Continued)*

Behavior Assessment System for Children, Second Edition (BASC-2), Parent Report	**T-Score**
Clinical Scales	
Hyperactivity	47
Aggression	44
Conduct Problems	48
Anxiety	52
Depression	47
Somatization	42
Atypicality	44
Withdrawal	56
Attention Problems	45
Adaptive Scales	
Adaptability	50
Social Skills	54
Leadership	51
Activities of Daily Living	49
Functional Communication	47
Composites	
Externalizing Problems	46
Internalizing Problems	46
Behavioral Symptoms Index	46
Adaptive Skills	50
Behavior Assessment System for Children, Second Edition (BASC-2), Teacher Report	
Clinical Scales	
Hyperactivity	53
Aggression	43
Conduct Problems	47
Anxiety	42
Depression	42
Somatization	43
Atypicality	46
Withdrawal	39
Attention Problems	46
Learning Problems	60
Adaptive Scales	
Adaptability	64
Social Skills	61
Leadership	59
Study Skills	53
Functional Communication	57
Composites	
Externalizing Problems	48
Internalizing Problems	40
School Problems	49
Behavioral Symptoms Index	44
Adaptive Skills	60

Processing Speed

Processing speed is the ability to quickly and efficiently process simple or routine visual information without making errors. Speed of mental processing provides a foundation for more complex problem-solving skills, enabling the rapid switching of attentional resources between various sources of information. Structured assessment of Vinnie's processing speed revealed mildly impaired ability to process quickly and efficiently simple or routine visual information without making errors (WISC-IV Processing Speed Index Standard Score = 75).

Language Skills

In conversation, Vinnie's speech was fluent, with normal pace and prosody; results of language processing and development assessment are presented in Table 17.6. Auditory comprehension was observed to be grossly intact as he readily and accurately supplied a response to verbal directions. Structured assessment of receptive language-related skills revealed low-average ability to supply a nonverbal response (pointing) to increasingly difficult multistep instructions (NEPSY-2 Comprehension of Instructions SS = 80). Structured assessment of expressive language-related skills revealed average word knowledge and general fund of verbal information. Verbal reasoning was borderline, and knowledge of social conventions was low average, yielding an overall composite score in the low average range (WISC-IV Verbal Comprehension Index Standard Score = 85). Verbal fluency was average. Vinnie demonstrated evenly developed ability to automatically and efficiently retrieve linguistic information according to both phonemic (initial letter) and semantic (category) cues (D-KEFS Verbal Fluency Test, Letter Fluency SS = 95 and Category Fluency SS = 100).

Language-related skills are critically important for the reading acquisition process. In this regard, Vinnie demonstrated average phonological awareness, or understanding that individual units of sound comprise words (NEPSY-2 Phonological Processing SS = 95). Phonological awareness is critically important for reading acquisition. In contrast, on measures requiring automatic retrieval of linguistic information, Vinnie's performance was in the borderline range (NEPSY-2 Speeded Naming, Combined SS = 75). Qualitative analysis of his performance on this rapid-naming task revealed low-average naming speed and borderline naming accuracy (NEPSY-2 Speeded Naming, Completion Time SS = 85 versus Total Correct = 2nd–5th %ile rank). Rapid naming is requisite for reading fluency. Taken together, the basic linguistic skills requisite for reading fluency were weak for Vinnie (see Table 17.6).

Visual-Motor Functioning

Visual-spatial skills help Vinnie make sense of what he sees. These skills are necessary for completing patterns that are made up of parts, such as jigsaw puzzles. Structured assessment revealed average visual discrimination on the Developmental Test of Visual Motor Integration, Fifth Edition (DTVMI-V, Visual Perception SS = 98). Similarly, Vinnie demonstrated average perception of subtle visual detail (WISC-IV Picture Completion SS = 90) and high-average visual scanning (D-KEFS Trail Making Test, Visual Scanning SS = 110).

Vinnie used his right hand for graphomotor and constructional tasks. He evidenced an awkward extended-fingers pencil grip and poor pencil control. Qualitative analysis of his handwriting revealed large and poorly formed letters. Structured assessment revealed low-average fine motor control on a timed tracing task (DTVMI-V Motor Coordination

SS = 88). On a timed tracing task that placed fewer demands on fine motor precision, Vinnie demonstrated average psychomotor speed (D-KEFS Trail Making Test, Motor Speed SS = 100). When a motor component was added to visual-spatial tasks, such as block assembly or figure copying, Vinnie demonstrated average constructional praxis (WISC-IV Block Design SS = 90) and average visual-motor integration (DTVMI-V SS = 97).

Memory

Vinnie demonstrated average ability to learn and remember visual information that was presented in a social context (NEPSY-2 Memory for Faces, Total SS = 100). Following a time delay, he also demonstrated average ability to recall this contextualized visual information (NEPSY-2 Memory for Faces, Delayed SS = 95). Vinnie demonstrated low-average ability to learn and remember rote auditory/verbal information that was presented with repetition (CVLT-C List A Total Trials 1–5 T-score = 39). After a short time delay, Vinnie demonstrated average recall of the words from the list (CVLT-C List A Short-Delay Free Recall T-score = 45). Following a longer time delay, he demonstrated low-average recall of the words from the list (CVLT-C List A Long-Delay Free Recall T-score = 40). He recalled fewer words when provided with cues/reminders as compared to free recall (CVLT-C List A Long-Delay Cued Recall T-score = 30), suggesting that he has difficulty using semantic strategies to remember auditory/verbal information. In addition, his perseveration rate was significantly elevated (CVLT-C Perseverations T-score = 70), indicating that he is likely not self-monitoring during recall and, as a result, repeated many of the words (see Table 17.6).

Attention and Executive Function

Vinnie demonstrated adequate ability to focus and sustain his attention during this highly structured evaluation. As previously noted, he was mildly restless but responded readily and appropriately to redirection. Structured assessment revealed average focused auditory attention (WISC-IV Digit Span Forward SS = 95). His performance on a visual cancellation task revealed indicators of inattention (D-KEFS Trail Making Test, Visual Scanning: Omission Errors = 10th cumulative %ile rank) without significant impulsivity (D-KEFS Trail Making Test, Visual Scanning: Commission Errors = 100th cumulative %ile rank). Sustained visual attention varied from borderline to high average (D-KEFS Trail Making Test, Number Sequencing SS = 110, and Letter Sequencing SS = 70). His performance on the letter sequencing task was slowed by sequencing errors. On a computerized sustained vigilance task, in which he was required to inhibit a response to target stimuli, his performance better matched a clinical profile (CPT-II Clinical, Confidence Index = 92.0%). Moreover, his performance revealed indicators of inattention (CPT-II Omissions T-score = 63.28, Hit Reaction Time Standard Error T-score = 72.70, and Variability T-score = 67.74) and impulsivity (CPT-II Perseverations T-score = 66.27). His reaction times became slower and less consistent in response to longer interstimulus intervals (CPT-II Hit Reaction Time with Interstimulus Interval Change T-score = 71.93 and Hit Standard Error for Interstimulus Interval Change T-score = 65.77), suggesting that Vinnie's attention quickly wanes during prolonged, tedious tasks.

Executive function is a name for brain processes that guide, direct, and manage thinking, feeling, and behaving. Examples of executive functions include the ability to start and stop actions; plan and organize a means of solving a problem; shift problem-solving strategies flexibly when necessary; and monitor and evaluate behavior, emotion, and thoughts. Structured assessment revealed high-average nonverbal concept formation (NEPSY-2 Animal Sorting Total Correct Sorts SS = 110) but many rule violations (NEPSY-2 Animal

Sorting, Total Errors = 6th–10th %ile). He demonstrated average cognitive flexibility on a task that required alternation of two over-learned sequences (D-KEFS Trail Making Test, Number-Letter Sequencing SS = 95). On a verbal fluency task, he also demonstrated average cognitive flexibility (D-KEFS Verbal Fluency Test, Total Switching Accuracy SS = 105). Nonverbal/abstract reasoning was average (WISC-IV Matrix Reasoning SS = 105). On those subtests that required a sturdy working memory, or ability to "hold" information in mind for the purpose of multistep problem solving, Vinnie demonstrated average auditory working memory (WISC-IV Working Memory Scale SS = 94). In contrast, Vinnie demonstrated mildly impaired verbal concept formation (WISC-IV Similarities SS = 75).

Academic Achievement

In order to assess academic achievement, the Woodcock-Johnson III Normative Update, Tests of Academic Achievement (WJ III NU) were administered. On a standard administration of the WJ III NU, Vinnie demonstrated average single-word reading skills, which was commensurate with his average phonological awareness (NEPSY-2 Phonological Processing SS = 95). On a measure of reading fluency, in which he was required to determine the correctness of short sentences within a time limit, he demonstrated an average reading rate. Reading comprehension also was average and grade appropriate. Taken together, Vinnie's average basic reading skills and reading comprehension were generally commensurate with his verbal functioning (WISC-IV Verbal Comprehension Scale SS = 85).

Vinnie demonstrated average spelling skills, which were commensurate with his average phonological awareness (NEPSY-2 Phonological Processing SS = 95). On a measure of writing fluency, in which he was required to construct simple sentences using three target words within a time limit, he obtained a score in the low-average range. He demonstrated average written expression. Qualitative analysis of his written responses, which were not penalized for errors in spelling or punctuation, revealed grammatical errors and poor inferential thinking (e.g., supplying a missing sentence based on two provided sentences). In general, Vinnie's average spelling and writing skills were commensurate with his verbal functioning (WISC-IV Verbal Comprehension Index SS = 85).

Vinnie's math calculation skills were in the upper limits of the low-average range. Qualitative analysis of his written calculations revealed generally accurate completion of single-step addition and subtraction problems but difficulty on multistep problems involving carrying and borrowing. On a measure of math fluency, in which he was required to solve single-step math calculations within a time limit, he obtained a score in the low-average range. His errors on this task were suggestive of carelessness or inattention (i.e., adding instead of subtracting). Finally, Vinnie demonstrated average ability to apply basic math facts within the context of word problems. Taken together, Vinnie's low-average math calculation skills and average mathematics reasoning were generally commensurate with his average nonverbal/abstract reasoning skills (WISC-IV Perceptual Reasoning Index SS = 96).

Behavior Rating Scales

In order to assess Vinnie's social/emotional and behavioral functioning, his mother and teacher completed the Behavior Assessment System for Children, Second Edition (BASC-2), a broad-band measure of child behavior problems. Inspection of the validity scales indicated valid response patterns for both informants. The results of the BASC-2 are described in terms of T-scores. T-scores compare a child's behavior to the behavior of typical children his or her age. Clinical scale T-scores have an average of 50 and an average range between 40 and 60. T-scores falling in the range of 60 to 69 are generally indicative of behaviors that are considered "at risk" or "borderline clinically significant." T-scores of 70 and above generally are considered indicative of behaviors that are "clinically significant." Adaptive scale T-scores of 31 to 40 are considered to fall within the "at-risk" range while scores of 30 and below are indicative of "clinically significant" adaptive skills deficits.

On this administration, Vinnie's mother and teacher both reported that he does not evidence significant internalizing symptoms, externalizing behavior problems, or inattention in the home or classroom settings (see Table 17.6). Similarly, no concerns were reported for problems with adaptive behavioral functioning. To the contrary, Vinnie's teacher reported that he adapts very well to most situations, recovers quickly from situations that are difficult, and is socially adept, courteous, polite, and generally helpful to others.

Vinnie's mother and teacher also completed the Behavior Rating Inventory of Executive Function (BRIEF), a narrow-band measure designed to assess various executive functions. Inspection of the validity scales indicated valid response patterns for both informants. The results of the BRIEF are described in terms of T-scores, in order to compare Vinnie's behavior to the behavior of typical children his age. T-scores have a mean of 50 and standard deviation of 10. BRIEF T-scores that are 65 and higher generally are considered indicative of behaviors that are "clinically significant." On this administration, Vinnie's mother and teacher both reported that he does not evidence any everyday behaviors associated with executive dysfunction.

Summary and Recommendations

In summary, Vinnie is an 8-year-old boy with phenylketonuria (PKU). Due to recent onset of academic difficulty and disruptive behaviors in the classroom coinciding with rising phenylalanine (Phe) levels, he was referred for comprehensive evaluation of cognitive functioning by his geneticist. The results of this neuropsychological evaluation revealed general intellectual functioning in the low-average range. The range of Vinnie's cognitive abilities is best captured by examining his performance across specific neurocognitive domains. In this regard, Vinnie demonstrated relative strengths in the areas of visual-perceptual skills, constructional praxis, visual memory, and many executive functions (cognitive flexibility, nonverbal concept generation, auditory working memory, and nonverbal/abstract reasoning), which were average. Receptive and expressive language skills and auditory/verbal memory ranged from low average to average. In contrast, Vinnie demonstrated relative weaknesses in processing speed (including psychomotor speed and rapid naming), sustained attention, and some executive functions (verbal concept formation, use of semantic clustering strategies when learning and remembering rote auditory/verbal information, and self-monitoring), which were mildly impaired.

PKU represents one possible etiology for Vinnie's neurocognitive profile. Research reports generally positive outcomes for early-treated children with PKU; however, subtle neurocognitive deficits may be evident even in those children who receive optimal dietary interventions, including deficits in reaction times and speed of information processing, sustained attention, and executive functions (problem solving, abstract reasoning, planning/organization, working memory, and inhibition). Vinnie's neurocognitive profile was consistent with these findings reported in the literature.

In academic areas, Vinnie demonstrated average basic reading skills, reading comprehension, spelling skills, and written expression, which were commensurate with his average phonological awareness and low-average to average verbal functioning. Mathematics reasoning also was average and commensurate with his average nonverbal/abstract reasoning skills. His low-average writing fluency and math fluency likely reflected his mildly impaired psychomotor speed and/or fluctuations in sustained attention on these timed tasks. Taken together, Vinnie does not evidence a learning disability as traditionally defined (IQ-achievement discrepancy); however, his neurocognitive weaknesses in processing speed, sustained attention, and executive function may exert a global and adverse impact on his academic progress, particularly as the complexity and volume of work increases. As such, he would benefit from accommodations in order to ensure his academic success.

According to his mother and teacher, Vinnie does not currently evidence significant internalizing symptoms, externalizing behavior problems, inattention, hyperactivity, or everyday behaviors associated with executive dysfunction in the home or classroom setting. Additionally, his teacher reported that Vinnie adapts very well to most situations and is socially adept. It is difficult to determine the source of Vinnie's disruptive classroom behaviors during the past school year. Behavioral dysregulation may have been secondary to executive dysfunction associated with rising Phe levels. It will be important to monitor the impact of his neurocognitive status in the context of his PKU management and to intervene when appropriate.

Medical Management of PKU

Based on the results of this evaluation, Vinnie would continue to benefit from follow-up with medical specialists who can monitor optimal dietary interventions for the management of PKU. His geneticist will receive a copy of this report, and all medical management decisions are deferred to his expertise. Serial neuropsychological evaluation also may assist with the monitoring of Vinnie's neurocognitive status as he matures. Vinnie's parents may obtain more information about PKU from the National Institute of Child Health and Human Development web site: www.nichd.nih.gov/health/topics/phenylketonuria.cfm.

Recommendations for School

Vinnie's mother is encouraged to share a copy of this report with the school psychologist who serves Vinnie's school. His current placement in a regular education classroom appears to be appropriate, and he is making good academic progress. Educators should be mindful that his neurocognitive weaknesses may exert an adverse impact on his academic progress as he advances in school. As such, development of a 504 Accommodation Plan may be considered. These recommendations may assist with the development of appropriate accommodations in the regular education setting:

To accommodate Vinnie's deficits in sustained attention and executive function:

- Consider preferential seating for Vinnie away from bulletin boards, doorways, windows, or other students, if necessary, where excessive stimuli might prove distracting. Also, seat Vinnie in close proximity to the teacher. Provide classroom instruction in small-group settings.
- Consider alternating more passive activities (such as listening) with more active tasks (such as hands-on, collaborative projects) to facilitate interest and sustained attention.

- It may be helpful to frequently check in with Vinnie in order to ensure his understanding of verbal directions by asking him to repeat what was stated. Similarly, have Vinnie rehearse learning tasks or assignments.
- Vinnie may evidence difficulty following multistep instructions. Thus, he would benefit from cues, organizing assistance, and reminders. Auditory/verbal cues tend to be more effective than visual cues because they are more likely to capture Vinnie's attention. In addition, cognitive cues, checklists, and written reminders will facilitate his completion of multistep instructions or multi-element problem solving.
- Vinnie's executive dysfunction may adversely affect organizational aspects of written expression. Therefore, he would benefit from such prewriting techniques as cognitive mapping, webbing, and graphic organizers to help him organize his thoughts prior to writing.
- Teach Vinnie how to be an active reader. That is, encourage him to underline key points while reading and to re-read the underlined text when he has reached the end of each page. In addition to underlining, he should asterisk very important points, write words or brief comments in the margins, and in general use many different ways of indicating different degrees of importance (e.g., double underlining, circling, etc.).
- Given his poor self-monitoring skills, Vinnie would benefit from frequent prompts to check his work for errors.

To accommodate Vinnie's slow processing speed:

- Educators should be made aware that Vinnie's slow cognitive tempo may masquerade as inattention. For example, he may be thinking about a previous set of instructions or lessons when the teacher and classmates already have moved onto the next material. He may appear to be daydreaming when he is unable to keep pace with the information. Therefore, frequent repetition of information will be helpful.
- Permit more time for academic tasks, including note taking, copying, and test taking. A reduction in the amount, but not the difficulty level, of assignments is recommended in order to assist Vinnie in completing classroom tasks and homework in a timely manner. Consider providing tests in multiple-choice/matching format instead of essay/short-answer format, with additional time and a reduction in the number of questions/answer choices.
- Completion of academic tasks may be tiring and frustrating for Vinnie, as he processes more slowly than his peers. Because it takes him more time to process and complete assignments, encourage him to take frequent breaks.
- There should be a strong emphasis on the review of material, especially in those subject areas that are causing Vinnie difficulty. He may have difficulty assimilating important concepts, vocabulary, and procedures initially if the material is presented too rapidly.

Further Discussion of Case Study

Vinnie's neurocognitive profile was consistent with research on children with PKU. As would be expected, he has generally low-average abilities in most areas, with sluggish cognitive tempo, inattention, and some problems with executive function. His low-average writing fluency and math fluency likely reflected his mildly impaired psychomotor speed and/or fluctuations in sustained attention on these timed tasks. The immediate referral was precipitated by academic difficulties that coincided with increased Phe levels. This is also a frequent finding in the literature. His relative strengths in the areas of visual-perceptual skills, constructional praxis, visual memory, and many executive functions (cognitive flexibility, nonverbal concept generation, auditory working memory, and nonverbal/abstract reasoning) are somewhat surprising, as is his average ability in mathematics. It will be interesting to see if this continues to be the case over time.

MUCOPOLYSACCHARIDE DISORDERS

Definition and Etiology

Mucopolysaccharide disorders comprise a group of rare disorders that affect mucopolysaccharide metabolism; mucopolysaccharides are long molecular chains of sugar that are used by the body in the building of connective tissues (M. B. Brown, 1999). The group of disorders include:

Type I—Hurler syndrome, Scheie syndrome, and Hurler-Scheie syndrome
Type II—Hunter syndrome
Type III—Sanfilippo syndrome
Type IV—Morquio syndrome

Type I—Hurler, Scheie, and Hurler-Scheie—are autosomal recessive, and rare; all three occur in both males and females and have skeletal effects referred to as dysostosis multiplex (M. J. Goldberg, 1996). These effects include an enlarged head, progressive curvature of the lower spine, significant shortening of stature, shortened neck with widened collarbones and ribs, clawlike hands, contractions of joints, flattening of the bridge of the nose with wide nostrils, thick lips, protruding tongue, thick hair, and excessive body hair. Hurler syndrome is the most severe and occurs in 1 in 100,000 live births. Children appear normal at birth, with problems evident between 6 and 18 months of age (M. B. Brown & Trivette, 1998). Learning peaks at about 2 or 3 years of age, followed by a loss of skills and progressive mental retardation. The maximum functional age with Hurler syndrome is approximately the 2- to 4-year age level. Medical complications, including cardiovascular disease and respiratory problems, generally lead to death early in adolescence.

Of the Type I disorders, Scheie syndrome is the least severe and occurs in 1 in 600,000 live births (M. B. Brown & Trivette, 1998). With Scheie, stature is usually normal; facial appearance is coarse with large tongue, and there is an excess of body hair (A. M. Murphy, Lambert, Treacy, O'Meara, & Lynch, 2009). Joint stiffness is the predominant symptom; vision may or may not be affected with clouding or glaucoma. Because the characteristics are relatively mild, Scheie usually is not diagnosed until the teenage years. Scheie is associated with normal life expectancy. Hurler-Scheie is the intermediate form of Type I. Its incidence is unknown (M. B. Brown & Trivette, 1998). It presents with mild facial deformities, corneal clouding, and hearing loss. Children with Hurler-Scheie are of short stature, but not as short as those with Hurler. As is the case with Scheie syndrome, with Hurler-Scheie, the joints become stiff and contracted. Hurler-Scheie usually is evident by 3 to 8 years of age; children with Hurler-Scheie may have average cognitive ability or may be mildly impaired cognitively (M. B. Brown & Trivette, 1998; A. M. Murphy et al., 2009).

Type II—Hunter syndrome—is an X-linked disorder with several alleles implicated (M. B. Brown & Trivette, 1998). It occurs in 1 in 130,000 to 150,000 male births; it occurs primarily in Caucasians, but rarely in other racial groups. Skeletal features are similar to the Type I versions and severity ranges from mild to severe. With the mild or late-onset form, development initially is normal with abnormalities evident by early childhood. Cognitive functioning usually is not impaired with the mild or late-onset type. Life expectancy is early 20s, but some live until their 40s. With severe or early-onset form, average age of onset is 2.5 years with marked progressive neurological involvement. Learning and developmental skills level out at about 2 to 6 years functionally, with progressive mental retardation. Seizure disorder is common by age 10; the mean life expectancy is 11 to 12 years of age (M. B. Brown, 1999).

Less is known about the other types of mucopolysaccharide disorders. Type III—Sanfilippo syndrome—is defined by four different enzyme deficiencies designated as type A, B, C, or D (M. B. Brown, 1999). Type A is the most common form found in most populations; there is no difference in presentation despite differences in the enzymes. The incidence of Sanfilippo syndrome is 1 in 85,000, and the severity varies. Type IV—Morquio syndrome—is autosomal recessive with an incidence of 3 in 1 million. Infants look normal at birth, but abnormalities develop during infancy or early childhood. These children are generally of average or near-average cognitive ability. Additional types of mucopolysaccharide disorders have been identified with limited case studies available for review. These include Maroteaux-Lamy disease (Type VI), with five babies identified with this form over a 10-year period in Britain, and Sly disease (Type VII), which was identified in the 1970s and is estimated to occur in 1 in 250,000 births (M. B. Brown, 1999).

Course and Prognosis

As noted, the overall prognosis is guarded, with varying severity and progressive course depending on the specific form. Optimal care requires frequent follow-up by various health care specialists (vision, hearing, dental, general medical). Care focuses on management and complications for each individual. Cardiovascular and pulmonary issues are common. Intervention for hearing and vision loss may be needed as well (M. J. Goldberg, 1996). Life expectancy with Hunter disease is markedly reduced and may be limited to 12 years of age in more severe cases (Sawaf, Mayatepek, & Hoffmann, 2008). Complications include airway obstruction and cardiac failure; neurological complications may include hydrocephalus, spinal cord compression, cervical myelopathy, optic nerve compression, and hearing impairment (Sawaf et al., 2008).

Educational Implications

Early intervention is helpful in maximizing functional levels. Careful evaluation of cognitive functioning, achievement, and behavior is needed in order to develop appropriate intervention. Focus should be on short-term goals with frequent monitoring due to rapid regression of skills. Teachers need to be educated about the child's condition, ability level, and needs; teachers will need support as the child's condition deteriorates. Because of the disease's potential effects on hearing function and speech, these areas require monitoring as well (Cho et al., 2008).

Psychological Implications

It is common for children with these disorders to be described as anxious or fearful (Bax & Colville, 1995). In addition, 41% evidence overactivity or restlessness;

aggressive-destructive behavior is common in early childhood. Behavior support and management with emphasis on reinforcement and simplification of task demands is helpful (M. B. Brown & Trivette, 1998). Many children with these disorders (63%) have trouble with sleep; many have difficulty with toilet training. High levels of stress are common within the family; parents are very anxious about the child coupled with medical expenses and demands of having a child with a chronic condition. Parental stress increases with the child's decreased communication skills. It is important to encourage the child's independence to the extent possible.

Evidence-Based Treatment

Because of the concerns for basic survival and relatively short life expectancy, the majority of evidence-based treatment research has addressed the physiological aspects of the mucopolysaccharidoses (see Table 17.7). In some cases, enzyme replacement can help in management, but it is not a cure. Results of a 26-week, randomized, open-label, multinational dose-optimization trial of laronidase (Aldurazyme) revealed that laronidase had an acceptable safety profile across dose regimen groups. Infusion-associated reactions were the most common drug-related adverse events across dose regimens; the approved 0.58 mg/kg/week laronidase dose regimen provided near-maximal reductions in glycosaminoglycan storage and the best benefit-to-risk ratio; however, long-term effects of this regimen are unknown (Giugliani et al., 2009). Only one study has begun to look at long-term effects with positive results (L. A. Clarke et al., 2009). Recombinant human arylsulfatase B (rhASB) treatment of mucopolysaccharidosis type VI (MPS VI: Maroteaux-Lamy syndrome) has been found to result in sustained improvements in endurance up to 5 years and has an acceptable safety profile (Harmatz et al., 2008).

Bone marrow transplantation can modify effects and increase survival but is not a cure either (Gassas et al., 2003; Polgreen et al., 2008; Weisstein et al., 2004). Data from at least one study indicated a lack of social competency and a tendency toward inhibition and withdrawal in children with mucopolysaccharidosis I Hurler disease after bone marrow transplant (Pitt, Lavery, & Wager, 2009). Alternatively, existing research also suggests that early hematopoietic stem cell transplantation in Hurler syndrome preserves an affected child's cognitive functions (G. Malm et al., 2008).

Table 17.7 Evidence-Based Status for Interventions for Mucopolysaccharidoses

Interventions	Target	Status
Enzyme replacement	Metabolic control	Emerging (L. A. Clarke et al., 2009; Giugliani et al., 2009; Harmatz et al., 2008)
Bone marrow transplant	Metabolic control	Emerging (Gassas, Sung, Doyle, Clarke, & Saunders, 2003; Polgreen et al., 2008; Weisstein, Delgado, Steinbach, Hart, & Packman, 2004)
Stem cell transplant	Metabolic control	Emerging (G. Malm et al., 2008)

CONCLUDING COMMENTS

Children with metabolic disorders and their parents need ongoing education with a focus on self-management (Brink, 1996). This process involves collaboration and cooperation of school personnel as well as health professionals. One approach to support and management of metabolic disorders is the increased education of teachers, psychologists, and school nurses. Continuing education is most evident in the school nursing literature in conjunction with diabetes (Bachman & Hsueh, 2008), but it would seem equally appropriate for the other metabolic disorders and for other professionals who work with affected children. Educational and psychoeducational approaches with affected children and families also would seem to be important to enhance treatment compliance, but most current evidence suggests limited effectiveness of these approaches. Future research may focus on the development of programs based on specific outcomes for children and families affected by metabolic disorders.

As evident with the growing concerns with obesity, additional research to determine if there are divergent neurocognitive effects for Type 1 and Type 2 diabetes will be needed, particularly with regard to educational and psychological implications. Similarly, little research has addressed the educational needs and psychological impact of PKU. As interventions and prognosis improve, research with regard to educational implications and interventions, as well as psychosocial outcomes for individuals with mucopolysaccharidoses, in particular, will be needed.

Chapter 18

LOOKING BACK, LOOKING FORWARD

ASSESSMENT TO INTERVENTION PLANNING IN PEDIATRIC NEUROPSYCHOLOGY

As stated in Chapter 1, as a field, pediatric neuropsychology has made significant growth in the area of assessment and identification of individual strengths and weaknesses. Pediatric neuropsychology has added to the literature and understanding of children in the context of special education decision making and intervention planning as well as to the understanding of specific disorders (Augustyniak, Murphy, & Phillips, 2005; Feagans, Short, & Meltzer, 1991; S. Goldstein & Naglieri, 2008; Hendriksen et al., 2007; S. A. Peters, Fox, Weber, & Llorente, 2005; Riccio, Gonzales, & Hynd, 1994; Riccio & Hynd, 1995a; Schwarte, 2008). With recent trends toward the response to intervention (RtI) approach to identification of children with learning disabilities, there has been increased discussion of how neuropsychology will fit in this model (Fletcher-Janzen & Reynolds, 2008). The RtI model is not used solely for identification of learning disabilities but is expanding to identification of Attention-Deficit/Hyperactivity Disorder (ADHD) and other disorders. At its core, the model does not focus on a specific disorder, syndrome, or disease but aims to monitor progress, with interventions as needed, to attain at least minimal adequacy. As such, the model, theoretically, can be applied to children with any disorder (Fuchs & Deshler, 2007; Fuchs, Mock, Morgan, & Young, 2003; Gresham, 2006). The RtI model uses a multitier system for identification of disabilities. In the context of the multitier system, a student who is identified as at risk or who is struggling is supposed to receive remediation services; a disability is evidenced by the student's lack of response to intervention (Riccio, 2008a). The question unanswered by RtI, however, is *why* the child did not respond to the intervention. Thus, the RtI approach may be adequate for *describing* the child's performance but may fall short in terms of *explaining* the child's performance or deficits.

Neuropsychological assessment is intended to aid in the understanding of the student, predict student behavior, and improve student behavior and development (A. J. Schmitt & Wodrich, 2008). There is evidence to suggest that cognitive abilities are relevant as part of both the identification and the intervention process, with environmental and psychosocial factors more salient for those children with lower ability (S. J. Wadsworth, Olson, Pennington, & DeFries, 2000). The arguments for the incorporation of neuropsychological methods in the assessment process focus on the desire to integrate cognitive and behavioral data, thus increasing the ability to deal with the multidimensionality of individuals (Reynolds, 2008; Riccio & Reynolds, 1998b) and creating a unified or holistic picture of the student's functioning. Whether applying Luria's model (Luria, 1980), the Cattell-Horn-Carroll model (Floyd et al., 2007; Hale et al., 2001), or the Cognitive Hypothesis Testing model (Hale & Fiorello, 2004) as the comprehensive framework for examining individual differences in cognitive abilities, it is clear that the range of cognitive abilities and functional systems impact both achievement and adjustment (Kaufman, 2008a). Despite, and in conjunction with, RtI, neurology and neuropsychology are the keys for understanding learning problems and treating them (Kaufman, 2008a). Ultimately, it is important to evaluate the cognitive-processing deficits that help explain the learning deficits, as this information may help point us in the appropriate direction for intervention (D. C. Miller, 2008).

Across disorders, the learning deficits may be in reading, math, or written expression, but the underlying areas that are impaired most often include language, learning and memory, attention, executive functions of problem-solving and planning, and processing speed. In addition, subsequent psychological and adjustment issues associated with learning deficits, regardless of the disorder or syndrome, are possible. Unfortunately, these areas may not be addressed as part of progress monitoring, yet the problems in these neurocognitive areas may, in fact, need to be considered as an integral part of the identification and strategic intervention process. The design of intervention programs should not be limited to the designation that the individual has or does not have a specific disorder. Silver et al. (2006) asserted that neuropsychological evaluation answers not only "what" is going on academically or behaviorally but the "why," or causal features; again, this is where RtI falls short. Treatment or intervention planning from a neuropsychological perspective includes the identification of both specific management or rehabilitation techniques and environmental modifications that need to be addressed (Silver, Blackburn, Arffa, Barth, Bush, & Koffler, 2006). The neuropsychological perspective also leads to an increased ability to develop appropriate interventions or circumvent future problems. In other words, the decision of which intervention to implement and monitor as part of the RtI process can be based on data from neuropsychological assessment in order to ensure a good fit between the intervention and the child's individual needs.

An emphasis on individual strengths (intact functions) in conjunction with compensatory strategies leads to alternative approaches to instruction (Riccio & Reynolds, 1998b). A critical issue that has gained in visibility is the evidence base for interventions used. There is a paucity of research to confirm that the same methods used, for example, to address a language problem in one child will work when the target child has a different disorder or syndrome. Chapters 2 and 3 covered interventions used for reading and math in detail. Other areas and domains are covered across chapters to differing degrees. Because of the frequency of deficits in areas of language, memory, attention, executive function, and processing speed, regardless of syndrome or disorder, additional research related to these domains, assessment, and evidence-based interventions follows. Notably, the empirical research available most often has a medical context rather than an educational or real-life context. In addition, trials often are limited by short follow-up times, restrictions in sampling, and limited assessment (Gingras et al., 2006).

Language

Language is an essential means of communication from the time a child is born. It is through language that the child interacts with the world; it is also through language that the world interacts with the child (Riccio & Hynd, 1993). Not only is language a means of communication; language itself is an important social behavior. In many disorders, for example, it is the pragmatic aspects of language that are impaired, not the general vocabulary skills of the individual (Vallecorsa & Garriss, 1990). Pragmatic language affects not only social areas (presupposition, initiation, humor, sarcasm), but reading and written language as well (M. Lahey, 1988b). A number of suggested strategies for children with specific language impairment are discussed in Chapter 4 and elsewhere, and are listed in Table 18.1. Some additional suggestions to enhance language development include ensuring that the child has a language- and experience-rich environment, with frequent exposure and practice with words (B. Hart & Risley, 1995). Direct and explicit word instruction and instruction in morphology (National Institute of Child Health and Human Development, 2000) are applicable to language development as well as reading.

Table 18.1 Evidence-Based Status of Interventions for Language Development and Functional Communication

Interventions	Target	Status
Fast ForWord	Language	Promising practice (W. Cohen et al., 2005; Gillam et al., 2008b; Merzenich et al., 1999; Tallal, 2000)
Functional communication training	Communication	Promising practice with autism spectrum disorders (H. Goldstein, 2002)
Visual systems and supports (e.g., Picture Exchange Communication System; PECS)	Communication	Emerging to promising practice with autism spectrum and other disorders (Odom et al., 2003)
Facilitated communication	Communication	Ineffective (American Academy of Pediatrics Committee on Children with Disabilities, 1998; Simpson, 2005a; Zimmer & Molloy, 2007)
Vocal stimulation, articulation exercises, reinforcement	Early intervention for speech production	Emerging with specific populations (Rondal et al., 2003)
Sign language or other alternative visual communication strategy	Fostering communication	Emerging with specific populations (J. E. Roberts et al., 2007; Rondal et al., 2003)

Learning and Memory

As evidenced across the chapters in this book, the assessment of learning and memory in the comprehensive evaluation of children with suspected or identified neurological involvement is critical. Memory processes are complex, and this complexity reflects the intricate nature of the underlying functional systems; difficulties may occur at any point in the process: encoding, storage, manipulation, or retrieval (Ewing-Cobbs, Fletcher, & Levin, 1986; Lezak, 1986, 1995). The status of evidence-based interventions for deficits in memory and learning are summarized in Table 18.2. A number of these are included in the recommendations for the case studies across multiple chapters.

Attention

Some of the most frequent symptoms associated with neurodevelopmental disorders often include problems with attention/concentration. As with memory, attention is multifaceted,

Table 18.2 Evidence-Based Status of Interventions for Learning and Memory

Interventions	Target	Status
Rehearsal	Short- and long-term memory	Promising practice (Wendling & Mather, 2009)
Elaboration	Short- and long-term memory	Promising practice (Squire & Schacter, 2003; Wendling & Mather, 2009)
Chunking	Short- and long-term memory	Promising practice (Dehn, 2008)
Imagery, visual representations	Short- and long-term memory	Promising practice (Wendling & Mather, 2009)
Mnemonics	Short- and long-term memory; computation/ algorithms	Promising practice (Maccini & Hughes, 2000; Mastropieri & Scruggs, 1998; Wendling & Mather, 2009)
Attention remediation programs (e.g., Amsterdam Memory and Training Program for Children)	Memory	Positive practice with traumatic brain injury (Laatsch et al., 2007)

including selective attention, sustained attention, shifting of attention, alertness, and so on (Barkley, 1997). Although a focus of assessment for ADHD, research suggests that many of the measures used to assess attention (e.g., continuous performance tests) often are sensitive to any disruption in central nervous system function (Riccio & Reynolds, 2001). This is due most likely to the presence of attentional problems across neurologically based disorders. The need to address problems with attentional skills is based on the premise that adequate attention (i.e., selective attention, sustained attention, shifting of attention) is necessary in order for efficient information processing to occur (Ewing-Cobbs et al., 1986); it has been suggested that other more overt problems (i.e., in memory or processing speed) may be the result of underlying deficits in attention (Sohlberg & Mateer, 1987). It also has been suggested that by developing a taxonomy of attentional deficits, it may be possible to differentiate the types of attentional problems associated with specific neurodevelopmental disorders, with possible identification of endophenotypes (Dennis, Sinopoli, Fletcher, & Schachar, 2008). Such endophenotypes then would facilitate intervention development and implementation.

Interventions specific to attentional function are summarized in Table 18.3; these are discussed in more detail and in conjunction with ADHD in Chapter 6; the review by Riccio and French (2004) reviews intervention studies for attentional problems in more detail. In general, stimulant medications are seen as a first-line treatment option for ADHD, but these medications also have been found effective at improving attention among children with traumatic brain injuries (TBIs), Tourette syndrome, and other disorders. At the same time, children using stimulants must be monitored closely for adverse side effects, including onset or exacerbation of tics. More recently, the development of nonstimulant medications has expanded the possible psychopharmacological approaches to attentional problems. As noted in Table 18.3, a number of approaches aside from medication can be considered, with limited evidence as yet to support their use across disorders. In addition to interventions that are intended to change or alter the child's behavior, often environmental modifications, such as preferential seating, quiet and uncluttered environment, frequent prompting or cues, and self-monitoring, are suggested to address

Table 18.3 Evidence-Based Status of Interventions for Attentional Problems

Interventions	Target	Status
Stimulant medications (e.g., methylphenidate, Ritalin, Concerta)	Attention; on-task behavior	Positive to promising practice depending on disorder (Conklin et al., 2007; Daly & Brown, 2007; Mautner et al., 2002; Nickels et al., 2008; S. J. Thompson et al., 2001; Torres et al., 2008; Wernicke et al., 2007)
Nonstimulant medications (e.g., atomoxetine [Strattera])	Attention	Positive practice with ADHD (Cheng et al., 2007)
Dietary modifications (e.g., elimination of refined sugar, Feingold diet)	Attention	Ineffective with ADHD (N. L. Rojas & Chan, 2005)
Attention remediation programs (e.g., Amsterdam Memory and Training Program for Children)	Attention	Positive practice with TBI (Galbiati et al., 2009; Laatsch et al., 2007)
Attention process training	Vigilance and concentration	Emerging (R. W. Butler & Copeland, 2002; Murray, Keeton, & Karcher, 2006)
Behavioral classroom management/Classroom modifications (e.g., point systems, daily report card, self-monitoring)	On-Task behaviors	Positive practice with ADHD (Chronis et al., 2006; Daly et al., 2007; Pelham & Fabiano, 2008)
Electroencephalogram biofeedback	Attention	Inconclusive with ADHD (Riccio & French, 2004; Rojas & Chan, 2005)
Cognitive remediation program	Attention, academic achievement	Emerging with specific disorders (R. W. Butler & Copeland, 2002; R. W. Butler, Copeland et al., 2008; R. W. Butler, Sahler et al., 2008)

attentional problems. Many of these modifications do not have an evidence base to support them (e.g., quiet setting) but may be helpful for any student. Specific educational interventions that involve increasing stimulus conditions that affect the actual task (e.g., changing the task to eliminate irrelevant cues, highlighting relevant information) as well as instruction/sequencing (e.g., beginning with a simple format, allowing the child to set his or her own goals, use of self-instructional strategies) are among those considered evidence based (Zentall, 2005). In addition, additional practice and cues for self-monitoring of the child's own performance may be helpful. Finally, provision of visual feedback to an auditory task (or auditory feedback to a visual task) has resulted in more normalized attention (Zentall, 2005).

Executive Function

The domain of executive function has been defined in many ways but generally is presumed to involve those higher-order processes associated with planning, organization, and problem-solving as well as behaviors that are needed to maintain an appropriate problem-solving set (Luria, 1980; Zelazo, Carter, Reznick, & Frye, 1997). Executive function is not a unitary concept; it is a multifaceted construct comprised of multiple component functions (Miyake et al., 2000). A broad definition of executive function is "the control or self-regulatory functions that organize and direct all cognitive activity, emotional response, and overt behavior" (Gioia, Isquith, & Guy, 2001, p. 320). Executive function traditionally is associated with frontal and prefrontal function but is not limited to frontal function (Denckla, 1996). Typically, development of executive function unfolds predictably with increasing independence, maturation of self-regulation, and development of self-generated productivity from childhood to adulthood. This development appears to be intertwined with the development of the prefrontal cortex and other subcortical brain structures (Gioia, Isquith, & Guy, 2001; M. C. Welsh, Pennington, & Groisser, 1991). It is these same structures that often are compromised in neurodevelopmental disorders.

A review of the chapters in this volume suggests that executive function is involved in a variety of disorders, which is consistent with the research on the executive function construct (e.g., Sullivan, Riccio, & Castillo, 2009). As such, interventions for executive function likely will be applicable for a range of diagnoses. Some of the specific behaviors associated with impaired executive function include procrastination or difficulty initiating new or challenging tasks, difficulty prioritizing or self-pacing, difficulty transitioning or shifting from one activity to another, difficulty multitasking, disorganization, and difficulty regulating emotional state (K. B. Powell & Voeller, 2004). In educational settings, these problems manifest as children's difficulty with organizing and regulating themselves in class, failure to complete work on time, failure to prioritize assigned tasks, failure to allocate time and energy accordingly, frequent off-task behavior, and failure to bring home what is needed to finish homework assignments. Such difficulties often will extend to the home and other environments, affecting not only academic but everyday functioning as well. With regard to decision making, two aspects ("cool" and "hot") have been identified; a given individual may be impaired in one or both types of processing (Hendriksen et al., 2007). Based on their study, Hendriksen et al. concluded that assessment of both types of processes would facilitate treatment planning, particularly for those with more behavioral or regulatory (hot, or affective and emotional) problems. Unfortunately, many of the laboratory measures frequently used in the assessment of executive function do not correlate well with parent- or teacher-reported behaviors (e.g., Anderson, Anderson, Northam, Jacobs, & Mikiewicz, 2002; Vriezen & Pigott, 2002). The Behavior Rating Inventory of Executive Function (BRIEF) is one of the few measures that allows for comparison of perceptions of a child's executive function skills (self-regulatory and metacognitive) from multiple sources.

Several accommodations and modifications have been suggested to address the specific executive function deficits that an individual may exhibit. For example, it has been suggested that an adult serve as a coach, or "prosthetic frontal lobe" (K. B. Powell & Voeller, 2004), providing guidelines and monitoring, eventually leading to increased self-monitoring. Education about the individual's difficulties for parents and teachers, as well as the individual, also is seen as an important component. Behavioral strategies that focus on manipulating or modifying the antecedents (i.e., breaking down complex tasks into simpler components, providing an outline of how components fit together, teaching the child to use organizational systems and aids when possible, using repetitive training to make routines automatic, using positive behavioral supports) as opposed to imposing negative consequences also are suggested in the literature (K. B. Powell & Voeller, 2004).

Four broadly defined approaches to intervention for executive dysfunction have been proposed: pharmacological, consequence-focused, antecedent-focused, and self-instructional/metacognitive strategies. Pharmacological intervention (i.e., use of stimulants) is clearly supported for the management of significant attention problems regardless of the disorder; however, there is no evidence to suggest that medications alter executive thinking strategies (W. B. Marlowe, 2000). Thus, although medication is considered a viable option for the management of executive problems, it may best be used as a potentially helpful adjunct to other interventions rather than as an isolated treatment strategy (Ozonoff, 1998).

Behavioral interventions may be consequence focused or antecedent focused. With consequence-focused interventions, behavior that is considered desirable ("executive") is systematically rewarded; behavior that is considered undesirable ("dysexecutive") is ignored or followed by punishment or removal from reinforcement. This approach has been used with children with ADHD (Lerner, Lowenthal, & Lerner, 1995), and well-designed consequence-focused programs have been found effective for reducing a variety of behavioral problems and for increasing work productivity and accuracy among school-age children with ADHD (P. A. Teeter, 1998). It is not clear if consequence-focused intervention improves executive function processes or if the behavior change can be maintained when the contingencies are removed. Further, although consequence-focused behavioral interventions may be appropriate to help individuals initiate executive problem-solving processes and shape target behaviors, many researchers have indicated that emphasis on consequences is questionable when applied to individuals with executive disorders because of the necessary link between the behavior and the consequence (DeBonis, Ylvisaker, & Kundert, 2000). For example, it has been argued that because impairment in ventromedial prefrontal regions interferes with attachment of feeling states to stored memories, punishments or rewards do not have lasting effects on behavior (Bechara, Damasio, & Damasio, 2000). Clinical observation of individuals with prefrontal impairment suggests that consequence-focused approaches can, in fact, create or exacerbate behavior problems (Ylvisaker & Feeney, 1998). Others argue that levels of motivation and drive (Stuss & Benson, 1986) or working memory deficits (Alderman, Fry, & Youngson, 1995) that are associated with prefrontal damage may account for the inefficiency of this approach.

Also a behavioral approach, antecedent-focused approaches involve modifications in the child's home and school environments to circumvent or prevent problems. Antecedent-focused approaches tend to involve either direct environmental management (i.e., classroom modifications) or direct teaching of external compensatory systems (Ozonoff, 1998). Environmental management is considered as a critical approach for managing dysexecutive symptoms (Sohlberg & Mateer, 2001). Lerner and colleagues (1995) identified a number of characteristics of teachers and classrooms that are associated with the successful management of executive function disorders, including consistency in schedule, consistency in routine and rules, clear presentation of directions, and frequent monitoring by the teacher. Alternatively, the direct teaching component includes teaching children with executive problems to use external devices and written reminders/cues that will help with organization. Some specific suggestions include the use of weekly assignment logs, day planners or appointment books, to-do lists, and a timer or alarm to cue the child for self-monitoring.

Another group of interventions include metacognitive interventions, or strategies that the individual is trained to use. These strategies typically involve teaching the student systematic problem-solving processes and/or how to monitor and regulate their behavior via self-talk. The foundation of this approach lies in the early work of Vygotsky and Luria, who suggested that volitional behavior originates not in mental acts but rather is mediated by inner speech (Sohlberg & Mateer, 2001). This approach has been widely espoused by many researchers and clinicians in cognitive rehabilitation to address executive function impairments, particularly those due to traumatic brain injury (e.g., Alderman, Fry,

& Youngson, 1995; Cicerone & Wood, 1986; Duke, Weathers, Caldwell, & Novack, 1992; Levine et al., 2000; Sohlberg, Mateer, & Stuss, 1993). Ylvisaker, Szekeres, and Feeney (1998) described an ecological metacognitive approach to executive function intervention. Although consistent with more traditional metacognitive training, they emphasized ecological elements, such as using everyday tasks as the context for exercising self-regulation and the role of everyday people in the child's environment in creating a culture that facilitates development of executive function. The procedures include modeling and coaching within the context of everyday routines and everyday conversational interaction, including classroom, therapeutic, and recreational activities, and activities of daily living at home (Ylvisaker & Feeney, 1998; Ylvisaker, Szekeres, & Feeney, 1998). Unfortunately, relatively little research has been published on specific interventions for executive function; the status of evidence-based interventions specific to aspects of executive function are provided in Table 18.4.

Table 18.4 Evidence-Based Status of Interventions for Executive Function

Interventions	Target	Status
Attention remediation programs (e.g., Amsterdam Memory and Training Program for Children)	Executive function, self-regulation	Positive practice with TBI (Laatsch et al., 2007)
Metacognitive strategy instruction	Executive function, problem solving, decision making	Emerging with some populations (M. R. T. Kennedy et al., 2008; Limond & Leeke, 2005; Montague, 2008; Ylvisaker et al., 1998)
Behavioral approaches (chaining, use of contingencies)	Means-end thinking, problem-solving	Emerging with some populations (Fidler, 2006)
Behavioral approaches: consequence-focused	Executive function, self-regulation	Emerging with TBI (Ylvisaker & Feeney, 1998)
Behavioral approaches: antecedent-focused	Problem-solving, self-regulation	Emerging with some populations (Ozonoff, 1998)

Processing Speed

Across disorders, the terms *slowed reaction time, decreased processing speed*, or *sluggish cognitive tempo* are used to describe individuals with the disorder. The use of a fluency-based measure as part of the assessment process also is important from a neuropsychological perspective in that slow processing or difficulty retrieving information rapidly may be one effect of some neurological disorders, including problems with executive function (Blair & Razza, 2007; Gaskins, Satlow, & Pressley, 2007). Further, this slow rate of processing or decreased level of automaticity likely has cumulative effects on the educational process, not only in the area being assessed but across areas and skills. For example, speed of processing has been useful in differentiating fluent from nonfluent readers (D. Powell, Stainthorp, Stuart, Garwood, & Quinlan, 2007; Semrud-Clikeman, Guy, & Griffin, 2000). Some common accommodations for impaired processing speed include time extensions, particularly on standardized tests, and adjusting length of assignments as well as eliminating or limiting unnecessary copying of information from a book or board (Wendling & Mather, 2009). No specific evidence-based interventions for processing speed were identified in the literature. Although the use of methylphenidate (e.g., Ritalin,

Concerta) may enhance processing speed among children with TBI (see Chapter 8), this may in fact be the result of effects on attentional aspects of processing rather than on processing speed itself.

Adjustment and Behavioral Problems

Consistent research findings suggest that adjustment and behavioral problems often are associated with or secondary to neurological impairment, regardless of the etiology (Adab et al., 2001; Benasich et al., 1993; Conti-Ramsden & Botting, 2008; R. S. Dean, 1986; Riccio & Hynd, 1993; Snowling et al., 2006). The high frequency of comorbidity of emotional and behavioral disorders with ADHD, autism, Tourette syndrome, and learning disabilities is particularly notable. The field of pediatric psychology has contributed greatly to our understanding of the psychological implications of medical illness in children, with depression, anxiety, and conduct problems often the result of experiencing stress, fear, and loss of control in response to chronic medical conditions such as diabetes and sickle cell disease (see Roberts, 2003). Further, the chronic academic and social struggles associated with the disorders discussed in this volume likely contribute to low self-efficacy and poor emotional and behavioral outcomes.

Interventions that address social, emotional, and behavioral adjustment are summarized in Table 18.5. One issue that is of increasing interest is the effect on parents or siblings of the child with a neurodevelopmental or genetic disorder. Although the effects may be most salient at the time of initial diagnosis, there is some indication that, for mothers at least, there is improved coping and family functioning over time (Barnett et al., 2006). While there is not sufficient evidence to support a specific therapeutic approach for families and children, helping parents and siblings to cope with the affected child's disorder may be beneficial for all family members and for the family system as a whole (Barnett et al., 2006).

SUMMARY OF INTERVENTION ISSUES

Although the research evidence on the effectiveness of a treatment always should be considered, often this information is inconclusive, unavailable, or confusing for families and caregivers of children with disabilities; it also does not necessarily relate to compliance or treatment fidelity in real-world settings. In addition to the need for empirical support for interventions being recommended and implemented, it is important to consider issues of social validity and treatment acceptability (Kazdin, 1994). *Treatment acceptability* is defined as "judgments by laypersons, clients, and others of whether the treatment procedures are appropriate, fair, and reasonable for the problem that is to be treated" (Kazdin, 1994, p. 402). Treatment acceptability has been studied with several different populations, including those with ADHD (D. S. Bennett, Power, Rostain, & Carr, 1996; Power, Hess, & Bennett, 1995), and with specific behaviors, such as self-injury (Rasnake, Martin, Tarnowski, & Mulick, 1993). At the same time, there is a paucity of research examining the treatment acceptability of differing interventions for individuals with many of the neurodevelopmental and genetic disorders.

Further, it is vital to prioritize the importance of specific intervention targets or the salience of the behavior being targeted in various settings. For example, parents of children with Down syndrome indicated improvements in speech and reading as salient targets (Fidler, Lawson, & Hodapp, 2003). In contrast, Fidler and colleagues reported

Table 18.5 Evidence-Based Status of Interventions for Overall Adjustment

Interventions	Target	Status
Creating Opportunities for Parent Empowerment (COPE) program	Cognitive development, maternal coping, mother-infant interactions	Emerging with specific populations (Melnyk et al., 2001)
Behavioral parent training	Parent-child interactions	Positive practice with some disorders (Chronis et al., 2006; Daly et al., 2007; Pelham & Fabiano, 2008)
Parent training programs	Caregiving skills, parent-child interactions	Promising practice with LBW (Achenbach et al., 1993; Patteson & Barnard, 1990)
Traditional counseling approaches (e.g., individual counseling, play therapy, cognitive therapy)	Comprehensive psychological issues	Ineffective with some disorders but understudied with many disorders (Pelham & Fabiano, 2008)
Cognitive-behavioral therapy in a family systems context	Stress, trauma of diagnosis and treatment	Emerging with childhood cancer (Kazak et al., 2004)
Family-centered rehabilitation programs (i.e., family members involved in planning and providing treatment)	Comprehensive	Positive practice (Laatsch et al., 2007)
Social skills training (generic)	Social interaction	Inconclusive (Barakat et al., 2003; Rao et al., 2008)
Self-monitoring	Social interaction	Emerging (Odom et al., 2003)
Positive behavior support	Problem behaviors, functional communication	Promising practice (Odom et al., 2003)
Inclusive education	Socialization, communication	Inconclusive (S. Rogers & Vismara, 2008)
General behavioral interventions (e.g., functional analysis of behavior, operant conditioning approaches, contingency management systems, positive behavior supports)	Disruptive behaviors, compliance, aggression	Positive practice (Gurdin et al., 2005; Ylvisaker et al., 2007)
Coping skills training	Psychosocial outcome	Emerging with specific populations (M. Davidson et al., 1997; Grey et al., 1999)
Educational or informational interventions (e.g., using informational booklets about the effects and symptoms of disorder to facilitate the family's understanding)	Comprehensive	Promising practice with TBI (Laatsch et al., 2007)
Infant health and development program	Cognitive development, behavior problems, mother-child interactions	Positive practice with LBW (McCormick et al., 1998, 2006)
Office-based social skills training groups	Social skills	Inconclusive (Chronis et al., 2006; Pelham & Fabiano, 2008)

that parents of children with Prader-Willi syndrome were more concerned with exercise and adaptive physical education services; parents of children with Williams syndrome expressed an interest in increased provision of music-related services. Taking these preferences into consideration likely will increase treatment acceptability and compliance.

Finally, although the constructs highlighted in this chapter are involved in multiple disorders, generalizability of related interventions often has not been established. For example, interventions that address attention problems may be well established with children with ADHD, but we cannot assume that these same interventions would be equally effective at treating attention problems among children with autism, learning disabilities, Tourette syndrome, and so on. Although the attention problems may "look the same" across these different disorders, the differing etiological, neurological, and environmental factors may lead to differential effects of interventions. Thus, interventions designed to address the cross-cutting constructs discussed in this chapter need to be established with each distinct disorder.

CONCLUSION AND FUTURE DIRECTIONS

A critical issue that continues to be problematic is the translation of knowledge from neuropsychology (the science component) to the contexts in which children function (the practice piece). There is a clear need to ensure that the information gained from neuropsychological assessment is useful to the consumers receiving the information: parents, schools, and physician. The assessment methods and approaches may vary, but results need to be translated across disorders easily. There has been found to be overall consensus that parents find the information worthwhile (Bodin et al., 2007). The same cannot be said, however, with regard to the ability to link information on neurocognitive functioning and the disorder to appropriate interventions (Kanne et al., 2008).

There has been much discussion of the "Matthew effect" in reading (Stanovich, 1986). Although not usually described in these terms, a generalized decline as a result of initial deficits also has been noted for math disability (see Chapter 3), specific language impairment (see Chapter 4), and other disorders. The Matthew effect (or its equivalent) underlies the need for early intervention with evidenced-based methods that are selected individually based on each child's needs.

The increased, and very appropriate, interest in neuropsychological perspectives by school personnel is evident and may be attributed to increased appreciation of the importance of these individual differences in treatment planning. Further, with medical advances, more and more children with neurodevelopmental and genetic disorders are surviving; with the movement for inclusive education, children with disorders are now more likely to be served in their public school setting. In translating the information gained from the neuropsychological evaluation as well as medical information, it may be helpful for a liaison to be developed between school personnel and other professionals functioning outside of the school (medical personnel, neuropsychologist). It has been suggested that neuropsychologists working with children become more cognizant of the environment in which children function and with the administrative and legal aspects specific to school settings (W. J. Ernst, Pelletier, & Simpson, 2008). In fact, Ernst et al. provided a summary of the major components (and potential obstacles) that neuropsychologists need to be aware of in order to effectively work in or with school settings (i.e., Individuals with Disabilities Education Act, the team approach, RtI, and the concept of educational rather than medical need).

In treatment planning, regardless of setting, it is important to prioritize treatment recommendations and to indicate clearly the domain or targeted behaviors for each component. Kanne et al. (2008) provided a format to facilitate this process specifically in relation to autism, but the same format would apply regardless of the disorder. In addition, the process Kanne and colleagues suggested includes a bridge between the report and the individualized educational plan, with possible methods for monitoring progress identified. This would ensure that the recommendations generated from the neuropsychological evaluation are in a format that student support teams can use in the development of intervention planning (Kanne et al., 2008). Also from the autism area, the Ziggurat model (Aspy & Grossman, 2007) suggests development of interventions and treatment plans based on the needs of the individual, the supports available, and task demands. Again, although proposed specifically for autism, the individual differences and changing targets of all children with neurodevelopmental disorders also would seem to benefit from this type of approach. These approaches are consistent with a recurring theme throughout this volume: the importance of assessing constructs that go beyond traditional evaluation of intelligence and academic achievement. Although intellectual and academic abilities certainly are important to understanding the child's current functioning, relying solely on these measures likely will lead the practitioner to miss subtle deficits in narrower areas of function, such as memory, language, and executive skills, that can better inform comprehensive intervention programs.

Finally, one major contribution of RtI as a process is the frequent monitoring of performance (Fuchs & Deshler, 2007), and this should be incorporated into all intervention planning. As was evident across chapters, for children with neurodevelopmental and genetic disorders, the manifestation of the syndrome may vary over time. Frequent monitoring and modification of the treatment plan is needed, whether through the use of neuropsychological assessment measures or curriculum-based measures, to document changes in behavior and development.

References

Aaron, P., Joshi, R. M., & Phipps, J. (2004). A cognitive tool to diagnose predominantly inattentive ADHD behaviour. *Journal of Attention Disorders, 7*, 125–135.

Aaron, P. G., Joshi, R. M., Gooden, R., & Kentum, K. E. (2008). Diagnosis and treatment of reading disabilities based on the component model of reading. *Journal of Learning Disabilities, 41*, 67–84.

Aarons, M., & Gittens, T. (1999). *The handbook of autism: A guide for parents and professionals* (2nd ed.). New York: Routledge.

Aarsen, F. K., van Dongen, H. R., Paquier, P. F., van Mourik, M., & Catsman-Berrevoets, C. E. (2004). Long-term sequelae in children after cerebellar astrocytoma surgery. *Neurology, 62*, 1311–1316.

Abbeduto, L., Murphy, M. M., Cawthon, S. W., Richmond, E., Weissman, M. D., Karadottir, S., et al. (2003). Receptive language skills of adolescents and young adults with Down or fragile X syndrome. *American Journal of Mental Retardation, 108*, 149–160.

Abbeduto, L., Pavetto, M., Kesin, E., Weissman, M., Karadottir, S., O'Brien, A., et al. (2001). The linguistic and cognitive profile of Down syndrome: Evidence from a comparison with fragile X syndrome. *Down Syndrome: Research and Practice, 7*, 9–15.

Abbeduto, L., Warren, S. F., & Conners, F. A. (2007). Language development in Down syndrome: From the prelinguistic period to the acquisition of literacy. *Mental Retardation and Developmental Disabilities Research Reviews, 13*, 247–261.

Abel, E. L., & Sokol, R. J. (1987). Incidence of fetal alcohol syndrome and economic impact of FAS-related anomalies. *Drug and Alcohol Dependence, 19*, 51–70.

Abell, F., Krams, M., Ashburner, J., Passingham, R., Friston, K., Frackowiaki, R., et al. (1999). The neuroanatomy of autism: A voxel-based whole brain analysis of structural scans. *NeuroReport, 10*, 1647–1651.

Accornero, V. H., Amado, A. J., Morrow, C. E., Xue, L., Anthony, J. C., & Bandstra, E. S. (2007). Impact of prenatal cocaine exposure on attention and response inhibition as assessed by continuous performance tests. *Journal of Developmental & Behavioral Pediatrics, 28*, 195–205.

Achenbach, T. M., Howell, C. T., Aoki, M. F., & Rauh, V. A. (1993). Nine-year outcome of the Vermont Intervention Program for low birth weight infants. *Pediatrics, 91*, 45–55.

Ackerman, P. T., Anhalt, J. M., Holcomb, P. J., & Dykman, R. A. (1986). Presumably innate and acquired automatic processes in children with attention and/or reading disorders. *Journal of Child Psychology and Psychiatry, 27*, 513–529.

Ackermann, H., Gräber, S., Hertrich, I., & Daum, I. (1999). Phonemic vowel length contrasts in cerebellar disorders. *Brain and Language, 67*(2), 95–109.

Ackermann, H., Mathiak, K., & Ivry, R. B. (2004). Temporal organization of "internal speech" as a basis for cerebellar modulation of cognitive functions. *Behavioral and Cognitive Neuroscience Reviews, 3*, 14–22.

Adab, N., Jacoby, A., Smith, D., & Chadwick, D. (2001). Additional educational needs in children born to mothers with epilepsy. *Journal of Neurology, Neurosurgery & Psychiatry, 70*, 15–21.

Adab, N., Kini, U., Vinten, J., Ayres, J., Baker, G., Clayton-Smith, J., et al. (2004). The longer term outcome of children born to mothers with epilepsy. *Journal of Neurology, Neurosurgery & Psychiatry, 11*, 1575–1583.

Adab, N., Tudur, S. C., Vinten, J., Williamson, P., & Winterbottom, J. (2004). Common antiepileptic drugs in pregnancy in women with epilepsy. *Cochrane Database of Systematic Reviews (Online), 3*, CD004848.

Adams, A., & Gathercole, S. E. (2000). Limitations in working memory: Implications for language development. *International Journal of Language & Communication Disorders, 35*, 95–116.

Adams, M. E., Aylett, S. E., Squier, W., & Chong, W. (2009). A spectrum of unusual neuroimaging findings in patients with suspected Sturge-Weber syndrome. *American Journal of Neuroradiology, 30*, 276–281.

Adgate, J. L., Barr, D. B., Clayton, C. A., Eberly, L. E., Freeman, N. C. G., Lioy, P. J., et al. (2001). Measurement of children's exposure to pesticides: Analysis of urinary metabolite levels in a probability-based sample. *Environmental Health Perspectives, 109*, 583–590.

Agency for Toxic Substances and Disease Registry. (1999). *ToxFAQs for Cadmium*. Retrieved January 13, 2008, from www.atsdr.cdc.gov/tfacts5.html.

Agency for Toxic Substances and Disease Registry. (2001). *ToxFAQs for Manganese*. Retrieved January 13, 2008, from www.atsdr.cdc.gov/tfacts151.html.

Ahmed, R., & Varghese, T. (2006). Unusual presentation of absence seizures: A case report. *Journal of Pediatric Neurology, 4*, 45–47.

Akefeldt, A., Akefeldt, B., & Gillberg, C. (1997). Voice, speech and language characteristics of children with Prader-Willi syndrome. *Journal of Intellectual Disability Research, 41*, 302–311.

Akefeldt, A., & Gillberg, C. (1999). Behavior and personality characteristics of children and young adults with Prader-Willi syndrome: A controlled study. *Journal of the American Academy of Child and Adolescent Psychiatry, 38*, 761–769.

Akshoomoff, N., Farid, N., Courchesne, E., & Haas, R. H. (2007). Abnormalities on the neurological examination and EEG in young children with pervasive developmental disorders. *Journal of Autism and Developmental Disorders, 37*, 887–893.

Alarcón, M., DeFries, J. C., & Pennington, B. F. (1997). A twin study of mathematics disability. *Journal of Learning Disabilities, 30*, 617–623.

Alarcón, M., Knopik, V. S., & DeFries, J. C. (2000). Covariation of mathematics achievement and general cognitive ability in twins. *Journal of School Psychology, 38*, 63–77.

Aldridge, J. E., Meyer, A., Seidler, F. J., & Slotkin, T. (2005). Alteration in central nervous system serotonergic and dopaminergic synaptive activity in adulthood after prenatal or neonatal chlorpyrifos exposure. *Environmental Health Perspective, 113*, 1027–1031.

Aldridge, J. E., Seidler, F. J., Meyer, A., Thillai, I., & Slotkin, T. (2003). Serotonergic systems targeted by developmental exposure to chlorpyrifos: Effects during different critical periods. *Environmental Health Perspective, 111*, 1736–1743.

Alexander, A., Anderson, H., Heilman, P., Voeller, K., & Torgesen, J. (1991). Phonological awareness training and the remediation of analytic decoding deficits in a group of severe dyslexics. *Annals of Dyslexia, 41*, 193–206.

Alexander, M. P. (1995). Mild traumatic brain injury: Pathophysiology, natural history, and clinical management. *Neurology, 45*, 1253–1260.

Ali, S., & Frederickson, N. (2006). Investigating the evidence base of social stories. *Educational Psychology in Practice, 22*, 355–377.

Allanson, J. E. (2007). Noonan syndrome. *American Journal of Medical Genetics, 145C*, 274–279.

Allen, D., Evans, C., Hider, A., Hawkins, S., Peckett, H., & Morgan, H. (2008). Offending behavior in adults with Asperger syndrome. *Journal of Autism and Developmental Disorders, 38*, 748–758.

Allen, J. W., Mutkus, L. A., & Aschner, M. (2001). Mercuric chloride, but not methylmercury, inhibits glutamine synthetase activity in primary cultures of cortical astrocytes. *Brain Research, 891*, 148–157.

Als, H., Gilkerson, L., Duffy, F. H., McAnulty, G. B., Buehler, D. M., VandenBerg, K., et al. (2003). A three-center, randomized, controlled trial of individualized developmental care for very low birth weight preterm infants: Medical, neurodevelopmental, parenting, and caregiving effects. *Journal of Developmental and Behavioral Pediatrics, 24,* 399–408.

Alsdorf, R., & Wyszynski, D. F. (2005). Teratogenicity of sodium valproate. *Expert Opinion on Drug Safety, 4*, 345–353.

Alsobrook, J. P., & Pauls, D. L. (2002). A factor analysis of tic symptoms in Gilles de la Tourette's syndrome. *American Journal of Psychiatry, 159*, 291–296.

Altemeier, L., Abbott, R. D., & Berninger, V. W. (in press). Contribution of executive functions to reading and writing in typical literacy development and dyslexia. *Journal of Clinical and Experimental Neuropsychology*.

Altiay, S., Kaya, M., Karasalihoglu, S., Gultekin, A., Oner, N., & Biner, B. (2006). 99mTc-HMPAP brain perfusion single-photon emission computed tomography in children with Down syndrome: Relationship to epilepsy, thyroid functions, and congenital heart disease. *Journal of Child Neurology, 21*, 610–614.

Amar, A. P. (2007). Vagus nerve stimulation for the treatment of intractable epilepsy. *Expert Review of Neurotherapeutics, 7*, 1763–1773.

Amaral, D. G., Schumann, C. M., & Nordahl, C. W. (2008). Neuroanatomy of autism. *Trends in Neurosciences, 31*, 137–145.

Amat, J. A., Bronen, R. A., Saluja, S., Sato, N., Zhu, H., Gorman, D. A., et al. (2006). Increased number of subcortical hyperintensities on MRI in children and adolescents with Tourette's syndrome, obsessive compulsive disorder, and attention deficit hyperactivity disorder. *American Journal of Psychiatry, 163*, 1106–1108.

American Academy of Pediatrics. (2000). Clinical practice guideline: Diagnosis and evaluation of the child with ADHD. *Pediatrics, 105*, 1158–1170.

American Academy of Pediatrics Committee on Children with Disabilities. (1998). Auditory integration training and facilitated communication for autism. *Pediatrics, 102*, 431–433.

American Cancer Society. (2006). *Cancer facts and figures*. Atlanta: Author.

American Diabetes Association. (2006). Total prevalence of diabetes and prediabetes. Retrieved December 19, 2008, from http://www.diabetes.org/diabetes-statistics/prevalence.jsp.

American Psychiatric Association (2000). *Diagnostic and statistical manual of mental disorders, 4th ed.: Text revision*. Washington, DC: Author.

American Speech-Language-Hearing Association. (1996). Central auditory processing: Current status of research and implications for clinical practice. *American Journal of Audiology, 5*, 41–54.

Anderson, G. M. (2004). Peripheral and central neurochemical effects of the selective serotonin reuptake inhibitors (SSRIs) in humans and nonhuman primates: Assessing bioeffect and mechanisms of action. *International Journal of Developmental Neuroscience, 22*, 397–404.

Anderson, G. M., Czarkowski, K., Ravski, N., & Epperson, C. N. (2004). Platelet serotonin in newborns and infants: Ontogeny, heritability, and effect of in utero exposure to selective serotonin reuptake inhibitors. *Pediatric Research, 56*, 418–422.

Anderson, P. J., Wood, S. J., Francis, D. E., Coleman, L., Anderson, V., & Boneh, A. (2007). Are neuropsychological impairments in children with early-treated phenylketonuria (PKU) related to white matter abnormalities or elevated phenylalanine levels? *Developmental Neuropsychology, 32*, 645–668.

Anderson, V., Godber, T., Smibert, E., & Ekert, H. (1997). Neurobehavioral sequelae following cranial irradiation and chemotherapy in children: An analysis of risk factors. *Pediatric Rehabilitation, 1*, 63–76.

Anderson, V. A., Anderson, P. Northam, E., Jacobs, R., Mikiewicz, O. (2002). Relationships between cognitive and behavioral measures of executive function in children with brain disease. *Child Neuropsychology, 8*, 231–240.

Andrews, T. K., Rose, F. D., & Johnson, D. A. (1998). Social and behavioural effects of traumatic brain injury in children. *Brain Injury, 12,* 133–138.

Angastiniotis, M., & Modell, B. (1998). Global epidemiology of hemoglobin disorders. *Annals of New York Academy of Science, 850*, 251–269.

Angelman, H. (1965). Puppet children: A report on three cases. *Developmental Medicine & Child Neurology, 7*, 681–688.

Angulo-Barroso, R. M., Wu, J., & Ulrich, D. A. (2008). Long-term effect of different treadmill interventions on gait development in new walkers with Down syndrome. *Gait & Posture, 27*, 231–238.

Antshel, K. M., & Waisbren, S. E. (2003). Timing is everything: Executive functions in children exposed to elevated levels of phenylalanine. *Neuropsychology, 17*, 458–468.

Apperly, I. A., Samson, D., & Humphreys, G. W. (2005). Domain-specificity and theory of mind: Evaluating neuropsychological evidence. *Trends in Cognitive Science, 9*, 572–577.

Aprea, C., Strambi, M., Novelli, M. T., Lunghini, L., & Bozzi, N. (2000). Biologic monitoring of exposure to organophosphorus pesticides in 195 Italian children. *Environmental Health Perspectives, 108*, 521–525.

Apter, A., Farbstein, I., & Yaniv, I. (2003). Psychiatric aspects of pediatric cancer. *Child and Adolescent Psychiatric Clinics of North America, 12*, 473–492.

Aram, D. M., Ekelman, B., & Nation, J. (1984). Preschoolers with language disorders: 10 years later. *Journal of Speech and Hearing Research, 27*, 232–245.

Aram, D. M., Hack, M., Hawkins, S.,Weissman, B. M., & Borawski-Clark, E. (1991). Very-low-birthweight children and speech and language development. *Journal of Speech & Hearing Research, 34,* 1169–1179.

Aram, D. M., & Hall, N. (1989). Longitudinal follow-up of children with preschool communication disorders: Treatment implications. *School Psychology Review, 18*, 487–501.

Archibald, L. M. D., & Gathercole, S. E. (2007). The complexities of complex memory span: Storage and processing deficits in specific language impairment. *Journal of Memory and Language, 57*, 177–194.

Archibald, S. L., Fennema-Notestine, C., Gamst, A., Jernigan, T. L., Mattson, S. N., & Riley, E. P. (2001). Brain dysmorphology in individuals with severe prenatal alcohol exposure. *Developmental Medicine & Child Neurology, 43*, 148–154.

Ardesch, J. J., Buschman, H. P. J., Wagener-Schimmel, L. J. J. C., van der Aa, H. E., & Hageman, G. (2007). Vagus nerve stimulation for medically refractory epilepsy: A long-term follow-up study. *Seizure, 16*, 579–585.

Ardila, A., Galeano, L. M., & Rosselli, M. (1998). Toward a model of neuropsychological activity. *Neuropsychology Review, 8*(4), 171–190.

Ardila, A., & Rosselli, M. (2002). Acalculia and dyscalculia. *Neuropsychology Review, 12*(4), 179–231.

Ardinger, H. H., Atkin, J. F., Blackston, D., Elsas, L. J., Clarren, S. K., Livingstone, S., et al. (2005). Verification of the fetal valproate syndrome phenotype. *American Journal of Medical Genetics, 29*, 171–185.

Arendt, R. W., Short, E. J., Singer, L. T., Minnes, S., Hewitt, J., Flynne, S., et al. (2004). Children prenatally exposed to cocaine: Developmental outcomes and environmental risks at seven years of age. *Journal of Developmental and Behavioral Pediatrics, 25*, 83–90.

Argargün, M. Y., Öner, A. F., & Akbayram, S. (2001). Hypnotic intervention for pain management in a child with sickle cell anemia. *Sleep and Hypnosis, 3*(3), 127–128.

Armstrong, F. D., & Briery, B. G. (2004). Childhood cancer and the school. In R. T. Brown (Ed.), *Handbook of pediatric psychology in school settings* (pp. 263–281). New York: Erlbaum.

Armstrong, F. D., Thompson, R., Wang, W., Zimmerman, R., Pegalow, C. H., Miller, S., et al. (1996). Cognitive functioning and brain magnetic resonance imaging in children with sickle cell disease: Neuropsychology Committee of the Cooperative Study of Sickle Cell Disease. *Pediatrics, 97*, 864–870.

Arnon, J., Schechtman, S., & Ornaoy, A. (2000). The use of psychiatric drugs in pregnancy and lactation. *Israel Journal of Psychiatry and Related Sciences, 37*, 205–222.

Asbury, K., Wachs, T. D., & Plomin, R. (2005). Environmental moderators of genetic influence on verbal and nonverbal abilities in early childhood. *Intelligence, 33*, 643–661.

Ashcraft, M. H., Krause, J. A., & Hopko, D. R. (2007). Is math anxiety a mathematical learning disability? In D. B. Berch & M. M. M. Mazzocco (Eds.), *Why is math so hard for some children? The nature and origins of mathematical difficulties and disabilities* (pp. 329–348). Baltimore, MD: Brookes.

Askins, M. A., & Moore, B. D., III. (2008). Preventing neurocognitive late effects in childhood cancer survivors. *Journal of Child Neurology, 23*, 1160–1171.

Atkinson, D. E., Brice-Bennett, S., & D'Souza, S. W. (2007). Antiepileptic medication during pregnancy: Does fetal genotype affect outcome? *Pediatric Research, 62*, 120–127.

Austin, J., & Caplan, K. (in press). Behavioral and psychiatric comorbidities in pediatric epilepsy: Toward an integrative model. *Epilepsia.*

Austin, J., Huberty, T. J., Huster, G. A., & Dunn, D. W. (1998). Academic achievement in children with epilepsy or asthma. *Developmental Medicine & Child Neurology, 40*, 248–255.

Avesani, R., Salvi, L., Rigoli, G., & Gambini, M. G. (2005). Reintegration after severe brain injury: A retrospective study. *Brain Injury, 19,* 933–939.

Axton, J. M. H. (1972). Six cases of poisoning after a parenteral organic mercurial compound (merthiolate). *Postgraduate Medical Journal, 48*, 417–421.

Aydin, M., Kabakus, N., Balci, T. A., & Ayar, A. (2007). Correlative study of the cognitive impairment, regional cerebral blood flow, and electroencephalogram abnormalities in children with Down syndrome. *International Journal of Neuroscience, 117*, 327–336.

Aydinok, Y., Ulger, Z., Nart, D., Terzi, A., Cetiner, N., Ellis, G., et al. (2007). A randomized controlled 1-year study of daily deferiprone plus twice weekly desferrioxamine compared with daily deferiprone monotherapy in patients with thalassemia major. *Hematology, 92*, 1599–1606.

Aylward, E. H., Minshew, N. J., Goldstein, G., Honeycutt, N. A., Augustine, A. M., Yates, K. O., et al. (1999). MRI volumes of amygdale and hippocampus in non-mentally retarded autistic adolescents and adults. *Neurology, 53*, 2145–2150.

Aylward, E. H., Richards, T. L., Berninger, V. W., Nagy, W., Field, K. M., Grimme, A., et al. (2003). Instructional treatment associated with changes in brain activation in children with dyslexia. *Neurology, 61*, 212–219.

Aylward, G. P. (2002). Cognitive and neuropsychological outcomes: More than IQ scores. *Mental Retardation and Developmental Disabilities Research Reviews, 8*, 234–240.

Bach, L. J., Happé, F., Fleminger, S., & Powell, J. (2005). Theory of mind: Independence of executive function and the role of the frontal cortex in acquired brain injury. *Cognitive Neuropsychiatry, 5*, 175–192.

Bachevalier, J. (1994). Medial temporal lobe structures and autism: A review of clinical and experimental findings. *Neuropsychologia, 32*, 627–648.

Bachevalier, J., & Loveland, K. A. (2006). The orbitofrontal-amygdala circuit and self-regulation of social-emotional behavior in autism. *Neuroscience & Biobehavioral Reviews, 30*, 97–117.

Bachman, J. A., & Hsueh, K.-H. (2008). Evaluation of online education about diabetes management in the school setting. *Journal of School Nursing, 24*(3), 151–157.

Baddeley, A. D. (2000). Short-term and working memory. In E. Tulving & F. I. M. Craik (Eds.), *The Oxford handbook of memory* (pp. 77–92). Oxford: Clarendon Press.

Baddeley, A. D. (2007). *Working memory, thought, and action*. New York: Oxford University Press.

Baddeley, A. D., Gathercole, S. E., & Papagno, C. (1998). The phonological loop as a language learning device. *Psychological Review, 105*, 158–173.

Baddeley, A. D., Papagno, C., & Vallar, G. (1988). When long-term learning depends on short-term storage. *Journal of Memory and Language, 27*, 586–595.

Bagner, D. M., Williams, L. B., Geffken, G. R., Silverstein, J. H., & Storch, E. A. (2007). Type 1 diabetes in youth: The relationship between adherence and executive functioning. *Children's Health Care, 36*, 169–179.

Bailet, L. L., & Turk, W. R. (2000). The impact of childhood epilepsy on neurocognitive and behavioral performance: A prospective longitudinal study. *Epilepsia, 41*, 426–431.

Bailey, A., LeCouteur, A., Gottestmen, I., Bolton, P., Simonoff, E., Yuzda, E., et al. (1995). Autism as a strongly genetic disorder: Evidence from a British twin study. *Psychological Medicine, 25*, 63–77.

Bailey, A., Luthert, P., Dean, A., Harding, B., Janota, I., Montgomery, M., et al. (1998). A clinicopathological study of autism. *Brain, 121*, 889–905.

Bailey, A., Phillips, W., & Rutter, M. (1996). Autism: Towards an integration of clinical, genetic, neuropsychological, and neurobiological perspectives. *Journal of Child Psychology and Psychiatry, 37*, 86–126.

Bailey, D. B. J., Roberts, J. E., Hooper, S. R., Hatton, D., Mirrett, P., Roberts, J. E., et al. (2004). Research on fragile X syndrome and autism: Implications for the study of genes, environments, and developmental language disorders. In M. L. Rice & S. F. Warren (Eds.), *Developmental language disorders: From phenotypes to etiologies* (pp. 121–150). Mahwah, NJ: Erlbaum.

Baker, L., & Cantwell, D. P. (1990). The association between emotional/behavioral disorders and learning disorders in children with speech/language disorders. *Advances in Learning and Behavioral Disabilities, 6*, 27–46.

Baker, M. J. (2000). Incorporating the thematic ritualistic behaviors of children with autism into games: Increasing social play interactions with siblings. *Journal of Positive Behavior Interventions, 2*, 66–84.

Baker, S., Gersten, R., & Lee, D. (2002). A synthesis of empirical research on teaching mathematics to low-achieving students. *Elementary School Journal, 103*, 51–73.

Ball, J. D., & Zinner, E. S. (1994). Pediatric brain injury: Psychoeducation for parents and teachers. *Advances in Medical Psychotherapy, 7*, 39–50.

Ball, L. K., Ball, R., & Pratt, D. (2001). An assessment of thimerosal use in childhood vaccines. *Pediatrics, 107*, 1147–1154.

Ballantyne, A. O., Spilkin, A. M., Hesselink, J., & Trauner, D. A. (2008). Plasticity in the developing brain: Intellectual, language and academic functions in children with ischaemic perinatal stroke. *Brain, 131*, 2975–2985.

Ballantyne, A. O., Spilkin, A. M., & Trauner, D. A. (2007). Language outcome after perinatal stroke: Does side matter? *Child Neuropsychology, 13*, 494–509.

Ballas, S. K. (2002). Sickle cell anaemia: Progress in pathogenesis and treatment. *Drugs, 62*, 1143–1172.

Bandstra, E. S., Morrow, C. E., Anthony, J. C., Accornero, V. H., & Fried, P. A. (2001). Longitudinal investigation of task persistence and sustained attention in children with prenatal cocaine exposure. *Neurotoxicology and Teratology, 23*, 545–559.

Bangs, M. E., Emslie, G. J., Spencer, T. J., Ramsey, J. L., Carlson, C., Bartky, E. J., et al. (2007). Efficacy and safety of atomoxetine in adolescents with attention-deficit/hyperactivity disorder and major depression. *Journal of Child and Adolescent Psychopharmacology, 17*, 407–419.

Baptista-Neto, L., Dodds, A., Rao, S., Whitney, J., Torres, A. R., & Gonzalez-Heydrich, J. (2008). An expert opinion on methylphenidate treatment for attention deficit hyperactivity disorder in pediatric patients with epilepsy. *Expert Opinion on Investigational Drugs, 17*, 77–84.

Barakat, L. P., Hetzke, J. D., Foley, B., Carey, M. E., Gyato, K., & Phillips, P. C. (2003). Evaluation of a social-skills training group intervention with children treated for brain tumors: A pilot study. *Journal of Pediatric Psychology, 28*, 299–307.

Barbagallo, M., Ruggieri, M., Incorpora, G., Pavone, P., Nucifora, C., Spalice, A., et al. (2009). Infantile spasms in the setting of Sturge Weber syndrome. *Child's Nervous System, 25*, 111–118.

Barbarin, O., Whitten, C., & Bonds, S. (1994). Estimating rates of psychosocial problems in urban and poor children with sickle cell anemia. *Health and Social Work, 19*, 112–119.

Barbieri, F., & Ferioli, A. (1994). Morpholine derivatives. *Toxicology and Applied Pharmacology, 91*, 83–86.

Bard, K. A., Coles, C. D., Platzman, K. A., & Lynch, M. E. (2000). The effects of prenatal drug exposure, term status, and caregiving on arousal and arousal modulation in 8-week-old infants. *Developmental Psychobiology, 36*, 194–212.

Barkley, R. A. (1997). Behavioral inhibition, sustained attention, and executive functions: Constructing a unifying theory of ADHD. *Psychological Bulletin, 121*, 65–94.

Barkley, R. A. (1998). *Attention-deficit hyperactivity disorder: A handbook for diagnosis and treatment* (2nd ed.). New York: Guilford.

Barkley, R. A., Fischer, M., Smallish, L., & Fletcher, K. (2004). Young adult follow-up of hyperactive children: Antisocial activities and drug use. *Journal of Child Psychology and Psychiatry, 45*, 195–211.

Barnes, M. A., Fletcher, J., & Ewing-Cobbs, L. (2007). Mathematical disabilities in congenital and acquired neurodevelopmental disorders. In D. B. Berch & M. M. M. Mazzocco (Eds.), *Why is math so hard for some children? The nature and origins of mathematical learning difficulties and disabilities* (pp. 195–218). Baltimore, MD: Brookes.

Barnette, A. R., & Inder, T. E. (2009). Evaluation and management of stroke in the neonate. *Clinics in Perinatology, 36*, 125–136.

Baron, I. S. (2008). Growth and development of pediatric neuropsychology. In J. E. Morgan & J. H. Ricker (Eds.), *Textbook of clinical neuropsychology. Studies on neuropsychology, neurology and cognition* (pp. 91–104). New York: Psychology Press.

Baron-Cohen, S. (1988). Social and pragmatic deficits in autism: Cognitive or affective? *Journal of Autism and Developmental Disorders, 18*, 379–402.

Baron-Cohen, S. (1995). *Mindblindness: An essay on theory of mind and autism*. Cambridge, MA: MIT Press.

Baron-Cohen, S., Baldwin, D. A., & Crowson, M. (1997). Do children with autism use the speaker's direction of gaze strategy to crack the code of language? *Child Development, 68*, 48–57.

Baron-Cohen, S., Leslie, A. M., & Frith, U. (1985). Does the autistic child have a "theory of mind"? *Cognition, 21*, 37–46.

Baron-Cohen, S., Wheelwright, S., Hill, J., Raste, Y., & Plumb, I. (2001). The 'Reading the mind in the eyes' test, revised version: A study with normal adults, and adults with Asperger syndrome or high-functioning autism. *Journal of Child Psychology and Psychiatry, 42*, 241–253.

Barr, C. L., Wigg, K. G., Pakstis, A. J., Kurlan, R., Pauls, D. L., Kidd, K. K., et al. (1999). Genome scan for linkage to Gilles de la Tourette syndrome. *American Journal of Medical Genetics, 88*, 437–445.

Barr, H. M., Sampson, P. D., & Streissguth, A. P. (1990). Moderate prenatal alcohol exposure: Effects on child IQ and learning problems at age 7 years. *Alcoholism: Clinical and Experimental Research, 14*, 662–669.

Barrera, M. E., Rosenbaum, P. L., & Cunningham, C. E. (1986). Early home intervention with low-birth-weight infants and their parents. *Child Development, 57*, 20–33.

Barrois, L., Haynes, R., Riccio, C., & Haws, B. (2006). *Prediction of mathematical skills with the BRIEF in children.* Paper presented at the National Academy of Neuropsychology Conference, San Antonio, TX.

Barry, J. G., Yasin, I., & Bishop, D. V. M. (2007). Heritable risk factors associated with language impairment. *Genes, Brain & Behavior, 6*, 66–76.

Bartlett, C. W., Flax, J. F., Logue, M. W., Smith, B. J., Vieland, V. J., Tallal, P., et al. (2004). Examination of potential overlap in autism and language loci on chromosomes 2, 7, and 13 in two independent samples ascertained for specific language impairment. *Human Heredity, 57*, 10–20.

Bartlett, C. W., Flax, J. F., Logue, M. W., Vieland, V. J., Bassett, A. S., Tallal, P., et al. (2002). A major susceptibility locus for specific language impairment is located on 13q21. *American Journal of Human Genetics, 71*, 45–55.

Barton, B., & North, K. N. (2004). Social skills of children with neurofibromatosis type 1. *Developmental Medicine and Child Neurology, 46*, 553–563.

Barton, B., & North, K. N. (2007). The self-concept of children and adolescents with neurofibromatosis type 1. *Child: Care, Health and Development, 33*, 401–408.

Barton, M., & Volkmar, F. (1998). How commonly are known medical conditions associated with autism? *Journal of Autism and Developmental Disorders, 28*, 273–278.

Baskin, H. J. (2008). The pathogenesis and imaging of the tuberous sclerosis complex. *Pediatric Radiology, 38*, 936–952.

Batchelor, E. S. (1996). Neuropsychological assessment of children. In J. E. S Batchelor & R. S. Dean (Eds.), *Pediatric neuropsychology: Interfacing assessment and treatment for rehabilitation* (pp. 9–26). Boston: Allyn & Bacon.

Bates, E., Reilly, J., Wulfeck, B., Dronkers, N., Opie, M., Fenson, J., et al. (2001). Differential effects of unilateral lesions on language production in children and adults. *Brain and Language, 79*, 223–265.

Bates, E., Thal, D., Trauner, D., Fenson, J., Aram, D. M., Eisele, J., et al. (1997). From first words to grammar in children with focal brain injury. *Developmental Neuropsychology, 13*, 447–476.

Batista, C. E. A., Chugani, H. T., Hu, J., Haacke, E. M., Behen, M. E., Helder, E. J., et al. (2008). Magnetic resonance spectroscopic imaging detects abnormalities in normal-appearing frontal lobe of patients with Sturge-Weber syndrome. *Journal of Neuroimaging, 18*, 306–313.

Batista, C. E. A., Juhasz, C., Muzik, O., Chugani, D. C., & Chugani, H. T. (2007). Increased visual cortex glucose metabolism contralateral to angioma in children with Sturge-Weber syndrome. *Developmental Medicine & Child Neurology, 49*, 567–573.

Batshaw, M. L., Pellegrino, L., & Roizen, N. J. (2007). *Children with disabilities* (6th ed.). Baltimore, MD: Brookes.

Bauermeister, J. J., Matos, M., Reina, G., Salas, C. C., Martinez, J. V., Cumba, E., et al. (2005). Comparison of the DSM-IV combined and inattentive types of ADHD in a school-based sample of Latino/Hispanic children. *Journal of Child Psychology and Psychiatry, 46*, 166–179.

Bauman, M. (1991). Microscopic neuroanatomic abnormalities in autism. *Pediatrics, 87*, 791–796.

Bauman, M., & Kemper, T. L. (1985). Histoanatomic observations of the brain in early infantile autism. *Neurology, 35*, 866–874.

Bauman, M., & Kemper, T. L. (2005). Neuroanatomic observations of the brain in autism: A review and future directions. *International Journal of Developmental Neuroscience, 23*, 183–187.

Bauman, M., & Kemper, T. L. (2007). The neuroanatomy of the brain in autism: Current thoughts and future directions. In J. M. Pérez, P. M. González, M. Llorente Comí, & C. Nieto (Eds.), *New developments in autism: The future is today* (pp. 259–267). London: Jessica Kingsley.

Baumer, J. H., Hunt, L. P., & Shield, J. P. H. (1998). Social disadvantage, family composition, and diabetes mellitus: Prevalence and outcomes. *Archives of Diseases in Children, 79*, 427–430.

Baumert, M., Brozek, G., Paprotny, M., Walencka, Z., Sodowska, H., Cnota, W., et al. (2008). Epidemiology of peri/intraventricular haemorrhage in newborns at term. *Journal of Physiology and Pharmacology, 59* (Suppl. 4), 67–75.

Baumgartel, A., Wolraich, M., & Dietrich, M. (1995). Comparison of diagnostic criteria for attention deficit disorders in a German elementary school sample. *Journal of the American Academy of Child and Adolescent Psychiatry, 34*, 629–638.

Bawden, H. N., Stokes, A., Camfield, C. S., Camfield, P. R., & Salisbury, S. (1998). Peer relationship problems in children with Tourette's disorder or diabetes mellitus. *Journal of Child Psychology and Psychiatry, 39*, 663–668.

Bax, M. C., & Colville, G. A. (1995). Behavior in mucopolysaccharide disorders. *Archives of Disease in Childhood, 73*, 77–81.

Baxter, A. J., & Krenzelok, E. P. (2008). Pediatric fatality secondary to EDTA chelation. *Clinical Toxicology, 46*, 1083–1084.

Baym, C. L., Corbett, B. A., Wright, S. B., & Bunge, S. A. (2008). Neural correlates of tic severity and cognitive control in children with Tourette syndrome. *Brain, 131*, 165–179.

Bazarian, J. J., McClung, J., Shah, M. N., Cheng, Y. T., Flesher, W., & Kraus, J. (2005). Mild traumatic brain injury in the United States, 1998–2000. *Brain Injury, 19,* 85–91.

Bazylewicz-Walckzak, B., Majkzakova, W., & Szymczak, M. (1999). Behavioral effects of occupational exposure to organophosphorous pesticides in female greenhouse planting workers. *Neurotoxicology and Teratology, 20*, 819–826.

Becker, P. T., Grunwald, P. C., & Brazy, J. E. (1999). Motor organization in very low birth weight infants during caregiving: Effects of a developmental intervention. *Journal of Developmental and Behavioral Pediatrics, 20,* 344–354.

Beckung, E., Steffenburg, S., & Kyllerman, M. (2004). Motor impairments, neurological signs, and developmental level in individuals with Angelman syndrome. *Developmental Medicine and Child Neurology, 46*, 239–243.

Beebe, D. W., Ris, M. D., Armstrong, F. D., Fontanesi, J., Mulhern, R. K., Holmes, E., et al. (2005). Cognitive and adaptive outcome in low-grade pediatric cerebellar astrocytomas: Evidence of diminished cognitive and adaptive functioning in national collaborative studies. *Journal of Clinical Oncology, 23*, 5198–5204.

Beilock, S. L., Rydell, R. J., & McConnell, A. R. (2007). Stereotype threat and working memory: Mechanisms, alleviation, and spillover. *Journal of Experimental Psychology: General, 136*, 256–276.

Beitchman, J. H., Brownlie, E. B., Inglis, A., Wild, J., Ferguson, B., Schachter, D., et al. (1996). Seven-year follow-up of speech/language impaired and control children: Psychiatric outcome. *Journal of Child Psychology and Psychiatry, 37*, 961–970.

Beitchman, J. H., Brownlie, E. B., & Wilson, B. (1996). Linguistic impairment and psychiatric disorder: Pathways to outcome. In J. H. Beitchman, N. J. Cohen, M. M. Konstantareas, & R. Tannock (Eds.), *Language, learning, and behavior disorders: Developmental, biological, and clinical perspectives* (pp. 493–514). New York: Cambridge University Press.

Beitchman, J. H., Hood, J., & Inglis, A. (1990). Psychiatric risk in children with speech and language disorders. *Journal of Abnormal Child Psychology, 18*, 283–296.

Belanger, H. G., Vanderploeg, R. D., Curtiss, G., & Warden, D. L. (2007). Recent neuroimaging techniques in mild traumatic brain injury. *Journal of Neuropsychiatry and Clinical Neurosciences, 19,* 5–20.

Bell, N. (1991). Gestalt imagery: A critical factor in language comprehension. *Annals of Dyslexia, 41,* 246–260.

Bellinger, D., Leviton, A., Waternaux, C., Needleman, H., & Rabinowitz, M. (1987). Longitudinal analyses of prenatal and postnatal lead exposure and early cognitive development. *New England Journal of Medicine, 316,* 1037–1043.

Bellinger, D., Leviton, A., Waternaux, C., Needleman, H., & Rabinowitz, M. (1988). Low-level lead exposure, social class, and infant development. *Neurotoxicology and Teratology, 10,* 497–503.

Bellinger, D., Stiles, K. M., & Needleman, H. A. (1992). Low-level lead exposure, intelligence and academic achievement: A long-term follow-up study. *Pediatrics, 90,* 855–861.

Bellini, S., & Akullian, J. (2007). A meta-analysis of video modeling and video self-modeling interventions for children and adolescents with autism spectrum disorders. *Exceptional Children, 73,* 264–287.

Bellini, S., & Peters, J. K. (2008). Social skills training for youth with autism spectrum disorders *Child and Adolescent Psychiatric Clinics of North America, 17,* 857–873.

Bellugi, U., Järvinen-Pasley, A., Doyle, T. F., Reilly, J., Reiss, A. L., & Korenberg, J. (2007). Affect, social behavior, and the brain in Williams syndrome. *Current Directions in Psychological Science, 16,* 99–104.

Bellugi, U., Lichtenberger, L., Mills, D., Galaburda, A., & Korenberg, J. R. (1999). Bridging cognition, the brain, and molecular genetics: Evidence from Williams syndrome. *Trends in Neurosciences, 22,* 197–207.

Bellugi, U., Lichtenberger, L., Jones, W., Lai, Z., & St. George, M. (2000). The neurocognitive profile of Williams syndrome: A complex pattern of strengths and weaknesses. *Journal of Cognitive Neuroscience, 12* (Suppl. 1), 7–29.

Belmonte, M. K., Mazziotta, J. C., Minshew, N. J., Evans, A. C., Courchesne, E., Dager, S. R., et al. (2008). Offering to share: How to put heads together in autism neuroimaging. *Journal of Autism and Developmental Disorders, 38,* 2–13.

Belser, R. C., & Sudhalter, V. (2001). Conversational characteristics of children with fragile X syndrome: Repetitive speech. *American Journal on Mental Retardation, 106,* 28–38.

Benasich, A. A., Curtiss, S., & Tallal, P. (1993). Language, learning, and behavioral disturbances in childhood: A longitudinal perspective. *Journal of the American Academy of Child and Adolescent Psychiatry, 32,* 585–594.

Benbadis, S. R., Tatum, I. V., & William, O. (2001). Advances in the treatment of epilepsy. *American Family Physician, 64,* 91–99.

Bender, H. A., Auciello, D., Morrison, C. E., MacAllister, W. S., & Zaroff, C. M. (2008). Comparing the convergent validity and clinical utility of the Behavior Assessment System for Children—Parent Rating Scales and Child Behavior Checklist in children with epilepsy. *Epilepsy & Behavior, 13,* 237–242.

Bender, H. A., Marks, B. C., Brown, E. R., Zach, L., & Zaroff, C. M. (2007). Neuropsychologic performance of children with epilepsy on the NEPSY. *Pediatric Neurology, 36,* 312–317.

Benifla, M., Rutka, J. T., Logan, W., & Donner, E. J. (2006). Vagal nerve stimulation for refractory epilepsy in children: Indications and experience at the Hospital for Sick Children. *Child's Nervous System, 22*, 1018–1026.

Bennett, K., & Cavanaugh, R. A. (1998). Effects of immediate self-correction, delayed self-correction, and no correction on the acquisition and maintenance of multiplication facts by a fourth grade student with learning disabilities. *Journal of Applied Behavior Analysis, 31*, 303–306.

Bennett, P. H. (1994). Definition, diagnosis, and classification of diabetes mellitus and impaired glucose tolerance. In C. R. Kahn & G. C. Weir (Eds.), *Joslin's diabetes mellitus* (pp. 193–200). Philadelphia: Lea & Febiger.

Bennett, T., Szatmari, P., Bryson, S., Volden, J., Zwaigenbuam, L., Vaccarella, L., et al. (2008). Differentiating autism and Asperger syndrome on the basis of language delay or impairment. *Journal of Autism and Developmental Disorders, 38*, 616–625.

Bennett, T. L., & Ho, M. R. (2009). The neuropsychology of pediatric epilepsy and antiepileptic drugs. In C. R. Reynolds & E. Fletcher-Janzen (Eds.), *Handbook of clinical child neuropsychology* (3rd ed., pp. 505–528). New York: Springer.

Bennetto, L., Pennington, B., & Rogers, S. (1996). Intact and impaired memory function in autism. *Child Development, 67*, 1816–1835.

Bercovici, E. (2005). Prenatal and perinatal effects of psychotropic drugs on neuro-cognitive development in the fetus. *Journal on Developmental Disabilities, 11*(2), 1–20.

Berg, R. A., & Linton, J. C. (1997). Neuropsychological sequelae of chronic medical disorders in children and youth. In C. R. Reynolds & E. Fletcher-Janzen (Eds.), *Handbook of clinical child neuropsychology* (2nd ed., pp. 663–687). New York: Plenum.

Bergqvist, A. G., Schall, J. J., Gallagher, P. R., Cnaan, A., & Stallings, V. A. (2005). Fasting versus gradual initiation of the ketogenic diet: A prospective, randomized clinical trial of efficacy. *Epilepsia, 46*, 1810–1819.

Berkelhammer, L. D. (2008). Pediatric neuropsychological evaluation. In M. Herson & A. M. Gross (Eds.), *Handbook of clinical psychology* (pp. 497–519). Hoboken, NJ: Wiley.

Berkelhammer, L. D., Williamson, A. L., Sanford, S. D., Dirkson, C. L., Sharp, W., Margulies, A. S., et al. (2007). Neurocognitive sequelae of pediatric sickle cell disease: A review of the literature. *Child Neuropsychology, 13*, 120–131.

Bernard, L., Muldoon, K., Hasan, R., O'Brien, G., & Steward, M. (2008). Profiling executive dysfunction in adults with autism and comorbid learning disability. *Autism, 12*, 125–141.

Bernard, S., Enayati, A., Redwood, L., Roger, H., & Binstock, T. (2001). Autism: A novel form of mercury poisoning. *Medical Hypotheses, 56*, 462–471.

Berninger, V. W., Nielsen, K. H., Abbott, R., D., Wijsman, E., & Raskind, W. (2008a). Gender differences in severity of writing and reading disabilities. *Journal of School Psychology, 46*, 151–172.

Berninger, V. W., Nielsen, K. H., Abbott, R., D., Wijsman, E., & Raskind, W. (2008b). Writing problems in developmental dyslexia: Under-recognized and under-treated. *Journal of School Psychology, 46*, 1–21.

Berninger, V. W., Raskind, W., Richards, T. L., Abbott, R. D., & Stock, P. S. (2008). A multidisciplinary approach to understanding developmental dyslexia within working-memory architecture: Genotypes, phenotypes, brain, and instruction. *Developmental Neuropsychology, 33*, 707–744.

Berry-Kravis, E., Hessl, D., Coffey, S., Hervey, C., Schneider, A., Yuhas, J., et al. (2009). A pilot open label, single dose of fenobam in adults with fragile X syndrome. *Journal of Medical Genetics, 46*, 266–271.

Berry-Kravis, E., & Potanos, K. (2004). Psychopharmacology in fragile X syndrome: Present and future. *Mental Retardation and Developmental Disabilities Research Reviews, 10*, 42–48.

Berry-Kravis, E., Sumis, A., Hervery, C., Nelson, M., Porges, S. W., Weng, N., et al. (2008). Open-label treatment trial of lithium to target the underlying defect in fragile X syndrome. *Journal of Developmental & Behavioral Pediatrics, 29*, 293–302.

Besag, F. M. C. (1995). Myoclonus and infantile spasms. In M. M. Robertson & V. Eapen (Eds.), *Movement and allied disorders in childhood* (pp. 149–175). Oxford: Wiley.

Besag, F. M. C. (2004). Behavioral aspects of pediatric epilepsy syndromes. *Epilepsy and Behavior, 5*(Suppl.), S3–S13.

Best, C. S., Moffat, V. J., Power, M. J., Owens, D. G. C., & Johnstone, E. C. (2008). The boundaries of the cognitive phenotype of autism: Theory of mind, central coherence, and ambiguous figure perception in young people with autistic traits. *Journal of Autism and Developmental Disorders, 38*, 840–847.

Bhat, S. R., Goodwin, T. L., Burwinkle, T. M., Lansdale, M. F., Dahl, G. V., Huhn, S. L., et al. (2005). Profile of daily life in children with brain tumors: An assessment of health-related quality of life. *Journal of Clinical Oncology, 23*, 5493–5500.

Bhattacharya, A., & Ehri, L. C. (2004). Graphosyllabic analysis helps adolescent struggling readers read and spell words. *Journal of Learning Disabilities, 37*, 331–348.

Bhattacharya, A., Shukla, R., Auyang, E. D., Dietrich, K. N., & Bornschein, R. L. (2007). Effect of succimer chelation therapy on postural balance and gait outcomes in children with early exposure to environmental lead. *Neurotoxicology, 28*, 686–695.

Bhattacharya, A., Shukla, R., Dietrich, K. N., & Bornschein, R. L. (2006). Effect of early lead exposure on the maturation of children's postural balance: A longitudinal study. *Neurotoxicology and Teratology, 28*, 376–385.

Bhutta, A. T., Cleves, M. A., Casey, P. H., Cradock, M. M., & Anand, K. J. S. (2002). Cognitive and behavioral outcomes of school-aged children who were born preterm: A meta-analysis. *Journal of the American Medical Association, 288*, 728–737.

Bialystok, E. (2001). *Bilingualism in development: Language, literacy, and cognition*. New York: Cambridge University Press.

Biederman, J. (2005). Attention-deficit/hyperactivity disorder: A selective overview. *Biological Psychiatry, 57*, 1215–1220.

Biessels, G. J., Kerssen, A., de Haan, E. H. F., & Kappelle, L. J. (2007). Cognitive dysfunction and diabetes: Implications for primary care. *Primary Care Diabetes, 1*(4), 187–193.

Bigel, G. M., & Smith, M. L. (2001). The impact of different neuropathologies on pre- and postsurgical neuropsychological functioning in children with temporal lobe epilepsy. *Brain and Cognition, 46*, 46–49.

Bigler, E. D. (1999). Neuroimaging in pediatric traumatic head injury: Diagnostic considerations and relationships to neurobehavioral outcome. *Journal of Head Trauma Rehabilitation, 14*, 406–423.

Bigler, E. D., Tate, D. F., Neeley, E. S., Wolfson, L. J., Miller, M. J., Rice, S. A., et al. (2003). Temporal lobe, autism, and macrocephaly. *American Journal of Neuroradiology, 24*, 2066–2076.

Billingsley, R. L., Jackson, E. F., Slopis, J. M., Swank, P. R., Mahankali, S., & Moore, B. D. (2004). Functional MRI of visual-spatial processing in neurofibromatosis, type I. *Neuropsychologia, 42*, 395–404.

Billingsley, R. L., Jackson, E. F., Slopis, J. M., Swank, P. R., Mahankali, S., & Moore, B. D., III. (2003). Functional magnetic resonance imaging of phonologic processing in neurofibromatosis 1. *Journal of Child Neurology, 18*, 731–740.

Billingsley, R. L., Schrimsher, G. W., Jackson, E. F., Slopis, J. M., & Moore, B. D., III. (2002). Significance of planum temporale and planum parietale morphologic features in neurofibromatosis type 1. *Archives of Neurology, 59*, 616–622.

Billingsley, R. L., Slopis, J. M., Swank, P. R., Jackson, E. F., & Moore, B. D., III. (2003). Cortical morphology associated with language function in neurofibromatosis, type I. *Brain and Language, 85*, 125–139.

Billstedt, E., Gillberg, I. C., & Gillberg, C. (2005). Autism after adolescence: Population-based 13- to 22-year follow-up study of 120 individuals with autism diagnosed in childhood. *Journal of Autism and Developmental Disorders, 35*, 351–360.

Bishop, D. V. M. (1992). The underlying nature of specific language impairment. *Journal of Child Psychology and Psychiatry, 33*, 1–64.

Bishop, D. V. M. (2002). The role of genes in the etiology of specific language impairment. *Journal of Communication Disorders, 35*, 311–328.

Bishop, D. V. M., & Hayiou-Thomas, M. E. (2008). Heritability of specific language impairment depends on diagnostic criteria. *Genes, Brain & Behavior, 7*, 365–372.

Bishop, D. V. M., Laws, G., Adams, C., & Norbury, C. F. (2006). High heritability of speech and language impairments in 6-year-old twins demonstrated using parent and teacher report. *Behavior Genetics, 36*, 173–184.

Bishop, D. V. M., & McArthur, G. M. (2005). Individual differences in auditory processing in specific language impairment: A follow-up study using event-related potentials and behavioural thresholds. *Cortex, 41*, 327–341.

Bishop, D. V. M., & Norbury, C. F. (2002). Exploring the borderlands of autistic disorder and specific language impairment: A study using standardized diagnostic instruments. *Journal of Child Psychology and Psychiatry, 43*, 917–929.

Blaauwbroek, R., Groenier, K. H., Kamps, W. A., Meyboom-de Jong, B., & Postma, A. (2007). Late effects in adult survivors of childhood cancer: The need for life-long follow-up. *Annals of Oncology, 18*, 1898–1902.

Blacher, J., Kraemer, B., & Schalow, M. (2003). Asperger syndrome and high-functioning autism: Research concerns and emerging foci. *Current Opinion in Psychiatry, 16,* 535–542.

Blair, C. (2002). Early intervention for low birth weight, preterm infants: The role of negative emotionality in the specification of effects. *Development and Psychopathology, 14,* 311–332.

Blaney, S. M., Kun, L. E., Hunter, J., Rorke-Adams, L. B., Lau, C., Strother, D., et al. (2006). Tumors of the central nervous system. In P. A. Pizzo & D. G. Poplack (Eds.), *Principles and practice of pediatric oncology* (5th ed., pp. 786–864). Philadelphia: Lippincott.

Bleyer, W. A. (1990). The impact of childhood cancer on the United States and the world. *Cancer: A Cancer Journal for Clinicians, 40*, 355–367.

Bleyer, W. A. (1999). Epidemiologic impact of children with brain tumors. *Child's Nervous System 15*, 758–763.

Blischak, D. M., Shah, S. D., Lombardino, L. J., & Chiarella, K. (2004). Effects of phonemic awareness instruction on the encoding skills of children with severe speech impairment. *Disability and Rehabilitation, 26*, 1295–1304.

Bliss, L. S., Allen, D. V., & Walker, G. (1978). Sentence structures of trainable and educable mentally retarded subjects. *Journal of Speech and Hearing Research, 21*, 722–731.

Bloch, M. H., Leckman, J. F., Zhu, H., & Peterson, B. (2005). Caudate volumes in childhood predict symptom severity in adults with Tourette syndrome. *Neurology, 65*, 1253–1258.

Bloch, M. H., Sukhodolsky, D. G., Leckman, J. F., & Schultz, R. T. (2006). Fine-motor skill deficits in childhood predict adulthood tic severity and global psychosocial functioning in Tourette's syndrome. *Journal of Child Psychology and Psychiatry, 47*, 551–559.

Bloss, C. S., & Courchesne, E. (2007). MRI neuroanatomy in young girls with autism: A preliminary study. *Journal of the American Academy of Child & Adolescent Psychiatry, 46*, 515–523.

Boake, C. (2008). Clinical neuropsychology. *Professional Psychology: Research and Practice, 39*, 234–239.

Bodansky, H. J., Beverley, D. W., Gelsthorpe, K., Saunders, A., Bottazzo, G. F., & Haigh, D. (1987). Insulin dependent diabetes in Asians. *Archives of Diseases in Children, 62*, 227–230.

Boddaert, N., Mochel, F., Meresse, I., Seidenwurm, D., Cachia, A., Brunelle, F., et al. (2005). Parieto-occipital grey matter abnormalities in children with Williams syndrome. *NeuroImage, 30*, 721–725.

Bodin, D., Beetar, J. T., Yeates, K. O., Boyer, K., & Colvin, A. N. (2007). A survey of parent satisfaction with pediatric neuropsychological evaluations. *Clinical Neuropsychologist, 21*, 884–898.

Boll, T. J., & Stanford, L. D. (1997). Pediatric brain injury: Brain mechanisms and amelioration. In C. R. Reynolds and E. Fletcher-Janzen (Eds.), *Handbook of clinical child neuropsychology* (2nd ed., pp. 140–156). New York: Plenum.

Bolman, W. M., & Richmond, J. A. (1999). A double-blind, placebo-controlled, crossover pilot trial of low-dose dimethylglycine in patients with autistic disorder. *Journal of Autism and Developmental Disorders, 29*, 191–194.

Boman, U. W., Hanson, C. A., Hijelmquist, E., & Möller, A. (2006). Personality traits in women with Turner syndrome. *Scandinavian Journal of Psychology, 47*, 219–223.

Bonneau, F., Lenherr, E. D., Pena, V., Hart, D. J., & Scheffzek, K. (2009). Solubility survey of fragments of the neurofibromatosis type 1 protein neurofibromin. *Protein Expression and Purification, 65*, 30–37.

Booth, J. L., & Siegler, R. S. (2008). Numerical magnitude representations influence arithmetic learning. *Child Development, 79*, 1016–1031.

Borg, E. (2007). If mirror neurons are the answer, what was the question? *Journal of Consciousness Studies, 14*, 5–19.

Bornstein, R. A. (1990). Neuropsychological performance in children with Tourette's syndrome. *Psychiatry Research, 33*, 73–81.

Bortz, J. J., Prigatano, G. P., Blum, D., & Fisher, R. S. (1995). Differential response characteristics in the nonepileptic and epileptic seizure patients on a test of verbal learning and memory. *Neurology, 45*, 2029–2034.

Bourgeois, B. F. (1998). Antiepileptic drugs, learning, and behavior in childhood epilepsy. *Epilepsia, 39*, 913–921.

Bourgeois, B. F., Prensky, A. L., Palkes, H. S., Talent, B. K., & Busch, G. B. (1983). Intelligence in epilepsy: A prospective study in children. *Annals of Neurology, 14*, 438–444.

Bowen, J. M. (2005). Classroom interventions for students with traumatic brain injuries. *Preventing School Failure, 49*, 34–41.

Boyce, G. C., Saylor, C. F., & Price, C. L. (2004). School-age outcomes for early intervention participants who experienced intraventricular hemorrhage and low birth weight. *Children's Health Care, 33*, 257–274.

Boyd, S. G., Harden, A., & Patton, M. A. (1988). The EEG in early diagnosis of the Angelman (Happy Puppet) syndrome. *European Journal of Pediatrics, 147*, 508–513.

Boyle, J., McCartney, E., Forbes, J., & O'Hare, A. (2007). A randomised controlled trial and economic evaluation of direct versus indirect and individual versus group modes of speech and language therapy for children with primary language impairment. *Health Technology Assessment, 11*, 1–139.

Braden, J. S., & Obrzut, J. E. (2002). Williams syndrome: Neuropsychological findings and implications for practice. *Journal of Developmental and Physical Disabilities, 14*, 203–213.

Bradley, L., & Bryant, P. E. (1983). Categorizing sounds and learning to read: A causal connection. *Nature, 301*, 419–421.

Bradley, R. H., Whiteside, L., Mundfrom, D. J., Casey, P. H., Caldwell, B. M., & Barrett, K. (1994). Impact of the Infant Health and Development Program (IHDP) on the home environments of infants born prematurely and with low birthweight. *Journal of Educational Psychology, 86*, 531–541.

Brambati, S. M., Termine, C., Ruffino, M., Danna, M., Lanzi, G., Stella, G., et al. (2006). Neuropsychological deficits and neural dysfunction in familial dyslexia. *Brain Research, 1113*, 174–185.

Brand, N., Geenen, R., Oudenhoven, M., Lindenborn, B., van der Ree, A., Cohen-Kettenis, P., et al. (2002). Brief report: Cognitive functioning in children with Tourette's syndrome with and without comorbid ADHD. *Journal of Pediatric Psychology, 27*, 203–208.

Brandling-Bennett, E. M., White, D. A., Armstrong, M., Christ, S. E., & DeBaun, M. R. (2003). Patterns of verbal long-term and working memory performance reveal deficits in strategic processing in children with frontal infarcts related to sickle cell disease. *Developmental Neuropsychology, 24*, 423–434.

Brandt, I., Sticker, E. J., Gausche, R., & Lentze, M. J. (2005). Catch-up growth of supine length/height of very low birth weight, small for gestational age preterm infants to adulthood. *Journal of Pediatrics, 147*, 662–668.

Breen, M. J. (2006). Cognitive and behavioral differences in ADHD boys and girls. *Journal of Child Psychology and Psychiatry, 30*, 711–716.

Breslau, N., & Chilcoat, H. D. (2000). Psychiatric sequelae of low birth weight at 11 years of age. *Biological Psychiatry, 47*, 662–668.

Brickman, A. M., Cabo, R., & Manly, J. J. (2006). Ethical issues in cross-cultural neuropsychology. *Applied Neuropsychology, 13*, 91–100.

Brieber, S., Neufang, S., Bruning, N., Kamp-Becker, I., Remschmidt, H., Herpertz-Dahlmann, B., et al. (2007). Structural brain abnormalities in adolescents with autism spectrum disorder and patients with attention deficit/hyperactivity disorder. *Journal of Child Psychology and Psychiatry, 48*, 1251–1258.

Brink, J. (1996). Diabetes camping and youth support programs. In F. Lifshitz (Ed.), *Pediatric endocrinology* (3rd ed., pp. 671–676). New York: Marcel Dekker.

Brink, J. D., Garrett, A. L., Hale, W. R., Woo-Sam, J., & Nickel, V. C. (1970). Recovery of motor and intellectual function in children sustaining severe head injuries. *Developmental Medicine and Child Neurology, 12,* 545–571.

Britten, A. C., Mijovic, C. H., Barnett, A. H., & Kelly, M. A. (2009). Differential expression of HLA-DQ alleles in peripheral blood mononuclear cells: Alleles associated with susceptibility to and protection from autoimmune type 1 diabetes. *International Journal of Immunogenetics, 36*, 47–57.

Brockel, B. J., & Cory-Shlechta, D. A. (1999). Lead-induced decrements in waiting behavior: Involvement of D2-like dopamine receptors. *Pharmacological Biochemical Behavior, 63*, 423–434.

Brookes, R. L., & Stirling, J. (2005). The cerebellar deficit hypothesis and dyslexic tendencies in a non-clinical sample. *Dyslexia: An International Journal of Research and Practice, 11*, 174–185.

Brooks-Gunn, J., Klebanov, P. K., Liaw, F., & Spiker, D. (1993). Enhancing the development of low-birthweight, premature infants: Changes in cognition and behavior over the first three years. *Child Development, 64,* 736–753.

Brouwer, O. F., Okenhout, W., Edelbroek, P. M., de Kom, J. F. M., de Wolff, F. A., & Peters, A. C. B. (1992). Increased neurotoxicity of arsenic in methylenetetrahydrofolate reductase deficiency. *Clinical Neurology and Neurosurgery, 94*, 307–310.

Brown, A. L., Palincsar, A. S., & Armbruster, B. B. (1994). Instructing comprehension-fostering activities in interactive learning situations. In R. B. Ruddell, M. R. Ruddell, & H. Singer (Eds.), *Theoretical models and processes of reading* (4th ed., pp. 757–787). Newark, DE: International Reading Association.

Brown, J. K. (1988). Valproate toxicity. *Developmental Medicine and Child Neurology, 80*, 115–125.

Brown, M. B. (1999). The mucopolysaccharidoses. In G. W. Goldstein & C. R. Reynolds (Eds.), *Handbook of neurodevelopmental and genetic disorders in children* (pp. 317–336). New York: Guilford.

Brown, M. B., & Trivette, P. S. (1998). Mucopolysaccharide disorders (Hurler, Scheie, Hurler- Scheie, Hunter, Morquio, and Sanfilippo syndromes). In L. Phelps (Ed.), *Health-related disorders in children and adolescents: A guidebook for understanding and educating* (pp. 442–452). Washington, DC: American Psychological Association.

Brown, R. T., Amler, R. W., Freeman, W. S., Perrin, J. M., Stein, M. T., Feldman, H. M., et al. (2005). Treatment of attention-deficit/hyperactivity disorder: Overview of the evidence. *Pediatrics, 115*, 749–757.

Brown, R. T., Armstrong, F. D., & Eckman, J. R. (1993). Neurocognitive aspects of pediatric sickle cell disease. *Journal of Learning Disabilities, 26*, 33–45.

Brown, R. T., Davis, P. C., Lambert, R. G., Hsu, L., Hopkins, K., & Eckman, J. (2000). Neurocognitive functioning and magnetic resonance imaging in children with sickle cell disease. *Journal of Pediatric Psychology, 25*, 503–513.

Brown, R. T., Doepke, K., & Kaslow, N. J. (1993). Risk-resistance-adaptation model for pediatric chronic illness: Sickle cell syndrome as an example. *Clinical Psychology Review, 13*, 119–132.

Brownlie, E. B., Beitchman, J. H., Escobar, M., Young, A., Atkinson, L., Johnson, C., et al. (2004). Early language impairment and young adult delinquent and aggressive behavior. *Journal of Abnormal Child Psychology, 32*, 453–467.

Bruggeman, R., van der Linden, C., Buitelaar, J. K., Gericke, G. S., Hawkridge, S. M., & Temlett, J. A. (2001). Risperidone versus pimozide in Tourette's disorder: A comparative double-blind parallel-group study. *Journal of Clinical Psychiatry, 62*, 50–56.

Bruns, J., & Hauser, W. A. (2003). The epidemiology of traumatic brain injury: A review. *Epilepsia, 44*(Supplement 10), 2–10.

Bryson, S. E. (1996). Brief report: Epidemiology of autism. *Journal of Autism and Developmental Disorders, 26*, 165–167.

Bryson, S. E., & Smith, I. (1998). Epidemiology of autism: Prevalence, associated characteristics, and implications for research and service delivery. *Mental Retardation and Developmental Disabilities Research Reviews, 4*, 97–103.

Buccino, G., & Amore, M. (2008). Mirror neurons and the understanding of behavioural symptoms in psychiatric disorders. *Current Opinion in Psychiatry, 21*, 281–285.

Buccino, G., Binkofski, F., Fink, G. R., Fadiga, L., Fogassi, L., Gallese, V., et al. (2001). Action observation activates premotor and parietal areas in a somatotropic manner: An fMRI study. *European Journal of Neuroscience, 13*, 400–404.

Buchsbaum, M. S., Siegel, B. V., Wu, J. C., Hazlett, E., Sicotte, N., Haier, R., et al. (1992). Brief report: Attention performance in autism and regional brain metabolic rate assessed by positron emission tomography. *Journal of Autism and Developmental Disorders, 22*, 115–125.

Buck, G. M. (1996). Epidemiologic perspective of the developmental neurotoxicity of PCBs in humans. *Neurotoxicology and Teratology, 18*, 239–241.

Budman, C. L., Rockmore, L., Stokes, J., & Sossin, M. (2003). Clinical phenomenology of episodic rage in children with Tourette syndrome. *Journal of Psychosomatic Research, 55*, 59–65.

Buizer, A. I., de Sonneville, L. M. J., van den Heuvel-Eibrink, M. M., & Veerman, A. J. P. (2006). Behavioral and educational limitations after chemotherapy for childhood acute lymphoblastic leukemia or Wilms tumor. *Cancer, 106*, 2067–2075.

Bull, R., Espy, K. A., & Wiebe, S. A. (2008). Short-term, working memory, and executive functioning in preschoolers: Longitudinal predictors of mathematical achievement at age 7 years. *Developmental Neuropsychology, 33*, 205–228.

Bull, R., & Johnston, R. S. (1997). Children's arithmetical difficulties: Contributions from processing speed, item identification, and short-term memory. *Journal of Experimental Child Psychology, 65*, 1–24.

Bull, R., Johnston, R. S., & Roy, J. A. (1999). Exploring the roles of visuospatial sketch pad and central executive in children's arithmetic's skills: Views from cognition and developmental neuropsychology. *Developmental Neuropsychology, 15*, 421–442.

Bull, R., & Scerif, G. (2001). Executive functioning as a predictor of children's mathematical ability: Inhibition, switching, and working memory. *Developmental Neuropsychology, 19*, 273–293.

Bulteau, C., Jambaque, I., Viguier, D., Kieffer, V., Dellatolas, G., & Dulac, O. (2000). Epileptic syndromes, cognitive assessment and school placement: A study of 251 children. *Developmental Medicine & Child Neurology, 42*, 319–327.

Bunn, L., Roy, E. A., & Elliott, D. (2007). Speech perception and motor control in children with Down syndrome. *Child Neuropsychology, 13*, 262–275.

Bunn, L., Welsh, T. N., Simon, D. A., Howarth, K., & Elliott, D. (2003). Dichotic ear advantages in adults with Down's syndrome predict speech production errors. *Neuropsychology, 17*, 32–38.

Buntinx, I. M., Hennekam, R. C. M., Brouwer, O. F., Stroink, H., Beuten, J., Mangelschots, K., et al. (1995). Clinical profile of Angelman syndrome at different ages. *American Journal of Medical Genetics, 56*, 176–183.

Burd, L., Freeman, R. D., Klug, M. G., & Kerbeshian, J. (2005). Tourette syndrome and learning disabilities. *BMC Pediatrics, 5*(34), 1–6.

Burd, L., Kauffman, D. W., & Kerbeshian, J. (1992). Tourette syndrome and learning disabilities. *Journal of Learning Disabilities, 25*, 598–604.

Burd, L., Kerbeshian, J., Barth, A., Klug, M. G., Avery, K., & Benz, B. (2001). Long-term follow-up of an epidemiologically defined cohort of patients with Tourette syndrome. *Journal of Child Neurology, 16*, 431–437.

Burd, L., Leech, C., Kerbeshian, J., & Gascon, G. G. (1994). A review of the relationship between Gilles de la Tourette syndrome and speech and language. *Journal of Developmental & Physical Disabilities, 6*, 271–289.

Burke, C., Howard, L., & Evangelou, T. (2005). A Project of Hope: Lindamood-Bell Center in a School Project Final Evaluation Report. Retrieved November 11, 2008, from www.sandag.org.

Burlina, A., & Blau, N. (2009). Effect of BH(4) supplementation on phenylalanine tolerance. *Journal of Inherited Metabolic Disease, 32*, 40–45.

Burnette, C. P., Mundy, P. C., Meyer, J. A., Sutton, S. K., Vaughan, A. E., & Charak, D. (2005). Weak central coherence and its relations to theory of mind and anxiety in autism. *Journal of Autism and Developmental Disorders, 35*, 63–73.

Bush, S. S., & Martin, T. A. (2008). Confidentiality in neuropsychological practice. In A. M. Horton & D. Wedding (Eds.), *The neuropsychology handbook* (3rd ed., pp. 515–530). New York: Springer.

Bustos, R. R., & Goldstein, S. (2008). Including blood lead levels of all immigrant children when evaluating for ADHD. *Journal of Attention Disorders, 11*, 425–426.

Butler, F. M., Miller, S. P., Crehan, K., Babbitt, B., & Pierce, T. (2003). Fraction instruction for students with mathematics disabilities: Comparing two teaching sequences. *Learning Disabilities Research & Practice, 18*, 99–111.

Butler, R. W., & Copeland, D. R. (2002). Attentional processes and their remediation in children treated for cancer: A literature review and the development of a therapeutic approach. *Journal of International Neuropsychological Society, 8*, 115–124.

Butler, R. W., Copeland, D. R., Fairclough, D. L., Mulhern, R. K., Katz, E. R., Kazak, A. E., et al. (2008). A multicenter, randomized clinical trial of a cognitive remediation program for childhood survivors of a pediatric malignancy. *Journal of Consulting and Clinical Psychology, 76*, 367–378.

Butler, R. W., & Haser, J. K. (2006). Neurocognitive effects of treatment for childhood cancer. *Mental Retardation and Developmental Disabilities, 12*, 184–191.

Butler, R. W., & Mulhern, R. K. (2005). Neurocognitive interventions for children and adolescents surviving cancer. *Journal of Pediatric Psychology, 30*, 65–78.

Butler, R. W., Sahler, O. J. Z., Askins, M. A., Alderfer, M. A., Katz, E. R., Phipps, S., et al. (2008). Interventions to improve neuropsychological functioning in childhood cancer survivors. *Developmental Disabilities Research Reviews, 14*, 251–258.

Butterworth, B. (2005). Developmental dyscalculia. In J. I. D. Campbell (Ed.), *Handbook of mathematical cognition* (pp. 455–467). New York: Psychology Press.

Bystritsky, A., Ackerman, D. L., Rosen, R. M., Vapnik, T., Gorbis, E., Maidment, K. M., et al. (2004). Augmentation of serotonin reuptake inhibitors in refractory obsessive-compulsive disorder using adjunctive olanzapine: A placebo-controlled trial. *Journal of Clinical Psychiatry, 65*, 565–568.

Caine, C., Delis, D. C., Goodman, A. M., Mattson, S. N., & Riley, E. P. (1999). Executive functioning in children with heavy prenatal alcohol exposure. *Alcoholism: Clinical and Experimental Research, 23*, 1808–1815.

Calderón, J., Navarro, M., Jimenez-Capdeville, M., Santos-Diaz, M. A., Golden, A., Rodriguez-Leyva, I., et al. (2001). Exposure to arsenic and lead and neurodevelopmental development in Mexican children. *Environmental Research, 85*, 69–76.

Callahan, K., Henson, R. K., & Cowan, A. K. (2008). Social validation of evidence-based practices in autism by parents, teachers, and administrators. *Journal of Autism and Developmental Disorders, 38*, 678–692.

Camfield, P., & Camfield, C. (2003). Childhood epilepsy: What is the evidence for what we think and what we do? *Journal of Child Neurology, 18*, 272–278.

Campbell, D., Gonzales, M. S., & Sullivan, J. B. (1992). Mercury. In J. B. Sullivan & G. R. Krieger (Eds.), *Hazardous materials toxicology: Clinical principles of environmental health* (pp. 824–833). Baltimore: Williams & Wilkins.

Campbell, J. M. (2003). Efficacy of behavioral interventions for reducing problem behavior in persons with autism: A quantitative synthesis of single subject research. *Research in Developmental Disabilities, 24*, 120–138.

Campbell, J. M., Herzinger, C. V., & James, C. L. (2008). Evidence-based therapies for autistic disorder and pervasive developmental disorders. In R. Steele, D. Elkin, & M. Roberts (Eds.), *Handbook of evidence-based therapies for children and adolescents: Bridging science and practice* (pp. 373–388). New York: Springer.

Campbell, L. K., Scaduto, M., Sharp, W., Dufton, L., Van Slyke, D., & Compas, B. (2007). A meta-analysis of the neurocognitive sequelae of treatment for childhood acute lymphocytic leukemia. *Pediatric Blood and Cancer, 49*, 65–73.

Campbell, L. K., Scaduto, M., Van Slyke, D., Niarhos, F., Whitlock, J. A., & Compas, B. (2009). Executive function, coping, and behavior in survivors of childhood acute lymphocytic leukemia. *Journal of Pediatric Psychology, 34,* 317–327.

Campbell, L. K., Scaduto, M., Van Slyke, D., Niarhos, F., Whitlock, J. A., & Compas, B. E. (2008). Executive function, coping and behavior in survivors of childhood acute lymphocytic leukemia. *Journal of Pediatric Psychology, 33*, 1–11.

Canfield, R. L., Gendle, M. H., & Cory-Slechta, D. A. (2004). Impaired neuropsychological functioning in lead-exposed children. *Developmental Neuropsychology, 26*, 513–540.

Canfield, R. L., Kreher, D. A., Cornwell, C., & Henderson, C. R. J. (2003). Low-level lead exposure, executive functioning, and learning in early childhood. *Child Neuropsychology, 9*, 35–53.

Canitano, R., & Vivanti, G. (2007). Tics and Tourette syndrome in autism spectrum disorders. *Autism, 11*, 19–28.

Cantwell, D. P., & Baker, L. (1991). Association between attention deficit hyperactivity disorder and learning disorders. *Journal of Learning Disabilities, 24*, 88–94.

Cao, F., Bitan, T., Chou, T.-L., Burman, D. D., & Booth, J. R. (2006). Deficient orthographic and phonological representations in children with dyslexia revealed by brain activation patterns. *Journal of Child Psychology and Psychiatry, 47*, 1041–1050.

Caplan, R., Siddarth, P., Gurbani, S., Hanson, R., Sankar, R., & Shields, W. D. (2005). Depression and anxiety disorders in pediatric epilepsy. *Epilepsia 46*, 720–730.

Cardon, L. R., Smith, S. D., Fulker, D. W., Kimberling, W. J., Pennington, B. F., & DeFries, J. C. (1994). Quantitative trait locus for reading disability on chromosome 6. *Science, 266*, 276–279.

Carey, M. E., Barakat, L. P., Foley, B., Gyato, K., & Phillips, P. C. (2001). Neuropsychological functioning and social functioning of survivors of pediatric brain tumors: Evidence of nonverbal learning disability. *Child Neuropsychology, 7*, 265–272.

Carey, M. E., Haut, M. W., Reminger, S. L., Hutter, S. L., Theilmann, R., & Kaemingke, K. L. (2008). Reduced frontal white matter volume in long-term childhood leukemia survivors: A voxel-based morphometry study. *American Journal of Neuroradiology, 29*, 792–797.

Carlson, C. L., Lahey, B. B., & Neeper, R. J. (1986). Direct assessment of the cognitive correlates of attention deficit disorders with and without hyperactivity. *Journal of Psychopathology and Behavioral Assessment, 8*, 69–86.

Carlson, C. L., Tamm, L., & Gaub, M. (1997). Gender differences in children with ADHD, ODD, and co-occurring ADHD/ODD identified in a school population. *Journal of the American Academy of Child and Adolescent Psychiatry, 36*, 1706–1715.

Carmichael, O. H., Feldman, J. J., Streissguth, A. P., & Gonzalez, R. D. (1992). Neuropsychological deficits and life adjustment in adolescents and adults with fetal alcohol syndrome. *Alcoholism: Clinical and Experimental Research, 16*, 380.

Carper, R., Moses, P., Tigue, Z., & Courchesne, E. (2002). Cerebral lobes in autism: Early hyperplasia and abnormal age effects. *NeuroImage, 16*, 1038–1051.

Carr, J. E., & Chong, I. M. (2005). Habit reversal treatment of tic disorders: A methodological critique of the literature. *Behavior Modification, 29*, 858–875.

Carreño, M., Gil-Nagel, A., Sánchez, J. C. E., Elices, E., Serratosa, J. M., Salas-Puig, J., Villanuyeva, V., et al. (2008). Strategies to detect adverse effects of antiepileptic drugs in clinic practice. *Epilepsy & Behavior, 13*, 178–183.

Carrillo-Zuniga, G., Coutinho, C., Shalat, S. L., Freeman, N. C. G., Black, K., Jimenez, W., et al. (2004). Potential sources of childhood exposure to pesticides in an agricultural community. *Journal of Children's Health, 2*, 1–11.

Carrim, Z. I., McKay, L., Sidiki, S. S., & Lavy, T. E. (2007). Early intervention for the ocular and neurodevelopmental sequelae of fetal valproate syndrome. *Journal of Paediatrics and Child Health, 43*, 643–645.

Carroll, J. M., & Snowling, M. J. (2004). Language and phonological skills in children at high risk of reading difficulties. *Journal of Child Psychology and Psychiatry, 45*, 631–640.

Carter, A. S., O'Donnell, D. A., Schultz, R. T., Scahill, L., Leckman, J. F., & Pauls, D. L. (2000). Social and emotional adjustment in children affected with Gilles de la Tourette's syndrome: Associations with ADHD and family functioning. *Journal of Child Psychology and Psychiatry, 41*, 215–223.

Carter, C. M. (2001). Using choice with game play to increase language skills and interactive behaviors in children with autism. *Journal of Positive Behavior Interventions, 3*, 131–151.

Carter, J. C., Capone, G. T., Kaufmann, W. E. (2008). Neuroanatomic correlates of autism and stereotypy in children with Down syndrome. *NeuroReport, 19*, 653–656.

Casanova, M. F., Araque, J., Giedd, J., & Rumsey, J. M. (2004). Reduced brain size and gyrification in the brains of dyslexic patients. *Journal of Child Neurology, 19*, 275–281.

Casanova, M. F., Buxhoeveden, D. P., Cohen, M. J., Switala, A. E., & Roy, E. L. (2002). Minicolumnar pathology in dyslexia. *Annals of Neurology, 52*, 108–110.

Casanova, M. F., Buxhoeveden, D. P., Switala, A. E., & Roy, E. (2002). Minicolumnar pathology in autism. *Neurology, 58*, 428–432.

Casanova, M. F., van Kooten, A. J., Switala, A. E., van Engeland, H., Heinsen, H., Steinbusch, H. M., et al. (2006). Minicolumnar abnormalities in autism. *Acta Neuropathologica, 112*, 287–303.

Casey, B. J. (2004). Mathematics problem-solving adventures: A language arts based supplementary series for early childhood that focuses on spatial sense. In D. H. Clements, J. Sarama, & A. DiBiase (Eds.), *Engaging young children in mathematics: Standards for early childhood mathematics education* (pp. 377–389). Mahwah, NJ: Erlbaum.

Casey, P. H., Whiteside-Mansell, L., Barrett, K., Bradley, R. H., & Gargus, R. (2006). Impact of prenatal and/or postnatal growth problems in low birth weight preterm infants on school-age outcomes: An 8-year longitudinal evaluation. *Pediatrics, 118*, 1078–1086.

Casper, R. C., Fleischer, B. E., Lee-Ancalas, J. C., Gilles, A., Gaylor, E., DeBattista, A., et al. (2003). Follow-up of children of depressed mothers exposed or not exposed to antidepressant drugs during pregnancy. *Journal of Pediatrics, 142*, 402–408.

Cass, M., Cates, D., Smith, M., & Jackson, C. (2003). Effects of manipulative instruction on solving area and perimeter problems by students with learning disabilities. *Learning Disabilities Research & Practice, 18*, 112–120.

Castellanos, F. X., Giedd, J. N., Berquin, P. C., Walter, J. M., Sharp, W., Tran, T., et al. (2001). Quantitative brain magnetic resonance imaging in girls with attention-deficit/hyperactivity disorder. *Archives of General Psychiatry, 58*, 289–295.

Castellanos, F. X., Sharp, W. S., Gottesman, R. F., Greenstein, D. K., Giedd, J. N., & Rapoport, J. L. (2003). Anatomic brain abnormalities in monozygotic twins discordant for attention deficit hyperactivity disorder. *American Journal of Psychiatry, 160*, 1693–1696.

Castoldi, A. F., Candura, S. M., Costa, P., Manzo, L., & Costa, L. G. (1996). Interaction of mercury compounds with muscarinic receptor subtypes in the rat brain. *Neurotoxicology, 17*, 735–741.

Catroppa, C., & Anderson, V. (1999). Recovery of educational skills following pediatric head injury. *Pediatric Rehabilitation, 3*, 167–175.

Catroppa, C., & Anderson, V. (2007). Recovery in memory function, and its relationship to academic success, at 24 months following pediatric TBI. *Child Neuropsychology, 13*, 240–261.

Catroppa, C., Anderson, V. A., Morse, S. A., Haritou, F., & Rosenfeld, J. V. (2007). Children's attentional skills 5 years post-TBI. *Journal of Pediatric Psychology, 32*, 354–369.

Catroppa, C., Anderson, V. A., Morse, S. A., Haritou, F., & Rosenfeld, J. V. (2008). Outcome and predictors of functional recovery 5 years following pediatric traumatic brain injury (TBI). *Journal of Pediatric Psychology, 33*, 707–718.

Catts, H., Fey, M., Tomblin, J. B., & Zhang, X. (2002). A longitudinal investigation of reading outcomes in children with language impairments. *Journal of Speech Language and Hearing Research, 45*, 1142–1157.

Catts, H. W., Hogan, T. P., & Adlof, S. M. (2005). Developmental changes in reading and reading disabilities. In H. W. Catts & A. G. Kamhi (Eds.), *The connection between language and reading disabilities* (pp. 25–40). Mahwah, NJ: Erlbaum.

Cavanna, A. E., Robertson, M. M., & Critchley, H. D. (2007). Schizotypal personality traits in Gilles de la Tourette syndrome. *Acta Neurologica Scandinavica, 116*, 385–391.

Cawthon, R. M., Weiss, R., Xu, G. F., Viskochil, D., Colver, M., Stevens, J., et al. (1990). A major segment of the neurofibromatosis type 1 gene: cDNA sequence, genomic structure, and point mutations. *Cell, 62*, 193–201.

Censabella, S., & Noël, M.-P. (2008). The inhibition capacities of children with mathematical disabilities. *Child Neuropsychology, 14*, 1–20.

Centers for Disease Control (2002). Delayed diagnosis of fragile X syndrome: United States, 1990–1999. *Morbidity and Mortality Weekly Report, 51,* 740–742.

Centers for Disease Control. (2003). Second national report on human exposure to environmental chemicals (NCEH Pub. No. 03–0022). Retrieved from www.cdc.gov/exposurereport.

Centers for Disease Control. (2005). National diabetes fact sheet. Retrieved from http://www.cdc.gov/diabetes/pubs/estimates05.htm#prev.

Chaix, Y., Laguitton, V., Lauwers-Cances, V., Daquin, G., Cances, C., Demonet, J., et al. (2006). Reading abilities and cognitive functions of children with epilepsy: Influence of epileptic syndrome. *Brain & Development, 28*, 122–130.

Chalhub, E. G. (1976). Neurocutaneous syndromes in children. *Pediatric Clinics of North America, 23*, 499–516.

Chambers, C. D., Johnson, K. A., Dick, L. M., Felix, R. J., & Jones, K. J. (1996). Birth outcomes in pregnant women taking fluoxetine. *New England Journal of Medicine, 335*, 1010–1015.

Chambliss, D. L., & Ollendick, T. H. (2001). Empirically supported psychological interventions: Controversies and evidence. *Annual Review of Psychology, 52*, 685–716.

Chang, H., Tu, M., & Wang, H. (2004). Tourette's syndrome: Psychopathology in adolescents. *Psychiatry and Clinical Neurosciences, 58*, 353–358.

Chang, P., Tsau, Y. K., Tsai, W. Y., Tsai, W. S., Hour, J. W., Hsiao, P. H., et al. (2000). Renal malformations in children with Turner's syndrome. *Journal of the Formosan Medical Association, 99*, 823–826.

Chang, S. W., McCracken, J. T., & Piacentini, J. C. (2007). Neurocognitive correlates of child obsessive compulsive disorder and Tourette syndrome. *Journal of Clinical and Experimental Neuropsychology, 29*, 724–733.

Channon, S., Goodman, G., Zlotowitz, S., Mockler, C., & Lee, P. J. (2007). Effects of dietary management of phenylketonuria on long-term cognitive outcome. *Archives of Diseases in Children, 92*, 213–218.

Channon, S., Pratt, P., & Robertson, M. M. (2003). Executive function, memory, and learning in Tourette's syndrome. *Neuropsychology, 17*, 247–254.

Chapieski, L., Friedman, A., & Lachar, D. (2000). Psychological functioning in children and adolescents with Sturge-Weber syndrome. *Journal of Child Neurology, 15*, 660–665.

Chapman, N. H., Igo, R. P., Thomson, J. B., Matsushita, M., Brkanac, Z., Holzman, T., et al. (2004). Linkage analyses of four regions previously implicated in dyslexia: Confirmation of a locus on chromosome 15q. *American Journal of Medical Genetics, 131B*(1), 67–75.

Chapman, S. B., Levin, H. S., Wanek, A., Weyrauch, J., & Kufera, J. (1998). Discourse after closed head injury in young children. *Brain and Language, 61,* 420–449.

Chapman, S. B., Sparks, G., Levin, H. S., Dennis, M., Roncadin, C., Zhang, L., et al. (2004). Discourse macrolevel processing after severe pediatric traumatic brain injury. *Developmental Neuropsychology, 25,* 37–60.

Chapman, S. S., Ewing, C. B., & Mozzoni, M. P. (2005). Precision teaching and fluency training across cognitive, physical, and academic tasks in children with traumatic brain injury: A multiple baseline study. *Behavioral Interventions, 20,* 37–49.

Charlop-Christy, M. H., Carpenter, M., Le, L., LeBlanc, L. A., & Keller, K. (2002). Using the Picture Exchange Communication Systems (PECS) with children with autism: Assessment of PECS acquisition, speech, social communicative behavior, and problem behavior. *Journal of Applied Behavior Analysis, 35*, 213–231.

Charman, T., Baron-Cohen, S., Swettenbaum, J., Cox, A., Baird, G., & Drew, A. (1997). Infants with autism: An investigation of empathy, pretend play, joint attention, and imitation. *Developmental Psychiatry, 33*, 781–789.

Chavez, B., Chavez-Brown, M., & Rey, J. A. (2006). Role of risperidone in children with autism spectrum disorder. *Annals of Pharmacotherapy, 40*, 909–916.

Chen, A., Cai, B., Dietrich, K. N., Radcliffe, J., & Rogan, W. (2007). Lead exposure, IQ, and behavior in urban 5- and 7-year olds: Does lead affect behavior only by lowering IQ? *Pediatrics, 119*, 650–658.

Chen, A., Dietrich, K. N., Ware, J. H., Radcliffe, J., & Rogan, W. (2005). IQ and blood lead from 2 to 7 years of age: Are the effects in older children the residual of high blood lead concentrations in 2-year-olds? *Environmental Health Perspective, 113*, 597–601.

Chen, J., & Millar, W. J. (1999). Birth outcome, the social environment and child health. *Health Reports, 10*(4), 57–67.

Cheng, J. Y. W., Chen, R. Y. L., Ko, J. S. N., & Ng, E. M. L. (2007). Efficacy and safety of atomoxetine for attention-deficit/hyperactivity disorder in children and adolescents: Meta-analysis and meta-regression analysis. *Psychopharmacology, 194*, 197–209.

Cherniske, E. M., Carpenter, T. O., Klaiman, C., Young, E., Bregman, J., Isongna, K., et al. (2004). Multisystem study of 20 older adults with Williams syndrome. *American Journal of Medical Genetics, 131*, 255–264.

Chiarello, C., Kacinik, N., Manowitz, B., Otto, R., & Leonard, C. (2004). Cerebral asymmetries for language: Evidence for structural-behavioral correlations. *Neuropsychology, 18*, 219–231.

Ch'ng, S., & Tan, S. T. (2008). Facial port-wine stains—clinical stratification and risks of neuro-ocular involvement. *Journal of Plastic, Reconstructive & Aesthetic Surgery, 61*, 889–893.

Cho, Y.-S., Kim, J. H., Kim, T. W., Chung, S. C., Chang, S.-A., & Jin, D.-K. (2008). Otologic manifestations of Hunter syndrome and their relationship with speech development. *Audiology & Neurotology, 13*, 206–212.

Choi, I. S. (1983). Delayed neurologic sequelae in carbon monoxide intoxification. *Archives of Neurology, 40*, 433–435.

Christensen, A. L. (1975). *Luria's neuropsychological investigation*. New York: Spectrum.

Christianson, A. L., Cheslar, N., & Kromber, J. G. (1994). Fetal valproate syndrome: Clinical and neuro-developmental features in two sibling pairs. *Developmental Medicine and Child Neurology, 36*, 361–369.

Chronis, A. M., Jones, H. A., & Raggi, V. L. (2006). Evidence-based psychosocial treatments for children and adolescents with attention-deficit/hyperactivity disorder. *Clinical Psychology Review, 26*, 486–502.

Chugani, D. C. (2002). Role of altered brain serotonin mechanisms in autism. *Molecular Psychiatry, 7*(Suppl. 2), S16–S17.

Chugani, D. C., Muzik, O., Rothermel, R., Behen, M., Chakraborty, P., Mang de Silva, E. A., et al. (1997). Altered serotonin synthesis in the dentatothalamocortical pathway in autistic boys. *Annals of Neurology, 42*, 666–669.

Church, J. A., Fair, D. A., Dosenbach, N. U. F., Cohen, A. L., Miezin, F. M., Peterson, S. E., et al. (2009). Control networds in paediatric Tourette syndrome show immature and anomalous patterns of functional connectivity. *Brain, 132*, 225–238.

Ciaranello, A., & Ciaranello, R. D. (1995). The neurobiology of infantile autism. *Annual Review of Neuroscience, 18*, 101–128.

Cicchetti, D. V. (1994). Multiple comparison methods: Establishing guidelines for their valid application in neuropsychological research. *Journal of Clinical and Experimental Neuropsychology, 16*, 155–161.

Cicchetti, D. V., Kaufman, A. S., & Sparrow, S. S. (2004). The relationship between prenatal and postnatal exposure to polychlorinated biphenyls (PCBs) and cognitive, neuropsychological, and behavioral deficits: A critical appraisal. *Psychology in the Schools, 41*, 589–624.

Cicerone, K. D., Dahlberg, C., Kalmar, K., Langenbahn, D. M., Malec, J. F., Bergquist, T. F., et al. (2000). Evidence-based cognitive rehabilitation: Recommendations for clinical practice. *Archives of Physical Medicine and Rehabilitation, 81,* 1596–1615.

Cirino, P. T., Morris, M. K., & Morris, R. D. (2002). Neuropsychological concomitants of calculation skills in college students referred for learning disabilities. *Developmental Neuropsychology, 21*, 201–218.

Clark, A., O'Hare, A., Watson, J., Cohen, W., Cowie, H., Elton, R., et al. (2007). Severe receptive language disorder in childhood—familial aspects and long-term outcomes: Results from a Scottish study. *Archives of Disease in Childhood, 92*, 614–619.

Clark, C. M., Conry, J., Conry, R., Li, D., & Loock, C. (2000). Structural and functional brain integrity of fetal alcohol syndrome in nonretarded cases. *Pediatrics, 105*, 1096–1099.

Clark, C. M., Conry, J. L., Li, D., & Loock, C. (1993). Disregulation of caudate/cortical metabolism in FAS: A case study. *Alcoholism: Clinical and Experimental Research, 17*, 485.

Clark, M. M., & Plante, E. (1998). Morphology of the inferior frontal gyrus in developmentally language-disordered adults. *Brain and Language, 61,* 288–303.

Clarke, D. J., & Marston, G. (2000). Problem behaviors associated with 15q—Angelman syndrome. *American Journal of Mental Retardation, 105*(1), 25–31.

Clarke, L. A., Wraith, J. E., Beck, M., Kolodny, E. H., Pastores, G. M., Muenzer, J., et al. (2009). Long-term efficacy and safety of laronidase in the treatment of mucopolysaccharidosis I. *Pediatrics, 123*, 229–240.

Clarke, M. A., Bray, M. A., Kehle, T. J., & Truscott, S. D. (2001). A school-based intervention designed to reduce the frequency of tics in children with Tourette's syndrome. *School Psychology Review, 30*, 11–22.

Clarke, S., Heussler, H., & Kohn, M. R. (2005). Attention deficit disorder: Not just for children. *Internal Medicine Journal, 35*, 721–725.

Claudio, L., Kiva, W. C., Russell, A. L., & Wallinga, D. (2000). Testing methods for developmental neurotoxicity of environmental chemicals. *Toxicology and Applied Pharmacology, 164*, 1–14.

Clay, O. J., & Telfair, J. (2007). Evaluation of a disease-specific self-efficacy instrument in adolescents with sickle cell disease and its relationship to adjustment. *Child Neuropsychology, 13*, 188–203.

Clayton Smith, J. (2001). Angelman syndrome: Evolution of the phenotype in adolescents and adults. *Developmental Medicine & Child Neurology, 43*, 476–480.

Clayton Smith, J., & Donnai, D. (1995). Fetal valproate syndrome. *Journal of Medical Genetics, 32*, 724–727.

Cleary, M. A., Walter, J. H., Wraith, J. E., & Jenkins, J. (1995). Magnetic resonance imaging in phenylketonuria: Reversal of cerebral white matter change. *Journal of Pediatrics, 127*, 251–255.

Clegg, J., Hollis, C., Mawhood, L., & Rutter, M. (2005). Developmental language disorders—a follow-up in later adult life. Cognitive, language and psychosocial outcomes. *Journal of Child Psychology and Psychiatry, 46*, 128–149.

Clements-Stephens, A. M., Rimrodt, S. L., Gaur, P., & Cutting, L. E. (2008). Visuospatial processing in children with neurofibromatosis type 1. *Neuropsychologia, 46*, 690–697.

Clinton, W. (1997). Executive Order 13045: Protection of Children from Environmental Health Risks and Safety Risks. *Federal Register, April 21, 1997*, 19883–19888.

Coben, R., Clarke, A. R., Hudspeth, W., & Barry, R. J. (2008). EEG power and coherence in autistic spectrum disorder. *Clinical Neurophysiology, 119*, 1002–1009.

Coderre, J. A., Morris, G. M., Micca, P. L., Hopewell, J. W., Verhagen, I., Kleiboer, B. J., et al. (2006). Late effects of radiation on the central nervous system: Role of vascular endothelial damage and glial cell survival. *Radiation Research, 186*, 495–503.

Cody, H., & Hynd, G. W. (1998). Sturge Weber syndrome. In L. Phelps (Ed.), *Health-related disorders in children and adolescents: A guidebook for understanding and educating* (pp. 624–628). Washington, DC: American Psychological Association.

Cody, H., & Hynd, G. W. (1999). Klinefelter syndrome. In S. Goldstein & C. R. Reynolds (Eds.), *Handbook of neurodevelopmental and genetic disorders in children* (pp. 406–432). New York: Guilford.

Cody, H., & Kamphaus, R. W. (1999). Down syndrome. In S. Goldstein & C. R. Reynolds (Eds.), *Handbook of neurodevelopmental and genetic disorders in children* (pp. 385–405). New York: Guilford.

Coffey, B. J., Biederman, J., Geller, D. A., Spencer, T. J., Park, K. S., Shapiro, S. J., et al. (2000). The course of Tourette's disorder: A literature review. *Harvard Review of Psychiatry, 8*, 192–198.

Cohen, D. J., Caparulo, B., & Shaywitz, B. (1976). Primary childhood aphasia and childhood autism: Clinical, biological and conceptual observations. *Journal of the American Academy of Child and Adolescent Psychiatry, 15*, 604–605.

Cohen, E., Sade, M., Benarroch, F., Pollak, Y., & Gross-Tsur, V. (2008). Locus of control, perceived parenting style, and symptoms of anxiety and depression in children with Tourette's syndrome. *European Child and Adolescent Psychiatry, 17*, 299–305.

Cohen, M. J. (1992). Auditory/verbal and visual/spatial memory in children with complex partial epilepsy of temporal lobe origin. *Brain and Cognition, 20*, 315–326.

Cohen, M. J., Branch, W. B., McKie, V. C., & Adams, R. J. (1994). Neuropsychological impairment in children with sickle cell anemia and cerebrovascular accidents. *Clinical Pediatrics, 33*, 517–524.

Cohen, M. J., Campbell, R., & Gelardo, M. (1987). Hyperlexia: A variant of aphasia or dyslexia. *Pediatric Neuropsychology, 3*, 22–28.

Cohen, M. J., Campbell, R. C., & Yaghmai, F. (1989). Neuropathological abnormalities in developmental dysphasia. *Annals of Neurology, 25*, 567–570.

Cohen, M. J., Hall, J., & Riccio, C. A. (1997). Neuropsychological profiles of children diagnosed as specific language impaired with and without hyperlexia. *Archives of Clinical Neuropsychology, 12*, 223–229.

Cohen, M. J., Holmes, G. L., Campbell, R., Smith, J. R., & Flanigin, H. F. (1991). Cognitive functioning following anterior two-thirds corpus callosotomy in children and adolescents: A one-year prospective report. *Journal of Epilepsy, 4*(2), 63–65.

Cohen, M. J., Riccio, C. A., & Hynd, G. W. (1999). Children with specific language impairment: Quantitative analysis of dichotic listening performance. *Developmental Neuropsychology, 16*, 243–252.

Cohen, N. J., Vallance, D. D., Barwick, M., Im, N., Menna, R., Horodezky, N. B., et al. (2000). The interface between ADHD and language impairments: An examination of language, achievement, and cognitive processing. *Journal of Child Psychology and Psychiatry and Allied Disciplines, 41*, 353–362.

Cohen, W., Hodson, A., O'Hare, A., Boyle, J., Durani, T., McCartney, E., et al. (2005). Effects of computer-based intervention through acoustically modified speech (Fast ForWord) in severe mixed receptive-expressive language impairment: Outcomes from a randomized controlled trial. *Journal of Speech, Language, and Hearing Research, 48*, 715–729.

Cohen Hubal, E. A. C., Sheldon, L. S., Burke, J. M., McCurdy, T. R., Berry, M. R., Rigas, M. L., et al. (2000). Children's exposure assessment: A review of factors influencing children's exposure, and the data available to characterize and assess that exposure. *Environmental Health Perspectives, 108*, 475–486.

Colborn, T. (2006). A case for revisiting the safety of pesticides: A closer look at neurodevelopment. *Environmental Health Perspective, 114*, 10–17.

Coldren, J. T., & Halloran, C. (2003). Spatial reversal as a measure of executive functioning in children with autism. *Journal of Genetic Psychology, 164*, 29–41.

Coles, C. D., Bard, K. A., Platzman, K. A., & Lynch, M. E. (1999). Attentional response at eight weeks in prenatally drug exposed and preterm infants. *Neurotoxicology and Teratology, 21*, 527–537.

Colle, L., Baron-Cohen, S., Wheelwright, S., & van der Lely, H. K. J. (2008). Narrative discourse in adults with high-functioning autism or Asperger syndrome. *Journal of Autism and Developmental Disorders, 38*, 28–40.

Colletti, L. (2007). Beneficial auditory and cognitive effects of auditory brainstem implantation in children. *Acta Oto-laryngologica, 127*, 943–946.

Collins, C. T., Ryan, P., Crowther, C. A., McPhee, A. J., Paterson, S., & Hiller, J. E. (2004). Effect of bottles, cups, and dummies on breast feeding in preterm infants: A randomised controlled trial. *British Medical Journal, 329,* 193–198.

Collins, M., Kaslow, N., Doepke, K., Eckman, J., & Johnson, M. (1998). Psychosocial interventions for children and adolescents with sickle cell disease (SCD). *Journal of Black Psychology, 24*, 432–454.

Colosio, C., Tiramani, M., & Maroni, M. (2003). Neurobehavioral effects of pesticides: State of the art. *Neurotoxicology and Teratology, 24*, 577–591.

Comi, A. M. (2003). Pathophysiology of Sturge-Weber syndrome. *Journal of Child Neurology, 18*, 509–516.

Comi, A. M., Bellamkonda, S., Ferenc, L. M., Cohen, B. A., & Germain-Lee, E. L. (2008). Central hypothyroidism and Sturge-Weber syndrome. *Pediatric Neurology, 39*, 58–62.

Comings, B. G., & Comings, D. E. (1987). A controlled study of Tourette syndrome. V: Depression and mania. *American Journal of Human Genetics, 41*, 804–821.

Comings, D. E., & Comings, B. G. (1987a). A controlled study of Tourette syndrome I: Attention-deficit disorder, learning disorders, and school problems. *American Journal of Human Genetics, 41*, 701–741.

Comings, D. E., & Comings, B. G. (1987b). A controlled study of Tourette syndrome. II: Conduct. *American Journal of Human Genetics, 41*, 742–760.

Comings, D. E., & Comings, B. G. (1987c). A controlled study of Tourette syndrome. III: Phobias and panic attacks. *American Journal of Human Genetics, 41*, 761–781.

Comings, D. E., & Comings, B. G. (1987d). A controlled study of Tourette syndrome. IV: Obsessions, compulsions, and schizoid behaviors. *American Journal of Human Genetics, 41*, 782–803.

Comings, D. E., & Comings, B. G. (1987e). A controlled study of Tourette syndrome. VI: Early development, sleep problems, allergies, and handedness. *American Journal of Human Genetics, 41*, 822–838.

Comper, P., Bisschop, S. M., Carnide, N., & Tricco, A. (2005). A systematic review of treatments for mild traumatic brain injury. *Brain Injury, 19,* 863–880.

Conelea, C. A., & Woods, D. W. (2008a). Examining the impact of distraction on tic suppression in children and adolescents with Tourette syndrome. *Behaviour Research and Therapy, 46*, 1193–1200.

Conelea, C. A., & Woods, D. W. (2008b). The influence of contextual factors on tic expression in Tourette's syndrome: A review. *Journal of Psychosomatic Research, 65*, 487–496.

Conklin, H. M., Khan, R. B., Reddick, W. E., Helton, S., Howard, S. C., Bonner, M., et al. (2007). Acute neurocognitive response to methylphenidate among survivors of childhood cancer: A randomized, double-blind, cross-over trial. *Journal of Pediatric Psychology, 32*, 1127–1139.

Conners, C. K. (1997). *Conners' Rating Scales Revised manual.* North Tonawanda, NY: Multi-Health Systems.

Conners, C. K. (2008). *Conners' Rating Scales III manual.* North Tonawanda, NY: Multi-Health Systems.

Conners, F. A., Rosenquist, C. J., Atwell, J. A., & Klinger, L. G. (2000). Cognitive strengths and weaknesses associated with Prader-Willi syndrome. *Education and Training in Mental Retardation and Developmental Disabilities, 35*, 441–448.

Connolly, M. B., Hendson, G., & Steinbok, P. (2006). Tuberous sclerosis complex: A review of the management of epilepsy with emphasis on surgical aspects. *Child's Nervous System, 22*, 896–908.

Connor, J. M. (1990). Epidemiology and genetic approaches in tuberous sclerosis. In Y. Ishibasi & Y. Hori (Eds.), *Tuberous sclerosis and neurofibromatosis: Epidemiology, pathophysiology, biology, and management* (pp. 55–62). Amsterdam: Elsevier.

Constantino, J. N., & Todd, R. D. (2003). Autistic traits in the general population: A twin study. *Archives of General Psychiatry, 60*, 524–530.

Constine, L. S., Konski, A., Ekholm, S., McDonald, S., & Rubin, P. (1988). Adverse effects of brain irradiation correlated with MR and CT imaging. *International Journal of Radiation Oncology, Biology, and Physics, 15*, 319–330.

Conti-Ramsden, G., & Botting, N. (2008). Emotional health in adolescents with and without a history of specific language impairment (SLI). *Journal of Child Psychology and Psychiatry, 49*, 516–525.

Conti-Ramsden, G., Falcaro, M., Simkin, Z., & Pickles, A. (2007). Familial loading in specific language impairment: Patterns of differences across proband characteristics, gender and relative type. *Genes, Brains, & Behavior, 6*, 216–228.

Conway, T., Heilman, P., Gonzalez-Rothi, L., Alexander, A., Adair, J., Crosson, B., et al. (1998). Treatment of a case of phonological alexia with agraphia using the Auditory Discrimination in Depth (ADD) program. *Journal of the International Neuropsychological Society, 4*, 608–620.

Cook, C. R., & Blacher, J. (2007). Evidence-based psychosocial treatments for tic disorders. *Clinical Psychology: Science and Practice, 14*, 252–267.

Cook, E. H., & Leventhal, B. L. (1995). Autistic disorder and other pervasive developmental disorders. *Child and Adolescent Psychiatric Clinics of North America, 42*, 389–399.

Cooper, G. P., Suszkiw, J. B., & Manalis, R. S. (1984). Heavy metals: Effects on synaptic transmission. *Neurotoxicity, 7*, 483–496.

Copeland, D. R., Dowell, R. E., Fletcher, J. M., Sullivan, M. P., Jaffe, N., Cangir, A., et al. (1988). Neuropsychological test performance of pediatric cancer patients at diagnosis and one year later. *Journal of Pediatric Psychology, 13*, 183–196.

Copeland, D. R., Moore, B. D., Francis, D. J., Jaffe, N., & Culbert, S. J. (1996). Neuropsychologic effects of chemotherapy on children with cancer: A longitudinal study. *Journal of Clinical Oncology, 14*, 2826–2835.

Cordier, S., Garel, M., Mandereau, L., Morcel, H., Coineua, P., Gosme-Seguret, S., et al. (2002). Neurodevelopmental investigations among methylmercury-exposed children in French Guiana. *Environmental Research, 89*, 2–11.

Cornaggia, C., & Gobbi, G. (2002). Epilepsy and learning disorders. In M. Trimble & B. Schmitz (Eds.), *The neuropsychiatry of epilepsy* (pp. 62–69). New York: Cambridge University Press.

Cornish, K. M., Levitas, A., & Sudhalter, V. (2007). Fragile X syndrome: The journey from genes to behavior. In M. M. M. Mazzocco & J. L. Ross (Eds.), *Neurogenetic developmental disorders: Variation of manifestation in childhood* (pp. 73–104). Cambridge, MA: MIT Press.

Cornish, K. M., Munir, F., & Wilding, J. (2001). A neuropsychological and behavioral profile of attention deficits in fragile X syndrome. *Revista de Neurologia, 33*, 24–29.

Cornoldi, C., Barbieri, A., Gaiani, C., & Zocchi, S. (1999). Strategic memory deficits in attention deficit disorder with hyperactivity participants: The role of executive processes. *Developmental Neuropsychology, 15*, 53–71.

Cory-Slechta, D. A. (1994). Bridging human and experimental animal studies of lead neurotoxicity: Moving beyond IQ. *Neurotoxicology and Teratology, 17*, 219–222.

Coscia, J. M., Ris, M. D., Succop, P. A., & Dietrich, K. N. (2003). Cognitive development of lead exposed children from ages 6 to 15 years: An application of growth curve analysis. *Child Neuropsychology, 9*, 10–21.

Costa, E. T., Savage, D. D., & Valenzuela, F. (2000). A review of the effects of prenatal or early postnatal ethanol exposure on brain ligand-gated ion channels. *Alcoholism: Clinical and Experimental Research, 24*, 706–715.

Coudé, F. X., Mignot, C., Lyonnet, S., & Munnich, A. (2006). Academic impairment is the most frequent complication of neurofibromatosis type-1 (NF1) in children. *Behavior Genetics, 36*, 660–664.

Coudé, F. X., Mignot, C., Lyonnet, S., & Munnich, A. (2007). Early grade repetition and inattention associated with neurofibromatosis type 1. *Journal of Attention Disorders, 11*, 101–105.

Counter, S. A., Ortega, F., Shannon, M. W., & Buchanan, L. H. (2003). Succimer (meso-2, 3-dimercaptuosuccinic acid [DMSA]) treatment of Andean children with environmental lead exposure. *International Journal of Occupational and Environmental Health, 9*, 164–168.

Courchesne, E. (1987). A neurophysiological view of autism. In E. Schopler & G. B. Mesibov (Eds.), *Neurobiological issues in autism. Current issues in autism* (pp. 285–324). New York: Plenum.

Courchesne, E. (1997). Brainstem, cerebellar and limbic neuroanatomical abnormalities in autism. *Current Opinion in Neurobiology, 7*, 269–278.

Courchesne, E., Courchesne, R. Y., Hicks, G., & Lincoln, A. J. (1985). Functioning of the brain-stem auditory pathway in non-retarded autistic individuals. *Electroencephalography & Clinical Neurophysiology, 61*, 491–501.

Courchesne, E., Pierce, K., Schumann, C. M., Redcay, E., Buckwalter, J. A., Kennedy, D. P., et al. (2007). Mapping early brain development in autism. *Neuron, 56*, 399–413.

Courchesne, E., Townsend, J., & Saitoh, O. (1994). The brain in infantile autism: Posterior fossa structures are abnormal. *Neurology, 44*, 214–223.

Cowan, N. (1996). Short-term memory, working memory, and their importance in language processing. *Topics in Language Disorders, 17*, 1–18.

Cowell, P. E., Jernigan, T. L., Denenberg, V. H., & Tallal, P. (1995). Language and learning impairment and prenatal risk: An MRI study of the corpus callosum and cerebral volume. *Journal of Medical Speech-Language Pathology, 3*, 1–13.

Cox, S., Posner, S. F., Kourtis, A. P., & Jamieson, D. J. (2008). Hospitalizations with amphetamine abuse among pregnant women. *Obstetrics and Gynecology, 111*, 341–347.

Cozzi, L., Tryon, W. W., & Sedlacek, K. (1987). The effectiveness of biofeedback-assisted relaxation in modifying sickle cell crises. *Biofeedback and Self-Regulation, 12*, 51–61.

Craft, S., Schatz, J., Glauser, T. A., Lee, B., & DeBaun, M. R. (1993). Neuropsychological effects of stroke in children with sickle cell anemia. *Journal of Pediatrics, 123*, 712–717.

Craggs, J. G., Sanchez, J., Kibby, M. Y., Gilger, J. W., & Hynd, G. W. (2006). Brain morphology and neuropsychological profiles in a family displaying dyslexia and superior nonverbal intelligence. *Cortex, 42*, 1107–1118.

Crawford, A. H., & Schorry, E. K. (2006). Neurofibromatosis update. *Journal of Pediatric Orthopedics, 26*, 413–423.

Crawford, D. C., Acuña, J. M., & Sherman, S. L. (2001). FMR1 and the fragile X syndrome: Human genome epidemiology review. *Genetics in Medicine, 3*, 359–371.

Crawford, P. (2002). Epilepsy and pregnancy. *Seizure: Journal of the British Epilepsy Association, 11*(Suppl. A), 212–219.

Crawford, S., Channon, S., & Robertson, M. M. (2005). Tourette's syndrome: Performance on tests of behavioural inhibition, working memory and gambling. *Journal of Child Psychology and Psychiatry, 46*, 1327–1336.

Crenshaw, T. M., Kavale, K. A., Forness, S. R., & Reeve, R. E. (1999). Attention deficit hyperactivity disorder and the efficacy of stimulant medication: A meta-analysis. In T. E. Scruggs & M. A. Mastropieri (Eds.), *Advances in learning and behavioral disabilities* (Vol. 13, pp. 135–165). New York: Elsevier.

Croona, C., Kihlgren, M., Lundberg, S., Eeg-Olofsson, O., & Eeg-Olofsson, K. E. (1999). Neuropsychological findings in children with benign childhood epilepsy with centrotemporal spikes. *Developmental Medicine & Child Neurology, 41*, 813–818.

Cunningham, M., Tennis, P., & International Lamotrigine Pregnancy Registry Scientific Advisory Committee (2005). Lamotrigine and the risk of malformations in pregnancy. *Neurology, 64*, 955–960.

Cupples, L., & Iacono, T. (2002). The efficacy of "whole word" versus "analytic" reading instruction for children with Down syndrome. *Reading and Writing, 15*, 549–574.

Curatolo, P., Bombardieri, R., & Cerminara, C. (2006). Current management for epilepsy in tuberous sclerosis complex. *Current Opinion in Neurology, 19*, 119–123.

Curatolo, P., Cusmai, R., Cortesi, F., Chiron, C., Jambaque, I., & Dulac, O. (1991). Neuropsychiatric aspects of tuberous sclerosis. *Annals of the New York Academy of Sciences, 615*, 8–16.

Curatolo, P., D'Argenzio, L., Cerminara, C., & Bombardieri, R. (2008). Management of epilepsy in tuberous sclerosis complex. *Expert Review of Neurotherapeutics, 8*, 457–467.

Curfs, L. M. G., Hoondert, V., Van Lieshout, C. F. M., & Fryns, J. P. (1995). Personality profiles of youngsters with Prader-Willi syndrome and youngsters attending regular schools. *Journal of Intellectual Disability Research, 39*, 241–248.

Curl, C. L., Fenske, R., Kissel, J. C., Shirai, J. H., Griffith, T. W., Coronado, G., et al. (2002). Evaluation of take-home organophosphorous pesticide exposure among agricultural workers and their children. *Environmental Health Perspective, 110*, 787–792.

Curtis, L., & Patel, K. (2008). Nutritional and environmental approaches to preventing and treating autism and attention deficit hyperactivity disorder (ADHD): A review. *Journal of Alternative and Complementary Medicine, 14*, 79–85.

Curtis, M. E. (1980). Development of components of reading skill. *Journal of Educational Psychology, 72*, 656–669.

Cushner-Weinstein, S., Dassoulas, K., Salpekar, J., Henderson, S. E., Pearl, P. L., Gaillard, W. D., et al. (2008). Parenting stress and childhood epilepsy: The impact of depression, learning, and seizure-related factors. *Epilepsy & Behavior, 13*, 109–114.

Cutler, S. K., Handmaker, N. S., Handmaker, S. D., Kodituwakku, P. W., & Weathersby, E. K. (1995). Specific impairments in self-regulation in children exposed to alcohol prenatally. *Alcoholism: Clinical and Experimental Research, 19*, 1558–1564.

Cutter, W. J., Daly, E. M., Robertson, D. M. W., & Chitnis, X. A. (2006). Influence of X chromosome and hormones on human brain development: A magnetic resonance imaging and proton magnetic resonance spectroscopy study of Turner syndrome. *Biological Psychiatry, 59*, 273–283.

Cutting, L. E., Clements, A. M., Lightman, A. D., Yerby-Hammack, P. D., & Denckla, M. B. (2004). Cognitive profile of neurofibromatosis Type 1: Rethinking nonverbal learning disabilities. *Learning Disabilities Research & Practice, 19*, 155–165.

Cutting, L. E., Huang, G.-H., Zeger, S., Koth, C. W., Thompson, R. E., & Denckla, M. B. (2002). Growth curve analyses of neuropsychological profiles in children with neurofibromatosis Type 1: Specific cognitive tests remain "spared" and "impaired" over time. *Journal of the International Neuropsychological Society, 8*, 838–846.

Dahl, L. B., Kaaresen, P. I., Tunby, J., Handegard, B. H., Kvernmo, S., & Ronning, J. A. (2006). Emotional, behavioral, social, and academic outcomes in adolescents born with very low birth weight. *Pediatrics, 118*, e449-e459.

Dalens, B., Raynaud, E. J., & Gaulme, J. (1980). Teratogenicity of valproic acid. *Journal of Pediatrics, 97*, 332–333.

Daley, D. (2006). Attention deficit hyperactivity disorder: A review of the essential facts. *Child: Care, Health & Development, 32*, 193–204.

Daly, B. P., & Brown, R. T. (2007). Management of neurocognitive late effects with stimulant medication. *Journal of Pediatric Psychology, 32*, 1111–1126.

Daly, B. P., Creed, T., Xanthopoulos, M., & Brown, R. T. (2007). Psychosocial treatments for children with attention deficit/hyperactivity disorder. *Neuropsychology Review, 17*, 73–89.

Daly, B. P., Kral, M. C., & Brown, R. T. (2008). Cognitive and academic problems associated with childhood cancers and sickle cell disease. *School Psychology Quarterly, 23*, 230–242.

Damasio, A. R., & Maurer, R. G. (1978). A neurological model for childhood autism. *Archives of Neurology, 35*, 777–786.

D'Amato, R. C., Rothlisberg, B. A., & Rhodes, R. L. (1997). Utilizing neuropsychological paradigms for understanding common educational and psychological tests. In C. R. Reynolds & E. Fletcher-Janzen (Eds.), *Handbook of clinical child neuropsychology* (2nd ed., pp. 270–295). New York: Plenum.

Dampier, C., Ely, B., Brodecki, D., & O'Neal, P. (2002). Characteristics of pain managed at home in children and adolescents with sickle cell disease by using diary self-reports. *Journal of Pain, 3*, 461–470.

Daneman, M., & Merikel, P. M. (1996). Working memory and language comprehension: A meta-analysis. *Psychonomic Bulletin and Review, 3*, 422–433.

Danielsson, S., Gillberg, I. C., Billstedt, E., Gillberg, C., & Olsson, I. (2005). Epilepsy in young adults with autism: A prospective population-based follow-up study of 120 individuals diagnosed in childhood. *Epilepsia, 46*, 918–923.

Dapretto, M., Davies, M. S., Pfeifer, J. H. S., A. A., Sigman, M. D., Bookheimer, S. Y., & Iacoboni, M. (2006). Understanding emotions in others: Mirror neuron dysfunction in children with autism spectrum disorders. *Nature Neuroscience, 9*, 28–30.

Das, S. K., Sharma, N. K., Chu, W. S., Wang, H., & Elbein, S. C. (2008). Aryl hydrocarbon receptor nuclear translocator (ARNT) gene as a positional and functional candidate for type 2 diabetes and prediabetic intermediate traits: Mutation detection, case-control studies, and gene expression analysis. *BMC Medical Genetics, 9*, 16.

Dasgupta, B., & Gutmann, D. H. (2005). Neurofibromin regulates neural stem cell proliferation, survival, and astroglial differentiation in vitro and in vivo. *Journal of Neuroscience, 25*, 5584–5594.

Davenport, M. L. (2008). Moving toward an understanding of hormone replacement therapy in adolescent girls. *Annals of the New York Academy of Sciences, 1135*, 126–137.

Davenport, M. L., Hooper, S. R., & Zeger, M. (2007). Turner syndrome in childhood. In M. M. M. Mazzocco & J. L. Ross (Eds.), *Neurogenetic developmental disorders: Variation of manifestation in childhood* (pp. 3–46). Cambridge, MA: MIT Press.

David, N., Gawronski, A., Santos, N. S., Huff, W., Lehnhardt, F.-G., Newen, A., et al. (2008). Dissociation between key processes of social cognition in autism: Impaired mentalizing but intact sense of agency. *Journal of Autism and Developmental Disorders, 38*, 593–605.

Davidson, M., Boland, E. A., & Grey, M. (1997). Teaching teens to cope: Coping skills training for adolescents with insulin-dependent diabetes mellitus. *Journal of the Society of Pediatric Nurses, 2*, 65–72.

Davidson, M., Dorris, L., O'Regan, M., & Zuberi, S. M. (2007). Memory consolidation and accelerated forgetting in children with idiopathic generalized epilepsy. *Epilepsy & Behavior, 11*, 394–400.

Davidson, M. A. (2008). Primary care for children and adolescents with Down syndrome. *Pediatric Clinics of North America, 55*, 1099–1111.

Davidson, P. W., Myers, G. J., Cox, C., Wilding, G. E., Shamlaye, C. F., Huang, L. S., et al. (2006). Methylmercury and neurodevelopment: Longitudinal analysis of the Seychelles child development cohort. *Neurotoxicology and Teratology, 28*, 529–535.

Davidson, P. W., Weiss, B., Myers, G. J., Cory-Slechta, D. A., Brockel, B. J., Young, E. C., et al. (2000). Evaluation of techniques for assessing neurobehavioral development in children. *Neurotoxicology, 21*, 957–972.

Davies, M., Udwin, O., & Howlin, P. (1998). Adults with Williams syndrome: Preliminary study of social, emotional and behavioral difficulties. *British Journal of Psychiatry, 172*, 273–276.

Davies, S., Heyman, L., & Goodman, R. (2003). A population survey of mental health problems in children with epilepsy. *Developmental Medicine & Child Neurology, 45*, 553–564.

Davis, A. S. (2008). Children with Down syndrome: Implications for assessment and intervention in the school. *School Psychology Quarterly, 23*, 271–281.

Davis, A. S., & Dean, R. S. (2005). Lateralization of cerebral functions and hemispheric specialization: Linking behavior, structure, and neuroimaging. In R. C. D'Amato, E. Fletcher-Janzen, & C. R. Reynolds (Eds.), *Handbook of school neuropsychology* (pp. 120–141). Hoboken, NJ: Wiley.

Davis, A. S., & Phelps, L. (2008). Psychoeducational implications of neurodevelopmental genetic disorders. *School Psychology Quarterly, 23*, 243–245.

Davis, D. D., McIntyre, C. W., Murray, M. E., & Mims, S. S. (1986). Cognitive styles in children with dietary treated phenylketonuria. *Educational & Psychological Research, 6*, 9–15.

Davis, J. R., Brownson, R. C., & Garcia, R. (1992). Family pesticide use in the home, garden, orchard, and yard. *Archives of Environmental Contamination and Toxicology, 22*, 260–266.

Dawson, G., & Adams, A. (1984). Imitation and social responsiveness in autistic children. *Journal of Abnormal Child Psychology, 12*, 209–225.

Dawson, G., Klinger, L. G., Panagiotides, H., Lewy, A., & Castelloe, P. (1995). Subgroups of autistic children based on social behavior display distinct patterns of brain activity. *Journal of Abnormal Child Psychology, 23*, 569–583.

de Groot, C. M., Yeates, K. O., Baker, G. B., & Bornstein, R. A. (1997). Impaired neuropsychological functioning in Tourette's syndrome subjects with co-occurring obsessive-compulsive and attention deficit symptoms. *Journal of Neuropsychiatry and Clinical Neurosciences, 9*, 267–272.

de Lind van Wijngaarden, R. F. A., de Klerk, L. W. L., Festen, D. A. M., Duivenvoorden, H. J., Otten, B. J., & Hokken-Koelega, A. C. S. (2009). Randomized controlled trial to investigate the effects of growth hormone treatment on scoliosis in children with

Prader-Willi syndrome. *Journal of Clinical Endocrinology and Metabolism, 94*, 1274–1280.

de Vasconcelos Hage, S. R., Cendes, F., Montenegro, M. A., Abramides, D. V., Guimarães, C. A., & Guerreiro, M. M. (2006). Specific language impairment: Linguistic and neurobiological aspects. *Arqueves Neuropsiquitria, 64*(2-A), 173–180.

de Vries, P., Gardiner, J., & Bolton, P. (2009). Neuropsychological attention deficits in tuberous sclerosis complex (TSC). *American Journal of Medical Genetics, 149*, 387–395.

de Vries, P., Humphrey, A., McCartney, D., Prather, P., Bolton, P., Hunt, A., et al. (2005). Consensus clinical guidelines for the assessment of cognitive and behavioral problems in tuberous sclerosis. *European Child and Adolescent Psychiatry, 14*(4), 183–190.

de Vries, P., Hunt, A., & Bolton, P. F. (2007). The psychopathologies of children and adolescents with tuberous sclerosis complex (TSC): A postal survey of UK families. *European Child & Adolescent Psychiatry, 16*, 16–24.

Dean, J., Hailey, H., Moore, S. J., Lloyd, D. J., Turnpenny, P. D., & Little, J. (2002). Long-term health and neurodevelopment in children exposed to antiepileptic drugs before birth. *Journal of Medical Genetics, 39*, 251–259.

Dean, J., Roberston, Z., Reid, V., Wang, Q. D., Hailey, H., Moore, S., et al. (2007). Fetal anticonvulsant syndromes and polymorphisms in MTHFR, MTR, and MTRR. *American Journal of Medical Genetics, 143A*, 2303–2311.

Dean, R. S. (1986). Lateralization of cerebral functions. In D. Wedding, A. M. Horton, & J. S. Webster (Eds.), *The neuropsychology handbook: Behavioral and clinical perspectives* (pp. 80–102). Berlin: Springer-Verlag.

Dean, R. S., & Gray, J. W. (1990). Traditional approaches to neuropsychological assessment. In C. R. Reynolds (Ed.), *Handbook of psychological and educational assessment of children* (pp. 317–388). New York: Guilford.

DeBaun, M. R., Schatz, J., Siegel, M. J., Koby, M., Craft, S., Resar, L., et al. (1998). Cognitive screening examinations for silent cerebral infarcts in sickle cell disease. *Neurology, 50*, 1678–1682.

Debes, F., Budtz-Jorgensen, E. B., Weihe, P., White, R. F., & Grandjean, P. (2006). Impact of prenatal methylmercury exposure on neurobehavioral function at age 14 years. *Neurotoxicology and Teratology, 28*, 363–375.

Decety, J., Chaminade, T., Grezes, J., & Meltzoff, A. (2002). A PET exploration of the neural mechanisms involved in reciprocal imitation. *NeuroImage, 15*, 265–272.

Decety, J., & Grezes, J. (1999). Neural mechanisms subserving the perception of human actions. *Trends in Cognitive Science, 3*, 172–178.

Decety, J., Grezes, J., Costes, N., Perani, D., Jeannerod, M., Procyk, E., et al. (1997). Brain activity during observation of actions. *Brain, 120*, 1763–1777.

DeFries, J. C. (1988). Colorado Reading Project: Longitudinal analyses. *Annals of Dyslexia, 38*, 120–130.

DeFries, J. C., Fulker, D. W., & Labuda, M. C. (1987). Evidence for a genetic aetiology in reading disability of twins. *Nature 329*, 537–539.

Dehaene, S., & Changeux, J.-P. (1993). Development of elementary numerical abilities: A neuronal model. *Journal of Cognitive Neuroscience, 5*, 390–407.

Dehaene, S., Cohen, L., & Changeux, J.-P. (1998). Neuronal network models of acalculia and prefrontal deficits. In R. W. Parks, D. S. Levine, & D. L. Long (Eds.), *Fundamentals of neural network modeling: Neuropsychology and cognitive neuroscience* (pp. 233–255). Cambridge, MA: MIT Press.

Dehaene, S., Molko, N., Cohen, L., & Wilson, A. J. (2004). Arithmetic and the brain. *Current Opinion in Neurobiology, 14*(2), 218–224.

Dehaene, S., Spelke, E., Pinel, P., Stanescu, R., & Tsivkin, S. (1999). Sources of mathematical thinking: Behavioral and brain imaging evidence. *Science, 284*, 970–974.

Delacato, D. F., Szegda, D. T., & Parisi, A. (1994). Neurophysiological view of autism: Review of recent research as it applies to the Delacato theory of autism. *Developmental Brain Dysfunction, 7*(2–3), 129–131.

Delazer, M., Domahs, F., Bartha, L., Brenneis, C., Lochy, A., Trieb, T., et al. (2003). Learning complex arithmetic—an fMRI study. *Cognitive Brain Research, 18*, 76–88.

Delis, D. C., Jones, K. L., Mattson, S. N., & Riles, E. P. (1998). Neuropsychological comparison of alcohol-exposed children with or without physical features of fetal alcohol syndrome. *Neuropsychology, 12*, 146–153.

DeLong, G. R. (1992). Autism, amnesia, hippocampus, and learning. *Neuroscience & Biobehavioral Reviews, 16*, 63–70.

DeLong, G. R., Teague, L. A., & Kamran, M. M. (1998). Effects of fluoxetine treatment in young children with idiopathic autism. *Developmental Medicine & Child Neurology, 40*, 551–562.

Deltour, L., Quaglino, V., Barathon, M., De Broca, A., & Berquin, P. (2007). Clinical evaluation of attentional processes in children with benign childhood epilepsy with centrotemporal spikes (BCECTS). *Epileptic Disorders, 9*, 424–431.

Denckla, M. B. (1996). A theory and model of executive function: A neuropsychological approach. In G. R. Lyon & N. A. Krasnegor (Eds.), *Attention, memory, and executive function* (pp. 263–278). Baltimore, MD: Paul H. Brookes.

Dennis, M. (2000). Developmental plasticity in children: The role of biological risk, development, time, and reserve. *Journal of Communication Disorders, 33,* 321–332.

Dennis, M., & Barnes, M. A. (2000). Speech acts after mild or severe childhood head injury. *Aphasiology, 14,* 391–405.

Dennis, M., & Barnes, M. A. (2001). Comparison of literal, inferential, and intentional text comprehension in children with mild or severe closed head injury. *Journal of Head Trauma Rehabilitation, 16,* 456–468.

Denson, L. A. (2008). Growth hormone therapy in children and adolescents: Pharmacokinetic/pharmacodynamic considerations and emerging indications. *Expert Opinion on Drug Metabolism and Toxicology, 4*, 1569–1580.

Denys, D., de Geus, F., van Megen, H. J. G. M., & Westenberg, H. G. M. (2004). A double-blind, randomized, placebo-controlled trial of quetiapine addition in patients with obsessive-compulsive disorder refractory to serotonin reuptake inhibitors. *Journal of Clinical Psychiatry, 65*, 1040–1048.

DeRoche, K., & Welsh, M. (2008). Twenty-five years of research on neurocognitive outcomes in early-treated phenylketonuria: Intelligence and executive function. *Developmental neuropsychology, 33*, 474–504.

Descheemaeker, M.-J., Ghesquière, P., Symons, H., Fryns, J. P., & Legius, E. (2005). Behavioural, academic and neuropsychological profile of normally gifted neurofibromatosis type 1 children. *Journal of Intellectual Disability Research, 49*, 33–46.

Descheemaeker, M.-J., Vogels, A., Govers, V., Borghgraef, M., Willekens, D., Swillen, A., et al. (2002). Prader-Willi syndrome: New insights in the behavioural and psychiatric spectrum. *Journal of Intellectual Disability Research, 46*, 41–50.

Després, C., Beuter, A., Richer, F., Poitras, K., Veilleux, A., Ayotte, P., et al. (2005). Neuromotor functions in Inuit preschool children exposed to Pb, PCBs, and Hg. *Neurotoxicology and Teratology, 27*, 245–257.

deVeber, G., MacGregor, D., Curtis, R., & Mayank, S. (2000). Neurologic outcome in survivors of childhood arterial ischemic stroke and sinovenous thrombosis. *Journal of Child Neurology, 15*, 316–324.

Devlin, B., Cook, E. H. Jr., Coon, H., Dawson, G., Grigorenko, E. L., McMahon, W., et al. (2005). Autism and the serotonin transporter: The long and short of it. *Molecular Psychiatry, 10*, 1110–1116.

Devlin, J. T., Jamison, H. L., Gonnerman, L. M., & Matthews, P. M. (2006). The role of the posterior fusiform gyrus in reading. *Journal of Cognitive Neuroscience, 18*, 911–922.

Devlin, L. A., Shepherd, C. H., Crawford, H., & Morrison, P. J. (2006). Tuberous sclerosis complex: Clinical features, diagnosis, and prevalence within Northern Ireland. *Developmental Medicine and Child Neurology, 48*, 495–499.

Diabetes Control and Complication Trial Research Group. (1993). The effect of intensive treatment of diabetes on the development and progression of long-term complications in insulin-dependent diabetes mellitus. *New England Journal of Medicine, 329*, 977–986.

Diamond, A., Prevor, M. B., Callender, G., & Druin, D. (1997). Prefrontal cortex cognitive deficits in children treated early and continuously for PKU. *Monographs of the Society for Research in Child Development, 62*, 1–206.

Diamond, R., Barth, J. T., & Zillmer, E. A. (1988). Emotional correlates of mild closed head trauma: The role of the MMPI. *International Journal of Clinical Neuropsychology, 10*, 35–40.

Dibbets, P., Bakker, K., & Jolles, J. (2006). Functional MRI of task switching in children with specific language impairment (SLI). *Neurocase, 12*, 71–79.

Dichter, M. A. (1997). Basic mechanisms of epilepsy. *Epilepsia, 9*, 2–6.

DiCicco-Bloom, E., Lord, C., Zwaigenbaum, L., Courchesne, E., Dager, S. R., Schmitz, C., et al. (2006). The developmental neurobiology of autism spectrum disorder. *Journal of Neuroscience, 26*, 6897–6906.

Dickinson, D. K., & Tabors, P. O. (1991). Early literacy: Linkages between home, school and literacy achievement at age five. *Journal of Research in Childhood Education, 6*, 30–46.

Didden, R., Sigafoos, J., Green, V. A., Korzilius, H., Mouws, C., Lancioni, G. E., et al. (2008). Behavioural flexibility in individuals with Angelman syndrome, Down syndrome, non-specific intellectual disability and autism spectrum disorder. *Journal of Intellectual Disabilities Research, 52*, 503–509.

Dietrich, K. N. (2000). Environmental neurotoxicants and psychological development. In K. O. Yeates, M. D. Ris, & H. G. Taylor (Eds.), *Pediatric neuropsychology: Research, theory, and practice* (pp. 206–234). New York: Guilford.

Dietrich, K. N., Berger, O. B., & Succop, P. A. (1993). Lead exposure and the motor developmental status of urban six-year-old-children in the Cincinnati prospective study. *Pediatrics, 91*, 301–307.

Dietrich, K. N., Eskenazi, B., Schantz, S. L., Yolton, K., Rauh, V. A., Johnson, C. B., et al. (2005). Principles and practices of neurodevelopmental assessment in children: Lessons learned from the Centers for Children's Environmental Health and Disease Prevention Research. *Environmental Health Perspective, 113*, 1437–1446.

Dietrich, K. N., Ris, M. D., Succop, P. A., Berger, O. G., & Bornschein, R. L. (2001). Early exposure to lead and juvenile delinquency. *Neurotoxicology and Teratology, 23*, 511–518.

Dietrich, K. N., Succop, P. A., Berger, O. G., & Keith, R. W. (1992). Lead exposure and the central auditory processing abilities and cognitive development of urban children: The Cincinnati Lead Study cohort at age 5 years. *Neurotoxicology and Teratology, 14*, 51–56.

Dietrich, K. N., Ware, J. H., Salganik, M., Radcliffe, J., Rogan, W., Rhoads, G. G., et al. (2004). Effect of chelation therapy on the neuropsychological and behavioral development of lead-exposed children after school entry. *Pediatrics, 114*, 19–26.

Dilberti, J. H., Farndon, P. A., Dennis, N. R., & Curry, C. J. R. (1984). The fetal valproate syndrome. *American Journal of Medical Genetics, 19*, 473–481.

Dilworth-Bart, J. E., & Moore, C. F. (2006). Mercy mercy me: Social injustice and the prevention of environmental pollutant exposures among ethnic minority and poor children. *Child Development, 77*, 247–265.

Dindot, S. V., Antalffy, B. A., Bhattacharjee, M. B., & Beaudet, A. L. (2007). The Angelman syndrome ubiquitin ligase localizes to the synapse and nucleus, and maternal deficiency results in abnormal dendritic spine morphology. *Human Molecular Genetics, 17*, 111–118.

Dinges, D. F., Whitehouse, W. G., Orne, E. C., Bloom, P. B., Carlin, M. M., Bauer, N. K., et al. (1997). Self-hypnosis training as an adjunctive treatment in the management of pain associated with sickle cell disease. *International Journal of Clinical and Experimental Hypnosis, 45*, 417–432.

Dodrill, C. B. (1993). Neuropsychology. In J. Laidlaw, A. Richens, & D. Chadwick (Eds.), *A textbook of epilepsy* (pp. 459–473). New York: Churchill Livingstone.

Dolan, M. C. (1985). Carbon monoxide poisoning. *Canadian Medical Association Journal, 133*, 392.

Donders, J., & Warschausky, S. (2007). Neurobehavioral outcomes after early versus late childhood traumatic brain injury. *Journal of Head Trauma Rehabilitation, 22*, 296–302.

D'Onofrio, B. M., Van Hulle, C. A., Waldman, I. D., Rodgers, J. L., Rathouz, P. J., & Lahey, B. B. (2007). Causal inferences regarding prenatal alcohol exposure and childhood externalizing problems. *Archives of General Psychiatry, 64,* 1296–1304.

Donze, J. R., & Tercyak, K. P. (2006). The Survivor Health and Resilience Education (SHARE) program: Development and evaluation of a health behavior intervention for adolescent survivors of childhood cancer. *Journal of Clinical Psychology in Medical Settings, 13*, 169–176.

Drasgow, E., Halle, J. W., & Phillips, B. (2001). Effects of different social partners on the discriminated requesting of a young child with autism and severe language delays. *Research in Developmental Disabilities, 22*, 125–139.

Dreux, S., Olivier, C., Dupont, J.-M., Leporrier, N., Study Group, Oury, J.-F., et al. (2008). Maternal serum screening in cases of mosaic and translocation Down syndrome. *Prenatal Diagnosis, 28*, 699–703.

Duara, R., Kushch, A., Gross-Glenn, K., Barker, W., Jallad, B., Pascal, S., et al. (1991). Neuroanatomic differences between dyslexic and normal readers on magnetic resonance imaging scans. *Archives of Neurology, 48*, 410–416.

Ducharme, J. M., Lucas, H., & Pontes, E. (1994). Errorless embedding in the reduction of severe maladaptive behavior during interactive and learning tasks. *Behavior Therapy, 25*, 489–501.

Duff, F. J., Fieldsend, E., Bowyer-Crane, C., Hulme, C., Smith, G., Gibbs, S., et al. (2008). Reading with vocabulary intervention: Evaluation of an instruction for children with poor response to reading intervention. *Journal of Research in Reading, 31*, 319–336.

Duff, M. C., Proctor, A., & Haley, K. (2002). Mild traumatic brain injury (MTBI): Assessment and treatment procedures used by speech-language pathologists (SLPs). *Brain Injury, 16,* 773–787.

Duffy, F. H., Denckla, M. B., Bartels, P. H., & Sandini, G. (1980). Dyslexia: Regional differences in brain electrical activity by topographic mapping. *Annals of Neurology, 7*, 412–420.

Dufour, O., Serniclaes, W., Sprenger-Charolles, L., & Démonet, J.-F. (2007). Top-down processes during auditory-phoneme categorization in dyslexia: A PET study. *NeuroImage, 34*, 1692–1707.

Duke, D. C., Geffken, G. R., Lewin, A. B., Williams, L. B., Storch, E. A., & Silverstein, J. H. (2008). Glycemic control in youth with type 1 diabetes: Family predictors and mediators. *Journal of Pediatric Psychology, 33*, 719–727.

Duncan, J. S., Sander, J. W., Sisodiya, S. M., & Walker, M. C. (2006). Adult epilepsy. *Lancet, 367*, 1087–1187.

Duncan, S. (2007). Teratogenesis of sodium valproate. *Current Opinion in Neurology, 20*, 175–180.

Dunlap, G., & Fox, L. (1999). A demonstration of behavioral support for young children with autism. *Journal of Positive Behavior Interventions, 1*, 77–87.

DuPaul, G. J. (2007). School-based interventions for students with attention deficit hyperactivity disorder: Current status and future directions. *School Psychology Review, 36*, 183–194.

DuPaul, G. J., & Stoner, G. (2003). *ADHD in the schools: Assessment and intervention strategies* (2nd ed.). New York: Guilford.

Durham-Shearer, S. J., Judd, P. A., Whelan, K., & Thomas, J. E. (2008). Knowledge, compliance and serum phenylalanine concentrations in adolescents and adults with phenylketonuria and the effect of a patient-focused educational resource. *Journal of Human Nutrition and Dietetics, 21*, 474–485.

Dykens, E., Leckman, J., Riddle, M., Hardin, M., Schwartz, S., & Cohen, D. (1990). Intellectual, academic, and adaptive functioning of Tourette syndrome children with and without attention deficit disorder. *Journal of Abnormal Child Psychology, 18*, 607–615.

Dykens, E. M., & Cassidy, S. B. (1999). Prader-Willi Syndrome. In S. Goldstein & C. R. Reynolds (Eds.), *Handbook of neurodevelopmental and genetic disorders in children* (pp. 525–554). New York: Guilford.

Dykens, E. M., Hodapp, R. M., & Evans, D. W. (2006). Profiles and development of adaptive behavior in children with Down syndrome. *Down Syndrome: Research and Practice, 9*, 45–50.

Dykens, E. M., Hodapp, R. M., & Finucane, B. (2000). *Genetics and mental retardation syndromes: A new look at behavior and interventions*. Baltimore, MD: Brooks.

Dykens, E. M., Hodapp, R. M., Walsh, K., & Nash, L. J. (1992). Profiles, correlates, and trajectories of intelligence in Prader-Willi syndrome. *Journal of the American Academy of Child and Adolescent Psychiatry, 31*, 1131–1136.

Dykens, E. M., & Kasari, C. (1997). Maladaptive behavior in children with Prader-Willi syndrome, Down syndrome, and nonspecific mental retardation. *American Journal on Mental Retardation, 102*, 228–237.

Eapen, V., & Robertson, M. M. (2000). Comorbid obsessive-compulsive disorder and Tourette syndrome. *CNS Drugs, 13*, 173–183.

Eaves, L. C., & Ho, H. H. (2008). Young adult outcome of autism spectrum disorders. *Journal of Autism and Developmental Disorders, 38*, 739–747.

Eberhard-Gran, M., Eskild, A., & Opjordsmoen, S. (2005). Treating mood disorders during pregnancy: Safety considerations. *Drug Safety, 28*, 695–706.

Eberhard-Gran, M., Eskild, A., & Opjordsmoen, S. (2006). Use of psychotropic medications in treating mood disorders during lactation: Practical recommendations. *CNS Drugs, 20*, 187–198.

Eckert, M. A., Hu, D., Eliez, S., Bellugi, U., Galaburda, A., Korenberg, J., et al. (2005). Evidence for superior parietal impairment in Williams syndrome. *Neurology, 64*, 152–153.

Efron, R. (1957). The conditioned inhibition of uncinate fits. *Brain, 80*, 251–262.

Egger, H. L., Kondo, D., & Angold, A. (2006). The epidemiology and diagnostic issues in preschool attention-deficit/hyperactivity disorder: A review. *Infants & Young Children, 19*, 109–122.

Eggleston, B., Patience, M., Edwards, S., Adamkiewicz, T., Buchanan, G. R., Davies, S. C., et al. (2007). Effect of myeloablative bone marrow transplantation on growth in children with sickle cell anaemia: Results of the multicenter study of haematopoietic cell transplantation for sickle cell anaemia. *British Journal of Haematology, 136*, 673–676.

Ehlers, S., & Gillberg, C. (1993). The epidemiology of Asperger syndrome: A total population study. *Journal of Child Psychology and Psychiatry, 34*, 1327–1350.

Ehlers, S., Nyden, A., Gillberg, C., Sandberg, A. D., Dahlgren, S., Hjelmquist, E., et al. (1997). Asperger syndrome, autism and attention disorders: A comparative study of the cognitive profiles of 120 children. *Journal of Autism and Developmental Disorders, 38*, 207–217.

Eidlitz-Markus, T., Gorali, O., Haimi-Cohen, Y., & Zeharia, A. (2008). Symptoms of migraine in the paediatric population by age group. *Cephalalgia, 28*, 1259–1263.

Eigenmann, P. A., & Haenggeli, C. A. (2004). Food colourings and preservatives: Allergy and hyperactivity. *Lancet, 364*, 823–824.

Eike, M. C., Olsson, M., Undlien, D. E., Dahl-Jørgensen, K., Joner, G., Rønningen, K. S., et al. (2009). Genetic variants of the HLA-A, HLA-B and AIF1 loci show independent associations with type 1 diabetes in Norwegian families. *Genes and Immunity, 10*, 141–150.

Einfeld, S. L., Tonge, B. J., & Rees, V. W. (2001). Longitudinal course of behavioral and emotional problems in Williams syndrome. *American Journal of Mental Retardation, 106*, 73–81.

Eiraldi, R. B., Power, T. J., & Nezu, C. M. (1997). Patterns of comorbidity associated with subtypes of attention-deficit/hyperactivity disorder among 6- to 12-year-old children. *Journal of the American Academy of Child & Adolescent Psychiatry, 36*, 503–514.

Eiser, C., Hill, J. J., & Blacklay, A. (2000). Surviving cancer: What does it mean for you? An evaluation of a clinic-based intervention for survivors of childhood cancer. *Psycho-Oncology, 9*, 214–220.

Eiser, C., Hill, J. J., & Vance, Y. H. (2000). Examining the psychological consequences of surviving childhood cancer: Systematic review as a research method in pediatric psychology. *Journal of Pediatric Psychology, 25*, 449–460.

Elger, C. E., & Schmidt, D. (2008). Modern management of epilepsy: A practical approach. *Epilepsy and Behavior, 12*, 501–539.

Ellis, J. M., Tan, H. K., Muller, D. P. R., Henley, W., Moy, R., Pumphrey, R., et al. (2008). Supplementation with antioxidants and folinic acid for children with Down syndrome: Randomized controlled trial. *British Medical Journal, 336*, 594–597.

Eluvathingal, T. J., Behen, M. E., Chugani, H. T., Janisse, J., Bernardi, B., Chakraborty, P., et al. (2006). Cerebellar lesions in tuberous sclerosis complex: Neurobehavioral and neuroimaging correlates. *Journal of Child Neurology, 21*, 846–851.

Erickson, K. M., Syversen, T., Aschner, J. L., & Aschner, M. (2005). Interactions between excessive manganese exposures and dietary iron-deficiency in neurodegeneration. *Environmental Toxicology and Pharmacology, 19*, 415–421.

Erlanger, D. M., Kutner, K. C., Barth, J. T., & Barnes, R. (1999). Neuropsychology of sports-related head injury: Dementia pugilistica to post concussion syndrome. *Clinical Neuropsychologist, 13*, 193–209.

Ernst, A., & Zibrak, J. D. (1998). Carbon monoxide poisoning. *New England Journal of Medicine, 339*, 1603–1608.

Ernst, C. C., Grant, T. M., & Streissguth, A. P. (1999). Intervention with high-risk alcohol and drug-abusing mothers: II. Three-year finds from the Seattle model of paraprofessional advocacy. *Journal of Community Psychology, 27*(1), 19–38.

Eskenazi, B., Harley, K., Bradman, A., Weltzein, E., Jewell, N. B., Barr, D. B., et al. (2004). Association of *in utero* organophosphate pesticide exposure and fetal growth and length of gestation in an agricultural population. *Environmental Health Perspective, 112*, 1116–1124.

Espy, K. A., McDiarmid, M. M., Cwik, M. F., Stalets, M. M., Hamby, A., & Senn, T. E. (2004). The contribution of executive functions to emergent mathematic skills in preschool children. *Developmental Neuropsychology, 26*(1), 465–486.

Espy, K. A., Moore, I. M., Kaufmann, P. M., Kramer, J. H., Matthay, K., & Hutter, J. J. (2001). Chemotherapeutic CNS prophylaxis and neuropsychologic change in children with acute lymphoblastic leukemia: A prospective study. *Journal of Pediatric Psychology, 26*, 1–9.

Ettinger, A., Reed, M., & Cramer, J. (2004). Depression and comorbidity in community-based patients with epilepsy or asthma. *Neurology, 63*, 1008–1014.

Evans, D. W., & Gray, F. L. (2000). Compulsive-like behavior in individuals with Down syndrome: Its relation to mental age level, adaptive and maladaptive behavior. *Child Development, 71*, 288–300.

Ewart, A. K., Morris, C. A., Atkinson, D., Jin, W., Sternes, K., Spallone, P., et al. (1993). Hemizygosity at the elastin locus in developmental disorder: Williams syndrome. *Nature Genetics, 5*, 11–16.

Ewing-Cobbs, L., & Barnes, M. (2002). Linguistic outcomes following traumatic brain injury in children. *Seminars in Pediatric Neurology, 9*, 209–217.

Ewing-Cobbs, L., Barnes, M. A., & Fletcher, J. M. (2003). Early brain injury in children: Development and reorganization of cognitive function. *Developmental Neuropsychology, 24*, 669–704.

Ewing-Cobbs, L., & Fletcher, J. M. (1987). Neuropsychological assessment of head injury in children. *Journal of Learning Disabilities, 20*, 526–535.

Ewing-Cobbs, L., Fletcher, J. M., Levin, H. S., Iovino, I., & Miner, M. E. (1998). Academic achievement and academic placement following traumatic brain injury in children and adolescents: A two-year longitudinal study. *Journal of Clinical and Experimental Neuropsychology, 20*, 769–781.

Fabbro, F., Moretti, R., & Bava, A. (2000). Language impairments in patients with cerebellar lesions. *Journal of Neurolinguistics, 13*, 173–188.

Faden, V. B., & Graubard, B. I. (2000). Maternal substance use during pregnancy and developmental outcome at age three. *Journal of Substance Abuse, 12*, 329–340.

Fadiga, L., Craighero, L., & Oliver, E. (2005). Human motor cortex excitability during the perception of others' actions. *Current Opinion in Neurobiology, 15*, 213–218.

Falcaro, M., Pickles, A., Newbury, D. F., Addis, L., Banfield, E., Fisher, S. E., et al. (2008). Genetic and phenotypic effects of phonological short-term memory and grammatical morphology in specific language impairment. *Genes, Brain, and Behavior, 7*, 393–402.

Fan, Y., Rao, H., Hurt, H., Gainnetta, J., Korczykowski, M., Shera, D., et al. (2007). Multivariate examination of brain abnormality using both structural and functional MRI. *NeuroImage, 26*, 1189–1199.

Fantuzzo, J. W., King, J. A., & Heller, L. R. (1992). Effects of reciprocal peer tutoring on mathematics and school adjustment: A component analysis. *Journal of Educational Psychology, 84*, 331–339.

Faraone, S. V., & Biederman, J. (2002). Efficacy of Adderall for attention-deficit/hyperactivity disorder: A meta-analysis. *Journal of Attention Disorders, 6*, 69–75.

Faraone, S. V., Biederman, J., & Friedman, D. (2000). Validity of DSM-IV subtypes of attention-deficit/hyperactivity disorder: A family study perspective. *Journal of the American Academy of Child & Adolescent Psychiatry, 39*, 300–307.

Faraone, S. V., Biederman, J., Weber, W., & Russell, R. L. (1998). Psychiatric, neuropsychological, and psychosocial features of DSM-IV subtypes of attention-deficit/hyperactivity disorder: Results from a clinically referred sample. *Journal of the American Academy of Child & Adolescent Psychiatry, 37*, 185–193.

Fargo, J. D., Schefft, B. K., Szaflarski, J. P., Howe, S. R., Yeh, H.-S., & Privitera, M. D. (2008). Accuracy of clinical neuropsychological versus statistical prediction in the classification of seizure types. *Clinical Neuropsychologist, 22*, 181–194.

Farmer, J. E., Haut, J. S., Williams, J., Kapila, C., Johnstone, B., & Kirk, K. S. (1999). Comprehensive assessment of memory functioning following traumatic brain injury in children. *Developmental Neuropsychology, 15*, 269–289.

Farran, E. K., Jarrold, C., & Gathercole, S. E. (2001). Block design performance in the Williams syndrome phenotype: A problem with mental imagery. *Journal of Child Psychology and Psychiatry, 42*, 719–728.

Fastenau, P. S., Shen, J., Dunn, D. W., & Austin, J. K. (2008). Academic underachievement among children with epilepsy: Proportion exceeding psychometric criteria for learning disability and associated risk factors. *Journal of Learning Disabilities, 41*, 195–207.

Fastenau, P. S., Shen, J., Dunn, D. W., Perkins, S. M., Hermann, B. P., & Austin, J. K. (2004). Neuropsychological predictors of academic underachievement in pediatric epilepsy: Moderating roles of demographic, seizure, and psychosocial variables. *Epilepsia, 45*, 1261–1272.

Fawcett, A. J., Nicolson, R. I., & Dean, P. (1996). Impaired performance of children with dyslexia on a range of cerebellar tasks. *Annals of Dyslexia, 46*, 259–283.

Fawcett, A. J., Nicolson, R. I., & Maclagan, F. (2001). Cerebellar tests differentiate between groups of poor readers with and without IQ discrepancy. *Journal of Learning Disabilities, 34*, 119–135.

Fearon, P., O'Connell, P., Frangou, S., Aquino, P., Nosarti, C., Allin, M., et al. (2004). Brain volumes in adult survivors of very low birth weight: A sibling-controlled study. *Pediatrics, 114*, 367–371.

Feeley, K. M., & Jones, E. A. (2006). Addressing challenging behaviour in children with Down syndrome: The use of applied behaviour analysis for assessment and intervention. *Down's Syndrome, Research and Practice, 11*(2), 64–77.

Feng, W., Wang, M., Li, B., Liu, J., Chai, Z., Zhao, J., et al. (2004). Mercury and trace element distribution in organic tissues and regional brain of fetal rat after in utero and weaning exposure to low dose of inorganic mercury. *Toxicology Letters, 25*, 223–234.

Fennell, E. B., & Bauer, R. M. (1997). Models of inference in evaluating brain-behavior relationships in children. In C. R. Reynolds & E. Fletcher-Janzen (Eds.), *Handbook of clinical child neuropsychology* (pp. 167–177). New York: Plenum.

Fenske, R. A., Kissel, J. C., Lu, C., Kalman, D. A., Simcox, N. J., Allen, E. H., et al. (2000). Biologically based pesticide dose estimates for children in an agricultural community. *Environmental Health Perspectives, 108*, 515–520.

Fernell, E., Watanabe, Y., Adolfsson, I., Tani, Y., Hartvig, P., Lilja, A., et al. (1997). Possible effects of tetrahydrobiopterin treatment in six children with autism: Clinical and positron emission tomography data: A pilot study. *Developmental Medicine & Child Neurology, 39*, 313–318.

Ferraro, F. R., & Zevenbergen, A. A. (2001). Assessment and treatment of fetal alcohol syndrome in children and adolescents. *Journal of Developmental and Physical Disabilities, 13*(2), 123–136.

Fey, M., Warren, S. F., Brady, N. C., Finestack, L. H., Bredin-Oja, S. L., Fairchild, M., et al. (2006). Early effects of responsivity education/prelinguistic milieu teaching for children with developmental delays and their parents. *Journal of Speech, Language and Hearing Research, 49*, 526–547.

Fey, M. E. (2006). Commentary on "Making evidence-based decisions about child language intervention in schools" by Gillam and Gillam. *Language Speech and Hearing Services in the Schools, 37*, 316–319.

Fiala, C. L., & Sheridan, S. M. (2003). Parent involvement and reading: Using curriculum-based measurement to assess the effects of paired reading. *Psychology in the Schools, 40*, 613–626.

Fidler, D. J. (2005). The emerging Down syndrome behavioral phenotype in early childhood: Implications for practice. *Infants & Young Children, 18*, 86–103.

Fidler, D. J. (2006). The emergence of a syndrome-specific personality profile in young children with Down syndrome. *Down Syndrome: Research and Practice, 10*, 53–60.

Fidler, D. J., Philofsky, A., & Hepburn, S. L. (2007). Language phenotypes and intervention planning: Bridging research and practice. *Mental Retardation and Developmental Disabilities Research Reviews, 13*, 47–57.

Fido, A., & Al-Saad, S. (2005). Toxic trace elements in the hair of children with autism. *Autism, 9*, 290–298.

Fiedler, N., Kipen, H., Kelly-McNeil, K., & Fenske, R. (1997). Long-term use of organophosphates and neuropsychological performance. *American Journal of Industrial Medicine, 32*, 487–496.

Fiez, J. A., Raife, E. A., Balota, D. A., Schwarz, J. P., Raichle, M. E., & Petersen, S. E. (1996). A positron emission tomography study of the short-term maintenance of verbal information. *Journal of Neuroscience, 16*, 808–822.

Filipek, P. A., Accardo, P. J., Ashwal, S., Baranek, G. T., Cook, E. H. J., Dawson, G., et al. (2000). Practice parameter: Screening and diagnosis of autism: Report of the quality subcommittee of the American Academy of Neurology and the Child Neurology Society. *Neurology, 55*, 468–479.

Fine, C., Lumsden, J., & Blair, R. J. R. (2001). Dissociation between "theory of mind" and executive functions in a patient with early left amygdala damage. *Brain, 124*, 287–298.

Fine, J. G., Semrud-Clikeman, M., Keith, T. Z., Stapleton, L. M., & Hynd, G. W. (2007). Reading and the corpus callosum: An MRI family study of volume and area. *Neuropsychology, 21*, 235–241.

Finucane, B., McConkie-Rosell, A., & Cronister, A. (2002). *Fragile X syndrome: A handbook for families and professionals*. Newburyport, MA: National Fragile X Foundation.

Fisch, G. S., Carpenter, N., Howard-Peebles, P. N., Holden, J. J. A., Tarleton, J., Simensen, R., et al. (2007). Studies of age-correlated features of cognitive-behavioral development in children and adolescents with genetic disorders. *American Journal of Medical Genetics, 143A*, 2478–2489.

Fisch, G. S., Holden, J. J. A., Carpenter, N., Howard-Peebles, P. N., Maddalena, A., Pandya, A., et al. (1999). Age-related characteristics of children and adolescents with fragile X syndrome. *American Journal of Medical Genetics, 83*, 253–256.

Fischer, S., Mann, G., Konrad, M., Metzler, M., Ebetsberger, G., Jones, N., et al. (2007). Screening for leukemia- and clone-specific markers at birth in children with T-cell precursor ALL suggests a predominantly postnatal origin. *Blood, 110*, 3036–3038.

Fisher, R. S., van Emde, B. W., Blume, W., Elger, C. E., Genton, P., Lee, P., et al. (2005). Epileptic seizures and epilepsy: Definitions proposed by the International League Against Epilepsy (ILAE) and the International Bureau for Epilepsy (IBE). *Epilepsia, 46*, 470–472.

Fisher, S. E., & DeFries, J. C. (2002). Developmental dyslexia: Genetic dissection of a complex cognitive trait. *Nature and Neuroscience, 4*, 767–780.

Fishler, K., Azen, C. G., Friedman, E. G., & Koch, R. (1989). School achievement in treated PKU children. *Journal of Mental Deficiency Research, 33*, 493–498.

Flanagan, D. P., Ortiz, S. O., & Alfonso, V. C. (2007). *Essentials of cross-battery assessment*. Hoboken, NJ: Wiley.

Flanagan, D. P., Ortiz, S. O., Alfonso, V. C., & Mascolo, J. T. (2002). *The achievement test desk reference (ATDR): Comprehensive assessment and learning disabilities*. Boston: Allyn & Bacon.

Fletcher, J. M., Lyon, G. R., Fuchs, L. S., & Barnes, M. A. (2007). *Learning disabilities: From identification to intervention*. New York: Guilford.

Fletcher-Janzen, E., & Reynolds, C. R. (2008). *Neuropsychological perspectives on learning disabilities in the era of RTI: Recommendations for diagnosis and intervention*. Hoboken, NJ: Wiley.

Flowers, D. L. (1993). Brain basis for dyslexia. *Journal of Learning Disabilities, 26*, 575–582.

Floyd, R. G., Keith, T. Z., Taub, G. E., & McGrew, K. S. (2007). Cattell-Horn-Carroll cognitive abilities and their effects on reading decoding skills; g has indirect effects, more specific abilities have direct effects. *School Psychology Quarterly, 22*, 200–233.

Flynn, J. M., & Rahbar, M. H. (1994). Prevalence of reading failure in boys compared with girls. *Psychology in the Schools, 31*, 66–71.

Folstein, S. E., & Rosen-Sheidley, B. (2001). Genetics of autism: Complex aetiology for a heterogeneous disorder. *National Review of Genetics, 2*, 943–955.

Fombonne, E. (2003). The prevalence of autism. *Journal of the American Medical Association, 289*, 87–89.

Fombonne, E. (2005). The changing epidemiology of autism. *Journal of Applied Research in Intellectual Disabilities, 18*, 281–294.

Fombonne, E., Simmons, H., Ford, T., Meltzer, H., & Goodman, R. (2001). Prevalence of pervasive developmental disorders in the British Nationwide Survey of Child Mental Health. *Journal of the American Academy of Child and Adolescent Psychiatry, 40*, 820–827.

Ford, L., Riggs, K. S., Nissenbaum, M., & LaRaia, J. (1994). Facilitating desired behavior in the preschool child with autism: A case study. *Contemporary Educational Psychology, 65*, 148–151.

Foster, D. W. (1991). Diabetes mellitus. In J. D. Wilson, E. Braunwald, K. J. Isselbacher, R. G. Petersdorf, J. B. Martin, A. S. Fauci & R. K. Root (Eds.), *Harrison's principles of internal medicine* (12th ed., pp. 1739–1759). New York: McGraw-Hill.

Foster, L. M., Hynd, G. W., Morgan, A. E., & Hugdahl, K. (2002). Planum temporale asymmetry and ear advantage in dichotic listening in developmental dyslexia and attention-deficit/hyperactivity disorder (ADHD). *Journal of the International Neuropsychological Society, 8*, 22–36.

Fowler, M. G., Johnson, M. P., & Atkinson, S. S. (1985). School achievement and absence in children with chronic health conditions. *Journal of Pediatrics, 106*, 683–687.

Fowler, M. G., Whitt, J. K., Lallinger, R. R., Nash, K. B., Atkinson, S. S., Wells, R. J., et al. (1988). Neuropsychologic and academic functioning of children with sickle cell anemia. *Developmental and Behavioral Pediatrics, 9*, 213–220.

Francis, D. J., Shaywitz, S. E., Stuebing, K. K., Shaywitz, B. A., & Fletcher, J. M. (1996). Developmental delay versus deficit models of reading disability: A longitudinal, individual growth curve analysis. *Journal of Educational Psychology, 88*, 3–17.

Francis, R. B. Jr. (1991). Platelets, coagulation and fibrinolysis in sickle cell disease: Their possible role in vascular occlusion. *Blood Coagulation and Fibrinolysis, 2*, 341–353.

Franco, F., & Wishart, J. G. (1995). Use of pointing and other gestures by young children with Down syndrome. *American Journal on Mental Retardation, 100*, 160–182.

Franzen, M. D., Burgess, E. J., & Smith-Seemiller, L. (1997). Methods of estimating premorbid functioning. *Archives of Clinical Neuropsychology, 12*, 711–738.

Frassetto, F., Tourneur Martel, F., Barjhoux, C.-E., Villier, C., Bot, B. L., & Vincent, F. (2002). Goiter in a newborn exposed to lithium in utero. *Annals of Pharmacotherapy, 36*, 1745–1748.

Fredericksen, K. A., Cutting, L. E., Kates, W. R., Mostofsky, S. H., Singer, H. S., Cooper, K. L., et al. (2002). Disproportionate increases of white matter in right frontal lobe in Tourette syndrome. *Neurology, 58*, 85–89.

Freeman, J. M., Kossoff, E. H., & Hartman, A. L. (2007). The ketogenic diet: One decade later. *Pediatrics, 119*, 535–534.

Freeman, J. M., Vining, E. P., Pillas, D. J., Pysik, P. L., Casey, J. C., & Kelly, M. T. (1998). The efficacy of the ketogenic diet—1998: A prospective evaluation in 150 children. *Pediatrics, 102*, 1358–1363.

Freeman, R. D., Fast, D. K., Burd, L., Kerbeshian, J., Robertson, M. M., & Sandor, P. (2000). An international perspective on Tourette syndrome: Selected findings from 3500 individuals in 22 countries. *Developmental Medicine & Child Neurology, 42*, 436–447.

Freilinger, M., Reisel, B., Reiter, E., Zelenko, M., Hauser, E., & Seidl, R. (2006). Behavioral and emotional problems in children with epilepsy. *Journal of Child Neurology, 21*, 939–945.

Freund, L. S., Peebles, C. D., Aylward, E., & Reiss, A. L. (1995). Preliminary report on cognitive and adaptive behaviors of preschool-aged males with fragile X. *Developmental Brain Dysfunction, 8*, 242–251.

Friefeld, S., Rosenfield, J. V., Laframboise, K., MacGregor, D., Marcovitch, S., Teshima, I., et al. (1993). The fragile X syndrome: A multidisciplinary perspective on clinical features, diagnosis, and intervention. *Journal on Developmental Disabilities, 2*, 56–72.

Friefeld, S., Yeboah, O., Jones, J. E., & de Veber, G. (2004). Health-related quality of life and its relationship to neurological outcome in child survivors of stroke. *CNS Spectrums, 9*, 465–475.

Frith, U. (1989). *Autism: Explaining the enigma*. Oxford: Blackwell.

Frith, U., & Happé, F. (1994). Autism: Beyond “theory of mind.”*Cognition, 50*, 115–132.

Froehlich, T. W., Lanphear, B. P., Dietrich, K. N., Cory-Slechta, D. A., Wang, N., & Kahn, R. S. (2007). Interactive effects of a DRD4 polymorphism, lead, and sex on executive functions in children. *Biological Psychiatry, 62*, 243–249.

Fryns, J. P., Borghgraef, M., Brown, T. W., Chelly, J., Fisch, G. S., Hamel, B., et al. (2000). 9th international workshop on fragile X syndrome and X-linked mental retardation. *American Journal of Medical Genetics, 94*, 345–360.

Fürst, A. J., & Hitch, G. J. (2000). Separate roles for executive and phonological components of working memory in mental arithmetic. *Memory & Cognition, 28*, 774–782.

Gaddes, W. H., & Edgell, D. (1994). *Learning disabilities and brain function: A neuropsychological approach* (3rd ed.). New York: Springer-Verlag.

Gadow, K. D., Drabick, D. A., Loney, J., Sprafkin, J., Salisbury, H., Azizian, A., et al. (2004). Comparison of ADHD symptom subtypes as source-specific syndromes. *Journal of Child Psychology and Psychiatry, 45*, 1135–1149.

Gadow, K. D., Nolan, E., Litcher, L., Carlson, G., Panina, N., Golovakha, E., et al. (2000). Comparison of attention-deficit/hyperactivity disorder symptom subtypes in Ukrainian schoolchildren. *Journal of the American Academy of Child & Adolescent Psychiatry, 39*, 1520–1527.

Gaffney, G. R., Perry, P. J., Lund, B. C., Bever-Stille, K. A., Arndt, S., & Kuperman, S. (2002). Risperidone versus clonidine in the treatment of children and adolescents with Tourette’s syndrome. *Journal of the American Academy of Child and Adolescent Psychiatry, 41*, 330–336.

Galaburda, A. M. (1994). Developmental dyslexia and animal studies: At the interface between cognition and neurology. *Cognition, 50*, 133–149.

Galaburda, A. M., & Kemper, T. L. (1979). Cytoarchitectonic abnormalities in developmental dyslexia: A case study. *Annals of Neurology, 6*, 94–100.

Galaburda, A. M., Sherman, G. F., Rosen, G. D., Aboitiz, F., & Geschwind, N. (1985). Developmental dyslexia: Four consecutive patients with cortical anomalies. *Annals of Neurology, 18*, 222–233.

Gallese, V. (2003). The roots of empathy: The shared manifold hypothesis and the neural basis of intersubjectivity. *Psychopathology, 36*, 171–180.

Garber, H. J., & Ritvo, E. R. (1992). Magnetic resonance imaging of the posterior fossa in autistic adults. *American Journal of Psychiatry, 149*, 245–247.

Garchet-Beaudron, A., Dreux, S., Leporrier, N., Oury, J.-F., Muller, F., ABA Study Group, et al. (2008). Second-trimester Down syndrome maternal serum marker screening: A prospective study of 11,040 twin pregnancies. *Prenatal Diagnosis, 28*, 1105–1109.

Garcia, S. S., Ake, C., Clement, B., Huebner, H. J., Donnelly, K. C., & Shalat, S. L. (2001). Initial results of environmental monitoring in the Texas Rio Grande Valley. *Environment International, 26*, 465–474.

Garrison, W. T., & McQuiston, S. (1989). *Chronic illness during childhood and adolescence: Psychological aspects*. Thousand Oaks, CA: Sage.

Garry, V. F., Holland, S. E., Erickson, L. L., & Burroughs, B. L. (2003). Male reproductive hormones and thyroid function in pesticide applicators in the Red River Valley of Minnesota. *Journal of Toxicology and Environmental Health, 66*, 965–986.

Gassas, A., Sung, L., Doyle, J. J., Clarke, J. T. R., & Saunders, E. F. (2003). Life-threatening pulmonary hemorrhages post bone marrow transplantation in Hurler syndrome. Report of three cases and review of the literature. *Bone Marrow Transplantation, 32*, 213–215.

Gassió, R., Artuch, R., Vilaseca, M. A., Fusté, E., Colone, R., & Campistol, J. (2008). Cognitive functions and the antioxidant system in phenylketonuric patients. *Neuropsychology, 22*, 426–431.

Gassió, R., Fusté, E., López-Sala, A., Artuch, R., Vilaseca, M. A., & Campistol, J. (2005). School performance in early and continuously treated phenylketonuria. *Pediatric Neurology, 33*, 267–271.

Gathercole, S., & Baddeley, A. (1989). Evaluation of the role of phonological STM in the development of vocabulary in children: A longitudinal study. *Journal of Memory and Language, 28*, 200–213.

Gathercole, S., & Baddeley, A. (1990). The role of phonological memory in vocabulary acquisition: A study of young children learning new words. *British Journal of Psychology, 81*, 439–454.

Gathercole, S., Hitch, G. J., Service, E., & Martin, A. J. (1997). Phonological short-term memory and new word learning in children. *Developmental Psychology, 33*, 966–979.

Gathercole, S., & Pickering, S. J. (2001). Working memory deficits in children with special educational needs. *British Journal of Special Education, 28*, 89–107.

Gathercole, S., Willis, C., Emslie, H., & Baddeley, A. (1992). Phonological memory and vocabulary development during the early school years: A longitudinal study. *Developmental Psychology, 28*, 887–898.

Gathercole, S. E., & Pickering, S. J. (2000). Assessment of working memory in six- and seven-year-old children. *Journal of Educational Psychology, 92*, 377–390.

Gathercole, S. E., Pickering, S. J., Ambridge, B., & Wearing, H. (2004). The structure of working memory from 4 to 15 years of age. *Developmental Psychology, 40*, 177–190.

Gaub, M., & Carlson, C. L. (1997). Gender differences in ADHD: A meta-analysis and critical review. *Journal of the American Academy of Child & Adolescent Psychiatry, 36*, 1036–1045.

Gaudieri, P. A., Chen, R., Greer, T. F., & Holmes, C. S. (2008). Cognitive function in children with type 1 diabetes: A meta-analysis. *Diabetes Care, 31*, 1892–1897.

Gauger, L. M., Lombardino, L. J., & Leonard, C. M. (1997). Brain morphology in children with specific language impairment. *Journal of Speech, Language and Hearing Research, 40*, 1272–1284.

Gayan, J., & Olson, R. K. (2001). Genetic and environmental influences on orthographic and phonological skills in children with reading disabilities. *Developmental Neuropsychology, 20*, 483–507.

Gaze, C., Kepley, H. O., & Walkup, J. T. (2006). Co-occurring psychiatric disorders in children and adolescents with Tourette syndrome. *Journal of Child Neurology, 21*, 657–664.

Geary, D. C. (1993). Mathematical disabilities: Cognitive, neuropsychological, and genetic components. *Psychological Bulletin, 114*(2), 345–362.

Geary, D. C. (1994). *Children's mathematical development: Research and practical applications*. Washington, DC: American Psychological Association.

Geary, D. C., Brown, S. C., & Samaranayake, V. (1991). Cognitive addition: A short longitudinal study of strategy choice and speed of processing difficulties in normal and mathematically disabled children. *Developmental Psychology, 27*, 787–797.

Geary, D. C., Hamson, C. O., & Hoard, M. K. (2000). Numerical and arithmetical cognition: A longitudinal study of process and concept deficits in children with learning disability. *Journal of Experimental Child Psychology, 77*, 236–263.

Geary, D. C., & Hoard, M. K. (2001). Numerical and arithmetic weakness in learning disabled children: Relation to dsycalculia and dyslexia. *Aphasiology, 15*, 635–647.

Geary, D. C., Hoard, M. K., Byrd-Craven, J., & DeSoto, M. C. (2004). Strategy choices in simple and complex addition: Contributions of working memory and counting knowledge for children with mathematical disability. *Journal of Experimental Child Psychology, 88*, 121–151.

Geary, D. C., Hoard, M. K., & Hamson, C. O. (1999). Numerical and arithmetical cognition: Patterns of functions and weaknesses in children at risk for a mathematical disability. *Journal of Experimental Child Psychology, 74*, 213–239.

Gennarelli, T. A., Thibault, L. E., & Graham, D. I. (1998). Diffuse axonal injury: An important form of traumatic brain damage. *Neuroscientist, 4*, 202–215.

Gerard, E., & Peterson, B. S. (2003). Developmental processes and brain imaging studies in Tourette syndrome. *Journal of Child Neurology, 21*, 657–664.

Gerhardt, C. A., Dixon, M., Miller, K., Vannatta, K., Valerius, K. S., Correll, J., et al. (2007). Educational and occupational outcomes among survivors of childhood cancer during the transition to emerging adulthood. *Journal of Developmental & Behavioral Pediatrics., 28*, 448–455.

Gersten, R., Clarke, B., & Mazzocco, M. M. M. (2007). Historical and contemporary perspectives on mathematical learning disabilities. In D. B. Berch & M. M. M. Mazzocco (Eds.), *Why is math so hard for some children? The nature and origins of mathematical difficulties and disabilities* (pp. 7–27). Baltimore, MD: Brookes.

Gersten, R., Jordan, N. C., & Flojo, J. R. (2005). Early identification and interventions for students with mathematical difficulties. *Journal of Learning Disabilities, 38*, 293–304.

Geschwind, D. H., Boone, K. B., Miller, B. L., & Swerdloff, R. S. (2000). Neurobehavioral phenotype of Klinefelter syndrome. *Mental Retardation and Developmental Disabilities Research Reviews, 6*, 107–116.

Geurts, H. M., Grasman, R. P. P. P., Verté, S., Oosterlaan, J., Roeyers, H., van Kammen, S. M., et al. (2008). Intra-individual variability in ADHD, autism spectrum disorders and Tourette's syndrome. *Neuropsychologia, 46*, 3030–3041.

Ghajar, J. *(2000)*. Traumatic brain injury. *Lancet, 356, 923–929.*

Ghaziuddin, M., Tsai, L., & Ghaziuddin, N. (1991). Fluoxetine in autism with depression. *Journal of the American Academy of Child & Adolescent Psychiatry, 30*, 508–509.

Ghosh, S. S., Tourville, J. A., & Guenther, F. H. (2008). A neuroimaging study of premotor lateralization and cerebellar involvement in the production of phonemes and syllables. *Journal of Speech, Language, and Hearing Research, 51*, 1183–1202.

Giardina, P. J., & Grady, R. W. (2001). Chelation therapy in beta-thalassemia: An optimistic update. *Seminars in Hematology, 38*, 360–366.

Gibbs, D. P., & Cooper, E. B. (1989). Prevalence of communication disorders in students with learning disabilities. *Journal of Learning Disabilities, 22*, 60–63.

Giedd, J. N., Blumenthal, J., Jeffries, N. O., Rajapakse, J. C., Vaituzis, A. C., Liu, H., et al. (1999). Development of the human corpus callosum during childhood and adolescence: A longitudinal MRI study. *Progress in Neuro-Psychopharmacology and Biological Psychiatry, 23*, 571–598.

Gil, K. M., Wilson, J. J., Edens, J. L., Webster, D. A., Abrams, M. A., Orringer, E., et al. (1996). Effects of cognitive coping skills training on coping strategies and experimental pain sensitivity in African American adults with sickle cell disease. *Health Psychology, 15*, 3–10.

Gilbert, D. L. (2006). Treatment of children and adolescents with tics and Tourette syndrome. *Journal of Child Neurology, 21*, 690–700.

Gilbert, D. L., Batterson, J. R., Sethuraman, G., & Sallee, F. R. (2004). Tic reduction with risperidone versus pimozide in a randomized, double-blind, crossover trial. *Journal of the American Academy of Child and Adolescent Psychiatry, 43*, 206–214.

Gillam, R. B., Loeb, D. F., Hoffman, L.-V. M., Bohman, T., Champlin, C. A., Thibodeau, L., et al. (2008). The efficacy of Fast ForWord Language intervention in school-age children with language impairment: A randomized controlled trial. *Journal of Speech, Language, and Hearing Research, 51*, 97–119.

Gillberg, C. (1995a). *Clinical child neuropsychiatry*. London: Cambridge University Press.

Gillberg, C. (1995b). Endogenous opioids and opiate antagonists in autism: Brief review of empirical findings and implications for clinicians. *Developmental Medicine & Child Neurology, 37*, 239–245.

Gillberg, C. (1995c). *Clinical child neuropsychiatry*. London: Cambridge University Press.

Gillberg, C., & Svennerholm, L. (1987). CSF monoamines in autistic syndromes and other pervasive developmental disorders of early childhood. *British Journal of Psychiatry, 151*, 189–194.

Gillberg, G. (1993). Autism and related behaviors. *Journal of Intellectual Disability Research, 37*, 343–372.

Gillberg, I. C., Bjure, J., Uvebrant, P., Vestergren, E., & Gillberg, C. (1993). SPECT (single photon emission computed tomography) in 31 children and adolescents with autism and autistic-like conditions. *European Child & Adolescent Psychiatry, 2*, 50–59.

Gillberg, I. C., Gillberg, C., & Ahlsen, G. (1994). Autistic behavior and attention deficits in tuberous sclerosis: A population-based study. *Developmental Medicine & Child Neurology, 36*, 50–56.

Gillett, P. M., Gillett, H. R., Israel, D. M., Metzger, D. L., Stewart, L., Chanoine, J. P., et al. (2000). Increased prevalence of celiac disease in girls with Turner syndrome detected using antibodies to endomysium and tissue transglutaminase. *Canadian Journal of Gastroenterology, 14*, 915–918.

Gilstrap, L. C., & Little, B. B. (1998). *Drugs and pregnancy*. Toronto: Chapman and Hall.

Gingras, P., Santosh, P., & Baird, G. (2006). Development of an internet-based real-time system for monitoring pharmacological interventions in children with neurodevelopmental and neuropsychiatric disorders. *Child Care, Health, and Development, 32*, 591–600.

Ginsberg, M. D. (1995). Carbon monoxide intoxication: Clinical features, neuropathology, and mechanisms of injury. *Clinical Toxicology, 23*, 281.

Gioia, G. A., Isquith, P. K., Guy, S. C., & Kenworthy, L. (2000). *Behavior Rating Inventory of Executive Function Manual*. Odessa, FL: Psychological Assessment Resources.

Gioia, G. A., Isquith, P. K., Kenworthy, L., & Barton, R. M. (2002). Profiles of everyday executive function in acquired and developmental disorders. *Child Neuropsychology, 8*, 121–137.

Giovannini, M., Riva, E., Salvatici, E., Fiori, L., Paci, S., Verduci, E., et al. (2007). Treating phenylketonuria: A single-centre experience. *Journal of International Medical Research, 35*, 742–752.

Giraud, A.-L., Neumann, K., Bachoud-Levi, A.-C., von Gudenberg, A. W., Euler, H. A., Lanfermann, H., et al. (2008). Severity of dysfluency correlates with basal ganglia activity in persistent developmental stuttering. *Brain and Language, 104*, 190–199.

Girbau, D., & Schwartz, R. G. (2008). Phonological working memory in Spanish–English bilingual children with and without specific language impairment. *Journal of Communication Disorders, 41*, 124–145.

Giugliani, R., Rojas, V. M., Martins, A. M., Valadares, E. R., Clarke, J. T. R., Góes, J. E. C., et al. (2009). A dose-optimization trial of laronidase (Aldurazyme) in patients with mucopolysaccharidosis I. *Molecular Genetics and Metabolism, 96*, 13–19.

Gladen, B. C., & Rogan, W. (1991). Effects of perinatal polychlorinated biphenyls and dichlorodiphenyl dichloroethene on later development. *Journal of Pediatrics and Child Health, 113*, 58–63.

Glauser, T. A., & Packer, R. J. (1991). Cognitive deficits in long-term survivors of childhood brain tumors. *Child's Nervous System, 7*, 2–12.

Gleason, M. M., Egger, H. L., Emslie, G. J., Greenhill, L. L., Kowatch, R. A., Lieverman, A. F., et al. (2007). Psychopharmacological treatment for very young children: Contexts and guidelines. *Journal of American Academy of Child's and Adolescent Psychiatry, 46*, 1532–1572.

Glisky, E. L., & Glisky, M. L. (2002). Learning and memory impairments. In P. J. Eslinger (Ed.), *Neuropsychological interventions: Clinical research and practice* (pp. 137–162). New York: Guilford.

Glosser, G., Friedman, R. B., & Roeltgen, D. P. (1996). Clues to the cognitive organization of reading and writing from developmental hyperlexia. *Neuropsychology, 10*, 168–175.

Glosser, G., Grugan, P., & Friedman, R. B. (1997). Semantic memory impairment does not impact on phonological and orthographic processing in a case of developmental hyperlexia. *Brain and Language, 56*, 234–247.

Gloyn, A. L., & McCarthy, M. I. (2001). The genetics of type 2 diabetes. *Clinical Endocrinology & Metabolism, 15*, 293–308.

Godefroy, O., Lhullier, C., & Rousseaux, M. (1996). Non-spatial attention disorders in patients with frontal or posterior brain damage. *Brain: A Journal of Neurology, 119,* 191–202.

Goetz, K., Hulme, C., Brigstocked, S., Carroll, J. M., Nasir, L., & Snowling, M. (2008). Training reading and phoneme awareness skills in children with Down syndrome. *Reading and Writing, 21*, 395–412.

Goldberg, M. J. (1996). Syndromes of orthopaedic importance. In R. T. Morrissey & S. I. Weinstein (Eds.), *Lovell and Winter's pediatric orthopaedics* (pp. 237–276). Philadelphia: Lippincott.

Goldberg, T. E. (1987). On hermetic reading abilities. *Journal of Autism and Developmental Disorders, 17*, 29–44.

Golden, C. J. (1984). *Luria-Nebraska neuropsychological battery: Children's revision.* Los Angeles: Western Psychological Services.

Golden, C. J. (1997). The Nebraska neuropsychological children's battery. In C. R. Reynolds, & E. Fletcher-Janzen (Eds.), *Handbook of clinical child neuropsychology* (2nd ed., pp. 237–251). New York: Plenum.

Golden, C. J., Freshwater, S. M., & Vayalakkara, J. (2000). The Luria-Nebraska Neuropsychological Battery. In G. Groth-Marnat (Ed.), *Neuropsychological assessment in clinical practice: A guide to test interpretation and integration* (pp. 59–75). New York: Wiley.

Goldschmidt, L., Richardson, G. A., Willford, J., & Day, N. L. (2008). Prenatal marijuana exposure and intelligence test performance at age 6. *Journal of the American Academy of Child and Adolescent Psychiatry, 47*, 254–263.

Goldstein, H. (2002). Communication intervention for children with autism: A review of treatment efficacy. *Journal of Autism and Developmental Disorders, 32*, 373–396.

Goldstein, H., Kaczmarck, L., Pennington, R., & Shafer, K. (1992). Peer-mediated intervention: Attending to, commenting on, and acknowledging the behavior of preschoolers with autism. *Journal of Applied Behavior Analysis, 25*, 289–305.

Gomez, M. R. (1988). *Tuberous sclerosis: Neurologic and psychiatric features* (2nd ed.). New York: Raven.

Goodlet, A. Y., Greenough, W. T., Hungund, B. L., Klintsova, A. Y., Li, T., Powrozek,T., et al. (2001). Fetal alcohol effects: Mechanisms and treatment. *Alcoholism: Clinical and Experimental Research, 25*(5), 110–116.

Goodlet, C. R., Hannigan, J. H., Spear, L. P., & Spear, N. E. (1999). *Alcohol and alcoholism: Effects on brain and development*. Mahwah, NJ: Erlbaum.

Goodyear, P., & Hynd, G. W. (1992). Attention-deficit disorder with (ADD/H) and without (ADD/WO) hyperactivity: Behavioral and neuropsychological differentiation. *Journal of Clinical Child & Adolescent Psychology, 21*, 273–305.

Gordon, N. (2006). Williams syndrome. *Journal of Pediatric Neurology, 4*, 11–14.

Gothelf, D., Furfaro, J. A., Penniman, L. C., Glover, G. H., & Reiss, A. L. (2005). The contribution of novel brain imaging techniques to understanding the neurobiology of mental retardation and developmental disabilities. *Mental Retardation and Developmental Disabilities, 11*, 331–339.

Gottardo, N. G., & Gajjar, A. (2006). Current therapy for medulloblastoma. *Current Treatment Options in Neurology, 8*, 319–334.

Graf, A., Landolt, M. A., Mori, A. C., & Boltshauser, E. (2006). Quality of life and psychological adjustment in children and adolescents with neurofibromatosis type 1. *Journal of Pediatrics, 149*, 348–353.

Grafman, J., Kampen, D., Rosenberg, J., Salazar, A. M., & Boller, F. (1989). The progressive breakdown of number processing and calculation ability: A case study. *Cortex, 25*, 121–133.

Grandjean, P., Weihe, P., Burse, V. W., Needham, L. L., Storr-Hansen, E., Heinzow, B., et al. (2001). Neurobehavioral deficits associated with PCB in 7-year-old children prenatally exposed to neurotoxicants. *Neurotoxicology and Teratology, 23*, 305–317.

Grant, T. M., Ernst, C. C., & Streissguth, A. P. (1999). Intervention with high-risk alcohol and drug-abusing mothers: I. Administrative strategies of the Seattle model of paraprofessional advocacy. *Journal of Community Psychology, 27*(1), 19–38.

Greaves, M. (2006). Infection, immune responses and the aetiology of childhood leukemia. *National Review of Cancer, 6*(3), 193–203.

Green, J. H. (2007). Fetal alcohol spectrum disorders: Understanding the effects of prenatal alcohol exposure and supporting students. *Journal of School Health, 77*(3), 103–108.

Greene, R. W., & Ablon, J. S. (2001). What does the MTA study tell us about effective psychosocial treatment for ADHD? *Journal of Clinical Child Psychology, 30*, 114–121.

Greenswag, L. R., & Alexander, R. C. (1988). *Management of Prader-Willi syndrome*. New York: Springer-Verlag.

Greenwood, R. S., Tupler, L. A., Whitt, J. K., Buu, A. D., Dombeck, C. B., Harp, A. G., et al. (2005). Brain morphometry, T2-weighted hyperintensities, and IQ in children with neurofibromatosis type 1. *Archives of Neurology, 62*, 1904–1908.

Grey, M., Boland, E. A., Davidson, M., & Tamborlane, W. W. (1999). Coping skills training was effective in adolescents with type 1 diabetes. *Applied Nursing Research, 12*, 3–12.

Grey, M., Whittemore, R., & Tamborlane, W. (2002). Depression in Type 1 diabetes in children: Natural history and correlates. *Journal of Psychosomatic Research, 53*, 907–911.

Griffin, S. (2004). Number worlds: A research-based mathematics program for young children. In D. H. Clements & J. Sarama (Eds.), *Engaging young children in mathematics: Standards for early mathematics education* (pp. 325–342). Mahwah, NJ: Erlbaum.

Griffin, S. (2007). Early intervention for children at risk of developing mathematical learning difficulties. In D. B. Berch & M. M. M. Mazzocco (Eds.), *Why is math so hard for some children? The nature and origins of mathematical learning difficulties and disabilities* (pp. 373–414). Baltimore, MD: Brookes.

Griffith, E. M., Pennington, B. F., Wehner, E. A., & Rogers, S. J. (1999). Executive functions in young children with autism. *Child Development, 70*, 817–832.

Griffiths, S. Y., Sherman, E. M. S., Slick, D. J., Lautzenhiser, A., Westerveld, M., & Zaroff, C. M. (2006). The factor structure of the CVLT-C in pediatric epilepsy. *Child Neuropsychology, 12*, 191–203.

Grigg, W., Donahue, P., & Dion, G. (2007). *The Nation's Report Card™: 12th-Grade Reading and Mathematics, 2005*. Washington, DC: National Center for Education Statistics.

Grigorenko, E. L., Wood, F. B., Meyer, M. S., Hart, L. A., Speed, W. C., Shuster, A., et al. (1997). Susceptibility loci for distinct components of developmental dyslexia on chromosomes 6 and 15. *American Journal of Human Genetics 60*(1), 27–39.

Grigsby, J., Brega, A. G., Engle, K., Leehey, M. A., Hagerman, R. J., Tassone, F., et al. (2008). Cognitive profile of fragile X permutation carriers with and without fragile X associated tremor/ataxia syndrome. *Neuropsychology, 22*, 48–60.

Grigsby, J. P., Kemper, M. B., & Hagerman, R. J. (1987). Developmental Gerstmann syndrome without aphasia among fragile X syndrome. *Neuropsychologia, 25*, 881–891.

Gross-Glenn, K., Duara, R., Barker, W., Loewenstein, D., Chang, J. Y., Yoshii, F., et al. (1991). Positron emission tomographic studies during serial word reading by normal and dyslexic adults. *Journal of Clinical and Experimental Neuropsychology, 13*, 531–544.

Gross-Glenn, K., Duara, R., Yoshii, F., Barker, W., Chang, J. Y., Apicella, A. M., et al. (1986). PET-scan studies during reading in dyslexic and non-dyslexic adults. *Neuroscience Abstracts, 15*, 371.

Gross-Tur, V., Manor, O., & Shalev, R. S. (1996). Developmental dyscalculia: Prevalence and demographic features. *Developmental Medicine & Child Neurology, 38*, 25–33.

Grossman, H. (1983). *Classification in mental retardation*. Washington, DC: American Association on Mental Retardation.

Grueneich, R., Ris, M. D., Ball, W., Kalinyak, K. A., Noll, R. B., Vannatta, K., et al. (2004). Functional outcomes of children with sickle-cell disease affected by stroke. *Archives of Physical Medicine and Rehabilitation, 72*, 498–502.

Grunau, R. E., Whitfield, M. F., & Fay, T. B. (2004). Psychosocial and academic characteristics of extremely low birth weight (≤800 g) adolescents who are free of major impairment compared with term-born control subjects. *Pediatrics, 114*, e725–e732.

Grunau, R. V., & Low, M. D. (1987). Cognitive and task-related EEG correlates of arithmetic performance in adolescents. *Journal of Clinical and Experimental Neuropsychology, 9*, 563–574.

Gryiec, M., Grandy, S., & McLaughlin, T. F. (2004). The effects of the copy, cover, and compare procedure in spelling with an elementary student with fetal alcohol syndrome. *Journal of Precision Teaching & Celeration, 20*(1), 2–8.

Guerreiro, M. M., Hage, S. R. V., Guimarães, C. A., Abramides, D. V., Fernandes, W., Pacheco, P. S., et al. (2002). Developmental language disorder associated with polymicrogyria. *Neurology, 59*, 245–250.

Guerrini, R., Carrozzo, R., Rinaldi, R., & Bonanni, P. (2003). Angelman syndrome: Etiology, clinical features, diagnosis, and management of symptoms. *Paediatric Drugs, 5*, 647–661.

Guillette, E., Meza, M., Aquilar, M., Soto, A. D., & Garcia, I. E. (1998). An anthropological approach to the evaluation of preschool children exposed to pesticides in Mexico. *Environmental Health Perspectives, 106*, 347–352.

Guimarães, C. A., Li, L. M., Rzezak, P., Fuentes, D., Franzon, R. C., Montenegro, M. A., et al. (2007). Temporal lobe epilepsy in childhood: Comprehensive neuropsychological assessment. *Journal of Child Neurology, 22*, 836–840.

Gump, B. B., Reihman, J., Stewart, P., Lonky, E., Darvill, T., & Matthews, K. A. (2007). Blood lead (Pb) levels: A potential environmental mechanism explaining the relation between socioeconomic status and cardiovascular reactivity in children. *Health Psychology, 26*, 296–304.

Gündüz, E., Demirbilek, V., & Korkmaz, B. (1999). Benign rolandic epilepsy: Neuropsychological findings. *Seizure, 4*, 246–249.

Gurdin, L. S., Huber, S. A., & Cochran, C. R. (2005). A critical analysis of data-based studies examining behavioral interventions with children and adolescents with brain injuries. *Behavioral Interventions, 20,* 3–16.

Gurney, J. G. (2007). Neuroblastoma, childhood cancer survivorship, and reducing the consequences of cure. *Bone Marrow Transplantation, 40*, 721–722.

Gutmann, D. H. (1999). Learning disabilities in neurofibromatosis. *Archives of Neurology, 56*, 1322–1323.

Gutmann, D. H., Aylsworth, A., Carey, J. C., Korf, B., Marks, J., Pyeritz, R. E., et al. (1997). Diagnostic evaluation and multidisciplinary management of neurofibromatosis 1 and neurofibromatosis 2. *Journal of the American Medical Association, 278*(1), 51–57.

Ha, E., Hong, Y., Lee, B., Woo, B., Schwartz, J., & Christiani, D. C. (2001). Is air pollution a risk factor for low birth weight in Seoul? *Epidemiology, 12*, 643–648.

Hack, M., Cartar, L., Schluchter, M., Klein, N., & Forrest, C. B. (2007). Self-perceived health, functioning and well-being of very low birth weight infants at age 20 years. *Journal of Pediatrics, 151*, 635–641.

Hack, M., Flannery, D. J., Schluchter, M., Cartar, L., Borawski, E., & Klein, N. (2002). Outcomes in young adulthood for very-low-birth-weight infants. *New England Journal of Medicine, 346,* 149–157.

Hack, M., Schluchter, M., Cartar, L., & Rahman, M. (2005). Blood pressure among very low birth weight (<1.5 kg) young adults. *Pediatric Research, 58*, 677–684.

Hack, M., Schluchter, M., Cartar, L., Rahman, M., Cuttler, L., & Borawski, E. (2003). Growth of very low birth weight infants to age 20 years. *Pediatrics, 112*, 30–38.

Hack, M., Taylor, H. G., Drotar, D., Schluchter, M., Cartar, L., Andreias, L., et al. (2005). Chronic conditions, functional limitations, and special health care needs of school-aged children born with extremely low-birth-weight in the 1990s. *Journal of the American Medical Association, 294*, 318–325.

Hack, M., Taylor, H. G., Klein, N., Eiben, R., Schatschneider, C., & Mercuri-Minich, N. (1994). School-age outcomes in children with birth weights under 750 g. *New England Journal of Medicine, 331*, 753–759.

Haddad, P. M. (2001). Antidepressant discontinuation syndrome. *Drug Safety, 24*, 183–197.

Hadjikhani, N., Joseph, R. M., Snyder, J., & Tager-Flusberg, H. (2006). Anatomical differences in the mirror neuron system and social cognition network in autism. *Cerebral Cortex, 16*, 1276–1282.

Hagen, J. W., Barclay, C. R., Anderson, B. J., Feeman, D. J., Segal, S. S., Bacon, G., et al. (1990). Intellective functioning and strategy use in children with insulin-dependent diabetes mellitus. *Child Development, 61*, 1714–1727.

Hagerman, R. J. (2002). The physical and behavioral phenotype. In R. J. Hagerman & P. J. Hagerman (Eds.), *Fragile X syndrome: Diagnosis, treatment, and research* (3rd ed., pp. 3–109). Baltimore, MD: Johns Hopkins University Press.

Hagerman, R. J., & Hagerman, P. J. (2002). *Fragile X syndrome: Diagnosis, treatment, and research* (3rd ed.). Baltimore, MD: Johns Hopkins University Press.

Hagman, J., Wood, F., Buchsbaum, M., Flowers, L., Katz, W., & Tallal, P. (1992). Cerebral brain metabolism in adult dyslexics assessed with positron emission tomography during performance of an auditory task. *Archives of Neurology, 49*, 734–739.

Haier, R. J., Head, E., & Lott, I. T. (2008). Neuroimaging of individuals with Down syndrome at risk for dementia: Evidence for possible compensatory events. *NeuroImage, 39*, 1324–1332.

Hakimi, A. S., Spanaki, M. V., Schuh, L. A., Smith, B. J., & Schultz, L. (2008). A survey of neurologists' views on epilepsy surgery and medically refractory epilepsy. *Epilepsy & Behavior, 13*, 96–101.

Hale, J. B., & Fiorello, C. A. (2004). *School neuropsychology: A practitioner's handbook.* New York: Guilford.

Hale, J. B., Fiorello, C. A., Bertin, M., & Sherman, R. (2003). Predicting math achievement through neuropsychological interpretation of WISC-III variance components. *Journal of Psychoeducational Assessment, 21*(4), 358–380.

Hale, J. B., Fiorello, C. A., Kavanaugh, J. A., Hoepner, J. B., & Gaither, R. A. (2001). WISC-III predictors of academic achievement for children with learning disabilities: Are global and factor scores comparable? *School Psychology Quarterly, 16*, 31–55.

Hale, J. B., Fiorello, C. A., Miller, J. A., Wenrich, K., Teodori, A., & Henzel, J. N. (2008). WISC-IV interpretation for specific learning disabilities identification and intervention: A cognitive hypothesis testing approach. In A. Prifitera (Ed.), *WISC-IV Clinical assessment and intervention* (pp. 109–171). New York: Elsevier.

Haller, S., Klarhoefer, M., Schwarzbach, J., Radue, E. W., & Indefrey, P. (2007). Spatial and temporal analysis of fMRI data on word and sentence reading. *European Journal of Neuroscience, 26*, 2074–2084.

Hampson, M., Tokoglu, F., Sun, Z., Schafer, R. J., Skudlarski, P., Gore, J. C., et al. (2006). Connectivity-behavior analysis reveals that functional connectivity between left BA39 and Broca's area varies with reading ability. *NeuroImage, 31*, 513–519.

Hampson, S. E., Skinner, T. C., Hart, J., Story, L., Gage, H., Foxcroft, D., et al. (2000). Behavioral interventions for adolescents in type 1 diabetes: How effective are they? *Diabetes Care, 23*, 1416–1422.

Hanich, L. B., Jordan, N. C., Kaplan, D., & Dick, J. (2001). Performance across different areas of mathematical cognition in children with learning difficulties. *Journal of Educational Psychology, 93*, 615–626.

Hannay, H. J., Bielasukas, L. A., Crosson, B., Hammeke, T. A., Hamsher, K. D., & Koffler, S. P. (1998). Proceedings: The Houston conference on specialty education and training in clinical neuropsychology. *Archives of Clinical Neuropsychology, 13*, 157–250.

Hannonen, R., Tupola, S., Ahonen, T., & Riikonen, R. (2003). Neurocognitive functioning in children with type-1 diabetes with and without episodes of severe hypoglycaemia. *Developmental Medicine & Child Neurology, 45*, 262–268.

Hans, S. L. (1999). Demographic and psychosocial characteristics of substance-abusing pregnant women. *Clinical Perinatology, 26*, 55–74.

Hansen, O. M., Trillingsgaard, A., Beese, I., Lyngbye, T., & Grandjean, P. A. (1989). A neuropsychological study of children with elevated dentine lead level: Assessment of the effect of lead in different socio-economic groups. *Neurotoxicology and Teratology, 11*, 205–214.

Hanson, C. L., Henggeler, S. W., & Burghen, G. A. (1987). Social competence and parental support as mediators of the link between stress and metabolic control in adolescents with insulin-dependent diabetes mellitus. *Journal of Consulting and Clinical Psychology, 55*, 529–533.

Hanten, G., Dennis, M., Zhang, L., Barnes, M., Roberson, G., Archibald, J., et al. (2004). Childhood head injury and metacognitive processes in language and memory. *Developmental Neuropsychology, 25*, 85–106.

Happé, F. (1993). Communicative competence and theory of mind in autism: A test of relevance theory. *Cognition, 48*, 101–119.

Happé, F. (2005). The weak central coherence account of autism. In F. R. Volkmar, R. Paul, A. Klin & D. Cohen (Eds.), *Handbook of autism and pervasive developmental disorders: Diagnosis, development, neurobiology, and behavior* (3rd ed., Vol. 1, pp. 640–649). Hoboken, NJ: Wiley.

Happé, F., Briskman, J., & Frith, U. (2001). Exploring the cognitive phenotype of autism: Weak "central coherence" in parents and siblings of children with autism: I. Experimental tests. *Journal of Child Psychology and Psychiatry, 42*, 299–307.

Happé, F., Ehlers, P., Fletcher, P., Frith, U., Johansson, M., Gillberg, C., et al. (1996). "Theory of mind" in the brain. Evidence from a PET scan study of Asperger syndrome. *NeuroReport, 8*, 197–201.

Harcherik, D. F., Leckman, J. F., Detlor, J., & Cohen, D. J. (1984). A new instrument for clinical studies of Tourette's syndrome. *Journal of the American Academy of Child & Adolescent Psychiatry, 23*, 153–160.

Harden, A. Y., Grigis, R. R., Adams, J., Gilbert, A. R., Melhem, N. M., Keshavan, M. S., et al. (2007). Brief report: Abnormal association between the thalamus and brain size in Asperger's disorder. *Journal of Autism and Developmental Disorders, 38*, 390–394.

Harding, C. O. (2008). Progress toward cell-directed therapy for phenylketonuria. *Clinical Genetics, 74*, 97–104.

Hare, M. F., Rezazadeh, S. M., Cooper, G. P., Minnema, D. J., & Michaelson, I. A. (1990). Effects of inorganic mercury on [3^H] dopamine release and calcium homeostasis in rat striatal synaptosomes. *Toxicology and Applied Pharmacology, 102*, 316–330.

Hargis, E. R. (2008). Targeting epilepsy, one of the nation's most common disabling neurological conditions at a glance. Retrieved June 27, 2008, from www.cdc.gov.

Hariman, L. M., Griffith, E. R., Hurtig, A. L., & Keehn, M. T. (1991). Functional outcomes of children with sickle cell disease affected by stroke. *Archives of Physical Medicine and Rehabilitation, 72*, 498–502.

Harmatz, P., Giugliani, R., Schwartz, I. V. D., Guffon, N., Teles, E. L., Miranda, M. C. S., et al. (2008). Long-term follow-up of endurance and safety outcomes during enzyme replacement therapy for mucopolysaccharidosis. VI: Final results of three clinical studies of recombinant human N-acetylgalactosamine 4-sulfatase. *Molecular Genetics and Metabolism, 94*, 469–475.

Harris, E. L., Schuerholz, L. J., Singer, H. S., Reader, M. J., Brown, J. E., Cox, C., et al. (1995). Executive function in children with Tourette syndrome and/or attention deficit hyperactivity disorder. *Journal of the International Neuropsychological Society, 1*, 511–516.

Harris-Schmidt, G. (2003). What are some important teaching strategies? Retrieved December 1, 2008, from www.fragilex.org/html/teaching.htm.

Harris, J. G., Wagner, B., & Cullum, C. M. (2007). Symbol vs. digit substitution task performance in diverse cultural and linguistic groups. *Clinical Neuropsychologist, 21*, 800–810.

Hart, A. R., Whitby, E. W., Griffiths, P. D., & Smith, M. F. (2008). Magnetic resonance imaging and developmental outcome following preterm birth: Review of current evidence. *Developmental Medicine & Child Neurology, 50,* 655–663.

Hart, K., & Faust, D. (1988). Prediction of the effects of mild head injury: A message about the Kennard principle. *Journal of Clinical Psychology, 44,* 780–782.

Hart, S. J., Davenport, M. L., Hooper, S. R., & Belger, A. (2006). Visuospatial executive function in Turner syndrome: Functional MRI and neurocognitive findings. *Brain, 129*, 1125–1136.

Hashimoto, T., Tayama, M., Miyazaki, M., Murakawa, K., Shimakawa, S., Yoneda, Y., et al. (1993). Brainstem involvement in high-functioning autistic children. *Acta Neurologica Scandinavica, 88*, 123–128.

Hashimoto, T., Tayama, M., Murakawa, K., Yoshimoto, T., Miyazaki, M., Harada, M., et al. (1995). Development of the brainstem and cerebellum in autistic patients. *Journal of Autism and Developmental Disorders, 25*, 1–18.

Hathout, E., Lakey, J., & Shapiro, J. (2003). Islet transplant: An option for childhood diabetes. *Archives of Diseases in Children, 88*, 591–594.

Hatton, D. D., Bailey, D. B. J., Roberts, J. P., Skinner, M., Mayhew, L., Clark, R. D., et al. (2000). Early intervention services for young boys with fragile X syndrome. *Journal of Early Intervention, 23*, 235–251.

Hatton, D. D., Wheeler, A., Sideris, J., Sullivan, K., Reichardt, A., Roberts, J. E., et al. (2009). Developmental trajectories of young girls with fragile X syndrome. *American Journal on Intellectual and Developmental Disabilities, 114*, 161–171.

Haupt, R., Fears, T. R., Robison, L. L., Miklls, J. L., Nicholson, H. S., Zeltzer, L. K., et al. (1994). Educational attainment in long-term survivors of childhood acute lymphoblastic leukemia. *Journal of the American Medical Association, 272*, 1427–1432.

Hauser, W. A., Annegers, J. F., & Rocca, W. A. (1996). Descriptive epidemiology of epilepsy: Contributions of population-based studies from Rochester, Minnesota. *Mayo Clinic Proceedings. Mayo Clinic, 71*, 576–586.

Hawke, J. L., Wadsworth, S. J., & Defries, J. C. (2006). Genetic influences on reading difficulties in boys and girls: The Colorado twin study. *Dyslexia: An International Journal of Research and Practice, 12*, 21–29.

Hayden, J., & McLaughlin, T. F. (2004). The effects of cover, copy, and compare and flash card drill on correct rate of math facts for a middle school student with learning disabilities. *Journal of Precision Teaching & Celeration, 20*(1), 17–21.

Hayes, S. C., Gifford, E. V., & Ruckstuhl, L. E., Jr. (1996). Relational frame theory and executive function: A behavioral approach. In G. R. Lyon & N. A. Krasnegor (Eds.), *Attention, memory, and executive function* (pp. 279–305). Baltimore, MD: Brookes.

Haynes, E. N., Kalkwarf, H. J., Hornung, R. W., Wenstrup, R., Dietrich, K. N., & Lanphear, B. P. (2003). Vitamin D receptor Fok1 polymorphism and blood lead concentration in children. *Environmental Health Perspectives, 111*, 1665–1669.

Hayter, S., Scott, E., McLaughlin, T. F., & Weber, K. P. (2007). The use of a modified direct instruction flashcard system with two high school students with developmental disabilities. *Journal of Developmental and Physical Disabilities, 19*, 409–415.

Hazlett, H. C., Poe, M. D., Gerig, G., Smith, R. G., & Piven, J. (2006). Cortical gray and white brain tissue volume in adolescents and adults with autism. *Biological Psychiatry, 59*, 1–6.

Haznedar, M. M., Buchsbaum, M. S., Wei, T.-C., Hof, P. R., Cartwright, C., Bienstock, C. A., et al. (2000). Limbic circuitry in patients with autism spectrum disorders studied with positron emission tomography and magnetic resonance imaging. *American Journal of Psychiatry, 157*, 1994–2001.

He, P., Liu, D. H., & Zhang, G. Q. (1994). Effects of high-level manganese sewage irrigation on children's neurobehavior. *Zhonghua Yu Fong Yi Xue Za Zhi, 28*, 216–218.

Heath, M., Grierson, L., Binsted, G., & Elliott, D. (2007). Interhemispheric transmission time in persons with Down syndrome. *Journal of Intellectual Disability Research, 51*, 972–981.

Heath, M., Welsh, T. N., Simon, D. A., Tremblay, L., Elliott, D., & Roy, E. A. (2005). Relative processing demands influence cerebral laterality for verbal-motor integration in persons with Down syndrome. *Cortex, 41*, 61–66.

Hécaen, H., Angelergues, T., & Houiller, S. (1961). Les varietés cliniques des acalculies au cours des lesions retrorolandiques (The clinical varieties of acalculias during petrocolaudic lesions: Statistical approach to the problem). *Revue Neurologicue, 105*, 85–103.

Helgeson, V. S., Reynolds, K. A., Siminierio, L., Escobar, O., & Becker, D. (2007). Parent and adolescent distribution of responsibility for diabetes self-care: Links to health outcomes. *Journal of Pediatric Psychology, 33*, 497–508.

Henderson, C. B., Filloux, F. M., Alder, S. C., Lyon, J. L., & Caplin, D. A. (2006). Efficacy of the ketogenic diet as a treatment option for epilepsy: Meta-analysis. *Journal of Child Neurology, 21*, 193–198.

Henkin, Y., Sadeh, M., & Gadoth, N. (2007). Learning difficulties in children with epilepsy with idiopathic generalized epilepsy and well-controlled seizures. *Developmental Medicine & Child Neurology, 49*, 874–875.

Hennedige, A. A., Quaba, A. A., & Al-Nakib, K. (2008). Sturge-Weber syndrome and dermatomal facial port-wine stains: Incidence, association with glaucoma, and pulsed tunable dye laser treatment effectiveness. *Plastic and Reconstructive Surgery, 121*, 1173–1180.

Hérault, J., Pettit, E., Martineau, J., Cherpi, C., Perrot, A., Barthélémy, C., et al. (1996). Serotonin and autism: Biochemical and molecular biology features. *Psychiatry Research, 65*, 33–43.

Herbert, M. R., Ziegler, D. A., Deutsch, C. K., O'Brien, L. M., Lange, N., Bakardjiev, A., et al. (2003). Dissociations of cerebral cortex, subcortical and cerebral white matter volumes in autistic boys. *Brain, 126*, 1181–1192.

Herbert, M. R., Ziegler, D. A., Makris, N., Bakardjiev, A., Hodgson, J., Adrien, K. T., et al. (2003). Larger brain and white matter volumes in children with developmental language disorder. *Developmental Science, 6*(4), F11–F22.

Hernandez, M. T., Sauerwein, H. C., Jambaqué, I., De Guise, E., Lussier, F., Lortie, A., et al. (2002). Deficits in executive functions and motor coordination in children with frontal lobe epilepsy. *Neuropsychologia, 4*, 384–400.

Hersh, J. H. (2008). Health supervision for children with neurofibromatosis. *Pediatrics, 121*, 633–642.

Hershey, T., Perantie, D. C., Warren, S. L., Zimmerman, E. C., Sadler, M., & White, N. H. (2005). Frequency and timing of severe hypoglycemia affects spatial memory in children with type 1 diabetes. *Diabetes Care, 28*, 2372–2377.

Hertz-Picciotto, I., Croen, L. A., Hansen, R., Jones, C. R., van de Water, J., & Pessah, I. N. (2006). The CHARGE study: An epidemiologic investigation of genetic and environmental factors contributing to autism. *Environmental Health Perspectives, 114*, 1119–1125.

Hervey, A. S., Epstein, J. N., & Curry, J. F. (2004). Neuropsychology of adults with attention-deficit/hyperactivity disorder: A meta-analytic review. *Neuropsychology, 18*, 485–503.

Hetzler, B. E., & Griffin, J. L. (1981). Infantile autism and the temporal lobe of the brain. *Journal of Autism and Developmental Disorders, 11*, 317–330.

Heudorf, U., Angerer, J., & Drexler, H. (2004). Current internal exposure to pesticides in children and adolescents in Germany: Urinary levels of metabolites of pyrethroid and organophosphorous insecticides. *International Archives of Occupational and Environmental Health, 77*, 67–72.

Hiemenz, J. R., & Hynd, G. W. (2000). Sulcal/gyral pattern morphology of the perisylvian language region in developmental dyslexia. *Brain and Language, 74*, 113–133.

Hier, D. B., LeMay, M., & Rosenberger, P. B. (1979). Autism and unfavorable left-right asymmetries of the brain. *Journal of Autism and Developmental Disorders, 9*, 153–159.

Higley, A. M., & Morin, K. H. (2004). Behavioral responses of substance-exposed newborns: A retrospective study. *Applied Nursing Research, 17*, 32–40.

Hill, J. L., Brooks-Gunn, J., & Waldfogel, J. (2003). Sustained effects of high participation in an early intervention for low-birth-weight premature infants. *Developmental Psychology, 39,* 730–744.

Hille, E. T. M., Weisglas-Kuperus, N., van Goudoever, J. B., Jacobusse, G. W., Ens-Dokkum, M. H., de Groot, L., et al. (2007). Functional outcomes and participation in young adulthood for very preterm and very low birth weight infants: The Dutch project on preterm and small for gestational age infants at 19 years of age. *Pediatrics, 120*, 587–595.

Hillery, C. A., & Panepinto, J. A. (2004). Pathophysiology of stroke in sickle cell disease. *Microcirculation, 11*, 195–208.

Hillier, L. W., Fulton, R. S., Fulton, L. A., Graves, T. A., Pepin, K. H., Wanger-McPherson, C., et al. (2003). The DNA sequence of chromosome 7. *Nature, 424*, 157–164.

Himanen, L., Portin, R., Isoniemi, H., Helenius, H., Kurki, T., & Tenovuo, O. (2005). Cognitive functions in relation to MRI findings 30 years after traumatic brain injury. *Brain Injury, 19,* 93–100.

Himle, M. B., Woods, D. W., Piacentini, J. C., & Walkup, J. T. (2006). Brief review of habit reversal training for Tourette syndrome. *Journal of Child Neurology, 21*, 719–725.

Hindmarsh, J., McLetchie, O. R., Heffernan, L. P. M., Hayne, O. A., Ellenberger, H. A., McCurdy, R. F., et al. (1977). Electromyographic abnormalities in chronic environmental arsenicalism. In S. S. Brown (Ed.), *Clinical chemistry and chemical toxicology of metals* (pp. 287–293). Amsterdam: Elsevier.

Hinshaw, S. P., March, J. S., Abikoff, H., Arnold, L. E., Cantwell, D. P., Conners, C. K., et al. (1997). Comprehensive assessment of childhood attention-deficit hyperactivity disorder in the context of a multisite, multimodal clinical trial. *Journal of Attention Disorders, 1*, 217–234.

Hirshberg, L. M., Chui, S., & Frazier, J. A. (2005). Emerging brain-based interventions for children and adolescents: Overview and clinical perspective. *Child and Adolescent Pediatric Clinics of North America, 14*, 1–19.

Hiscock, M. (1988). Behavioral asymmetries in normal children. In D. L. Molfese & S. J. Segalowitz (Eds.), *Brain Lateralization in children: Developmental implications* (pp. 85–169). New York: Guilford.

Hitch, G. J., & McAuley, E. (1991). Working memory in children with specific arithmetical learning difficulties. *British Journal of Psychology, 82*, 375–386.

Ho-Turner, M., & Bennett, T. L. (1999). Seizure disorders. In S. Goldstein & C. R. Reynolds (Eds.), *Handbook of neurodevelopmental and genetic disorders in children* (pp. 499–524). New York: Guilford.

Ho, L. S., Gittelsohn, J., Rimal, R., Treuth, M. S., Sharma, S., Rosecrans, A., et al. (2008). An integrated multi-institutional diabetes prevention program improves knowledge and healthy food acquisition in northwestern Ontario First Nations. *Health Education & Behavior, 35*, 561–573.

Hodapp, R. M., & Fidler, D. J. (1999). Special education and genetics: Connections for the 21st century. *Journal of Special Education, 33*, 130–137.

Hodgens, J. B., Cole, J., & Boldizar, J. (2000). Peer-based differences among children with ADHD. *Journal of Clinical Child Psychology, 29*, 443–452.

Hoekstra, P. J., Anderson, G. M., Limburg, P. C., Korf, J., Kallenberg, C. G. M., & Minderaa, R. B. (2004). Neurobiology and neuroimmunology of Tourette's syndrome: An update. *Cellular and Molecular Life Sciences, 61*, 886–898.

Hoekstra, P. J., Kallenberg, C. G. M., Korf, J., & Minderaa, R. B. (2002). Is Tourette's syndrome an autoimmune disease? *Molecular Psychiatry, 7*, 437–445.

Hogan, A. M., Kirkham, F. J., Isaacs, E. B., Wade, A. M., & Vargha-Khadem, F. (2005). Intellectual decline in children with moyamoya and sickle cell anemia. *Developmental Medicine & Child Neurology, 47*, 824–829.

Hollander, E., Anagnostou, E., Chaplin, W., Esposito, K., Haznedar, M. M., Licalzi, E., et al. (2005). Striatal volume on magnetic resonance imaging and repetitive behaviors in autism. *Biological Psychiatry, 58*, 226–232.

Holmes, C. S., Cant, M. C., Fox, M. A., Lampert, N. L., & Greer, T. (1999). Disease and demographic risk factors for disrupted cognitive functioning in children with insulin-dependent diabetes mellitus (IDDM). *School Psychology Review, 28*, 215–227.

Holmes, C. S., Hayford, J. T., Gonzalez, J. L., & Weydert, J. A. (1983). A survey of cognitive functioning at different glucose levels in diabetic persons. *Diabetes Care, 6*, 180–185.

Holmes, C. S., O'Brien, B., & Greer, T. (1995). Cognitive functioning and academic achievement in children with insulin-dependent diabetes mellitus (IDDM). *School Psychology Quarterly, 10*, 329–344.

Holmes, J., & Adams, J. W. (2006). Working memory and children's mathematical skills: Implications for mathematical development and mathematics curricula. *Educational Psychology, 26*, 339–366.

Holsti, L., Grunau, R. E., & Whitfield, M. F. (2002). Developmental coordination disorder in extremely low birth weight children at nine years. *Journal of Developmental and Behavioral Pediatrics, 23*, 9–15.

Holttum, J. R., Minshew, N. J., Sanders, R. S., & Phillips, N. E. (1992). Magnetic resonance imaging of the posterior fossa in autism. *Biological Psychiatry, 32*, 1091–1101.

Holzapfel, M., Barnea-Goraly, N., Eckert, M., Kesler, S., & Reiss, A. L. (2006). Selective alterations of white matter associated with visuospatial and sensorimotor dysfunction. *Journal of Neuroscience, 26*, 7007–7013.

Hommet, C., Sauerwein, H. C., De Toffol, B., & Lassonde, M. (2005). Idiopathic epileptic syndromes and cognition. *Neuroscience and Biobehavioral Reviews, 30*, 85–96.

Hood, K. K., Huestis, S., Maher, A., Butler, D., Volkening, L., & Laffel, L. M. B. (2006). Depressive symptoms in children and adolescents with Type 1 diabetes. *Diabetes Care, 29*, 1389–1391.

Hoofien, D., Gilboa, A., Vakil, E., & Donovick, P. J. (2001). Traumatic brain injury (TBI) 10–20 years later: A comprehensive outcome study of psychiatric symptomatology, cognitive abilities and psychosocial functioning. *Brain Injury, 15,* 189–209.

Hook, P. E., Macaruso, P., & Jones, S. (2001). Efficacy of Fast ForWord training on facilitating acquisition of reading skills by children with reading difficulties—a longitudinal study. *Annals of Dyslexia, 51*, 75–96.

Hoon, A. H., & Reiss, A. L. (1992). The mesial-temporal lobe and autism: Case report and review. *Developmental Medicine & Child Neurology, 34*, 252–259.

Hooper, S. R., Hatton, D., Sideris, J., Sullivan, K., Hammer, J., Schaaf, J., et al. (2008). Executive functions in young males with fragile X syndrome in comparison to mental age-matched controls: Baseline findings from a longitudinal study. *Neuropsychology, 22*, 36–47.

Hooper, S. R., Hatton, D. D., Baranek, G. T., Roberts, J. P., & Bailey, D. B. J. (2000). Nonverbal assessment of IQ, attention and memory abilities in children with fragile X syndrome using the Leiter-R. *Journal of Psychoeducational Assessment, 18*, 255–267.

Horiguchi, T., & Takeshita, K. (2003). Neuropsychological developmental change in a case with Noonan syndrome: Longitudinal assessment. *Brain & Development, 25*, 291–293.

Horsler, K., & Oliver, C. (2006). Environmental influences on the behavioral phenotype of Angelman Syndrome. *American Journal of Mental Retardation, 111*, 311–321.

Hotz, G., Helm-Estabrooks, N., & Nelson, N. W. (2001). Development of the Pediatric Test of Brain Injury. *Journal of Head Trauma Rehabilitation, 16,* 426–440.

Houtveen, A. A. M., & van de Grift, W. J. C. M. (2007). Effects of metacognitive strategy instruction and instruction time on reading comprehension. *School Effectiveness and School Improvement, 18*, 173–190.

Howland, R. H. (2006). What is vagus nerve stimulation? *Journal of Psychosocial Nursing and Mental Health Services, 44*, 11–14.

Howlin, P., Davies, l. M., & Udwin, O. (1998). Cognitive functioning in adults with Williams syndrome. *Journal of Child Psychology and Psychiatry, 39*, 183–189.

Huberty, T. J., Austin, J. K., Huster, G. A., & Dunn, D. W. (2000). Relations of change in condition severity and school self-concept to change in achievement-related behavior in children with asthma or epilepsy. *Journal of School Psychology, 38*, 259–276.

Huckeba, W., Chapieski, L., Hiscock, M., & Glaze, D. (2008). Arithmetic performance in children with Tourette syndrome: Relative contribution of cognitive and attentional factors. *Journal of Clinical and Experimental Neuropsychology, 30*, 410–420.

Hudson, M. M., Mertens, A. C., Yasui, Y., Hobbie, W., Chen, H., Gurney, J. G., et al. (2003). Health status of adult long-term survivors of childhood cancers: A report from the Childhood Cancer Survivor Study. *Journal of the American Medical Association, 290*, 1583–1592.

Hugdahl, K., Gunderson, H., Brekke, C., Thomsen, T., Rimol, L. M., Ersland, M., et al. (2004). fMRI brain activation in a Finnish family with specific language impairment compared with a normal control group. *Journal of Speech Language and Hearing Research, 47*, 162–172.

Hughes, C. (1996). Brief report: Planning problems in autism at the level of motor control. *Journal of Autism and Developmental Disorders, 26*, 99–107.

Hughes, C. (1998). Finding your marbles: Does preschoolers' strategic behavior predict later understanding of the mind? *Developmental Psychology, 34*, 1326–1339.

Hughes, C., & Graham, A. (2002). Measuring executive functions in childhood: Problems and solutions? *Child and Adolescent Mental Health, 7*, 131–142.

Hughes, J. R. (2007). Autism: The first firm finding—underconnectivity? *Epilepsy and Behavior, 11*, 20–24.

Hughes, J. R., & Melyn, M. (2005). EEG and seizures in autistic children and adolescents: Further findings with therapeutic implications. *Journal of Clinical EEG & Neuroscience, 36*, 15–20.

Hunt, A. (1995). Gaining new understanding of tuberous sclerosis. *Nursing Times, 91*(33), 31–33.

Hunt, A. (2006). Guidelines for the assessment of cognitive and behavioral issues in tuberous sclerosis complex. Retrieved October 28, 2008, from www.tsalliance.org.

Hurtig, A. L., & White, L. (1986). Psychosocial adjustment in children and adolescents with sickle cell disease. *Journal of Pediatric Psychology, 11*, 180–196.

Hussain, J., Woolf, A. D., Sandel, M., & Shannon, M. W. (2007). Environmental evaluation of a child with developmental disability. *Pediatric Clinics of North America, 54*, 47–62.

Hussman, J. P. (2001). Suppressed GABAergic inhibition as a common factor in suspected etiologies of autism. *Journal of Autism and Developmental Disorders, 31*, 247–248.

Huttenlocher, P. R., & Huttenlocher, J. (1973). A study of children with hyperlexia. *Neurology, 23*, 1107–1116.

Hyde, J. S. (2005). The gender similarities hypothesis. *American Psychologist, 60*, 582–589.

Hyman, S. L., Shores, A., & North, K. N. (2005). The nature and frequency of cognitive deficits in children with neurofibromatosis type 1. *Neurology, 65*, 1037–1044.

Hyman, S. L., Shores, E. A., & North, K. N. (2006). Learning disabilities in children with neurofibromatosis type 1: Subtypes, cognitive profile, and attention-deficit-hyperactivity disorder. *Developmental Medicine & Child Neurology, 48*, 973–977.

Hynd, G. W., & Cohen, M. J. (1983). *Dyslexia: Neuropsychological theory, research, and clinical differentiation*. New York: Grune & Stratton.

Hynd, G. W., Hynd, C. R., Sullivan, H. G., & Kingsbury, T. B. (1987). Regional cerebral blood flow in developmental dyslexia: Activation during reading in a surface and deep dyslexic. *Journal of Reading Disabilities, 20*, 294–300.

Hynd, G. W., Lorys, A. R., Semrud-Clikeman, M., Nieves, N., Huettner, M. I. S., & Lahey, B. B. (1991). Attention deficit disorder without hyperactivity: A distinct behavioral and neurocognitive syndrome. *Journal of Child Neurology, 6*(Suppl.), S37–S43.

Iacoboni, M. (2007). Face to face: The neural basis of social mirroring and empathy. *Psychiatric Annals, 37*, 236–241.

Iacoboni, M., & Mazziotta, J. C. (2007). Mirror neuron system: Basic findings and clinical applications. *Annals of Neurology, 62*, 213–218.

Iacoboni, M., Woods, R. P., Brass, M., Bekkering, H., Mazziotta, J. C., & Rizzolatti, G. (1999). Cortical mechanisms of human imitation. *Science, 286*, 2526–2528.

Iarocci, G., Virji-Babul, N., & Reebye, P. (2006). The Learn at Play Program (LAPP): Merging family, developmental research, early intervention, and policy goals for children with Down syndrome. *Journal of Policy and Practice in Intellectual Disabilities, 3*(1), 11–16.

Im, S.-H., Park, E. S., Kim, D. Y., Song, D. H., & Lee, J. D. (2007). The neuroradiological findings of children with developmental language disorder. *Yonsei Medical Journal, 48*, 405–411.

Im-Bolter, N., Johnson, J., & Pascual-Leone, J. (2006). Processing limitations in children with specific language impairment: The role of executive function. *Child Development, 77*, 1822–1841.

Individuals with Disabilities Education Improvement Act, P.L. 105–17 C.F.R. (2004).

Indredavik, M. S., Skranes, J. S., Vik, T., Heyerdahl, S., Romundstad, P., Myhr, G. E., et al. (2005). Low-birth-weight adolescents: Psychiatric symptoms and cerebral MRI abnormalities. *Pediatric Neurology, 33*, 259–266.

Indredavik, M. S., Vik, T., Heyerdahl, S., Kulseng, S., Fayers, P., & Brubakk, A. M. (2004). Psychiatric symptoms and disorders in adolescents with low birth weight. *Archives of Disease in Childhood Fetal and Neonatal Edition, 89,* 445–450.

Institute of Educational Sciences (2007). Institute of Educational Sciences. What Works Clearinghouse. Retrieved October 24, 2008, from http://ies.ed.gov/ncee/wwc/.

Institute of Medicine (2001). *Thimerosal-containing vaccines and neurodevelopmental disorders*. Washington, DC: National Academy Press.

Iovannone, R., Dunlap, G., Huber, H., & Kincaid, D. (2003). Effective educational practices for students with autism spectrum disorders. *Focus on Autism and Other Developmental Disabilities, 18*, 150–165.

Iqbal, M. M., Sobhan, T., & Ryals, T. (2002). Effects of commonly used benzodiazepines on the fetus, the neonate, and the nursing infant. *Psychiatric Services, 53*, 39–49.

Isaacs, E. B., Edmonds, C. J., Lucas, A., & Gadian, D. G. (2001). Calculation difficulties in children of very low birthweight: A neural correlate. *Brain, 124*, 1701–1707.

Isaacs, E. B., Lucas, A., Chong, W. K., Wood, S. J., Johnson, C. L., Marshall, C., et al. (2000). Hippocampal volume and everyday memory in children of very low birth weight. *Pediatric Research, 47*, 713–720.

Iverson, G. L., Brooks, B. L., & Holdnack, J. A. (2008). Misdiagnosis of cognitive impairment in forensic neuropsychology. In R. L. Heilbronner (Ed.), *Neuropsychology in the courtroom: Expert analysis of reports and testimony* (pp. 243–266). New York: Guilford.

Jackowski, A. P., & Schultz, R. T. (2005). Foreshortened dorsal extension of the central sulcus in Williams syndrome. *Cortex, 41*, 282–290.

Jackson, D., Turner-Stokes, L., Murray, J., & Leese, M. (2007). Validation of the Memory and Behavior Problems Checklist-1990R for use in acquired brain injury. *Brain Injury, 21,* 817–824.

Jacobs, J., Rohr, A., Moeller, F., Boor, R., Kobayashi, E., LeVan Meng, P., et al. (2008). Evaluation of epileptogenic networks in children with tuberous sclerosis complex using EEG-fMRI. *Epilepsia, 49*, 816–825.

Jacobs, S. E., Sokol, J., & Ohlsson, A. (2002). The Newborn Individualized Developmental Care and Assessment Program is not supported by meta-analyses of the data. *Journal of Pediatrics, 140,* 699–706.

Jacobson, S. W. (1998). Specificity of neurobehavioral outcomes associated with prenatal alcohol exposure. *Alcoholism: Clinical and Experimental Research, 22*, 313–320.

Jager-Roman, E., Deichl, A., Jakob, S., Koch, S., Rating, D., Steldinger, R., et al. (1986). Fetal growth, major malformation and minor anomalies in infants born to women receiving valproic acid. *Journal of Pediatrics, 108*, 997–1004.

Jahromi, L. B., Gulsrod, A., & Kasari, C. (2008). Emotional competence in children with Down syndrome: Negativity and regulation. *American Journal on Mental Retardation, 113*, 32–43.

Jambaqué, I., Dellatolas, G., Fohlen, M., Bulteau, C., Watier, L., Dorfmuller, G., et al. (2007). Memory functions following surgery for temporal lobe epilepsy in children. *Neuropsychologia, 45*, 2850–2862.

James, W. H. (2008). Further evidence that some male-based neurodevelopmental disorders are associated with high intrauterine testosterone concentrations. *Developmental Medicine and Child Neurology, 50*, 15–18.

Jäncke, L., Siegenthaler, T., Preis, S., & Steinmetz, H. (2007). Decreased white-matter density in a left-sided fronto-temporal network in children with developmental language disorder: Evidence for anatomical anomalies in a motor-language network. *Brain and Language, 102*, 91–98.

Jankovic, J. (2001). Tourette's syndrome. *New England Journal of Medicine, 345*, 1184–1192.

Jansen, M. W. J. C., Corral, L., van der Velden, V. H. J., Panzer-Gruemayer, R., Schrappe, M., Schrauder, A., et al. (2007). Immunobiological diversity in infant acute lymphoblastic leukemia is related to the occurrence and type of MLL gene rearrangement. *Leukemia, 21*, 633–641.

Jansiewicz, E. M., Goldberg, M. C., Newschaffer, C., Denckla, M. B., Landa, R., & Mostofsky, S. H. (2006). Motor signs distinguish children with high-functioning autism and Asperger syndrome from controls. *Journal of Autism and Developmental Disorders, 36*, 613–621.

Jarratt, K. P., Riccio, C. A., & Siekierski, B. (2005). Assessment of Attention Deficit Hyperactivity Disorder (ADHD) using the BASC and BRIEF. *Applied Neuropsychology, 12*, 83–93.

Jarrold, C., Baddeley, A., & Hewes, A. K. (2000). Verbal short-term memory deficits in Down syndrome: A consequence of problems in rehearsal? *Journal of Child Psychology and Psychiatry, 41*, 223–244.

Jarrold, C., Baddeley, A. D., Hewes, A. K., Leeke, T. C., & Phillips, C. E. (2004). What links verbal short-term memory performance and vocabulary level? Evidence of changing relationships among individuals with learning disability. *Journal of Memory and Language, 50*, 134–148.

Jarrold, C., Purser, H. R. M., & Brock, J. W. (2006). Short-term memory in Down syndrome. In T. P. Alloway & S. E. Gathercole (Eds.), *Working memory and developmental disorders* (pp. 239–266). New York: Psychology Press.

Järup, L., Berglund, M., Elinder, C. G., Nordberg, G., & Vahter, M. (1998). Health effects of cadmium exposure—a review of the literature and a risk estimate. *Scandinavian Journal of Work and Environmental Health, 24*(Suppl. 1), 1–51.

Jarvis, H. L., & Gathercole, S. E. (2003). Verbal and non-verbal working memory and achievements on National Curriculum tests at 11 and 14 years of age. *Educational and Child Psychology, 20*, 123–140.

Jauregi, J., Arias, C., Vegas, O., Alén, F., Martinez, S., Copet, P., et al. (2007). A neuropsychological assessment of frontal cognitive functions in Prader-Willi syndrome. *Journal of Intellectual Disability Research, 5*, 350–365.

Jefferson, I. G., Smith, M. A., & Baum, J. D. (1985). Insulin dependent diabetes in under 5 year olds. *Archives of Diseases in Children, 60*, 1144–1148.

Jenks, K. M., de Moor, J., van Lieshout, E. C. D. M., Maathuis, K. G. B., Keus, I., & Gorter, J. W. (2007). The effect of cerebral palsy on arithmetic accuracy is mediated by working memory, intelligence, early numeracy, and instruction time. *Developmental Neuropsychology, 32*, 861–880.

Jennekens-Schinkel, A., & Oostrom, K. J. (2005). Variables in childhood epilepsy and scholastic underachievement. *Epilepsia, 46*, 599.

Jensen, P. S., Arnold, L. E., Swanson, J. M., Vitiello, B., Abikoff, H. B., Greenhill, L. L., et al. (2007). 3-year follow-up of the NIMH MTA study. *Journal of the American Academy of Child and Adolescent Psychiatry, 46*, 989–1002.

Jensen, P. S., Hinshaw, S. P., Swanson, J. M., Greenhill, L. L., Conners, C. K., Arnold, L. E., et al. (2001). Findings from the NIMH multimodal treatment study of ADHD

(MTA): Implications and applications for primary care providers. *Journal of Developmental and Behavioral Pediatrics, 22*, 60–73.

Jensen, S. A., Elkin, T. D., Milker, K., Jordan, S., Iyer, R., & Smith, M. G. (2005). Caregiver knowledge and adherence in children with sickle cell disease: Knowing is not doing. *Journal of Clinical Psychology in Medical Settings, 12*, 333–337.

Jernigan, T. L., Hesselink, J., Sowell, E. R., & Tallal, P. (1991). Cerebral structure on magnetic resonance imaging in language- and learning-impaired children. *Archives of Neurology, 48*, 539–545.

Jernigan, T. L., Mattson, S. N., Riley, E. P., Sowell, E. R., Tessner, K. D., Thompson, P. M., et al. (2002). Regional brain shape abnormalities persist into adolescence after heavy prenatal alcohol exposure. *Cerebral Cortex, 12*, 856–865.

Jeste, S. S., Sahin, M., Bolton, P., Ploubidis, G. B., & Humphrey, A. (2008). Characterization of autism in young children with tuberous sclerosis complex. *Journal of Child Neurology, 23*, 520–525.

Jeyaratnam, J., & Maroni, M. (1994). Organophosphorous compounds. *Toxicology and Applied Pharmacology, 91*, 15–28.

Jimenez-Jimenez, F. J., & Garcia-Ruiz, P. J. (2001). Pharmacological options for the treatment of Tourette's disorder. *Drugs, 61*, 2207–2220.

Jocic-Jakubi, B., & Jovic, N. J. (2006). Verbal memory impairment in children with focal epilepsy. *Epilepsy & Behavior, 9*, 432–439.

Joffe, V. L., Cain, K., & Maric, N. (2007). Comprehension problems in children with specific language impairment: Does mental imagery training help? *International Journal of Language & Communication Disorders, 42*, 648–664.

Johannes, S., Wieringa, B. M., Nager, W., Rada, D., Muller-Vahl, K. R., Emrich, H. M., et al. (2003). Tourette syndrome and obsessive-compulsive disorder: Event-related brain potentials show similar mechanisms of frontal inhibition but dissimilar target evaluation processes. *Behavioural Neurology, 14*, 9–17.

Johnson-Glenberg, M. C. (2000). Training reading comprehension in adequate decoders/poor comprehenders: Verbal versus visual strategies. *Journal of Educational Psychology, 92*, 772–782.

Johnson, C. J., Beitchman, J. H., Young, A., Escobar, M., Atkinson, L., Wilson, B., et al. (1999). Fourteen-year follow-up of children with and without speech/language impairments: Speech/language stability and outcomes. *Journal of Speech, Language, and Hearing Research, 42*, 744–760.

Johnson, H., Wiggs, L., Stores, G., & Huson, S. M. (2005). Psychological disturbance and sleep disorders in children with neurofibromatosis type 1. *Developmental Medicine & Child Neurology, 47*, 237–242.

Johnson, M. H. (2003). Development of human brain functions. *Biological Psychiatry, 54,* 1312–1316.

Johnson, S., Ring, W., Anderson, P., & Marlow, N. (2005). Randomised trial of parental support for families with very preterm children: Outcome at 5 years. *Archives of Disease in Childhood, 90,* 909–915.

Joliffe, T., & Baron-Cohen, S. (1999). A test of central coherence theory: Linguistic processing in high-functioning adults with autism or Asperger syndrome—is local coherence impaired? *Cognition, 71*, 149–185.

Jolleff, N., Emmerson, F., Ryan, M., & McConachie, H. (2006). Communication skills in Angelman syndrome: Matching phenotype to genotype. *Advances in Speech Language Pathology, 8*, 28–33.

Jones, J. M., Lawson, M. I., Daneman, D., Olmsted, M. P., & Rodin, G. (2000). Eating disorders in adolescent females with and without type 1 diabetes: Cross sectional study. *British Medical Journal, 320*, 1563–1566.

Jones, K. L., & Smith, D. W. (1973). Recognition of the fetal alcohol syndrome in early infancy. *Lancet, 2*, 999–1001.

Jones, P. B., & Kerwin, E. J. (1990). Left temporal lobe damage in Asperger's syndrome. *British Journal of Psychiatry, 156*, 570–572.

Jones, W., Hesselink, J., Courchesne, E., Duncan, T., Matsuda, K., & Bellugi, U. (2002). Cerebellar abnormalities in infants and toddlers with Williams syndrome. *Developmental Medicine & Child Neurology, 44*, 688–694.

Jordan, N. C., & Hanich, L. B. (2000). Mathematical thinking in second-grade children with different forms of LD. *Journal of Learning Disabilities, 33*, 567–578.

Jordan, N. C., Kaplan, D., & Hanich, L. B. (2002). Achievement growth in children with learning difficulties in mathematics: Findings of a two-year longitudinal study. *Journal of Educational Psychology, 94*, 586–597.

Jordan, N. C., & Montani, T. O. (1997). Cognitive arithmetic and problem solving: A comparison of children with specific and general mathematics difficulties. *Journal of Learning Disabilities, 30*, 624–634.

Joseph, R. (1996). *Neuropsychiatry, neuropsychology, and clinical neuroscience: Emotion, evolution, cognition, language, memory, brain damage, and abnormal behavior* (2nd ed.). Baltimore, MD: Williams & Wilkins.

Joseph, R. (1999). Neuropsychological frameworks for understanding autism. *International Review of Psychiatry, 11*, 309–325.

Joseph, R., McGrath, L. M., & Tager-Flusberg, H. (2005). Executive dysfunction and its relation to language ability in verbal school-age children with autism. *Developmental Neuropsychology, 27*, 361–378.

Joshi, R. M., & Aaron, P. G. (2000). The component model of reading: Simple view of reading made a little more complex. *Reading Psychology, 21*, 85–97.

Juhász, C., Batista, C. E. A., Chugani, D. C., Muzik, O., & Chugani, H. T. (2007). Evolution of cortical metabolic abnormalities and their clinical correlates in Sturge-Weber syndrome. *European Journal of Paediatric Neurology, 11*, 277–284.

Juhász, C., Haacke, E. M., Hu, J., Xuan, Y., Makki, M., Behen, M. E., et al. (2007). Multimodality imaging of cortical and white matter abnormalities in Sturge-Weber syndrome. *American Journal of Neuroradiology, 28*, 900–906.

Juhász, C., Lai, C., Behen, M. E., Muzik, O., Helder, E. J., Chugani, D. C., et al. (2007). White matter volume as a major predictor of cognitive function in Sturge-Weber syndrome. *Archives of Neurology, 64*, 1169–1174.

Just, M. A., Cherkassky, V. L., Keller, T. A., Kana, R. K., & Minshew, N. J. (2007). Functional and anatomical cortical underconnectivity in autism: Evidence from an fMRI study of an executive function task and corpus callosum morphometry. *Cerebral Cortex, 17*, 951–961.

Justice, L., Chows, S., Capellini, C., Flanigan, K., & Colton, S. (2003). Emergent literacy intervention for vulnerable preschoolers: Relative effects of two approaches. *American Journal of Speech Language Pathology, 12*, 320–332.

Justice, L., Kaderavek, J., Bowles, R., & Grimm, K. (2005). Language impairment, parent-child shared reading and phonological awareness: A feasibility study. *Topics in Early Childhood Special Education, 25*, 143–156.

Justus, T. C., & Ivry, R. B. (2001). The cognitive neuropsychology of the cerebellum. *International Review of Psychiatry, 13*, 276–282.

Jyothy, A., Kumar, K. S., Mallikarjuna, G. N., Babu Rao, V., Uman Devi, B., Sujatha, M., et al. (2001). Parental age and origin of extra chromosome 21 in Down syndrome. *Journal of Human Genetics, 46*, 347–350.

Kaaja, E., Kaaja, R., & Hiilesmaa, V. (2003). Major malformations in offspring of women with epilepsy. *Neurology, 60*, 575–579.

Kaemingk, K. L., Carey, M. E., Moore, I. M., Herzer, M., & Hutter, J. J. (2004). Math weaknesses in survivors of acute lymphoblastic leukemia compared to healthy children. *Child Neuropsychology, 10*, 14–23.

Kaemingk, K. L., & Paquette, A. (1999). Effects of prenatal alcohol exposure on neuropsychological functioning. *Developmental Neuropsychology, 15*, 111–140.

Kalmar, M. (1996). The course of intellectual development in preterm and full-term children: An 8-year longitudinal study. *International Journal of Behavioral Development, 19*, 491–516.

Kamhi, A. G., Minor, J. J., & Mauer, D. (1990). Content analysis and intratest performance profiles on the Columbia and the TONI. *Journal of Speech and Hearing Research, 33*, 375–379.

Kamphaus, R. W., Petoskey, M. D., & Rowe, E. W. (2000). Current trends in psychological testing of children. *Professional Psychology: Research and Practice, 31*, 155–164.

Kanne, S. M., Randolph, J. K., & Farmer, J. E. (2008). Diagnostic and assessment findings: A bridge to academic planning for children with autism spectrum disorders. *Neuropsychology Review, 18*, 367–384.

Kanner, L. (1943). Autistic disturbances of affective contact. *Nervous Child, 2*, 217–250.

Kantola-Sorsa, E., Gaily, E., Tsoaho, M., & Korman, M. (2007). Neuropsychological outcomes in childhood of mothers with epilepsy. *Journal of the International Neuropsychological Society, 13*, 642–662.

Kaplan, E. (1988). A process approach to neuropsychological assessment. In T. Boll & B. K. Bryant (Eds.), *Clinical neuropsychology and brain function* (pp. 125–167). Washington, DC: American Psychological Association.

Kaplan, E. (1990). The process approach to neuropsychological assessment of psychiatric patients. *Journal of Neuropsychiatry, 2*(1), 72–87.

Karam, J. H. (1996). Diabetes mellitus and hypoglycemia. In J. L. Tierney, S. McPhee, & M. Apadakis (Eds.), *Current medical diagnosis and treatment* (35th ed., pp. 1030–1068). Stamford, CT: Appelton & Lange.

Karni, A., Morocz, I. A., Bitan, T., Shaul, S., Kushnir, T., & Breznitz, Z. (2005). An fMRI study of the differential effects of word presentation rates (reading acceleration) on dyslexic readers' brain activity patterns. *Journal of Neurolinguistics, 18*(2), 197–219.

Kates, W. R., Mostofsky, S. H., Zimmerman, A. W., Mazzocco, M. M. M., Landa, R., Warsofsky, I. S., et al. (1998). Neuroanatomical and neurocognitive differences in a pair of monozygous twins discordant for strictly defined autism. *Annals of Neurology, 43*, 782–791.

Katz, J., & Smith, P. S. (1991). The staggered spondaic word test: A ten-minute look at the central nervous system through the ears. *Annals of the New York Academy of Sciences, 620*, 233–251.

Katz, M. L., Smith-Whitley, K., Ruzek, S. B., & Ohene-Frempong, K. (2002). Knowledge of stroke risk, signs of stroke, and the need for stroke education among children with sickle cell disease and their caregivers. *Ethnicity and Health, 7*, 115–123.

Katzenstein, J. M., Fastenau, P. S., Dunn, D. W., & Austin, J. K. (2007). Teachers' ratings of the academic performance of children with epilepsy. *Epilepsy & Behavior, 10*, 426–431.

Katzir, T., Kim, Y.-S., Wolf, M., Morris, R., & Lovett, M. W. (2008). The varieties of pathways to dysfluent reading: Comparing subtypes of children with dyslexia at letter, word, and connected text levels of reading. *Journal of Learning Disabilities, 41*, 47–66.

Kau, A. S. M., Reider, E. E.., Payne, L., Meyer, W. A., & Freund, L. (2000). Early behavior signs of psychiatric phenotypes in fragile X syndrome. *American Journal on Mental Retardation, 105*, 286–299.

Kaufman, A. S. (2008). Neuropsychology and specific learning disabilities: Lessons from the past as a guide to present controversies and future clinical practice. In E. Fletcher-Janzen & C. R. Reynolds (Eds.), *Neuropsychological perspectives on learning disabilities in the era of RTI* (pp. 1–13). Hoboken, NJ: Wiley.

Kaul, D. K., Liu, X. D., Fabry, M. E., & Nagel, R. L. (2000). Impaired nitric oxide-mediated vasodilation in transgenic sickle mouse. *American Journal of Physiology—Heart and Circulatory Physiology, 278*, 1799–1806.

Kavale, K. A., & Forness, S. R. (1983). Hyperactivity and diet treatment: A meta-analysis of the Feingold hypothesis. *Journal of Learning Disabilities, 16*, 324–330.

Kazak, A. E. (2005). Evidence-based interventions for survivors of childhood cancer and their families. *Journal of Pediatric Psychology, 30*, 29–39.

Kazak, A. E., Alderfer, M. A., Streisand, R., Simms, S., Rourke, M. T., Barakat, L. P., et al. (2004). Treatment of posttraumatic stress symptoms in adolescent survivors of childhood cancer and their families: A randomized clinical trial. *Journal of Family Psychology, 18*, 493–504.

Kazak, A. E., Barakat, L. P., Alderfer, M., Rourke, M. T., Meeske, K., Gallagher, P. R., et al. (2001). Posttraumatic stress in survivors of childhood cancer and mothers:

Development and validation of the Impact of Traumatic Stressors Interview Schedule (ITSIS). *Journal of Clinical Psychology in Medical Settings, 8*, 307–323.

Kazak, A. E., Rourke, M. T., Alderfer, M. A., Pui, A., Reilly, A. F., & Meadows, A. T. (2007). Evidence-based assessment, intervention and psychosocial care in pediatric oncology: A blueprint for comprehensive services across treatment. *Journal of Pediatric Psychology, 32*, 1099–1110.

Kazak, A. E., Simms, S., Barakat, L., Hobbie, W., Foley, B., Golomb, V., et al. (1999). Surviving Cancer Competently Intervention Program (SCCIP): A cognitive-behavioral and family therapy intervention for adolescent survivors of childhood cancer and their families. *Family Process, 38*, 175–191.

Keen, D., Sigafoos, J., & Woodyatt, G. (2001). Replacing prelinguistic behaviors with functional communication. *Journal of Autism and Developmental Disorders, 31*, 385–398.

Keenan, J. M., Betjemann, R. S., Wadsworth, S. J., DeFries, J. C., & Olson, R. K. (2006). Genetic and environmental influences on reading and listening comprehension. *Journal of Research in Reading, 29*, 75–91.

Kehle, T. J., Clark, E., & Jenson, W. R. (1996). Interventions for students with traumatic brain injury: Managing behavioral disturbances. *Journal of Learning Disabilities, 29*, 633–642.

Kelch-Oliver, K., Smith, O. S., Diaz, D., & Collins, M. H. (2007). Individual and family contributions to depressive symptoms in African American children with sickle cell disease. *Journal of Clinical Psychology in Medical Settings, 14*, 376–384.

Keller, F., & Persico, A. M. (2003). The neurobiological context of autism. *Molecular Neurobiology, 28*, 1–22.

Keller, R. W., & Snyder-Keller, A. (2000). Prenatal cocaine exposure. *Annals of the New York Academy of Sciences, 909*, 217–232.

Kemper, T. L., & Bauman, M. (1993). The contribution of neuropathologic studies to the understanding of autism. *Neurologic Clinics, 11*, 175–187.

Kendrick, D., Elkan, R., Hewitt, M., Dewey, M., Blair, M., Robinson, J., et al. (2000). Does home visiting improve parenting and the quality of the home environment? A systematic review and meta analysis. *Archives of Disease in Childhood, 82,* 443–451.

Kennard, M. (1942). Cortical reorganization of motor function: Studies on series of monkeys of various ages from infancy to maturity. *Archives of Neurology and Psychiatry, 47,* 227–240.

Kennedy, D., & Courchesne, E. (2007). The intrinsic functional organization of the brain is altered in autism. *NeuroImage, 39*, 1877–1885.

Kennedy, E. J., & Flynn, M. C. (2003). Early phonological awareness and reading skills in children with Down syndrome. *Down Syndrome: Research and Practice, 8*, 100–109.

Kennedy, M. R. T., Coelho, C., Turkstra, L., Ylvisaker, M., Sohlberg, M. M., Yorkston, K., et al. (2008). Intervention for executive functions after traumatic brain injury: A systematic review, meta-analysis and clinical recommendations. *Neuropsychological Rehabilitation, 18,* 257–299.

Kent, L., Evans, J. E., Paul, M., & Sharp, M. (1999). Comorbidity of autistic spectrum disorders in children with Down syndrome. *Developmental Medicine & Child Neurology, 41*, 153–158.

Keri, S., Szlobodnyik, C., Benedek, G., Janka, Z., & Gadoros, J. (2002). Probabilistic classification learning in Tourette syndrome. *Neuropsychologia, 40*, 1356–1362.

Kern, J. K. (2003). Purkinje cell vulnerability and autism: A possible etiological connection. *Brain & Development, 25*, 377–382.

Kern, J. K., Miller, V. S., Cauller, L., Kendall, R., Mehta, J., & Dodd, M. (2001). Effectiveness of N,N-Dimethylglycine in autism and pervasive developmental disorder. *Journal of Child Neurology, 16*, 169–173.

Khong, P.-L., Leung, L. H. T., Fung, A. S. M., Fong, D. Y. T., Qiu, D., Kwong, D. L. W., et al. (2006). White matter anisotropy in post-treatment childhood cancer survivors: preliminary evidence of association with neurocognitive function. *Journal of Clinical Oncology, 24*, 884–890.

Khurana, D. S., Reumann, M., Hobdell, E. F., Neff, S., Valencia, I., Legido, A., et al. (2007). Vagus nerve stimulation in children with refractory epilepsy: Unusual complications and relationship to sleep-disordered breathing. *Child's Nervous System, 23*, 1309–1312.

Kibby, M. Y. (in press). There are multiple contributors to the verbal short-term memory deficit in children with developmental reading disabilities. *Child Neuropsychology*.

Kibby, M. Y., & Cohen, M. J. (2008). Memory functioning in children with reading disabilities and/or attention deficit/hyperactivity disorder: A clinical investigation of their working memory and long-term memory functioning. *Child Neuropsychology, 14*, 525–546.

Kibby, M. Y., Fancher, J. B., Markanen, R., & Hynd, G. W. (2008). A quantitative magnetic resonance imaging analysis of the cerebellar deficit hypothesis of dyslexia. *Journal of Child Neurology, 23*, 363–380.

Kibby, M. Y., Kroese, J. M., Krebbs, H., Hill, C. E., & Hynd, G. W. (in press). The pars triangularis in dyslexia and ADHD: A comprehensive approach. *Brain and Language*.

Kibby, M. Y., Kroese, J. M., Morgan, A. E., Hiemenz, J. R., Cohen, M. J., & Hynd, G. W. (2004). The relationship between perisylvian morphology and verbal short-term memory functioning in children with neurodevelopmental disorders. *Brain and Language, 89*, 122–135.

Kilbride, H. W., Thorstad, K., & Daily, D. K. (2004). Preschool outcome of less than 801-gram preterm infants compared with full-term siblings. *Pediatrics, 113*, 742–747.

Kini, U., Adab, N., Vinton, J., Fryer, A., Clayton-Smith, J., & Liverpool and Manchester Neurodevelopmental Study Group (2006). Dysmorphic features: An important clue to the diagnosis and severity of fetal anticonvulsant syndromes. *Archives of Disease in Childhood, 91*(2), F90–95.

Kinsbourne, M. (1968). Developmental Gerstmann syndrome. *Pediatric Clinics of North America, 15*, 771–778.

Kinsbourne, M., & Warrington, E. K. (1963). The developmental Gerstmann syndrome. *Archives of Neurology, 8*, 490–501.

Kirton, A., & deVeber, G. (2006). Cerebral palsy secondary to perinatal ischemic stroke. *Clinics in Perinatology, 33*, 367–386.

Kishino, T., Lalande, M., & Wagstaff, J. (1997). UBE3A/E6-AP mutations cause Angelman syndrome. *Nature Genetics, 15*, 70–73.

Kjelgaard, M. M., & Tager-Flusberg, H. (2001). An investigation of language impairment in autism: Implications for genetic subgroups. *Language and Cognitive Processes, 16*, 287–308.

Klebanov, P. K., Brooks-Gunn, J., & McCormick, M. C. (2001). Maternal coping strategies and emotional distress: Results of an early intervention program for low birth weight young children. *Developmental Psychology, 37,* 654–667.

Klein-Tasman, B. P., & Albano, A. M. (2007). Intensive, short-term cognitive behavioral treatment of OCD-like behavior with a young adult with Williams syndrome. *Clinical Case Studies, 6*, 483–492.

Klein-Tasman, B. P., Mervis, C. B., Lord, C., & Philips, K. D. (2007). Socio-communicative deficits in young children with Williams syndrome: Performance on the Autism Diagnostic Observation Schedule. *Child Neuropsychology, 13*, 444–467.

Kleinhans, N. M., Müller, R.-A., Cohen, D. N., & Courchesne, E. (2008). Atypical functional lateralization of language in autism spectrum disorders. *Brain Research, 1221*, 115–125.

Kleinhans, N. M., Richards, T., Weaver, K. E., Liang, O., Dawson, G., & Aylward, E. (2009). Brief report: Biochemical correlates of clinical impairment in high-functioning autism and Asperger's disorder. *Journal of Autism and Developmental Disorders, 39,* 1079–1086.

Kleppe, S. A., Katayama, K. M., Shipley, K. G., & Foushee, D. R. (1990). The speech and language characteristics of children with Prader-Willi syndrome. *Journal of Speech & Hearing Disorders, 55*, 300–309.

Klin, A., Jones, W., Schultz, R., Volkmar, F., & Cohen, D. (2001a). Defining and quantifying the social phenotype in autism. *American Journal of Psychiatry, 159*, 895–908.

Klin, A., Jones, W., Schultz, R., Volkmar, F., & Cohen, D. (2001b). Visual fixation patterns during viewing of naturalistic social situations as predictors of social competence in individuals with autism. *Archives of General Psychiatry, 159*, 809–816.

Klin, A., Saulnier, C., Tsatsanis, K., & Volkmar, F. (2005). Clinical evaluation in autism spectrum disorders: Psychological assessment within a transdisciplinary framework. In F. Volkmar, R. Paul, A. Klin, & D. Cohen (Eds.), *Handbook of autism and pervasive developmental disorders: Assessment, interventions, and policy* (3rd ed., Vol. 2, pp. 772–798). Hoboken, NJ: Wiley.

Klin, A., Saulnier, C. A., Sparrow, S. S., Cicchetti, D. V., Volkmar, F. R., & Lord, C. (2007). Social and communication abilities and disabilities in higher functioning individuals with autism spectrum disorders: The Vineland and the ADOS. *Journal of Autism and Developmental Disorders, 37*, 748–759.

Klin, A., Sparrow, S. S., de Bildt, A., Cicchetti, D. V., Cohen, D. J., & Volkmar, F. R. (1999). A normed study of face recognition in autism and related disorders. *Journal of Autism and Developmental Disorders, 29*, 499–508.

Klinger, L. G., & Dawson, G. (1996). Autistic disorder. In E. J. Mash & R. A. Barkley (Eds.), *Child psychopathology* (pp. 311–339). New York: Guilford.

Klingner, J. K., Vaughn, S., & Boardman, A. (2007). *Teaching reading comprehension to students with learning difficulties. What works for special needs learners.* New York: Guilford.

Knight, S., Northam, E., Donath, S., Gardner, A., Harkin, N., Taplin, C., et al. (2009). Improvements in cognition, mood and behaviour following commencement of continuous subcutaneous insulin infusion therapy in children with type 1 diabetes mellitus: A pilot study. *Diabetologia, 52*(2), 193–198.

Knobeloch, L. M., Zierold, K. M., & Anderson, H. A. (2006). Association of arsenic-contaminated drinking water with prevalence of skin cancer in Wisconsin's Fox River Valley. *Journal of Health and Popular Nutrition, 24*, 206–213.

Knopik, V. S., Alarcón, M., & DeFries, J. C. (1997). Comorbidity of mathematics and reading deficits: Evidence for a genetic etiology. *Behavior Genetics, 27*, 447–453.

Knoppert, K. D., Nimkar, R., Principi, T., & Yuen, D. (2006). Paroxetine toxicity in a newborn after in utero exposure: Clinical symptoms correlate with serum levels. *Therapeutic Drug Monitoring, 28*(1), 5–7.

Knops, N. B. B., Sneeuw, K. C. A., Brand, R., Hille, E. T. M., den Ouden, A. L., Wit, J., et al. (2005). Catch-up growth up to ten years of age in children born very preterm or with very low birth weight. *BMC Pediatrics, 5*(26), 1–9.

Koch, D., Lu, C., Fisker-Andersen, J., Jolley, L., & Fenske, R. A. (2002). Temporal association of children's pesticide exposure and agricultural spraying: Report of a longitudinal biological monitoring study. *Environmental Health Perspectives, 110*, 829–833.

Kodituwakku, P. W., Handmaker, N. S., Cutler, S. K., Weathersby, E. K., & Handmaker, S. D. (1995). Specific impairments in self-regulation in children exposed to alcohol prenatally. *Alcoholism: Clinical and Experimental Research, 19*, 1558–1564.

Koegel, L. K., Koegel, R. L., & McNerney, E. K. (2001). Pivotal areas in intervention for autism. *Journal of Clinical Child Psychology, 30*, 19–32.

Kogan, C. S., Boutet, I., Cornish, K. M., Graham, G. E., Berry-Kravis, E., Drouin, A., et al. (2009). A comparative neuropsychological test battery differentiates cognitive signatures of fragile X and Down syndrome. *Journal of Intellectual Disability Research, 53*, 125–142.

Koh, J. O., Cassidy, J. D., & Watkinson, E. J. (2003). Incidence of concussion in contact sports: A systematic review of the evidence. *Brain Injury, 17,* 901–917.

Kohler, F. W., Strain, P. S., & Goldstein, H. (2005). Learning experiences . . . An alternative program for preschoolers and parents: Peer mediated interventions for young children with autism. In E. D. Hibbs & P. S. Jensen (Eds.), *Psychosocial treatments for child and adolescent disorders: Empirically based strategies for clinical practice* (2nd ed., pp. 659–687). Washington, DC: American Psychological Association.

Kokiko, O. N., & Hamm, R. J. (2007). A review of pharmacological treatments used in experimental models of traumatic brain injury. *Brain Injury, 21*, 259–274.

Kokkonen, J., Kokkonen, E. R., Saukkonen, A. L., & Pennanen, P. (1997). Psychosocial outcome of young adults with epilepsy in childhood. *Journal of Neurology, Neurosurgery, and Psychiatry, 62*, 265–268.

Kollins, S. H., & Greenhill, L. (2006). Evidence base for the use of stimulant medication in preschool children with ADHD. *Infants & Young Children, 19*, 132–141.

Kong, J., Wang, C., Kwong, K., Vangel, M., Chua, E., & Gollub, R. (2005). The neural substrate of arithmetic operations and procedure complexity. *Cognitive Brain Research, 22*, 397–405.

Kono, Y., Mishina, J., Sato, N., Watanabe, T., & Honma, Y. (2008). Developmental characteristics of very low-birthweight infants at 18 months' corrected age according to birthweight. *Pediatrics International, 50*, 23–28.

Koponen, S., Taiminen, T., Portin, R., Himanen, L., Isoniemi, H., Heinonen, H., et al. (2002). Axis I and II psychiatric disorders after traumatic brain injury: A 30-year follow-up study. *American Journal of Psychiatry, 159,* 1315–1321.

Kopp, C. M. C., Muzykewicz, D. A., Staley, B. A., Thiele, E. A., & Pulsifer, M. B. (2008). Behavior problems in children with tuberous sclerosis complex and parental stress. *Epilepsy & Behavior, 13*, 505–510.

Kopp, C. M. C., Muzykewicz, D. A., Staley, B. A., Thiele, E. A., & Pulsifer, M. B. (in press). Brain oscillatory EEG event-related desynchronization (ERD) and synchronization (ERS) responses during an auditory memory task are altered in children with epilepsy. *Epilepsy & Behavior.*

Koren, G. (2001). *Maternal-fetal toxicology: A clinician's guide.* New York: Marcel Dekker.

Korkman, M., Kirk, U., & Kemp, S. (2007). *NEPSY* (2nd ed.). San Antonio, TX: Pearson.

Kosc, L. (1974). Developmental dyscalculia. *Journal of Learning Disabilities, 7,* 164–177.

Koshy, M., Thomas, C., & Goodwin, J. (1990). Vascular lesions in the central nervous system in sickle cell disease (neuropathology). *Journal of the Association for Academic Minority Physicians, 1*, 71–78.

Kossoff, E. H., Balasta, M., Hatfield, L. M., Lehmann, C. U., & Comi, A. M. (2007). Self-reported treatment patterns in patients with Sturge-Weber syndrome and migraines. *Journal of Child Neurology, 22*, 720–726.

Kossoff, E. H., Pyzik, P. L., Rubenstein, J. E., Bergqvist, A. G. C., Buchhalter, J. R., Donner, E. J., et al. (2007). Combined ketogenic diet and vagus nerve stimulation: Rational polytherapy? *Epilepsia, 48*, 77–81.

Kostanecka-Endress, T., Banaschewski, T., Kinkelbur, J., Wullner, I., Lichtblau, S., Cohrs, S., et al. (2003). Disturbed sleep in children with Tourette syndrome: A polysomnographic study. *Journal of Psychosomatic Research, 55*, 23–29.

Kotagal, P., & Rothner, A. (1993). Epilepsy in the setting of neurocutaneous syndromes. *Epilepsia, 34* (Suppl.), S71–S78.

Kotik-Friedgut, B. (2006). Development of the Lurian approach: A cultural neurolinguistic perspective. *Neuropsychology Review, 16*, 43–52.

Kouri, T., Selle, C., & Riley, S. (2006). Comparison of meaning and graphophonemic feedback strategies for guided reading instruction of children with language delays. *American Journal of Speech Language Pathology, 15*, 236–246.

Kovacs, M., Goldston, D., Obrosky, D. S., & Bonar, L. K. (1997). Psychiatric disorders in youths with IDM: Rates and risk factors. *Diabetes Care, 20*, 36–44.

Kovas, Y., Haworth, C. M. A., Harlaar, N., Petrill, S. A., Dale, P. S., & Plomin, R. (2007). Overlap and specificity of genetic and environmental influences on mathematics and reading disability in 10-year-old twins. *Journal of Child Psychology and Psychiatry, 48*, 914–922.

Kozák, L., Balzková, M., Kuhrová, V., Pijácková, A., Ruzicková, S., & St'astná, S. (1997). Mutation and haplotype analysis of phenylalanine hydroxylase alleles in classical PKU patients from the Czech republic: Identification of four novel mutations. *Journal of Medical Genetics, 34*, 893–898.

Kozma, C. (2001). Valproic acid embryopathy: Report of two siblings with further expansion of the phenotypic abnormalities and a review of the literature. *American Journal of Medical Genetics, 98*(2), 168–175.

Krab, L. C., Aarsen, F. K., de Goede-Bolder, A., Catsman-Berrevoets, C. E., Arts, W. F., Moll, H. A., et al. (2008). Impact of neurofibromatosis type 1 on school performance. *Journal of Child Neurology, 23*, 1002–1010.

Krab, L. C., de Goede-Bolder, A., Aarsen, F. K., Pluijm, S. M. F., Bouman, M. J., van der Geest, J. N., et al. (2008). Effect of simvastatin on cognitive functioning in children with neurofibromatosis type 1: A randomized controlled trial. *Journal of the American Medical Association, 300*, 287–294.

Krain, A. L., & Castellanos, F. X. (2006). Brain development and ADHD. *Clinical Psychology Review, 26*, 433–444.

Krause, C. M., Boman, P., Sillanmäki, L., Varho, T., & Holopainen, I. E. (2008). Brain oscillatory EEG event-related desynchronization (ERD) and synchronization (ERS) responses during an auditory memory task are altered in children with epilepsy. *Seizure, 17*, 1–10.

Kroesbergen, E. H., & Van Luit, J. E. H. (2003). Mathematics interventions for children with special educational needs: A meta-analysis. *Remedial and Special Education, 24*, 97–114.

Kroesbergen, E. H., Van Luit, J. E. H., & Maas, C. J. M. (2004). Effectiveness of explicit and constructivist mathematics instruction for low-achieving students in The Netherlands. *Elementary School Journal, 104*, 233–251.

Krueger, F., Spampinato, M. V., Pardini, M., Pajevic, S., Wood, J. N., Weiss, G. H., et al. (2008). Integral calculus problem solving: an fMRI investigation. *NeuroReport, 19*, 1095–1099.

Kulin, N. A., Pastuszak, A., & Koren, G. (1998). Are the new SSRIs safe for pregnant women? *Canadian Family Physician [Medecin de Famille Canadien], 44*, 2081–2083.

Kulin, N. A., Pastuszak, A., Sage, S. R., Schick-Boschetto, B., Spivey, G., Feldkamp, M., et al. (1998). Pregnancy outcome following maternal use of the new selective serotonin reuptake inhibitors: A prospective controlled multicenter study. *Journal of the American Medical Association, 279*, 609–610.

Kulkarni, M. L., Zaheeruddin, M., Shenoy, N., & Vani, H. N. (2006). Fetal valproate syndrome. *Indian Journal of Pediatrics* [serial online], *73*, 937–939.

Kumada, T., Ito, M., Miyajima, T., Fujii, T., Okuno, T., Go, T., et al. (2005). Multi-institutional study on the correlation between chromosomal abnormalities and epilepsy. *Brain and Development, 27*, 127–134.

Kushner, D. (1998). Mild traumatic brain injury: Toward understanding manifestations and treatment. *Archives of Internal Medicine, 158*, 1617–1624.

Kuypers, F. A., Lewis, R. A., Hua, M., Schott, M. A., Discher, D., Ernst, J. D., et al. (1996). Detection of altered membrane phospholipid asymmetry in subpopulations of human red blood cells using fluorescently labeled annexin V. *Blood, 87*, 1179–1187.

Kwan, P., & Brodie, M. J. (2000). Early identification of refractory epilepsy. *New England Journal of Medicine, 3*, 314–319.

Kwan, P., & Brodie, M. J. (2005). Provision of care. In W. H. Organization (Ed.), *Atlas of Epilepsy Care in the World* (pp. 34–35). Geneva, Switzerland: World Health Organization.

Kwiatkowski, J. L. (2008). Oral iron chelators. *Pediatric Clinics of North America, 55*, 461–482.

Kyttälä, M., Aunio, P., Lehto, J. E., Van Luit, J., & Hautamäki, J. (2003). Visuospatial working memory and early numeracy. *Educational and Child Psychology, 20*, 65–76.

Laan, L. A., van Haeringen, A., & Brouwer, O. F. (1999). Angelman syndrome: A review of clinical and genetic aspects. *Clinical Neurology and Neurosurgery, 101*, 161–170.

Laatsch, L., Harrington, D., Hotz, G., Marcantuono, J., Mozzoni, M. P., Walsh, V., et al. (2007). An evidence-based review of cognitive and behavioral rehabilitation treatment studies in children with acquired brain injury. *Journal of Head Trauma Rehabilitation, 22,* 248–256.

Lachiewicz, A., Dawson, D., & Spiridigliozzi, G. A. (2000). Physical characteristics of young boys with fragile X syndrome: Reasons for difficulties in making a diagnosis in young males. *American Journal of Medical Genetics, 92*, 229–236.

Laegreid, L., Olegard, R., Walstrom, J., & Conradi, N. (1992). Teratogenic effects of benzodiazepine use during pregnancy. *Journal of Pediatrics, 114*, 126–131.

Lahey, B. B., Pelham, W. E., Loney, J. L., S. S., & Willcutt, E. G. (2005). Instability of the DSM-IV subtypes of ADHD from preschool through elementary school. *Archives of General Psychiatry, 62*, 896–902.

Lahey, B. B., Schaughency, E. A., Hynd, G. W., Carlson, C. L., & Nieves, N. (1987). Attention deficit disorder with and without hyperactivity: Comparison of behavioral characteristics of clinic-referred children. *Journal of the American Academy of Child and Adolescent Psychiatry, 26*, 718–723.

Lahey, M. (1988). *Language disorders and language development*. New York: Macmillan.

Lahey, M., Edwards, J., & Munson, B. (2001). Is processing speed related to severity of language impairment? *Journal of Speech, Language, and Hearing Research, 44*, 1354–1361.

Lai, T. J., Lui, X., Guo, Y. L., Guo, N. W., Yu, M. L., Hsu, C. C., et al. (2002). A cohort study of behavioral problems and intelligence in children with high prenatal polychlorinated biphenyl exposure. *Archives of General Psychiatry, 59*, 1061–1066.

Laine, K., Heikkinen, T., Ekblad, U., & Kero, P. (2003). Effects of exposure to selective serotonin reuptake inhibitors during pregnancy on serotonergic symptoms in newborns and cord blood monamine and prolactin concentrations. *Archives of Psychiatry, 60*, 720–726.

Laing, E., Butterworth, G., Ansari, D., Gsödl, M., Longhi, E., Panagiotaki, G., et al. (2002). Atypical development of language and social communication in toddlers with Williams syndrome. *Developmental Science, 5*, 233–246.

Laing, E., & Jarrold, C. (2007). Comprehension of spatial language in Williams syndrome: Evidence for impaired spatial representation of verbal description. *Clinical Linguistics and Phonetics, 21*, 689–704.

Laing, S., & Espeland, W. (2003). Low-intensity phonological awareness training in a preschool classroom for children with communication impairments. *Journal of Communication Disorders, 38*, 65–82.

Lambert, W. E., Lasarev, M., Muniz, J., Scherer, J., Rothlein, J., Santana, J., et al. (2005). Variation in organophosphate pesticide metabolites in urine of children living in agricultural communities. *Environmental Health Perspective, 113*, 504–508.

Lannetti, P., Mastrangelo, M., & Di Netta, S. (2005). Neurological "soft signs" in children and adolescents. *Journal of Pediatric Neurology, 3*(3), 123–125.

Lanphear, B. P., Dietrich, K. N., Auinger, P., & Cox, C. (2000). Cognitive deficits associated with blood lead concentrations < 10 microg/dL in US children and adolescents. *Public Health, 115*, 521–529.

Lanphear, B. P., Hornung, R. W., Khoury, J., Yolton, K., Baghurst, P. A., Bellinger, D. C., et al. (2005). Low-level environmental lead exposure and children's intellectual function: An international pooled analysis. *Environmental Health Perspective, 113*, 894–899.

Larsen, J. P., Hoien, T., Lundberg, L., & Odegaard, H. (1990). MRI evaluation of the size and symmetry of the planum temporale in adolescents with developmental dyslexia. *Brain and Language, 39*, 289–301.

Larsen, S. C., & Hammill, D. D. (1975). The relationship of selected visual-perceptual abilities to school learning. *Journal of Special Education, 9*, 281–291.

Lasecki, K., Olympia, D., Clark, E., Jenson, W., & Heathfield, L. T. (2008). Using behavioral interventions to assist children with Type I diabetes manage blood glucose levels. *School Psychology Quarterly, 23*, 389–406.

Lasker, A. G., Mazzocco, M. M. M., & Zee, D. S. (2007). Ocular motor indicators of executive dysfunction in fragile X and Turner syndromes. *Brain and Cognition, 63*, 203–220.

Lathe, R. (2009). Fragile X and autism. *Autism, 13*, 194–197.

Lavoie, M. E., Thibault, G., Stip, E., & O'Connor, K. P. (2007). Memory and executive functions in adults with Gilles de la Tourette syndrome and chronic tic disorder. *Cognitive Neuropsychiatry, 12*, 165–181.

Lawrence, J. M., Standiford, D. A., Loots, B., Klingensmith, G. J., Williams, D. E., Ruggiero, A., et al. (2006). Prevalence and correlates of depresses mood among youth with diabetes: The SEARCH for Diabetes Youth Study. *Pediatrics, 117*, 1348–1358.

Laws, G., & Bishop, D. (2003). A comparison of language abilities in adolescents with Down syndrome and children with specific language impairment. *Journal of Speech, Language, and Hearing Research, 46*, 1324–1339.

Laws, G., Byrne, A., & Buckley, S. (2000). Language and memory development in children with Down syndrome at mainstream and special schools: A comparison. *Educational Psychology, 20*, 447–457.

Lazaro, C., Gaona, A., Ainsworth, P., Tenconi, R., Viduad, D., Kruyer, H., et al. (1996). Sex differences in mutational rate and mutational mechanisms in the NF1 gene in neurofibromatosis type 1 patients. *Human Genetics, 98*, 696–699.

Leach, L., Kaplan, E., Rewilak, D., Richards, P. M., & Proulx, G.-B. (2000). *Kaplan-Baycrest neurocognitive assessment manual.* San Antonio, TX: Psychological Corporation.

Leal, A. J. R., Dias, A. I., Vieira, J. P., Moreira, A., Távora, L., & Calado, E. (2008). Analysis of the dynamics and origin of epileptic activity in patients with tuberous sclerosis evaluated for surgery for epilepsy. *Clinical Neurophysiology, 119*, 853–861.

Learning Toolbox, The. (n.d.). The Learning Toolbox. Retrieved March 28, 2009, from http://coe.jmu.edu/Learningtoolbox/aboutus.htm.

LeBlanc, L. A., Coates, A. M., Daneshvar, S., Charlop-Christy, M. H., Morris, C., & Lancaster, B. M. (2003). Using video modeling and reinforcement to teach perspective-taking skills to children with autism. *Journal of Applied Behavior Analysis, 36*, 253–257.

Lebrun, Y. (2005). Gerstmann's syndrome. *Journal of Neurolinguistics, 18*, 317–326.

Leckman, J. F. (2002). Tourette's syndrome. *Lancet, 360*, 1577–1586.

Leckman, J. F. (2003). Phenomenology of tics and natural history of tic disorders. *Brain & Development, 25*(Suppl.), S24–S28.

Leckman, J. F., Peterson, B. S., Anderson, G. M., Arnsten, A. F. T., Pauls, D. L., & Cohen, D. J. (1997). Pathogenesis of Tourette's syndrome. *Journal of Child Psychology and Psychiatry, 38*, 119–142.

Leckman, J. F., Riddle, M. A., Hardin, M. T., Ort, S. I., Swartz, K. L., Stevenson, J., et al. (1989). The Yale Global Tic Severity Scale: Initial testing of a clinician-rated scale of tic severity. *Journal of the American Academy of Child & Adolescent Psychiatry, 28*, 566–573.

Leckman, J. F., Zhang, H., Vitale, A., Lahnin, F., Lynch, K., & Bondi, C. (1998). Course of tic severity in Tourette syndrome: The first two decades. *Pediatrics, 102*, 14–19.

Lee, A., Inch, S., & Finnigan, D. (2000). *Therapeutics in pregnancy and lactation.* Abingdon, UK: Radcliffe Medical Press.

Lee, D., & Riccio, C. A. (2005). Understanding and implementing cognitive neuropsychological retraining. In R. C. D'Amato, E. Fletcher-Janzen, & C. R. Reynolds (Eds.), *Handbook of school neuropsychology* (pp. 701–720). Hoboken, NJ: Wiley.

Lee, D. A., Portnoy, S., Hill, P., Gillberg, C., & Patton, M. A. (2005). Psychological profile of children with Noonan syndrome. *Developmental Medicine & Child Neurology, 47*, 35–38.

Legg, C., Penn, C., Temlett, J., & Sonnenberg, B. (2005). Language skills of adolescents with Tourette syndrome. *Clinical Linguistics & Phonetics, 19*, 15–33.

Lehto, J. E., Juujarvi, P., Kooistra, L., & Pulkkinen, L. (2003). Dimensions of executive functioning: Evidence from children. *British Journal of Developmental Psychology, 21*, 59–80.

Lemons, J. A., Bauer, C. R., Oh, W., Korones, S. B., Papile, L., Stoll, B. J., et al. (2001). Very low birth weight outcomes of the National Institute of Child Health and Human Development Neonatal Research Network, January 1995 through December 1996. *Pediatrics, 107*, 1–8.

Lendt, M., Helmstaedter, C., & Elger, C. E. (1999). Pre- and postoperative neuropsychological profiles in children and adolescents with temporal lobe epilepsy. *Epilepsia, 40*, 1543–1550.

Lenz, B. K., & Hughes, C. A. (1990). A word identification strategy for adolescents with learning disabilities. *Journal of Learning Disabilities, 23*, 149–158.

Leonard, B. J., Jang, Y., Savik, K., Plumbo, P. M., & Christensen, R. (2002). Psychosocial factors associated with levels of metabolic control in youth with type 1 diabetes. *Journal of Pediatric Nursing, 17*, 28–37.

Leonard, C. M., & Eckert, M. (2008). Asymmetry and dyslexia. *Developmental Neuropsychology, 33*, 663–681.

Leonard, C. M., Eckert, M., Given, B., Berninger, V., & Eden, G. (2006). Individual differences in anatomy predict reading and oral language impairments in children. *Brain, 129*, 3329–3342.

Leonard, C. M., Lombardino, L. J., Walsh, K., Eckert, M. A., Mockler, J. L., Rowe, L. A., et al. (2002). Anatomical risk factors that distinguish dyslexia from SLI predict reading skill in normal children. *Journal of Communication Disorders, 35*, 501–531.

Leonard, C. M., Voeller, K. K., Lombardino, L. J., Morris, M. K., Hynd, G. W., Alexander, A. W., et al. (1993). Anomalous cerebral structure in dyslexia revealed with magnetic resonance imaging. *Archives of Neurology, 50*, 461–469.

Leonard, L. B. (1998). *Children with specific language impairment*. Cambridge, MA: MIT Press.

Leonard, L. B., Weismer, S. E., Miller, C. A., Francis, D. J., Tomblin, J. B., & Kail, R. V. (2007). Speed of processing, working memory, and language impairment in children. *Journal of Speech, Language, and Hearing Research, 50*, 408–428.

Lerner, J. (1989). Educational interventions in learning disabilities. *Journal of American Academy of Child and Adolescent Psychiatry, 28*, 326–331.

Leslie, K. R., Johnson-Frey, S. H., & Grafton, S. T. (2004). Functional imaging of face and hand imitation: Towards a motor theory of empathy. *NeuroImage, 21*, 601–607.

Lester, B. M., Tronick, E. Z., LaGasse, L., Seifer, R., Bauer, C. R., Shankaran, S., et al. (2002). The maternal lifestyle study: Effects of substance exposure during pregnancy on neurodevelopmental outcome in 1-month-old infants. *Pediatrics, 110*, 1182–1192.

Levin, H. S. (1987). Neurobehavioral sequelae of head injury. In P. R. Cooper (Ed.), *Head injury* (2nd ed.). Baltimore, MD: Williams & Wilkins.

Levin, H. S., Benton, A. L., & Grossman, R. G. (1982). *Neurobehavioral consequences of closed head injury*. London: Oxford University Press.

Levin, H. S., Eisenberg, H. M., & Benton, A. L. (Eds.). (1989). *Mild head injury*. New York: Oxford University Press.

Levin, H. S., & Hanten, G. (2005). Executive functions after traumatic brain injury in children. *Pediatric Neurology, 33*, 79–93.

Levin, H. S., Zhang, L., Dennis, M., Ewing-Cobbs, L., Schachar, R., Max, J., et al. (2004). Psychosocial outcome of TBI in children with unilateral frontal lesions. *Journal of the International Neuropsychological Society, 10*, 305–316.

Levitt, J. G., Blanton, R. E., Smalley, S., Thompson, P. M., Guthrie, D., McCracken, J. T., et al. (2003). Cortical sulcal maps in autism. *Cerebral Cortex, 13*, 728–735.

Levy, S. E., & Hyman, S. L. (2003). Use of complementary and alternative treatments for children with autistic spectrum disorders is increasing. *Pediatric Annals, 32*, 685–691.

Levy, S. E., & Hyman, S. L. (2005). Novel treatments for autistic spectrum disorders. *Mental Retardation and Developmental Disabilities Research Reviews, 11*, 131–142.

Levy, S. E., & Hyman, S. L. (2008). Complementary and alternative medicine treatments for children with autism spectrum disorders. *Child and Adolescent Psychiatric Clinics of North America, 17*, 803–820.

Lew, Y., Smith, J., & Tager-Flusberg, H. (2003). Word reading and reading-related skills in adolescents with Williams syndrome. *Journal of Child Psychology and Psychiatry, 44*, 576–587.

Lewandowski, L. (2005). Providing neuropsychological services to learners with low-incidence disabilities. In R. C. D'Amato, E. Fletcher-Janzen, & C. R. Reynolds (Eds.), *Handbook of school neuropsychology* (pp. 614–636). Hoboken, NJ: Wiley.

Lewis, B. A., Freebairn, L. A., Heeger, S., & Casidy, S. B. (2002). Speech and language skills of individuals with Prader-Willi syndrome. *American Journal of Speech-Language Pathology, 11*, 285–294.

Lewis, B. A., Freebairn, L. A., & Taylor, H. G. (2000). Following-up of children with early expressive phonology disorders. *Journal of Learning Disabilities, 33*, 433–444.

Lewis, B. A., Singer, L. T., Short, E. J., Minnes, S., Arendt, R., Weishampel, P., et al. (2004). Four-year language outcomes of children exposed to cocaine in utero. *Neurotoxicology and Teratology, 26*, 617–627.

Lewis, C., Hitch, G. J., & Walker, P. (1994). The prevalence of specific arithmetic difficulties and specific reading difficulties in 9- to 10-year-old boys and girls. *Journal of Child Psychology and Psychiatry, 35*, 283–292.

Lewis, K. D., & Weiss, S. J., (2003). Psychometric testing of an infant risk assessment for prenatal drug exposure. *Journal of Pediatric Nursing, 18*, 371–378.

Lewitter, F. I., DeFries, J. C., & Elston, R. C. (1980). Genetic models of reading disability. *Behavior Genetics, 10*, 9–30.

Lezak, M. D. (1995). *Neuropsychological assessment*. New York: Oxford University Press.

Lezak, M. D., Howieson, D. B., & Loring, D. W. (2004). *Neuropsychological assessment*. New York: Oxford.

Li, Y., & Mogul, D. J. (2007). Electrical control of epileptic seizures. *Journal of Clinical Neurophysiology, 24*, 197–204.

Liberman, I. Y., & Liberman, A. M. (1990). Whole language vs. code emphasis: Underlying assumptions and their implications for reading instruction. *Annals of Dyslexia, 40*, 51–76.

Lidsky, T. I., Heaney, A. T., Schneider, J. S., & Rosen, J. F. (2007). Neurodevelopmental effects of childhood exposure to heavy metals: Lessons from pediatric lead poisoning. In M. M. M. Mazzocco & J. L. Ross (Eds.), *Neurogenetic developmental disorders: Variation of manifestation in childhood* (pp. 335–363). Cambridge, MA: MIT Press.

Light, J. G., & DeFries, J. C. (1995). Comorbidity of reading and mathematics disabilities: Genetic and environmental etiologies. *Journal of Learning Disabilities, 28*, 96–106.

Lim, H. H., Lenarz, T., Joseph, G., Battmer, R. D., Samii, A., Samii, M., et al. (2007). Electrical stimulation of the midbrain for hearing restoration: Insight into the functional organization of the human central auditory system. *Journal of Neuroscience, 27*, 13541–13551.

Limond, J., & Leeke, R. (2005). Practitioner review: Cognitive rehabilitation for children with acquired brain injury. *Journal of Child Psychology and Psychiatry, 46,* 339–352.

Lin, H., Katsovich, L., Ghebremichael, M., Findley, D. B., Grantz, H., Lombroso, P. J., et al. (2007). Psychosocial stress predicts future symptom severities in children and adolescents with Tourette syndrome and/or obsessive-compulsive disorder. *Journal of Child Psychology and Psychiatry, 48*, 157–166.

Litt, J., Taylor, H. G., Klein, N., & Hack, M. (2005). Learning disabilities in children with very low birthweight: Prevalence, neuropsychological correlates, and educational interventions. *Journal of Learning Disabilities, 38*, 130–141.

Liu, J., Nyholt, D. R., Magnussen, E. P., Pavone, P., Geschwind, D., Lord, C., et al. (2001). A genomewide screen for autism susceptibility loci. *American Journal of Human Genetics, 69*, 327–340.

Livingston, R. B., Pritchard, D. A., Moses, J. A., Jr., & Haak, R. A. (1997). Modal profiles for the Halstead Reitan Neuropsychological Battery for Children. *Archives of Clinical Neuropsychology, 12*, 459–476.

Livingstone, M. S., Rosen, G. D., Drislane, F. W., & Galaburda, A. M. (1991). Physiological and anatomical evidence for a magnocellular defect in developmental dyslexia. *Neurobiology, 88*, 943–947.

Lizardi, P., O'Rourke, M., & Morris, R. (2008). The effects of organophosphate pesticide exposure in Hispanic children's cognitive and behavioral functioning. *Journal of Pediatric Psychology, 33*, 91–101.

Llorente, A. M. (2008). *Principles of neuropsychological assessment with Hispanics: Theoretical foundations and clinical practice*. New York: Springer.

Lobaugh, N. J., Karaskov, V., Rombough, V., Rovet, J., Bryson, S., R., G., et al. (2001). Piracetam therapy does not enhance cognitive functioning in children with Down syndrome. *Archives of Pediatrics and Adolescent Medicine, 155*, 442–448.

Lobel, M., Cannella, D. L., Graham, J. E., DeVincent, C., Schneider, J., & Meyer, B. A. (2008). Pregnancy-specific stress, prenatal health behaviors, and birth outcomes. *Health Psychology, 27*, 604–615.

Loken, W. J., Thornton, A. E., Otto, R. L., & Long, C. J. (1995). Sustained attention after severe closed head injury. *Neuropsychology, 9,* 592–598.

London, L., Myers, J. E., Neil, V., Taylor, T., & Thompson, M. L. (1997). An investigation into neurologic and neurobehavioral effects of long-term agrochemical use among deciduous fruit farm workers in the Western Cape, South Africa. *Environmental Research, 73*, 132–145.

López, B., Leekam, S. R., & Arts, G. R. J. (2008). How central is central coherence? Preliminary evidence on the link between conceptual and perceptual processing in children with autism. *Autism, 12*, 159–171.

López, B. R., Lincoln, A. J., Ozonoff, S., & Lai, Z. (2005). Examining the relationship between executive functions and restricted, repetitive symptoms of autistic disorder. *Journal of Autism and Developmental Disorders, 35*, 445–460.

Lopez, N. J., Smith, P. C., & Gutierrez, J. (2002). Higher risk of preterm birth and low birth weight in women with periodontal disease. *Journal of Dental Research, 81*, 58–63.

Lord, C., & Risi, S. (2000). Diagnosis of autism spectrum disorders in young children. In A. M. Wetherby & B. M. Prizant (Eds.), *Autism spectrum disorders: A transactional developmental perspective* (pp. 11–30). Baltimore, MD: Brookes.

Loring, D. (1999). *INS Dictionary of Neuropsychology*. New York: Oxford University Press.

Loring, D. W., & Meador, K. J. (2004). Cognitive side effects of antiepileptic drugs in children. *Neurology, 62*, 872–877.

Lorsbach, T. C., Wilson, S., & Reimer, J. F. (1996). Memory for relevant and irrelevant information: Evidence for deficient inhibitory processes in language/learning disabled children. *Contemporary Educational Psychology, 21*, 447–466.

Lossie, A. C., Whitney, M. M., Armidon, D., Dong, H. J., Chen, P., Theriaque, D. W., et al. (2001). Distinct phenotypes distinguish the molecular classes of Angelman syndrome. *Journal of Medical Genetics, 38*, 834–845.

Loth, E., Gómez, J. C., & Happé, F. (2008). Event schemas in autism spectrum disorders: The role of theory of mind and weak central coherence. *Journal of Autism and Developmental Disorders, 38*, 449–463.

Lotter, V. (1978). Follow-up studies. In M. Rutter & E. Schopler (Eds.), *Autism: A reappraisal of concepts and treatment* (pp. 187–199). New York: Plenum.

Lovaas, O. I. (1987). Behavioral treatment and normal educational and intellectual functioning in young autistic children. *Journal of Consulting and Clinical Psychology, 55*, 3–9.

Loveland, K. A., Bachevalier, J., Pearson, D., & Lane, D. M. (2008). Fronto-limbic functioning in children and adolescents with and without autism. *Neuropsychologia, 46*, 49–62.

Loveland, K. A., & Tunali-Kotoski, B. (2005). The school-age child with an autistic spectrum disorder. In F. R. Volkmar, R. Paul, A. Klin, & D. Cohen (Eds.), *Handbook of autism and pervasive developmental disorders: Diagnosis, development, neurobiology, and behavior* (3rd ed., Vol. 1, pp. 247–287). Hoboken, NJ: Wiley.

Lu, C., & Fenske, R. A. (1999). Dermal transfer of chlorpyrifos residues from residential surfaces: Comparison of hand press, hand drag, wipe, and polyurethane foam roller measurements after broadcast and aerosol pesticide applications. *Environmental Health Perspectives, 107*, 463–467.

Lu, C., Fenske, R. A., Simcox, N. J., & Kalman, D. (2000). Pesticide exposure of children in an agriculture community: Evidence of household proximity to farmland and take home exposure pathways. *Environmental Research, 84*, 290–302.

Lu, Q., Lu, M. C., & Schetter, C. D. (2005). Learning from success and failure in psychosocial intervention: An evaluation of low birth weight prevention trials. *Journal of Health Psychology, 10,* 185–195.

Lubec, G., & Engidawork, E. (2002). The brain in Down syndrome (trisomy 21). *Journal of Neurology, 249*, 1347–1356.

Luby, J. L., Mrakotsky, C., Stalets, M. M., Belden, A., Heffelfinger, A., Williams, M., et al. (2006). Risperidone in preschool children with autistic spectrum disorders: An investigation of safety and efficacy. *Journal of Child and Adolescent Psychopharmacology, 16*, 575–587.

Luiselli, J., Cannon, B. O., Ellis, J. T., & Sisson, R. W. (2000). Home-based behavioral intervention for young children with autism/pervasive developmental disorder. *Autism, 4*, 426–438.

Luna, B., Minshew, N. J., Garver, K. E., Lazar, N. A., Thulborn, K. R., Eddy, W. F., et al. (2002). Neocortical system abnormalities in autism. An fMRI study of spatial working memory. *Neurology, 59*, 834–840.

Luo, F., Leckman, J. F., Katsovich, L., Findley, D., Grantz, H., Tucker, D. M., et al. (2004). Prospective longitudinal study of children with tic disorders and/or obsessive compulsive disorder: Relationship of symptom exacerbations to newly acquired streptococcal infections. *Pediatrics, 113*, 578–585.

Luria, A. R. (1966). *Higher cortical functions in man*. New York: Basic Books.

Luria, A. R. (1973). *The working brain*. New York: Basic Books.

Luria, A. R. (1980). *Higher cortical functions in man* (2nd ed.). New York: Basic Books.

Mabbott, D. J., & Bisanz, J. (2008). Computational skills, working memory, and conceptual knowledge in older children with mathematics learning disabilities. *Journal of Learning Disabilities, 41*, 15–28.

Mabbott, D. J., Noseworthy, M. D., Bouffet, E., Rockel, C., & Laughlin, S. (2006). Diffusion tensor imaging of white matter after cranial radiation in children for medulloblastoma: Correlation with IQ. *Neuro-Oncology, 8*, 244–252.

Mabbott, D. J., Penkman, L., Witol, A., Strother, D., & Bouffet, E. (2008). Core neurocognitive functions in children treated for posterior fossa tumors. *Neuropsychology, 22*, 159–168.

Mabbott, D. J., Spiegler, B. J., Greenberg, M. L., Rutka, J. T., Hyder, D. J., & Bouffet, E. (2005). Serial evaluation of academic and behavioral outcome after treatment with cranial radiation in childhood. *Journal of Clinical Oncology, 23*, 2256–2263.

MacAllister, W., & Schaffer, S. G. (2007). Neuropsychological deficits in childhood epilepsy syndromes. *Neuropsychological Review, 17*, 427–444.

Maccini, P., & Hughes, C. A. (2000). Effects of a problem solving strategy on the introductory algebra performance of secondary students with learning disabilities. *Learning Disabilities Research & Practice, 15*, 10–21.

MacDonald, A., Lilburn, M., Cochrane, B., Davies, P., Daly, A., Asplin, D., et al. (2004). A new, low-volume protein substitute for teenagers and adults with phenylketonuria. *Journal of Inherited Metabolic Disease, 27*(2), 127–135.

Machemer, L. H., & Pickel, M. (1994). Carbamate insecticides. *Toxicology and Applied Pharmacology, 91*, 29–36.

Maciag, D., Simpson, K. L., Coppinger, D., Lu, Y., Wang, Y., Lin, R. C. S., et al. (2006). Neonatal antidepressant exposure has lasting effects on behavior and serotonin circuitry. *Neuropsychopharmacology, 31*, 47–57.

Mackie, S., Shaw, P., Lenroot, R., Pierson, R., Greenstein, D. K., Nugent, T. F., et al. (2007). Cerebellar development and clinical outcome in attention deficit hyperactivity disorder. *American Journal of Psychiatry, 164*, 647–655.

Macmillan, M. (2000). Restoring Phineas Gage: A 150th retrospective. *Journal of the History of the Neurosciences, 9*, 46–66.

Madden, S. G., Loeb, S. J., & Smith, C. A. (2008). An integrative literature review of lifestyle interventions for the prevention of type II diabetes mellitus. *Journal of Clinical Nursing, 17*, 2243–2256.

Madhavan, D., Schaffer, S., Yankovsky, A., Arzimanoglou, A., Renaldo, F., Zaroff, C. M., et al. (2007). Surgical outcome in tuberous sclerosis complex: A multicenter survey. *Epilepsia, 48*, 1625–1628.

Madsen, K., Hvid, A., Vestergaard, M., Schendel, D., Wohlfahrt, J., Thorsen, P., et al. (2002). A population-based study of measles, mumps and rubella vaccination and autism. *New England Journal of Medicine, 347*, 1477–1482.

Madsen, K. M., Lauritsen, M. B., Pedersen, C. B., Thorsen, P., Plesner, A.-M., Andersen, P. H., et al. (2003). Thimerosal and the occurrence of autism: Negative ecological evidence from Danish population-based data. *Pediatrics, 112*, 604–606.

Maes, B., Fryns, J. P., Ghesquiére, P., & Borghgraef, M. (2000). Phenotypic checklist to screen for fragile X syndrome in people with mental retardation. *Mental Retardation, 38*, 207–215.

Maguire, C. M., Bruil, J., Wit, J. M., & Walther, F. J. (2007). Reading preterm infants' behavioral cues: An intervention study with parents of premature infants born <32 weeks. *Early Human Development, 83*, 419–424.

Mahone, E. M., Cirino, P. T., Cutting, L. E., Cerrone, P. M., Hagelthorn, K. M., Hiemenz, J. R., et al. (2002). Validity of the Behavior Rating Inventory of Executive Function in children with ADHD and/or Tourette syndrome. *Archives of Clinical Neuropsychology, 17*, 643–662.

Mahone, E. M., Koth, C. W., Cutting, L., Singer, H. S., & Denckla, M. B. (2001). Executive function in fluency and recall measures among children with Tourette syndrome or ADHD. *Journal of the International Neuropsychological Society, 7*, 102–111.

Mahoney, G., Perales, F., Wiggers, B., & Herman, B. (2006). Responsive teaching: Early intervention for children with Down syndrome and other disabilities. *Down Syndrome: Research and Practice, 11*, 18–28.

Maizlish, N., Schenker, M., Weisskopf, C., Seiber, J., & Samuels, A. (1987). A behavioral evaluation of pest control workers with short-term, low-level exposure to the organophosphate diazinon. *American Journal of Industrial Medicine, 12*, 153–172.

Majewicz-Hefley, A., & Carlson, J. S. (2007). A meta-analysis of combined treatments for children diagnosed with ADHD. *Journal of Attention Disorders, 10*, 239–250.

Malekpour, M. (2004). Low birth-weight infants and the importance of early intervention: Enhancing mother-infant interactions: A literature review. *British Journal of Developmental Disabilities, 50*, 78–88.

Malm, G., Gustafsson, B., Berglund, G., Lindström, M., Naess, K., Borgström, B., et al. (2008). Outcome in six children with mucopolysaccharidosis type IH, Hurler syndrome, after haematopoietic stem cell transplantation (HSCT). *Acta Paediatrica, 97,* 1108–1112.

Malm, H., Kajantie, E., Kivirikko, S., Kääriäen, H., Peippo, M., & Somer, M. (2002). Valproate embryopathy in three sets of siblings: Further proof of hereditary susceptibility. *Neurology, 59,* 630–633.

Mandelbaum, D. E., & Burack, G. D. (1997). The effect of seizure type and medication on cognitive and behavioral functioning in children with idiopathic epilepsy. *Developmental Medicine & Child Neurology, 39,* 731–735.

Mann, V. (1991). Language problems: A key to early reading problems. In B. Y. L. Wong (Ed.), *Learning about learning disabilities* (pp. 129–162). San Diego: Academic Press.

Manning, S. C., & Miller, D. C. (2001). Identifying ADHD subtypes using the parent and teacher rating scales of the Behavior Assessment Scale for Children. *Journal of Attention Disorders, 4,* 41–51.

Mannuzza, S., & Klein, R. G. (1999). Adolescent and adult outcomes in attention-deficit/hyperactivity disorder. In H. C. Quay & A. E. Hogan (Eds.), *Handbook of disruptive behavior disorders* (pp. 279–294). New York: Kluwer/Plenum.

Mansueto, C. S., & Keuler, D. J. (2005). Tic or compulsion? It's Tourettic OCD. *Behavior Modification, 29,* 784–799.

Margolin, J., Steuber, C., & Poplack, D. (2002). Acute lymphoblastic leukemia. In P. A. Pizzo & D. G. Poplack (Eds.), *Principles and practice of pediatric oncology* (4th ed., pp. 489–544). Philadelphia: Lippincott/Williams & Wilkins.

Marik, P. E., Varon, J., & Trask, T. (2002). Management of head trauma. *Chest, 122,* 699–711.

Markee, T. W., Moore, L. H., Brown, W. S., & Theberge, D. C. (1994). *Bilateral field advantage and evoked potential interhemispheric transfer time in dyslexic adults.* Paper presented at the International Neuropsychological Society.

Marler, J. A., Effenbein, J. L., Ryals, B. M., Urban, Z., & Netzloff, M. L. (2005). Sensorineural hearing loss in children and adults with Williams syndrome. *American Journal of Medical Genetics, 138,* 318–327.

Marlowe, M., Bliss, L., & Schneider, H. G. (1994). Hair trace element contract of violence prone male children. *Journal of Advances in Medicine, 7,* 5–18.

Marlowe, M., Errera, J., Ballowe, T., & Jacobs, J. (1983). Low metal levels in emotionally disturbed children. *Journal of Abnormal Psychology, 92,* 386–389.

Marlowe, M., Stellern, J., Moon, C., & Errera, J. (1985). Main and interaction effects of metallic toxins on aggressive classroom behavior. *Aggressive Behavior, 11,* 41–48.

Marsh, R., Alexander, G. M., Packard, M. G., Zhu, H., & Peterson, B. S. (2005). Perceptual-motor skill learning in Gilles de la Tourette syndrome: Evidence for multiple procedural learning and memory systems. *Neuropsychologia, 43,* 1456–1465.

Marsh, R., Alexander, G. M., Packard, M. G., Zhu, H., Wingard, J. C., Quackenbush, G., et al. (2004). Habit learning in Tourette syndrome: A translational neuroscience approach to a developmental psychopathology. *Archives of General Psychiatry, 61,* 1259–1268.

Marshall, R. M., Hynd, G. W., Handwerk, M. J., & Hall, J. (1997). Academic underachievement in ADHD subtypes. *Journal of Learning Disabilities, 30*, 635–642.

Marshall, R. M., Schafer, V. A., O'Donnell, L., Elliott, J., & Handwerk, M. L. (1999). Arithmetic disabilities and ADD subtypes: Implications for DSM-IV. *Journal of Learning Disabilities, 32*, 239–247.

Martel, M., Nikolas, M., & Nigg, J. T. (2007). Executive function in adolescents with ADHD. *Journal of the American Academy of Child and Adolescent Psychiatry, 46*, 1437–1444.

Martin, A. J., State, M. W., Koenig, K., Schultz, R. T., Dykens, E. M., Cassidy, S. B., et al. (1998). Prader-Willi syndrome. *American Journal of Psychiatry, 155*, 1265–1273.

Martin, J. A., Hamilton, B. E., Sutton, P. D., Ventura, S. J., Menacker, F., & Munson, M. L. (2005). Births: Final data for 2003 *National vital statistics reports* (Vol. 54, no.2). Hyattsville, MD: National Center for Health Statistics.

Martineau, J., Barthélémy, C., Jouve, J., & Müh, J. P. (1992). Monoamines (serotonin and catecholamines) and their derivatives in infantile autism: Age-related changes and drug effects. *Developmental Medicine and Child Neurology, 34*, 593–603.

Martineau, J., Hérault, J., & Petit, E. (1994). Catecholaminergic metabolism and autism. *Developmental Medicine and Child Neurology, 36*, 688–697.

Martinuik, A. L. C., Speechley, K. N., Seeco, M., Campbell, M. K., & Donner, A. (2007). Evaluation of an epilepsy education program for grade 5 students: A cluster randomized trial. *Epilepsy & Behavior, 9*, 58–67.

Martinussen, M., Fischl, B., Larsson, H. B., Skranes, J., Kulseng, S., Vangberg, T. R., et al. (2005). Cerebral cortex thickness in 15-year-old adolescents with low birth weight measured by an automated MRI-based method. *Brain, 128*, 2588–2596.

Marton, K. (2008). Visuo-spatial processing and executive functions in children with specific language impairment. *International Journal of Language & Communication Disorders, 43*, 181–200.

Masi, G., Cosenza, A., Mucci, M., & Brovedani, P. (2003). A 3-year naturalistic study of 53 preschool children with pervasive developmental disorder treated with risperidone. *Journal of Clinical Psychiatry, 64*, 1039–1047.

Mason, M. F., & Macrae, C. N. (2008). Perspective-taking from a social neuroscience standpoint. *Group Process and Intergroup Relations, 11*, 215–232.

Mason, R. A., Williams, D. L., Kans, R. K., Minshew, N. J., & Just, M. A. (2008). Theory of mind disruption and recruitment of the right hemisphere during narrative comprehension in autism. *Neuropsychologia, 46*, 269–280.

Mateer, C. A. (1999). The rehabilitation of executive disorders. In D. T. Stuss, G. Winocur, & I. H. Robertson (Eds.), *Cognitive rehabilitation* (pp. 314–322). Cambridge, UK: Cambridge University Press.

Matheson, D. S., Clarkson, T. W., & Gelfand, E. W. (1980). Mercury toxicity (acrodynia) induced by long-term injection of gamma-globulin. *Journal of Pediatrics, 97*, 153–155.

Mathews, T. J., & MacDorman, M. F. (2006). Infant mortality statistics from the 2003 period linked birth/infant death data set. *National vital statistics reports* (Vol. 54, no.16). Hyattsville, MD: National Center for Health Statistics.

Matson, J. L., & LoVullo, S. V. (2008). A review of behavioral treatments for self-injurious behaviors of persons with autism spectrum disorders. *Behavior Modification, 31*, 61–76.

Mattes, J. A. (1983). The Feingold diet: A current reappraisal. *Journal of Learning Disabilities, 16*, 319–323.

Mattson, A. J., Sheer, D. E., & Fletcher, J. M. (1992). Electrophysiological evidence of lateralized disturbances in children with learning disabilities. *Journal of Clinical and Experimental Neuropsychology, 14*, 707–716.

Mattson, S. N., Calarco, K. E., & Lang, A. R. (2006). Focused and shifting attention in children with heavy prenatal alcohol exposure. *Neuropsychology, 20*, 361–369.

Mattson, S. N., Goodman, A. M., Caine, C., Delis, D. C., & Riley, E. P. (1999). Executive functioning in children with heavy prenatal alcohol exposure. *Alcoholism: Clinical and Experimental Research, 23*, 1808–1815.

Mattson, S. N., Riley, E. P., Gramling, L., Delis, D. C., & Jones, K. L. (1998). Neuropsychological comparison of alcohol-exposed children with or without physical features of fetal alcohol syndrome. *Neuropsychology, 12*, 146–153.

Mattson, S. N., Riley, E. P., & Roebuck, T. M. (1998). A review of the neuroanatomical findings in children with fetal alcohol syndrome or prenatal exposure to alcohol. *Alcoholism: Clinical and Experimental Research, 22*, 339–344.

Mattson, S. N., Riley, E. P., & Schoenfeld, A. M. (2001). Teratogenic effects of alcohol on brain and behavior. *Alcohol Research and Health, 25*, 185–191.

Maurer, R. G. (1986). Neuropsychology of autism. *Psychiatric Clinics of North America, 9*, 367–380.

Mautner, V.-F., Kluwe, L., Thakker, S. D., & Leark, R. A. (2002). Treatment of ADHD in neurofibromatosis type 1. *Developmental Medicine & Child Neurology, 44*, 164–170.

Mayes, S. D., & Calhoon, S. L. (2008). WISC-IV and WIAT-II profiles in children with high-functioning autism. *Journal of Autism and Developmental Disorders, 38*, 428–439.

Mayes, S. D., & Calhoun, S. L. (2006). WISC-IV and WISC-III profiles in children with ADHD. *Journal of Attention Disorders, 9*, 486–493.

Mayo Clinic Staff. (n.d.). Stevens-Johnson syndrome. Definition retrieved April 24, 2009, from www.mayoclinic.com/health/stevens-johnson-syndrome/DS00940.

Mazzocco, M. M. M. (2001). Math learning disability and math LD subtypes: Evidence from studies of Turner syndrome, fragile x syndrome, and neurofibromatosis type 1. *Journal of Learning Disabilities, 34*, 520–533.

Mazzocco, M. M. M. (2007). Defining and differentiating mathematical learning disabilities and difficulties. In D. B. Berch & M. M. M. Mazzocco (Eds.), *Why is math so hard for some children? The nature and origin of mathematical learning difficulties and disabilities* (pp. 29–48). Baltimore, MD: Brookes.

Mazzocco, M. M. M., & Kover, S. T. (2007). A longitudinal assessment of executive function skills and their association with math performance. *Child Neuropsychology, 13*, 18–45.

Mazzoni, M., Pardossi, L., Cantini, R., Giornetti, V., & Arena, R. (1990). Gerstmann syndrome: A case report. *Cortex, 25*, 459–468.

McArthur, G. M., Ellis, D., Atkinson, C. M., & Coltheart, M. (2008). Auditory processing deficits in children with reading and language impairments: Can they (and should they) be treated? *Cognition, 107*, 946–977.

McBride, P., Anderson, G., Hertzig, M., Sweeney, J., Kream, J., Cohen, D., et al. (1989). Serotonergic responsivity in male young adults with autistic disorder. *Archives of General Psychiatry, 46*, 205–212.

McCandliss, B., Beck, I. L., Sandak, R., & Perfetti, C. A. (2003). Focusing attention on decoding for children with poor reading skills: Design and preliminary tests of the word building intervention. *Scientific Studies of Reading, 7*, 75–104.

McCarthy, A. M., Lindgren, S., Mengeling, M. A., Tsalikian, E., & Engvall, J. (2003). Factors associated with academic achievement in children with type 1 diabetes. *Diabetes Care, 26*, 112–117.

McCarton, C. M., Wallace, I. F., & Bennett, F. C. (1996). Early intervention for low-birth-weight premature infants: What can we achieve? *Annals of Medicine, 28,* 221–225.

McCauley, E., Kay, T., Ito, J., & Treder, R. (1987). The Turner syndrome: Cognitive deficits, affective discrimination, and behavior problems. *Child Development, 58*, 464–473.

McCloskey, M., Aliminosa, D., & Sokol, S. M. (1991). Models of arithmetic fact retrieval: An evaluation in light of findings from normal and brain-damaged subjects. *Journal of Experimental Psychology: Learning, Memory, and Cognition, 17*, 177–197.

McConnell, S. R. (2002). Interventions to facilitate social interaction for young children with autism: Review of available research and recommendations for educational intervention and future research. *Journal of Autism and Developmental Disorders, 32*, 351–371.

McCormick, M. C., Brooks-Gunn, J., Buka, S. L., Goldman, J., Yu, J., Salganik, M., et al. (2006). Early intervention in low birth weight premature infants: Results at 18 years of age for the Infant Health and Development Program. *Pediatrics, 117,* 771–780.

McCormick, M. C., McCarton, C., Brooks-Gunn, J., Belt, P., & Gross, R. T. (1998). The Infant Health and Development Program: Interim summary. *Journal of Developmental and Behavioral Pediatrics, 19,* 359–370.

McCrory, E. J., Mechelli, A., Frith, U., & Price, C. J. (2005). More than words: A common neural basis for reading and naming deficits in developmental dyslexia? *Brain, 128*, 261–267.

McDonald, C. R., Swartz, B. E., Halgren, E., Patell, A., Daimes, R., & Mandelkern, M. (2006). The relationship of regional frontal hypometabolism to executive function: A resting fluorodeoxyglucose PET study of patients with epilepsy and healthy controls. *Epilepsy & Behavior, 9*, 58–67.

McDougall, C. J., Scahill, L. D., Aman, M. G., McCracken, J. T., Tierney, E., Davies, M., et al. (2005). Risperidone for the core symptom domains of autism: Results from the study by the autism network of the research units on pediatric psychopharmacology. *American Journal of Psychiatry, 162*, 1142–1148.

McDougle, C. J., Price, L. H., & Goodman, W. K. (1990). Fluvoxamine treatment of coincident autistic disorder and obsessive-compulsive disorder: A case report. *Journal of Autism and Developmental Disorders, 20*, 537–543.

McGough, J. J., Wigal, S. B., Abikoff, H., Turnbow, J. M., Posner, K., & Moon, E. (2006). A randomized, double-blind, placebo-controlled, laboratory classroom assessment of methylphenidate transdermal system in children with ADHD. *Journal of Attention Disorders, 9*, 476–485.

McGrath, M. M., Sullivan, M. C., Lester, B. M., & Oh, W. (2000). Longitudinal neurologic follow-up in neonatal intensive care unit survivors with various neonatal morbidities. *Pediatrics, 106*, 1397–1405.

McHugh, J. C., Singh, H. W., Phillips, J., Murphy, K., Doherty, C. P., & Delanty, N. (2007). Outcome measurement after vagal nerve stimulation therapy: Proposal of a new classification. *Epilepsia, 48*, 375–378.

McKenzie, B., Bull, R., & Gray, C. (2003). The effects of phonological and visual-spatial interference on children's arithmetical performance. *Educational and Child Psychology, 20*, 93–108.

McKeown-Eyssen, G. E., Ruedy, J., & Neims, A. (1983). Methylmercury exposure in Northern Quebec: II. Neurologic findings in children. *American Journal of Epidemiology, 118*, 480–479.

McKinlay, A., Dalrymple-Alford, J. C., Horwood, L. J., & Fergusson, D. M. (2002). Long-term psychosocial outcomes after mild head injury in early childhood. *Journal of Neurology, Neurosurgery and Psychiatry, 73*, 281 288.

McLean, J. F., & Hitch, G. J. (1999). Working memory impairments in children with specific arithmetic learning difficulties. *Journal of Experimental Child Psychology. Special Issue: The development of mathematical cognition: Arithmetic, 74*, 240–260.

McLeod, T. M., & Crump, W. D. (1978). The relationship of visuospatial skills and verbal ability to learning disabilities in mathematics. *Journal of Learning Disabilities, 11*, 237–241.

McMahon, W. M., Carter, A. S., Fredine, N., & Pauls, D. L. (2003). Children at familial risk for Tourette's disorder: Child and parent diagnoses. *American Journal of Medical Genetics Part B (Neuropsychiatric Genetics), 121B*, 105–111.

Meaburn, E. L., Harlaar, N., Craig, I. W., Schalkwyk, L. C., & Plomin, R. (2008). Quantitative trait locus association scan of early reading disability and ability in pooled DNA and 100K SNP microarrays in a sample of 5760 children. *Molecular Psychiatry, 13*, 729–740.

Meador, K. J. (2002a). Cognitive outcomes and predictive factors in epilepsy. *Neurology, 58*(8), 21–26.

Meador, K. J. (2002b). Neurodevelopmental effects of antiepileptic drugs. *Current Neurology and Neuroscience Reports, 4*, 373–378.

Meador, K. J. (2007). The basic science of memory as it applies to epilepsy. *Epilepsia, 48*, 23–25.

Meador, K. J., Baker, G., Cohen, M. J., Gaily, E., & Westerveld, M. (2007). Cognitive/behavioral teratogenic effects of antiepileptic drugs. *Epilepsy & Behavior, 11*, 292–302.

Meador, K. J., Baker, G. A., Browning, N., Clayton-Smith, J., Combs-Cantrell, D. T., Cohen, M. J., et al. (2009). Cognitive function at 3 years of age after fetal exposure to antiepileptic drugs. *New England Journal of Medicine, 360*, 1597–1605.

Meador, K. J., Baker, G. A., Finnell, R. H., Kalayjian, L. A., Liporace, J. D., Loring, D. W., et al. (2006). In utero antiepileptic drug exposure: Fetal death and malformations. *Neurology, 67*, 407–412.

Medved, M., & Percy, M. (2001). Prader-Willi syndrome II: A literature review of behavioural and neuropsychological characteristics. *Journal on Developmental Disabilities, 8*, 41–55.

Meeks Gardner, J., Walker, S. P., Powell, C. A., & Grantham-McGregor, S. (2003). A randomized controlled trial of a home-visiting intervention on cognition and behavior in term low birth weight infants. *Journal of Pediatrics, 143,* 634–639.

Meharg, A. A. (2005). Arsenic in rice—Understanding a new disaster for South-East Asia. *Trends in Plant Science, 9*, 415–417.

Meidinger, A. L., Miltenberger, R. G., Himle, M., Omvig, M., Trainor, C., & Crosby, R. (2005). An investigation of tic suppression and the rebound effect in Tourette's disorder. *Behavior Modification, 29*, 716–745.

Melean, G., Sestini, R., Ammannati, F., & Papi, L. (2004). Genetic insights into familial tumors of the nervous system. *American Journal of Medical Genetics, 129C*, 74–84.

Mell, L. K., Davis, R. L., & Owens, D. (2005). Association between streptococcal infection and obsessive compulsive disorder. *Pediatrics, 116*, 56–60.

Melnyk, B. M., Alpert-Gillis, L., Feinstein, N. F., Fairbanks, E., Schultz-Czarniak, J., Hust, D., et al. (2001). Improving cognitive development of low-birth-weight premature infants with the COPE program: A pilot study of the benefit of early NICU intervention with mothers. *Research in Nursing & Health, 24,* 373–389.

Meltzoff, A. N. (2002). Imitation as a mechanism of social cognition: Origins of empathy, theory of mind, and the representation of action. In U. Goswami (Ed.), *Handbook of childhood cognitive development* (pp. 6–25). Malden, MA: Blackwell.

Meltzoff, A. N., & Moore, M. K. (1995). A theory of the role of imitation in the emergence of self. In P. Rochat (Ed.), *The self in infancy. Theory and research* (pp. 73–93). Amsterdam: Elsevier.

Mendola, P., Selevan, S. G., Gutter, S., & Rice, D. (2002). Environmental factors associated with a spectrum of neurodevelopmental deficits. *Mental Retardation and Developmental Disabilities Research Reviews, 8*, 188–197.

Ment, L. R., Bada, H. S., Barnes, P., Grant, P. E., Hirtz, D., Papile, L. A., et al. (2002). Practice parameter: Neuroimaging of the neonate. Report of the quality standards subcommittee of the American Academy of Neurology and the Practice Committee of the Child Neurology Society. *Neurology, 58,* 1726–1738.

Ment, L. R., Vohr, B., Allan, W., Katz, K. H., Schneider, K. C., Westerveld, M., et al. (2003). Change in cognitive function over time in very low-birth-weight infants. *Journal of the American Medical Association, 289*, 705–711.

Menyuk, P., & Looney, P. L. (1972). A problem of language disorder: Length vs. structure. *Journal of Speech and Hearing Research, 15*, 264–279.

Mervis, C. B., & Klein-Tasman, B. P. (2000). Williams syndrome: Cognition, personality, and adaptive behavior. *Mental Retardation and Developmental Disabilities Research Reviews, 6*, 148–158.

Mervis, C. B., & Morris, C. A. (2007). Williams syndrome. In M. M. M. Mazzocco & J. L. Ross (Eds.), *Neurogenetic developmental disorders: Variation in manifestation in childhood* (pp. 199–262). Cambridge, MA: MIT Press.

Mervis, C. B., Robinson, B. F., Bertrand, J., Morris, C. A., Klein-Tasman, B. P., & Armstrong, S. C. (2000). The Williams syndrome cognitive profile. *Brain and Cognition, 44*, 604–628.

Mervis, C. B., Robinson, B. F., Rowe, M. L., Becerra, A. M., & Klein-Tasman, B. P. (2004). Language abilities of individuals with Williams syndrome. In L. Abbeduto (Ed.), *International review of research in mental retardation: Language and communication in mental retardation* (Vol. 27, pp. 35–81). San Diego: Academic Press.

Merzenich, M. M., Saunders, G., Jenkins, W. M., Miller, S., Peterson, B., & Tallal, P. (1999). Pervasive developmental disorders: Listening training and language abilities. In S. H. Broman & J. M. Fletcher (Eds.), *The changing nervous system: Neurobehavioral consequences of early brain disorders.* (pp. 365–385). New York: Oxford.

Mesibov, G. B., Adams, L. W., & Klinger, L. G. (1997). *Autism: Understanding the disorder*. New York: Plenum.

Meyer-Lindenberg, A., Kohn, P., Mervis, C. B., Kippenhan, J. S., Olsen, R. K., Morris, C. A., et al. (2004). Neural basis of genetically determined visuospatial construction deficit in Williams syndrome. *Neuron, 43*, 623–631.

Meyer-Lindenberg, A., Mervis, C. B., & Berman, K. F. (2006). Neural mechanisms in Williams syndrome: A unique window to genetic influences on cognition and behavior. *Nature, 7*, 380–393.

Meyer-Lindenberg, A., Mervis, C. B., Sarpal, D., Koch, P., Steele, S., Kohn, P., et al. (2005). Functional, structural, and metabolic abnormalities of the hippocampal formation in Williams syndrome. *Journal of Clinical Investigation, 115*, 1888–1895.

Meyerson, M. D., & Frank, R. A. (1987). Language, speech and hearing in Williams syndrome: Intervention approaches and research needs. *Developmental Medicine & Child Neurology, 29*, 258–262.

Michelson, D., Allen, A. J., Busner, J., Casat, C., Dunn, D., Kratochvil, C., et al. (2002). Once-daily atomoxetine treatment for children and adolescents with attention deficit hyperactivity disorder: A randomized, placebo-controlled study. *American Journal of Psychiatry, 159*, 1896–1901.

Mickelwright, J. L., King, T. Z., Morris, R., & Morris, M., K. (2007). Attention and memory in children with brain tumors. *Child Neuropsychology, 13*, 522–527.

Mik, G., Gholve, P. A., Scher, D. M., Widmann, R. F., & Green, D. W. (2008). Down syndrome: Orthopedic issues. *Current Opinion in Pediatrics, 20*, 30–36.

Mikkola, K., Ritari, N., Tommiska, V., Salokorpi, T., Lehtonen, L., Tammela, O., et al. (2005). Neurodevelopmental outcome at 5 years of age of a national cohort of extremely low birth weight infants who were born in 1996–1997. *Pediatrics, 116*, 1391–1400.

Milberg, W., & Hebben, N. (2006). The historical antecedents of the Boston Process Approach. In A. M. Poreh (Ed.), *The quantified process approach to neuropsychological assessment. Studies on neuropsychology, neurology and cognition* (pp. 17–25). Philadelphia: Taylor & Francis.

Miller, C., Kail, R., Leonard, L., & Tomblin, B. (2001). Speed of processing in children with specific language impairment. *Journal of Speech, Language, and Hearing Research, 44*, 416–433.

Miller, C. J., & Hynd, G. W. (2004). What ever happened to developmental Gerstmann's syndrome? Links to other pediatric, genetic, and neurodevelopmental syndromes. *Journal of Child Neurology, 19*, 282–289.

Miller, C. J., Hynd, G. W., & Miller, S. R. (2005). Children with dyslexia: Not necessarily at risk for elevated internalizing symptoms. *Reading and Writing: An Interdisciplinary Journal, 18*, 425–436.

Miller, C. J., Sanchez, J., & Hynd, G. W. (2003). Neurological correlates of reading disabilities. In H. L. Swanson, K. R. Harris, & S. Graham (Eds.), *Handbook of learning disabilities* (pp. 242–255). New York: Guilford.

Miller, J. F., Leddy, M., Miolo, G., & Sedey, A. (1995). The development of early language skills in children with Down syndrome. In L. Nadel & D. Rosenthal (Eds.), *Down syndrome: Living and learning in the community* (pp. 115–120). New York: Wiley.

Miller, J. L., Couch, J. A., Schmalfuss, I., He, G., Liu, Y., & Driscoll, D. J. (2007). Intracranial abnormalities detected by three-dimensional magnetic resonance imaging in Prader-Willi syndrome. *American Journal of Medical Genetics, 143*, 476–483.

Miller, J. L., James, G. A., Goldstone, A. P., Couch, J. A., He, G., Driscoll, D. J., et al. (2007). Enhanced activation of reward mediating prefrontal regions in response to food stimuli in Prader-Willi syndrome. *Journal of Neurology, Neurosurgery, & Psychiatry, 78*, 615–619.

Miller, J. L., Kranzler, J., Liu, Y., Schmalfuss, I., Theriaque, D. W., Shuster, J. J., et al. (2006). Neurocognitive findings in Prader-Willi syndrome and early-onset morbid obesity. *Journal of Pediatrics, 149*, 192–198.

Miller, R. W., Young, J. L., & Novakovic, B. (1995). Childhood cancer. *Cancer: A Cancer Journal for Clinicians, 75*, 395–405.

Miller, V. S., & Bigler, E. D. (1982). Neuropsychological aspects of tuberous sclerosis. *Clinical Neuropsychology, 4*, 26–34.

Min, S. K. (1986). A brain syndrome associated with delayed neuropsychiatric sequelae following acute carbon monoxide intoxification. *Acta Psychiatrica of Scandinavia, 73*, 80–86.

Miniscalco, C., Nygren, G., Hagberg, B., Kadesjö, B., & Gillberg, C. (2006). Neuropsychiatric and neurodevelopmental outcome of children at age 6 and 7 years who screened positive language problems at 30 months. *Developmental Medicine & Child Neurology, 48*, 361–366.

Mink, J. W. (2001). Basal ganglia dysfunction in Tourette's syndrome: A new hypothesis. *Pediatric Neurology, 25*, 190–198.

Minshew, N. J. (1997). Pervasive developmental disorders: Autism and similar disorders. In T. E. Feinberg & M. J. Farah (Eds.), *Behavioral neurology and neuropsychology* (pp. 817–826). New York: McGraw-Hill.

Minshew, N. J., & Goldstein, G. (1993). Is autism an amnesic disorder? Evidence from the California Verbal Learning Test. *Neuropsychology, 7*, 209–216.

Minshew, N. J., Meyer, J., & Goldstein, G. (2002). Abstract reasoning in autism: A dissociation between concept formation and concept identification. *Neuropsychology, 16*, 327–334.

Minshew, N. J., Sung, K., Jones, B. L., & Furman, J. M. (2004). Underdevelopment of the postural control system in autism. *Neurology, 63*, 2056–2061.

Mirrett, P. L., Roberts, J. E., & Price, J. (2003). Early intervention practices and communication intervention strategies for young males with fragile X syndrome. *Language, Speech and Hearing Services in the Schools, 34*, 320–331.

Mitby, P. A., Robison, L. L., Whitton, J. A., Zevon, M. A., Gibbs, I. C., Tersak, J. M., et al. (2003). Utilization of special education services and educational attainment among long-term survivors of childhood cancer. *Cancer, 97*, 1115–1126.

Mitchell, W. G., Chavez, J. M., Lee, H., & Guzman, B. L. (1991). Academic underachievement in children with epilepsy. *Journal of Child Neurology, 6*, 65–72.

Mobbs, D., Eckert, M. A., Mills, D., Korenberg, J., Bellugi, U., Galaburda, A., et al. (2007). Frontostriatal dysfunction during response inhibition in Williams syndrome. *Biological Psychiatry, 62*, 256–261.

Mobbs, D., Garrett, A. S., Menon, V., Rose, F. E., Bellugi, U., & Reiss, A. L. (2004). Anomalous brain activation during face and gaze processing in Williams syndrome. *Neurology, 62*, 2070–2076.

Moberg, P. J., & Kniele, K. (2006). Evaluation of competency: Ethical considerations for neuropsychologists. *Applied Neuropsychology, 13*, 101–114.

Modahl, C., Green, L., Fein, D., Morris, M., Waterhouse, L., Feinstein, C., et al. (1998). Plasma oxytocin levels in autistic children. *Biological Psychiatry, 43*, 270–277.

Mody, R., Li, S., Dover, D. C., Sallan, S., Leisenring, W., Oeffinger, K. C., et al. (2008). Twenty-five year follow-up among survivors of childhood acute lymphoblastic leukemia: A report from the Childhood Cancer Survivor Study. *Blood, 111*, 5515–5523.

Moleski, M. (2000). Neuropsychological, neuroanatomical, and neurophysiological consequences of CNS chemotherapy for acute lymphoblastic leukemia. *Archives of Clinical Neuropsychology, 15*, 603–630.

Molfese, D. L., Molfese, V. J., Beswick, J., Jacobi-Vessels, J., Molfese, P. J., Key, A. P. F., et al. (2008). Dynamic links between emerging cognitive skills and brain processes. *Developmental Neuropsychology, 33*, 682–706.

Molfese, V. J., DiLalla, L. F., & Lovelace, L. (1996). Perinatal, home environment, and infant measures as successful predictors of preschool cognitive and verbal abilities. *International Journal of Behavioral Development, 19*, 101–119.

Molitor, A., Mayes, L. C., & Ward, A. (2003). Emotion regulation behavior during a separation procedure in 18-month-old children of mothers using cocaine and other drugs. *Development and Psychopathology, 15*, 39–54.

Molko, N., Cachia, A., Riviere, D., Mangin, J. F., Bruandet, M., LeBihan, D., et al. (2003). Functional and structural alternations of the intraparietal sulcus in a developmental dyscalculia of genetic origin. *Neuron, 40*, 847–858.

Momin, S., Flores, S., Angel, B., Codner, D., Carrasco, P., & Perez-Bravo, F. (2009). Interactions between programmed death 1 (PD-1) and cytotoxic T lymphocyte antigen 4 (CTLA-4) gene polymorphisms in type 1 diabetes. *Diabetes Research and Clinical Practice, 83*, 289–294.

Montague, M. (2008). Self-regulation strategies to improve mathematical problem solving for students with learning disabilities. *Learning Disability Quarterly, 31*, 37–44.

Montague, M., Applegate, B., & Marquard, K. (1993). Cognitive strategy instruction and mathematical problem-solving performance of students with learning disabilities. *Learning Disabilities Research & Practice, 8*, 223–232.

Moon, C., Marlowe, M., Stellern, J., & Errera, J. (1985). Main and interaction effects of metallic pollutants on cognitive functioning. *Journal of Learning Disabilities, 18*, 217–221.

Moore, B., III. (2000). Brain volume in children with neurofibromatosis type 1: Relation to neuropsychological status. *Neurology, 54*, 914–920.

Moore, S. J., Turnpenny, P. D., Quinn, A., Glover, S., Lloyd, D. J., Montgomery, T., et al. (2000). A clinical study of 57 children with fetal anticonvulsant syndrome. *Journal of Medical Genetics, 37*, 489–497.

Moretto, M. B., Lerman, C. L., Morsch, V. M., Bohrer, D., Ineu, R. P., da Silva, A. C., et al. (2004). Effect of subchronic treatment with mercury chloride on NTPDase, 5'-nucleotidase and acetylcholinesterase from cerebral cortex of rats. *Journal of Trace Elements in Medicine and Biology, 7*, 255–260.

Morgan, A. E., & Hynd, G. W. (1998). Dyslexia, neurolinguistic ability, and anatomical variation of the planum temporale. *Neuropsychology Review, 8*, 79–93.

Morgan, A. E., Hynd, G. W., Riccio, C. A., & Hall, J. (1996). Validity of DSM-IV ADHD predominantly inattentive and combined types: Relationship to previous DSM diagnoses/subtype differences. *Journal of the American Academy of Child & Adolescent Psychiatry, 35*, 325–333.

Morgan, S. A., & Jackson, J. (1986). Psychological and social concomitants of sickle cell anemia in adolescents. *Journal of Pediatric Psychology, 11*, 429–440.

Morris, C. A. (2006). The dysmorphology, genetics, and natural history of Williams-Beuren syndrome. In C. A. Morris, H. M. Lenhoff, & P. P. Wang (Eds.), *Williams-Beuren syndrome: Research, evaluation, and treatment* (pp. 3–17). Baltimore, MD: Johns Hopkins University Press.

Morris, D. W., Ivanov, D., Robinson, L., Williams, N., Stevenson, J., Owen, M. J., et al. (2004). Association analysis of two candidate phospholipase genes that map to the chromosome 15q15.1–15.3 region associated with reading disability. *American Journal of Medical Genetics, 129B*(1), 97–103.

Morris, R. J., & Morris, Y. P. (1998). Angelman syndrome. In L. Phelps (Ed.), *Health-related disorders in children and adolescents: A guidebook for understanding and educating* (pp. 50–55). Washington, DC: American Psychological Association.

Morrison, I., Lloyd, D., DiPellegrino, G., & Roberts, N. (2004). Vicarious responses to pain in anterior cingulate cortex: Is empathy a multisensory issue? *Cognitive, Affective, and Behavioral Neuroscience, 4*, 270–278.

Morrison, J. L., Riggs, K. W., & Rurak, D. W. (2005). Fluoxetine during pregnancy: Impact on fetal development. *Reproduction, Fertility, and Development, 17*, 641–650.

Morrow, C. E., Culbertson, J. L., Accornero, V. H., Xue, L., Anthony, J. C., & Bandstra, E. S. (2006). Learning disabilities and intellectual functioning in school-aged children with prenatal cocaine exposure. *Developmental Neuropsychology, 30*, 905–931.

Morse, S., Haritou, F., Ong, K., Anderson, V., Catroppa, C., & Rosenfeld, J. (1999). Early effects of traumatic brain injury on young children's language performance: A preliminary linguistic analysis. *Pediatric Rehabilitation, 3,* 139–148.

Moses, M., Johnson, E. S., Anger, W. K., Burse, V. W., Horstman, S. W., Jackson, R. J., et al. (1993). Environmental equity and pesticide exposure. *Toxicology and Industrial Health, 9*, 913–959.

Mostofsky, S. H., Burgess, M. P., & Larson, J. C. G. (2007). Increased motor cortex white matter volume predicts motor impairment in autism. *Brain, 130*, 2117–2122.

Mott, L. (1995). The disproportionate impact of environmental health threats on children of color. *Environmental Health Perspectives, 103*(Suppl. 6), 33–35.

Moyle, J. J., Fox, A. M., Arthur, M., Bynevelt, M., & Burnett, J. R. (2007). Meta-analysis of neuropsychological symptoms of adolescents and adults with PKU. *Neuropsychology Review, 17*(2), 91–101.

Moyle, J. J., Fox, A. M., Bynevelt, M., Arthur, M., & Burnett, J. R. (2006). Event-related potentials elicited during a visual go-no-go task in adults with phenylketonuria. *Clinical Neurophysiology, 117*, 2154–2160.

MTA Cooperative Group (1999a). A 14-month randomized clinical trial of treatment strategies for attention-deficit/hyperactivity disorder. *Archives of General Psychiatry, 56*, 1073–1086.

MTA Cooperative Group (1999b). Moderators and mediators of treatment response for children with attention-deficit/hyperactivity disorder. *Archives of General Psychiatry, 56*, 1088–1096.

MTA Cooperative Group (2004). National Institute of Mental Health multimodal treatment study of ADHD follow-up: 24-month outcomes of treatment strategies for attention-deficit/hyperactivity disorder. *Pediatrics, 113*, 754–761.

Mudrick, N. R. (2002). The prevalence of disability among children: Paradigms and estimates. *Physical Medical Rehabilitation Clinics of North America, 13*, 775–792.

Muhle, R., Trentacoste, S. V., & Rapin, I. (2004). The genetics of autism. *Pediatrics, 113*, 472–486.

Mula, M., Schmitz, B., & Sander, J. W. (2008). The pharmacological treatment of depression in adults with epilepsy. *Expert Opinion on Pharmacotherapy, 9*, 3159–3168.

Mulhern, R. K., & Butler, R. T. (2004). Neurocognitive sequelae of childhood cancers and their treatment. *Pediatric Rehabilitation, 7*, 1–14.

Mulhern, R. K., & Butler, R. T. (2006). Neuropsychological late effects. In R. T. Brown (Ed.), *Comprehensive handbook of childhood cancer and sickle cell disease: A biopsychosocial approach* (pp. 262–278). New York: Oxford University Press.

Mulhern, R. K., Reddick, W. E., Palmer, S. L., Glass, J. O., Elkin, T. D., Kun, L. E., et al. (1999). Neurocognitive deficits in medulloblastoma survivors are associated with white matter loss. *Annals of Neurology, 46*, 834–841.

Mulhern, R. K., White, H. A., Glass, J. O., Kun, L. E., Thompson, S. J., et al. (2004). Attentional functioning and white matter integrity among survivors of malignant brain tumors of childhood. *Journal of the International Neuropsychological Society, 10*, 180–189.

Muller, F., Reviffé, M., Taillandier, A., Oury, J.-F., & Mornet, E. (2000). Parental origin of the extra chromosome in prenatally diagnosed fetal trisomy 21. *Human Genetics, 106*, 340–344.

Müller, R.-A., Behen, M., Rothermel, R., Chugani, D. C., Muzik, T. J., & Chugani, H. T. (1999). Brain mapping of language and auditory perception in high-functioning autistic adults: A PET study. *Journal of Autism and Developmental Disorders, 29*, 19–31.

Müller, R. A., Pierce, K., Ambrose, J. B., Allen, G., & Courchesne, E. (2001). Atypical patterns of cerebral motor activation in autism: A functional magnetic resonance imaging study. *Biological Psychiatry, 49*, 665–676.

Muller, S. V., Johannes, S., Wieringa, B., Weber, A., Muller-Vahl, K., Matzke, M., et al. (2003). Disturbed monitoring and response inhibition in patients with Gilles de la Tourette syndrome and co-morbid obsessive compulsive disorder. *Behavioural Neurology, 14*, 29–37.

Mullis, I. V. S., Dossey, J. A., Owen, E. H., & Phillips, G. W. (1991). *The state of mathematics achievement: NAEP's 1990 assessment of the nation and the trial assessment of the states*. Washington, DC: U. S. Department of Education.

Muñoz-Yunta, J. A., Ortiz, T., Palau-Baduell, M., Martin-Muñoz, L., Salvadó-Salvadó, B., Valls-Sanasusana, A., et al. (2008). Magnetocephalographic pattern of epileptiform activity in children with early onset autism spectrum disorders. *Clinical Neurophysiology, 119*, 626–634.

Munro, N., Lee, K., & Baker, E. (2008). Building vocabulary knowledge and phonological awareness skills in children with specific language impairment through hybrid language intervention: A feasibility study. *International Journal of Language & Communication Disorders, 43*, 662–682.

Murdoch, B. E., & Whelan, B.-M. (2007). Language disorders subsequent to left cerebellar lesions. A case for bilateral cerebellar involvement in language? *Folia Phoniatrica et Logopaedica, 59*(4), 184–189.

Murphy, A. M., Lambert, D., Treacy, E. P., O'Meara, A., & Lynch, S. A. (2009). Incidence and prevalence of mucopolysaccharidosis type 1 in the Irish Republic. *Archives of Disease in Childhood, 94*, 52–54.

Murphy, C. C., Schei, B., Myhr, T. L., & Du Mont, J. (2001). Abuse: A risk factor for low birth weight? A systematic review and meta-analysis. *Canadian Medical Association Journal, 164*, 1567–1572.

Murphy, M. M., & Mazzocco, M. M. M. (2008). Mathematics learning disabilities in girls with fragile X or Turner syndrome during late elementary school. *Journal of Learning Disabilities, 41*, 29–46.

Murphy, M. M., & Mazzocco, M. M. M. (2008). Rote numeric skills may mask underlying mathematical disabilities in girls with fragile X syndrome. *Developmental Neuropsychology, 33*, 345–364.

Muzykewicz, D. A., Newberry, P., Danforth, N., Halpern, E. F., & Thiele, E. A. (2007). Psychiatric comorbid conditions in a clinic population of 241 patients with tuberous sclerosis complex. *Epilepsy & Behavior, 11*, 506–513.

Myers, G. J., Davidson, P. W., Cox, C., Shamlaye, C. F., Palumbo, D., Cernichiari, E., et al. (2003). Prenatal methylmercury exposure from ocean fish consumption in the Seychelles child development study. *Lancet, 961*, 1686–1692.

Myers, R. A. M., Snyder, S. K., & Emhoff, T. A. (1995). Sequelae of carbon monoxide poisoning. *Journal of Clinical Anesthesia, 7*, 87.

Myerson, M. D., & Frank, R. A. (1987). Language, speech and hearing in Williams syndrome: Intervention approaches and research needs. *Developmental Medicine & Child Neurology, 29*, 258–262.

Myles, B. S., Grossman, B. G., Aspy, R., Henry, S. A., & Coffin, A. B. (2007). Planning a comprehensive program for students with autism spectrum disorders using evidence-based practices. *Education and Training in Developmental Disabilities, 42*, 398–409.

Naber, F. B. A., Swinkels, S. H. N., Buitelaar, J. K., Dietz, C., van Daalen, E., Bakermans-Kranenburg, M. J., et al. (2007). Joint attention and attachment in toddlers with autism. *Journal of Abnormal Child Psychology, 35*, 899–911.

Nadebaum, C., Anderson, V., & Catroppa, C. (2007). Executive function outcomes following traumatic brain injury in young children: A five-year follow-up. *Developmental Neuropsychology, 32*, 703–728.

Nadel, L. (2003). Down's syndrome: A genetic disorder in biobehavioral perspective. *Genes, Brain & Behavior, 2*(3), 156–166.

Nadel, L., & Uecker, A. (1998). Spatial but not object memory impairments in children with fetal alcohol syndrome. *American Journal of Mental Retardation, 103*, 12–18.

Nagaraj, R., Singhi, P., & Malhi, P. (2006). Risperidone in children with autism: Randomized, placebo-controlled, double-blind study. *Journal of Child Neurology, 21*, 450–455.

Narita, T., & Koga, Y. (1987). Neuropsychological assessment of childhood autism. *Advances in Biological Psychiatry, 16*, 156–170.

Nass, R. D., & Trauner, D. (2004). Social and affective impairments are important recovery after acquired stroke in childhood. *CNS Spectrums, 9*, 420–434.

Nathan, P. C., Patel, S. K., Dilley, K., Goldsby, R., Harvey, J., Jacobsen, C., et al. (2007). Guidelines for identification of, advocacy for, and intervention in neurocognitive problems in survivors of childhood cancer: A report from the Children's Oncology Group. *Archives of Pediatrics & Adolescent Medicine, 161*, 798–806.

Nation, K., Clarke, P., Wright, B., & Williams, C. (2006). Patterns of reading ability in children with autism spectrum disorder. *Journal of Autism and Developmental Disorders, 36*, 911–919.

National Center for Environmental Health. (2001). *National Health and Nutrition Examination Survey (NHANES)*. Atlanta, GA: Centers for Disease Control and Prevention.

National Institute of Child Health and Human Development. (2000). *Report of the National Reading Panel. Teaching children to read: An evidence-based assessment of the scientific literature on reading and its implications for reading instruction (NIH Publication No. 004769).* Washington, DC: U. S. Government Printing Office.

National Institute of Mental Health (1999). *Autism.* Washington, DC: U. S. Government Printing Office.

Nattrass, M., & Hale, P. F. (1988). Diabetes mellitus. In M. C. Sheppard & J. A. Franklin (Eds.), *Clinical endocrinology and diabetes* (pp. 154–182). Edinburgh: Churchill Livingstone.

Needleman, H. L. (2002). Bone lead levels in adjudicated delinquents: A case control study. *Neurotoxicology and Teratology, 24*, 711–717.

Needleman, H. L., & Gatsonis, C. A. (1990). Low-level lead exposure and IQ of children: Meta-analysis of modern studies. *Journal of the American Medical Association, 263*, 673–678.

Neeley, E. S., Bigler, E. D., Krasny, L., Ozonoff, S., McMahon, W., & Lainhart, J. E. (2007). Quantitative temporal lobe differences: Autism distinguished from controls using classification and regression tree analysis. *Brain & Development, 29*, 389–399.

Neppe, V. M., & Tucker, G. J. (1994). Neuropsychiatric aspects of epilepsy and atypical spells. In S. C. Yudofsky & R. E. Hales (Eds.), *Synopsis of neuropsychiatry* (pp. 307–328). Washington, DC: American Psychiatric Association.

Newbury, D. F., Bishop, D. V. M., & Monaco, A. P. (2005). Genetic influences on language impairment and phonological short-term memory. *Trends in Cognitive Science, 9*, 528–534.

Newcorn, J. H., Kratochvil, C. J., Allen, A. J., Casat, C. D., Ruff, D. D., Moore, R. J., et al. (2008). Atomoxetine and osmotically released methylphenidate for the treatment of attention deficit hyperactivity disorder: Acute comparison and differential response. *American Journal of Psychiatry, 165*, 721–730.

Newman, T. M., Macomber, D., Naples, A. J., Babitz, T., Volkmar, F., & Grigorenko, E. L. (2007). Hyperlexia in children with autism spectrum disorders. *Journal of Autism and Developmental Disorders, 37*, 760–774.

Newport, D. J., Viguera, A. C., Beach, A. J., Ritchie, J. C., Cohen, L. S., & Stowe, Z. N. (2005). Lithium placental passage and obstetrical outcome: Implications for clinical management during late pregnancy. *American Journal of Psychiatry, 162*, 2162–2170.

Newschaffer, C. J., Croen, L. A., Daniels, J., Giarelli, E., Grether, J. K., Levy, S. E., et al. (2007). The epidemiology of autism spectrum disorders. *Annual Review of Public Health, 28*, 235–258.

Nicolson, R., Craven-Thuss, B., Smith, J., McKinlay, B. D., & Castellanos, F. X. (2005). A randomized, double-blind, placebo-controlled trial of metoclopramide for the treatment of Tourette's disorder. *Journal of the American Academy of Child and Adolescent Psychiatry, 44*, 640–646.

Nicolson, R. I., Fawcett, A. J., & Dean, P. (2001). Developmental dyslexia: The cerebellar deficit hypothesis. *Trends in Neurosciences, 24*, 508–511.

Nigg, J. T. (2005). Neuropsychologic theory and findings in attention-deficit/hyperactivity disorder: The state of the field and salient challenges for the coming decade. *Biological Psychiatry, 57*, 1424–1435.

Nilsson, D., & Bradford, L. W. (1999). Neurofibromatosis. In S. Goldstein & C. R. Reynolds (Eds.), *Handbook of neurodevelopmental and genetic disorders in children* (pp. 350–367). New York: Guilford.

Nittrouer, S., & Burton, L. T. (2005). The role of early language experience in the development of speech perception and phonological processing abilities: Evidence from 5-year-olds with histories of otitis media with effusion and low socioeconomic status. *Journal of Communication Disorders, 38*, 29–63.

Noeker, M., & Haverkamp, F. (2001). Successful cognitive-behavioral habituation training toward photophobia in photogenic partial seizures. *Epilepsia, 42*, 689–691.

Noland, J. S., Singer, L. T., Short, E. J., Minnes, S., Arendt, R. E., Kirchner, H. l. L., et al. (2005). Prenatal drug exposure and selective attention in preschoolers. *Neurotoxicology and Teratology, 27*, 429–438.

Noll, R. B., & Kupst, M. J. (2007). Commentary: The psychological impact of pediatric cancer hardiness, the exception or the rule? *Journal of Pediatric Psychology, 32*, 1089–1098.

Noll, R. B., Reiter-Purtill, J., Moore, B. D., Schorry, E. K., Lovell, A. M., Vannatta, K., et al. (2007). Social, emotional, and behavioral functioning of children with NF1. *American Journal of Medical Genetics, 143A*, 2261–2273.

Noll, R. B., Reiter-Purtill, J., Vannatta, K., & Gerhardt, C. A. (2007). Peer relationships and emotional well-being of children with sickle cell disease. *Child Neuropsychology, 13*, 173–187.

Nomura, Y., & Segawa, M. (2003). Neurology of Tourette's syndrome (TS): TS as a developmental dopamine disorder: A hypothesis. *Brain & Development, 25*, S37–S42.

Noordam, C., van der Burgt, I., Sengers, R. C., Delemarre-van de Waal, H. A., & Otten, B. J. (2001). Growth hormone treatment in children with Noonan's syndrome: Four-year results of a partly controlled trial. *Acta Paediatrica, 90*, 889–894.

Northam, E. A., Anderson, P. J., Jacobs, R., Hughes, M., Warne, G. L., & Werther, G. A. (2001). Neuropsychological profiles of children with type 1 diabetes 6 years after disease onset. *Diabetes Care, 24*, 1541–1546.

Nosarti, C., Al-Asady, M. H. S., Frangou, S., Stewart, A. L., Rifkin, L., & Murray, R. M. (2002). Adolescents who were born very preterm have decreased brain volumes. *Brain, 125*, 1616–1623.

Nussbaum, N. L., & Bigler, E. D. (1997). Halstead-Reitan neuropsychological test batteries for children. In C. R. Reynolds & E. Fletcher-Janzen (Eds.), *Handbook of clinical child neuropsychology* (2nd ed., pp. 219–236). New York: Plenum.

Nuzzolo-Gomez, R., Leonard, M. A., Ortiz, E., Rivera, C. M., & Greer, R. D. (2002). Teaching children with autism to prefer books or toys over stereotype or passivity. *Journal of Positive Behavior Interventions, 4*, 80–87.

Oakhill, J., & Kyle, F. (2000). The relation between phonological awareness and working memory. *Journal of Experimental Child Psychology, 75*, 152–164.

Oberman, L. M., Hubbard, E. M., McCleery, J. P., Altschuler, E. L., Ramachandran, V. S., & Pineda, J. A. (2005). EEG evidence for mirror neuron dysfunction in autism spectrum disorders. *Cognitive Brain Research, 24*, 190–198.

Oberman, L. M., & Ramachandran, V. S. (2007). The simulating social mind: The role of the mirror neuron system and simulation in the social communicative deficits of autism spectrum disorders. *Psychological Bulletin, 133*, 310–327.

Oberman, L. M., Ramachandran, V. S., & Pineda, J. A. (2008). Modulation of mu suppression in children with autism spectrum disorders in response to familiar and unfamiliar stimuli: The mirror neuron hypothesis. *Neuropsychologia, 46*, 1558–1565.

Obrzut, J. E., & Wacha, V. H. (2007). Effects of fetal alcohol syndrome on neuropsychological function. *Journal of Developmental Physical Disabilities, 19*, 217–226.

O'Connor, R., Jenkins, J., Leicester, N., & Slocum, T. (1993). Teaching phonological awareness to young children with learning disabilities. *Exceptional Children, 59*, 532–546.

Odom, S. L., Brown, W. H., Frey, T., Karasu, N., Smith-Canter, L. L., & Strain, P. S. (2003). Evidence-based practices for young children with autism: Contributions for single-subject design research. *Focus on Autism and Other Developmental Disabilities, 18*, 166–175.

O'Hare, A. E., Brown, J. K., & Aitken, K. (1991). Dyscalculia in children. *Developmental Medicine & Child Neurology, 33*, 356–361.

O'Hearn, K., & Landau, B. (2007). Mathematical skill in individuals with Williams syndrome: Evidence from a standardized mathematics battery. *Brain and Cognition, 64*, 238–246.

O'Keeffe, M. J., O'Callaghan, M., Williams, G. M., Najman, J. M., & Bor, W. (2003). Learning, cognitive, and attentional problems in adolescents born small for gestational age. *Pediatrics, 112*, 301–307.

O'Leary, D. S., Lovell, M. R., Sackellares, J. C., Berent, S., Giordani, B., Seidenberg, M., et al. (1983). Effects of age of onset of partial and generalized seizures on neuropsychological performance in children. *Journal of Nervous and Mental Disease, 171*, 623–629.

Olafsen, K. S., Ronning, J. A., Kaaresen, P. I., Ulvund, S. E., Handegard, B. H., & Dahl, L. B. (2006). Joint attention in term and preterm infants at 12 months corrected age: The significance of gender and intervention based on a randomized controlled trial. *Infant Behavior & Development, 29*, 554–563.

Oliveira, E. P. M., Hage, S. R. V., Guimarães, C. A., Brandão-Almeida, I., Lopes-Cendes, I., Guerreiro, C. A., et al. (2008). Characterization of language and reading skills in familial polymicrogyria. *Brain & Development, 30*, 254–260.

Oliver, C., Horsler, K., Berg, K., Bellamy, G., Dick, K., & Griffiths, E. (2007). Genomic imprinting and the expression of affect in Angelman syndrome: What's in a smile? *Journal of Child Psychology and Psychiatry, 48*, 571–579.

Olivieri, N. F., Brittenham, G. M., Matsui, D., Berkovitch, M., Blendis, L. M., Cameron, R. G., et al. (1995). Iron-chelation therapy with oral deferiprone in patients with thalassemia major. *New England Journal of Medicine, 332*, 918–922.

Olson, R. K. (2004). SSSR, environment, and genes. *Scientific Studies of Reading, 8*(2), 111–124.

Oostrom, K. J., Smeets-Schouten, A., Kruitwagen, C. L. J. J., Peters, A. C. B., Jennekens-Schinkel, A., & Dutch Study Group of Epilepsy in Childhood. (2003). Not only a matter of epilepsy: Early problems of cognition and behavior in children with "epilepsy only"—a prospective, longitudinal, controlled study starting at diagnosis. *Pediatrics, 112*, 1338–1344.

O'Reilly, M. F., & Lancioni, G. E. (2001). Treating food refusal in a child with Williams syndrome using the parent as therapist in the home setting. *Journal of Intellectual Disability Research, 45*, 41–46.

Ornitz, E. M., Atwell, C. W., Kaplan, A. R., & Westlake, J. R. (1985). Brain-stem dysfunction in autism: Results of vestibular stimulation. *Archives of General Psychiatry, 42*, 1018–1025.

Ortinski, P., & Meador, K. J. (2004). Cognitive side effects of antiepileptic drugs. *Epilepsy and Behavior, 5*, 560–565.

O'Shea, T. M., Washburn, L. K., Nixon, P. A., & Goldstein, D. J. (2007). Follow-up of a randomized, placebo-controlled trial of dexamethasone to decrease the duration of ventilator dependency in very low birth weight infants: Neurodevelopmental outcomes at 4 to 11 years of age. *Pediatrics, 120,* 594–602.

Osmon, D. C., & Smerz, J. M. (2005). Neuropsychological evaluation in the diagnosis and treatment of Tourette's syndrome. *Behavior Modification, 29*, 746–783.

Osmon, D. C., Smerz, J. M., Braun, M. M., & Plambeck, E. (2006). Processing abilities associated with math skills in adult learning disability. *Journal of Clinical and Experimental Neuropsychology, 28*, 84–95.

Osterling, J., Dawson, G., & Munson, J. (2002). Early recognition of one-year-old infants with autism spectrum disorder versus mental retardation: A study of first birthday party home videotapes. *Development and Psychopathology, 14*, 239–251.

Ott, D., Siddarth, P., Gurbani, S., Koh, S., Tournay, A., Shields, W. D., et al. (2003). Behavioral disorders in pediatric epilepsy: Unmet psychiatric need. *Epilepsia, 44*, 591–597.

Overstreet, S., Holmes, C. S., Dunlap, W. P., & Frentz, J. (1997). Sociodemographic risk factors to intellectual and academic functioning in children with diabetes. *Intelligence, 24*, 367–380.

Ozonoff, S. (1995). Reliability and validity of the Wisconsin Card Sorting Test in studies of autism. *Neuropsychology, 9*, 491–500.

Ozonoff, S., & Jensen, J. (1999). Specific executive function profiles in three neurodevelopmental disorders. *Journal of Autism and Developmental Disorders, 29*, 171–177.

Ozonoff, S., Pennington, B. F., & Rogers, S. J. (1991). Executive function deficits in high-functioning autistic individuals: Relationship to theory of mind. *Journal of Child Psychology and Psychiatry, 32*, 1081–1105.

Ozonoff, S., & Rogers, S. J. (2003). From Kanner to the millennium. In S. Ozonoff, S. Rogers, & R. Hendren (Eds.), *Autism spectrum disorders: A research review for practitioners* (pp. 3–33). Washington, DC: American Psychiatric Publishing.

Ozonoff, S., & Strayer, D. L. (2001). Further evidence of intact working memory in autism. *Journal of Autism and Developmental Disorders, 331*, 257–263.

Ozonoff, S., Strayer, D. L., McMahon, W. M., & Filloux, F. (1998). Inhibitory deficits in Tourette syndrome: A function of comorbidity and symptom severity. *Journal of Child Psychology and Psychiatry, 39*, 1109–1118.

Ozonoff, S., Young, G. S., Goldring, S., Greiss-Hess, L., Herrera, A. M., Steele, J., et al. (2008). Gross motor development, movement abnormalities, and early identification of autism. *Journal of Autism and Developmental Disorders, 38*, 644–656.

Packer, L. E. (2005). Tic-related school problems: Impact on functioning, accommodations, and interventions. *Behavior Modification, 29*, 876–899.

Packman, A., Code, C., & Onslow, M. (2006). On the cause of stuttering: Integrating theory with brain and behavioral research. *Journal of Neurolinguistics, 20*, 353–362.

Pai, A. L. H., Drotar, D., Zebracki, K., Moore, M., & Youngstrom, E. (2006). A meta-analysis of the effects of psychological interventions in pediatric oncology on outcomes of psychological distress and adjustment. *Journal of Pediatric Psychology, 31*, 978–988.

Pakalnis, A., Paolicchi, J., & Gilles, E. (2000). Psychogenic status epilepticus in children: Psychiatric and other risk factors. *Neurology, 54*, 969–970.

Palade, S., & Benga, I. (2007). Neuropsychological impairments on the CANTAB test battery: Case reports of children with frontal and temporal lobe epilepsy. *Cognition, Brain, & Behavior, 11*, 539–552.

Palermo, T. M., Schwartz, L., Drotar, D., & McGowan, K. (2002). Parental report of health-related quality of life in children with sickle cell disease. *Journal of Behavioral Medicine, 25*, 269–283.

Palmer, S. L., Gajjar, A., Reddick, W. E., Glass, J. O., Kun, L. E., Wu, S., et al. (2003). Predicting intellectual outcome among children treated with 35–40 by craniospinal irradiation for medulloblastoma. *Neuropsychology, 17*, 548–555.

Palmer, S. L., Goloubeva, O., Reddick, W. E., Glass, J. O., Gajjar, A., Kun, L. E., et al. (2001). Patterns of intellectual development in long-term survivors of pediatric medulloblastoma: A longitudinal analysis. *Journal of Clinical Oncology, 19*, 2302–2308.

Palmer, S. L., Hanson, C. A., Zent, C. S., Porrata, L. F., Laplant, B., Geyer, S. M., et al. (2008). Prognostic importance of T and NK-cells in a consecutive series of newly diagnosed patients with chronic lymphocytic leukaemia. *British Journal of Haematology, 141*, 607–614.

Palmer, S. L., Reddick, W. E., & Gajjar, A. (2007). Understanding the cognitive impact on children who are treated for medulloblastoma. *Journal of Pediatric Psychology, 32*, 1040–1049.

Palmer, S. L., Reddick, W. E., Glass, J. O., Goloubeva, O., Gajjar, A., & Mulhern, R. K. (2002). Decline in corpus callosum volume among pediatric patients with medulloblastoma: A longitudinal MR image study. *American Journal of Neuroradiology, 23*, 1088–1094.

Paneth, N. (1995). The problem of low birth weight. *Future of Children, 5*, 19–34.

Paolicchi, J. (2002). Epilepsy in adolescents: Diagnosis and treatment. *Adolescent Medicine, 13*, 443–459.

Paprocka, J., Jamroz, E., Szwed-Bialozyt, B., Jezela-Stanek, A., Kopyta, I., & Marszal, E. (2007). Angelman syndrome revisited. *Neurologist, 13*, 305–312.

Paré-Blagoev, J. (2007). The neural correlates of reading disorder: Functional magnetic resonance imaging. In K. W. Fischer, J. H. Bernstein, & M. H. Immordino-Yang (Eds.), *Mind, brain, and education in reading disorders* (pp. 148–167). New York: Cambridge University Press.

Parikh, M. S., Kolevzon, A., & Hollander, E. (2008). Psychopharmacology of aggression in children and adolescents with autism: A critical review of efficacy and tolerability. *Journal of Child and Adolescent Psychopharmacology, 18*, 157–178.

Parker, J. G., & Asher, S. R. (1987). Peer relations and later personal adjustment: Are low-accepted children at risk? *Psychological Bulletin, 102*, 357–389.

Parrish, J., Geary, E., Jones, J., Seth, R., Hermann, B., & Seidenberg, M. (2007). Executive functioning in childhood epilepsy: Parent-report and cognitive assessment. *Developmental Medicine & Child Neurology, 49*, 412–416.

Parsa, C. F. (2008). Sturge-Weber syndrome: A unified pathophysiologic mechanism. *Current Treatment Options in Neurology, 10*, 47–54.

Pascalicchio, T. F., de Araujo Filho, G. M., da Silva Noffs, M. H., Lin, K., Cabocio, L. O. S. F., Vidal-Dourado, M., et al. (2007). Neuropsychological profile of patients with juvenile myoclonic epilepsy: A controlled study of 50 patients. *Epilepsy and Behavior, 10*, 263–267.

Pascual-Castroviejo, I., Pascual-Pascual, S.-I., Velazquez-Fragua, R., & Viaño, J. (2008). Sturge-Weber syndrome: Study of 55 patients. *Canadian Journal of Neurological Sciences, 35*, 301–307.

Passolunghi, M. C., & Cornoldi, C. (2008). Working memory failures in children with arithmetical difficulties. *Child Neuropsychology, 14*, 387–400.

Passolunghi, M. C., Mammarella, I. C., & Altoé, G. (2008). Cognitive abilities as precursors of the early acquisition of mathematical skills. *Developmental Neuropsychology, 33*, 229–250.

Passolunghi, M. C., & Siegel, L. S. (2004). Working memory and access to numerical information in children with disability in mathematics. *Journal of Experimental Child Psychology, 88*, 348–367.

Patenaude, A. F., & Kupst, M. J. (2005). Psychosocial functioning in pediatric cancer. *Journal of Pediatric Psychology, 30*, 9–27.

Paterson, S. J., Girelli, L., Butterworth, B., & Karmiloff-Smith, A. (2006). Are numerical impairments syndrome specific? Evidence from Williams syndrome and Down's syndrome. *Journal of Child Psychology and Psychiatry, 47*, 190–204.

Patra, K., Wilson-Costello, D., Taylor, H. G., Mercuri-Minich, N., & Hack, M. (2006). Grades I–II intraventricular hemorrhage in extremely low birth weight infants: Effects on neurodevelopment. *Journal of Pediatrics, 149*, 169–173.

Patteson, D. M., & Barnard, K. E. (1990). Parenting of low birth weight infants: A review of issues and interventions. *Infant Mental Health Journal, 11*, 37–56.

Patterson, D., & Lott, I. T. (2008). Etiology, diagnosis and development in Down syndrome. In J. E. Roberts, R. S. Chapman, & S. F. Warren (Eds.), *Speech and language development and intervention in Down syndrome and fragile X syndrome* (pp. 3–25). Baltimore, MD: Brookes.

Pattison, H. M., Moledina, S., & Barrett, T. G. (2006). The relationship between parental perceptions of diabetes and glycemic control. *Archives of Diseases in Children, 91*, 487–490.

Paul, R. (1992). Language and speech disorders. In S. R. Hooper, G. W. Hynd & R. E. Mattison (Eds.), *Developmental disorders: Diagnostic criteria and clinical assessment* (pp. 209–238). Hillsdale, NJ: Erlbaum.

Paulesu, E., Frith, U., Snowling, M., Gallegher, A., Morton, J., Frackowiak, R. S., et al. (1996). Is developmental dyslexia a disconnection syndrome? Evidence from PET scanning. *Brain, 119*, 143–157.

Pauls, D. L. (2003). An update on the genetics of Gilles de la Tourette syndrome. *Journal of Psychosomatic Research, 55*, 712.

Pavlakis, S. G., Bello, J., Prohovnik, I., Sutton, M., Ince, C., Mohr, J. P., et al. (1988). Brain infarction in sickle cell anemia: Magnetic resonance imaging correlated. *Annals of Neurology, 23*, 125–130.

Pavol, M., Hiscock, M., Massman, P., Moore, B., III, Foorman, B., & Meyers, C. (2006). Neuropsychological function in adults with von Recklinghausen's neurofibromatosis. *Developmental Neuropsychology, 29*, 509–526.

Pavone, P., Bianchini, R., Trifiletti, R. R., Incorpora, G., Pavone, A., & Parano, E. (2001). Neuropsychological assessment in children with absence epilepsy. *Neurology, 56*, 1047–1051.

PeBenito, R., Fisch, B. C., & Fisch, M. L. (1988). Developmental Gerstmann syndrome. *Archives of Neurology, 45*, 977–982.

Peckham, V. C. (1991). Educational deficits in survivors of childhood cancer. *Pediatrician, 18*, 25–31.

Pediatric OCD Treatment Study Team (2004). Cognitive-behavior therapy, sertraline, and their combination for children and adolescents with obsessive-compulsive disorder: The Pediatric OCD Treatment Study (POTS) randomized controlled trial. *Journal of the American Medical Association, 292*, 1969–1976.

Pegalow, C. H., Macklin, E. A., Moser, F. G., & Names, N. M. (2002). Longitudinal changes in brain magnetic resonance imaging findings in children with sickle cell disease. *Blood, 99*, 3014–3018.

Pelham, W. E., & Fabiano, G. A. (2008). Evidence-based psychosocial treatments for attention-deficit/hyperactivity disorder. *Journal of Clinical Child and Adolescent Psychology, 37*, 184–214.

Pelham, W. E., Fabiano, G. A., & Massetti, G. M. (2005). Evidence-based assessment of attention deficit hyperactivity disorder in children and adolescents. *Journal of Clinical Child and Adolescent Psychology, 34*, 449–476.

Pelham, W. E., Gnagy, E. M., Greiner, A. R., Hoza, B., Hinshaw, S. P., Swanson, J. M., et al. (2000). Behavioral versus behavioral and pharmacological treatment in ADHD children attending a summer treatment program. *Journal of Abnormal Child Psychology, 28*, 507–525.

Pelicano, E., Maybery, M., & Durkin, K. (2005). Central coherence in typically developing preschoolers: Does it cohere and does it related to mindreading and executive control? *Journal of Child Psychology and Psychiatry, 46*, 533–547.

Pelios, L. V., & Lund, S. K. (2001). A selective overview of issues on classification, causation, and early intensive behavioral intervention for autism. *Behavior Modification, 25*, 678–697.

Pellicano, E. (2007). Links between theory of mind and executive function in young children with autism: Clues to developmental primacy. *Developmental Psychology, 43*, 974–990.

Pelphrey, K. A., Morris, J. P., & McCarthy, G. (2005). Neural basis of eye gaze processing deficits in autism. *Brain, 128*, 1038–1048.

Pennington, B., Moon, J., Edgin, J., Stedron, J., & Nadel, L. (2003). The neuropsychology of Down syndrome: Evidence for hippocampal dysfunction. *Child Development, 74*, 75–93.

Pennington, B. F., Gilger, J. W., Pauls, D., Smith, S. A., Smith, S. D., & DeFries, J. C. (1991). Evidence for a major gene transmission of developmental dyslexia. *Journal of the American Medical Association, 266*, 1527–1534.

Pennington, B. F., McGrath, L. M., Rosenberg, J., Barnard, H., Smith, S. D., Willcutt, E. G., et al. (2009). Gene–environment interactions in reading disability and attention-deficit/hyperactivity disorder. *Developmental Psychology, 45*, 77–89.

Perantie, D. C., Lim, A., Wu, J., Weaver, P., Warren, S. L., Sadler, M., et al. (2008). Effects of prior hypoglycemia and hyperglycemia on cognition in children with type 1 diabetes mellitus. *Pediatric Diabetes, 9*(2), 887–895.

Perfetti, C. A., Landi, N., & Oakhill, J. (2005). The acquisition of reading comprehension skill. In M. Snowling & C. Hulme (Eds.), *The science of reading: A handbook* (pp. 227–247). Oxford: Blackwell.

Perlo, V. P., & Rak, E. T. (1971). Developmental dyslexia in adults. *Neurology, 21*, 1231–1235.

Perner, J., & Lang, B. (2000). Theory of mind and executive function: Is there a developmental relationship? In S. Baron-Cohen, H. Tager-Flusberg, & D. Cohen (Eds.), *Understanding other minds: Perspectives from autism and developmental cognitive neuroscience* (2nd ed., pp. 150–181). Oxford: Oxford University Press.

Perret, E. (1974). The left frontal lobe of man and the suppression of habitual responses in verbal categorical behaviour. *Neuropsychologia, 12*, 323–330.

Perrin, E. M., Murphy, M. L., Casey, J. R., Pichichero, M. E., Runyan, D. K., Miller, W. C., et al. (2004). Does group A beta-hemolytic streptococcal infection increase risk for behavioral and neuropsychiatric symptoms in children? *Archives of Pediatrics & Adolescent Medicine, 158*, 848–856.

Perruca, E. (2005). Birth defects after prenatal exposure to antiepileptic drugs. *Lancet Neurology, 4*, 781–786.

Persad, V., Thompson, M. D., & Percy, M. (2002). Epilepsy and developmental disability. Part I: Developmental disorders in which epilepsy may be comorbid. *Journal on Developmental Disabilities, 9*, 123–151.

Persico, A. M., & Bourgeron, T. (2006). Searching for ways out of the autism maze: Genetic, epigenetic, and environmental clues. *Trends in Neurosciences, 29*, 349–358.

Peters, S. U., Beaudet, A. L., Madduri, N., & Bacino, C. A. (2004). Autism in Angelman syndrome: Implications for autism research. *Clinical Genetics, 66*, 530–536.

Peters, S. U., Goddard-Finegold, J., Beaudet, A. L., & Madduir, N. (2004). Cognitive and adaptive behavior profiles of children with Angelman syndrome. *American Journal of Medical Genetics, 128A*, 110–113.

Peterson, B. S., Choi, H. A., Hao, X., Amat, J. A., Zhu, H., Whiteman, R., et al. (2007). Morphologic features of the amygdala and hippocampus in children and adults with Tourette syndrome. *Archives of General Psychiatry, 64*, 1281–1291.

Peterson, B. S., & Cohen, D. J. (1998). The treatment of Tourette's syndrome: Multimodal, developmental intervention. *Journal of Clinical Psychiatry, 59*(Suppl. 1), 62–72.

Peterson, B. S., Skudlarksi, P., Anderson, A., Zhang, H., Gatenby, J. C., Lacadie, C. M., et al. (1998). A functional magnetic resonance imaging study of tic suppression in Tourette syndrome. *Archives of General Psychiatry, 55*, 326–333.

Peterson, B. S., Staib, L. H., Scahill, L., Zhang, H., Anderson, C., Leckman, J. F., et al. (2001). Regional brain and ventricular volumes in Tourette syndrome. *Archives of General Psychiatry, 58*, 427–440.

Peterson, B. S., Vohr, B., Staib, L. H., Cannistraci, C. J., Dolberg, A., Schneider, K. C., et al. (2000). Regional brain volume abnormalities and long-term cognitive outcome in preterm infants. *Journal of the American Medical Association, 284*, 1939–1947.

Peterson, C. C., Palermo, T. M., Swift, E., Beebe, A., & Drotar, D. (2005). Assessment of psycho-educational needs in a clinical sample of children with sickle cell disease. *Children's Health Care, 34*, 133–148.

Petit, T. L. (1986). Developmental effects of lead: Its mechanism, intellectual functioning, and neural plasticity. *Neurotoxicology and Teratology, 7*, 483–496.

Petridou, E. T., Pourtsidis, A., Dessypris, N., Katsiardanis, K., Baka, M., Moschovi, M., et al. (2008). Childhood leukaemias and lymphomas in Greece (1996–2006): A nationwide registration study. *Archives of Diseases in Children, 93*, 1027–1032.

Petrou, S., Sach, T., & Davidson, L. (2001). The long-term costs of preterm birth and low birth weight: Results of a systematic review. *Child: Care, Health and Development, 27*, 97–115.

Pfab, R., Muckter, H., Roider, G., & Zilker, T. (1996). Clinical course of severe poisoning with thiomersal. *Clinical Toxicology 34*, 453–460.

Pfaendner, N. H., Reuner, G., Pietz, J., Jost, G., Rating, D., Magnotta, V. A., et al. (2005). MR imaging-based volumetry in patients with early-treated phenylketonuria. *American Journal of Neuroradiology, 26*, 1681–1685.

Pfeifer, J. H., Iacoboni, M., Mazziotta, J. C., & Dapretto, M. (2008). Mirroring others' emotions relates to empathy and interpersonal competence in children. *NeuroImage, 39*, 2076–2085.

Phelps, L. (1999). Low level lead exposure: Implications for research and practice. *School Psychology Review, 28*, 477–492.

Phelps, L. (2008). Tourette's disorder: Genetic update, neurological correlates, and evidence-based interventions. *School Psychology Quarterly, 23*, 282–289.

Philip, R., & Turk, J. (2006). Neurofibromatosis and attentional deficits: An illustrative example of the common association of medical causes with behavioural syndromes, Implications for general child mental health services. *Child and Adolescent Mental Health, 11*, 89–93.

Philofsky, A., Fidler, D. J., & Hepburn, S. L. (2007). Pragmatic language profiles of school-age children with autism spectrum disorders and Williams syndrome. *American Journal of Speech Language Pathology, 16*, 368–380.

Philofsky, A., Hepburn, S. L., Hayes, A., Hagerman, R. J., & Rogers, S. J. (2004). Linguistic and cognitive function and autism symptoms in young children with fragile X syndrome. *American Journal of Mental Retardation, 109*, 208–218.

Phipps, S., Long, A., Hudson, M., & Rai, S. N. (2005). Symptoms of post-traumatic stress in children with cancer and their parents: Effects of informant and time from diagnosis. *Pediatric Blood & Cancer, 45*, 952–959.

Piacentini, J., & Chang, S. (2005). Habit reversal training for tic disorders in children and adolescents. *Behavior Modification, 29*, 803–822.

Piccinelli, P., Borgatti, R., Aldini, A., Bindelli, D., Ferri, M., Perna, S., et al. (2008). Academic performance in children with rolandic epilepsy. *Developmental Medicine & Child Neurology, 50*, 353–356.

Pickett, J., & London, E. (2005). The neuropathology of autism: A review. *Journal of Neuropathology and Experimental Neurology, 64*, 925–935.

Pierce, K., & Corchesne, E. (2001). Evidence for a cerebellar role in reduced exploration and stereotyped behavior in autism. *Biological Psychiatry, 49*, 655–664.

Pierce, K., Muller, R. A., Allen, J. A., & Courchesne, E. (2001). Face processing occurs outside the fusiform "face area" in autism: Evidence from functional MRI. *Brain, 124*, 2059–2073.

Pierik, F. H., Burdorf, A., Deddens, J. A., Juttmann, R. E., & Weber, R. F. A. (2004). Maternal and paternal risk factors for cryptorchidism and hypospadias: A case-control study in newborn boys. *Environmental Health Perspectives, 112*, 1570–1576.

Pieters, R., & Carroll, W. L. (2008). Biology and treatment of acute lymphoblastic leukemia. *Pediatric Clinics of North America, 55*, 1–20.

Pillard, R. C., Rosen, L. R., Meyer-Bahlburg, H., Weinrich, J. D., Feldman, J. F., Gruen, R., et al. (1993). Psychopathology and social functioning in men prenatally exposed to diethylstilbestrol (DES). *Psychosomatic Medicine, 55*, 485–491.

Pinter, J. D., Eliez, S., Schmitt, J. E., Capone, G. T., & Reiss, A. L. (2001). Neuroanatomy of Down's syndrome: A high-resolution MRI study. *American Journal of Psychiatry, 158*, 1659–1665.

Pisula, E. (2003). Parents of children with autism—review of current research. *Archives of Psychiatry and Psychotherapy, 5*, 51–63.

Pitt, C., Lavery, C., & Wager, N. (2009). Psychosocial outcomes of bone marrow transplant for individuals affected by mucopolysaccharidosis I Hurler disease: Patient social competency. *Child: Care, Health and Development, 35*, 271–280.

Piven, J., Arndt, S., Bailey, J., & Andreasen, N. (1996). Regional brain enlargement in autism: A magnetic resonance imaging study. *Journal of the American Academy of Child & Adolescent Psychiatry, 35*, 530–536.

Piven, J., Bailey, J., Ranson, B. J., & Arndt, S. (1997). An MRI study of the corpus callosum in autism. *American Journal of Psychiatry, 154*, 1051–1056.

Piven, J., Nelune, E., Simon, J., Barta, P., Pearlson, G., & Falstein, S. E. (1992). Magnetic resonance imagery in autism: Measurement of the cerebellum, pons, and fourth ventricle. *Biological Psychiatry, 31*, 491–504.

Plante, E., Swisher, L., & Vance, R. (1989). Anatomical correlates of normal and impaired language in a set of dizygotic twins. *Brain and Language, 37*, 643–655.

Plante, E., Swisher, L., Vance, R., & Rapcsak, S. (1991). MRI findings in boys with specific language impairment. *Brain and Language, 41*, 52–66.

Plante, W. A., & Lobato, D. J. (2008). Psychosocial group interventions for children and adolescents with Type I diabetes: The state of the literature. *Children's Health Care, 37*, 93–111.

Platt, M. J., Cans, C., Johnson, A., Surman, G., Topp, M., Torrioli, M. G., et al. (2007). Trends in cerebral palsy among infants of very low birthweight (<1500 g) or born prematurely (<32 weeks) in 16 European centres: A database study. *Lancet, 369*, 43–50.

Plessen, K. J., Wentzel-Larsen, T., Hugdahl, K., Feineigle, P., Klein, J., Staib, L. H., et al. (2004). Altered interhemispheric connectivity in individuals with Tourette's disorder. *American Journal of Psychiatry, 161*, 2028–2037.

Plioplys, S., Dunn, D. W., & Caplan, R. (2007). 10-year research update review: Psychiatric problems in children with epilepsy. *Journal of the American Academy of Child & Adolescent Psychiatry, 46*, 1389–1402.

Pliszka, S. R. (2007). Pharmacologic treatment of attention-deficit/hyperactivity disorder: Efficacy, safety and mechanisms of action. *Neuropsychology Review, 17*, 61–72.

Pocock, S. J., Smith, M., & Baghurst, P. A. (1994). Environmental lead and children's intelligence: A systematic review of the epidemiological evidence. *British Medical Journal, 309*, 1189–1197.

Pokorni, J. L., Worthington, C. K., & Jamison, P. J. (2004). Phonological Awareness Intervention: Comparison of Fast ForWord, Earobics, and LiPS. *Journal of Educational Research, 97*, 147–157.

Polgreen, L. E., Tolar, J., Plog, M., Himes, J. H., Orchard, P. J., Whitley, C. B., et al. (2008). Growth and endocrine function in patients with Hurler syndrome after hematopoietic stem cell transplantation. *Bone Marrow Transplantation, 41*, 1005–1011.

Poncin, Y., Sukhodolsky, D. G., McGuire, J., & Scahill, L. (2007). Drug and non-drug treatments of children with ADHD and tic disorders. *European Child and Adolescent Psychiatry, 16*(Suppl. 1), 78–88.

Poreh, A. M. (2006). Methodological quandaries of the Quantified Process Approach. In A. M. Poreh (Ed.), *The quantified process approach to neuropsychological assessment. Studies on neuropsychology, neurology and cognition* (pp. 27–41). Philadelphia: Taylor & Francis.

Posey, D. J., Aman, M. G., Arnold, L. E., Ramadan, Y., Witwer, A., Lindsay, R., et al. (2005). Randomized controlled, cross-over trial of methylphenidate in pervasive developmental disorders with hyperactivity. *Archives of General Psychiatry, 62*, 1266–1274.

Possl, J., Jurgensmeyer, S., Karlbauer, F., Wenz, C., & Goldenberg, G. (2001). Stability of employment after brain injury: A 7-year follow-up study. *Brain Injury, 15,* 15–27.

Post, Y. V. (2003). Reflections. Teaching the secondary language functions of writing, spelling, and reading. *Annals of Dyslexia, 53*, 128–148.

Potasová, A., & Biro, V. (1994). Retest of attention, memory performance, and galvanic skin response in children exposed to environmental toxins. *Studia Psychologica, 36*(4), 243–248.

Powell, M. P., & Schulte, T. (1999). Turner syndrome. In S. Goldstein & C. R. Reynolds (Eds.), *Handbook of neurodevelopmental and genetic disorders in children* (pp. 277–297). New York: Guilford.

Powell, T. W., & Germani, M. J. (1993). Linguistic, intellectual, and adaptive behavior skills in a sample of children with communication disorders. *Journal of Psychoeducational Assessment, 11*, 138–172.

Power, T., Catroppa, C., Coleman, L., Ditchfield, M., & Anderson, V. (2007). Do lesion site and severity predict deficits in attentional control after preschool traumatic brain injury (TBI)? *Brain Injury, 21,* 279–292.

Prassouli, A., Katsarou, E., Attilakos, A., & Antoniadou, L. (2007). Learning difficulties in children with epilepsy with idiopathic generalized epilepsy and well-controlled seizures. *Developmental Medicine & Child Neurology, 49*, 874.

Prather, P., & de Vries, P. (2004). Behavioral and cognitive aspects of tuberous sclerosis complex. *Journal of Child Neurology, 19*, 666–674.

Preis, S., Jäncke, L., Schittler, P., Huang, Y., & Steinmetz, H. (1998). Normal intrasylvian anatomical asymmetry in children with developmental language disorder. *Neuropsychologia, 36*, 849–855.

Prevatt, F. F., Heffer, R. W., & Lowe, P. A. (2000). A review of school reintegration programs for children with cancer. *Journal of School Psychology, 38*, 447–467.

Prevey, M. L., Delaney, R. C., Cramer, J. A., Cattanach, L., Collins, J. F., & Mattson, R. H. (1996). Effect of valproate on cognitive function: Comparison with carbamazepine. *Archives of Neurology, 53*, 1008–1016.

Price, C. J., & Mechelli, A. (2005). Reading and reading disturbance. *Current Opinion in Neurobiology, 15*, 231–238.

Price, J., Roberts, J. E., Vandergrift, N., & Martin, G. (2007). Language comprehension in boys with fragile X syndrome and boys with Down syndrome. *Journal of Intellectual Disabilities Research, 51*, 318–326.

Pritchard, P. B., Holmstrom, V. L., & Giacinto, J. (1985). Self-abatement of complex partial seizures. *Annals of Neurology, 18*, 265–267.

Proctor, B. E., Floyd, R. G., & Shaver, R. B. (2005). Cattell-Horn-Carroll broad ability profiles of low math achievers. *Psychology in the Schools, 42*, 1–12.

Pueschel, S. M., Louis, S., & McKnight, P. (1991). Seizure disorders in Down syndrome. *Archives of Neurology, 48*, 318–320.

Pui, C., & Evans, W. E. (1998). Acute lymphoblastic leukemia. *New England Journal of Medicine, 339*, 605–613.

Pulsifer, M. B., Butz, A. M., O'Reilly Foran, M., & Belcher, H. M. E. (2008). Prenatal drug exposure: Effects on cognitive functioning at 5 years of age. *Clinical Pediatrics, 47*, 58–65.

Puranek, C. S., Petscher, Y., Al Otaiba, S., Catts, H. W., & Lonigan, C. J. (2008). Development of oral reading fluency in children with speech or language impairments: A growth curve analysis. *Journal of Learning Disabilities, 41*, 545–560.

Purcell, A. E., Jeon, O. H., Zimmerman, A. W., Blue, M. E., & Pevsner, J. (2001). Postmortem brain abnormalities of the glutamate neurotransmitter system in autism. *Neurology, 57*, 1618–1628.

Quandt, S. A., Hernández-Valero, M. A., Grzywacz, J. G., Hovey, J. D., Gonzales, M., & Arcury, T. A. (2006). Workplace, household, and personal predictors of pesticide exposure for farmworkers. *Environmental Health Perspective, 114*, 943–952.

Rabin, L. A., Burton, L. A., & Barr, W. B. (2007). Utilization rates of ecologically oriented instruments among clinical neuropsychologists. *Clinical Neuropsychologist, 21*, 727–743.

Rabiner, D. L., Murray, D. W., Schmid, L., & Malone, P. (2004). An exploration of the relationship between ethnicity, attention problems, and academic achievement. *School Psychology Review, 33*, 498–509.

Ramakers-van Woerden, N. L., Pieters, R., Loonen, A. H., Hubeek, I., van Drunen, E., Beverloo, H. B., et al. (2000). TEL/AML1 gene fusion is related to in vitro drug sensitivity for L-asparaginase in childhood acute lymphoblastic leukemia. *Blood, 96*, 1094–1099.

Ramanjam, V., Adnams, C., Ndondo, A., Fieggen, G., Fieggen, K., & Wilmshurst, J. (2006). Clinical phenotype of South African children with neurofibromatosis 1. *Journal of Child Neurology, 21*, 63–70.

Ramus, F. (2004). Neurobiology of dyslexia: A reinterpretation of the data. *Trends in Neurosciences, 27*, 720–726.

Rao, P. A., Beidel, D. C., & Murray, M. J. (2008). Social skills interventions for children with Asperger's syndrome or high-functioning autism: A review and recommendations. *Journal of Autism and Developmental Disorders, 38*, 353–361.

Rapp, D. L., Ferber, P. S., & Bush, S. S. (2008). Unresolved issues about release of raw test data and test materials. In A. M. Horton & D. Wedding (Eds.), *The neuropsychology handbook* (3rd ed., pp. 469–497). New York: Springer.

Rasalam, A. D., Hailey, H., Williams, J. H. G., Moore, S. J., Turnpenny, P. D., Lloyd, D. J., et al. (2005). Characteristics of fetal anticonvulsant syndrome associated autistic disorder. *Developmental Medicine and Child Neurology, 47*, 551–555.

Raskind, W. H. (2004). Current understanding of the genetic basis of reading and spelling disability. *Learning Disabilities Quarterly, 24*, 141–157.

Rasmussen, C. (2005). Executive functioning and working memory in fetal alcohol spectrum disorder. *Alcoholism: Clinical and Experimental Research, 29*, 1359–1367.

Rathvon, N. (2008). *Effective school interventions* (2nd ed.). New York: Guilford.

Ravizza, S. M., McCormick, C. A., Schlerf, J. E., Justus, T., Ivry, R. B., & Fiez, J. A. (2006). Cerebellar damage produces selective deficits in verbal working memory. *Brain, 192*, 306–320.

Ready, R. E., Stierman, L., & Paulsen, J. S. (2001). Ecological validity of neuropsychological and personality measures of executive function. *Clinical Neuropsychologist, 15*, 314–323.

Reaser, A., Prevatt, F., Petscher, Y., & Proctor, B. (2007). The learning and study strategies of college students with ADHD. *Psychology in the Schools, 44*, 627–638.

Reber, M., Kazak, A. E., & Himmelberg, P. (1987). Phenylalanine control and family functioning in early-treated phenylketonuria. *Journal of Developmental & Behavioral Pediatrics, 8*, 311–317.

Records, N. L., Tomblin, J. B., & Buckwalter, P. R. (1995). Auditory learning and memory in young adults with specific language impairment. *Clinical Neuropsychologist, 9*, 187–193.

Redcay, E. (2008). The superior temporal sulcus performs a common function for social and speech perception: Implications for the emergence of autism. *Neuroscience & Biobehavioral Reviews, 32*, 123–142.

Redcay, E., & Courchesne, E. (2005). When is the brain enlarged in autism? A meta-analysis of all brain size reports. *Biological Psychiatry, 58*, 1–9.

Reddick, W. E., Glass, J. O., Palmer, S. L., Wu, S., Gajjar, A., Langston, J. W., et al. (2005). Atypical white matter volume development in children following craniospinal irradiation. *Neuro-Oncology, 7*, 12–19.

Reddick, W. E., Mulhern, R. K., Elkin, T. D., Glass, J. O., Merchant, T. E., & Langston, J. W. (1998). A hybrid neural network analysis of subtle brain volume differences in children surviving brain tumors. *Magnetic Resonance Imaging, 16*, 413–421.

Reddick, W. E., Shan, Z. Y., Glass, J. O., Helton, S., Xiong, X., Wu, S., et al. (2006). Smaller white-matter volumes are associated with larger deficits in attention and learning among long-term survivors of acute lymphoblastic leukemia. *Cancer, 106*, 941–949.

Reddy, L. A., & Pfeiffer, S. I. (2007). Behavioral and emotional symptoms of children and adolescents with Prader-Willi syndrome. *Journal of Autism and Developmental Disorders, 37*, 830–839.

Redondo, M. J., Fain, P. R., & Eisenbarth, G. S. (2001). Genetics of type 1A diabetes. *Recent Progress in Hormone Research, 56*, 69–89.

Reeb, R. N., & Regan, J. M. (1998). Survivors of pediatric cancer: Cognitive sequelae. *Journal of Psychological Practice, 4*(2), 61–76.

Rees, L., Marshall, S., Hartridge, C., Mackie, D., & Weiser, M. (2007). Cognitive interventions post acquired brain injury. *Brain Injury, 21*, 161–200.

Reeves, C. B., Palmer, S., Gross, A. M., Simonian, S. J., Taylor, L., Willingham, E., et al. (2007). Brief report: Sluggish cognitive tempo among pediatric survivors of acute lymphoblastic leukemia. *Journal of Pediatric Psychology, 32*, 1050–1054.

Reeves, C. B., Palmer, S. L., Reddick, W. E., Merchant, T. W., Buchanan, G. M., Gajjar, A., et al. (2006). Attention and memory functioning among pediatric patients with medulloblastoma. *Journal of Pediatric Psychology, 31*, 272–280.

Reich, J. N., Kaspar, C., Puczynski, M., Puczynski, S., Cleland, J. W., Angela, K. D., et al. (1990). Effect of a hypoglycemic episode on neuropsychological functioning in diabetic children. *Journal of Clinical and Experimental Neuropsychology, 12*, 613–626.

Reiss, A. L., Eckert, M. A., Rose, F. E., Karchemskiy, A., Kesler, S., Chang, M., et al. (2004). An experiment of nature: Brain anatomy parallels cognition and behavior in Williams syndrome. *Journal of Neuroscience, 24*, 5009–5015.

Reiss, A. L., Eliez, S., Schmitt, J. E., Straus, E., Lai, Z., Jones, W., et al. (2000). IV. Neuroanatomy of Williams syndrome: A high-resolution MRI study. *Journal of Cognitive Neuroscience, 12*(Suppl.), 65–73.

Reitan, R. M. (1969). *Manual for the administration of neuropsychological test batteries for adults and children*. Indianapolis, IN: Author.

Reitan, R. M. (1986). *Theoretical and methodological bases of the Halstead-Reitan Neuropsychological Test Battery.* Tucson, AZ: Neuropsychological Press.

Reitan, R. M. (1987). *Neuropsychological evaluation of children*. Tucson, AZ: Neuropsychological Press.

Reitan, R. M., & Davison, L. A. (1974). *Clinical neuropsychology: Current status and applications*. Washington, DC: V. H. Winston.

Reitan, R. M., & Wolfson, D. (1985). *The Halstead Reitan neuropsychological battery: Theory and clinical interpretation*. Tucson, AZ: Neuropsychological Press.

Remschmidt, H., & Kamp-Becker, I. (2006). *Asperger syndrome*. Heidelberg: Springer-Verlag.

Ressel, V., Wilke, M., Lidzba, K., Lutzenberger, W., & Krägeloh-Mann, I. (2008). Increases in language lateralization in normal children as observed using magnetoencephalography. *Brain and Language, 106*(3), 167–176.

Reynolds, C. R. (1982). The importance of norms and other traditional psychometric concepts to assessment in clinical neuropsychology. In R. N. Malathesha & L. C. Hartlage (Eds.), *Neuropsychology and cognition* (Vol. 3, pp. 55–76). The Hague: Nijhoff.

Reynolds, C. R. (1986a). Clinical acumen but psychometric naiveté in neuropsychological assessment of educational disorders. *Archives of Clinical Neuropsychology, 1*, 121–137.

Reynolds, C. R. (1986b). Transactional models of intellectual development, yes. Deficit models of process remediation, no. *School Psychology Review, 15*, 256–260.

Reynolds, C. R. (1997). Postscripts on premorbid ability estimation: Conceptual addenda and a few words on alternative and conditional approaches. *Archives of Clinical Neuropsychology, 12,* 769–778.

Reynolds, C. R. (2007). Subtest level profile analysis of intelligence tests: Editor's remarks and introduction. *Applied Neuropsychology, 14*, 1.

Reynolds, C. R., & Bigler, E. D. (1997). Clinical neuropsychological assessment of child and adolescent memory with the Test of Memory and Learning. In C. R. Reynolds & E. Fletcher-Janzen (Eds.), *Handbook of clinical child neuropsychology* (2nd ed., pp. 296–319). New York: Plenum.

Reynolds, C. R., & Kamphaus, R. W. (2004). *Behavior Assessment System for Children* (2nd ed.). San Antonio, TX: Pearson.

Reynolds, C. R., Kamphaus, R. W., Rosenthal, B. L., & Hiemenz, J. R. (1997). Application of the Kaufman assessment battery for children (KABC) in neuropsychological assessment. In C. R. Reynolds & E. Fletcher-Janzen (Eds.), *Handbook of clinical child neuropsychology* (2nd ed., pp. 252–269). New York: Plenum.

Reynolds, C. R., & Mason, B. A. (2009). Measurement and statistical problems in neuropsychological assessment of children. In C. R. Reynolds & E. Fletcher-Janzen (Eds.), *Handbook of clinical child neuropsychology* (pp. 203–230). New York: Springer.

Reynolds, C. R., & Mayfield, J. W. (1999). Neuropsychological assessment in genetically linked neurodevelopmental disorders. In S. Goldstein & C. R. Reynolds (Eds.), *Handbook of neurodevelopmental and genetic disorders in children* (pp. 9–37). New York: Guilford.

Ribas-Fito, N., Sala, M., Kobevinas, M., & Sunyer, J. (2001). Polychlorinated biphenyls (PCBs) and neurological development in children: A systematic review. *Journal of Epidemiology and Community Health, 55*, 537–546.

Riccio, C. A. (2008). A descriptive summary of essential neuropsychological tests. In R. C. D'Amato & L. C. Hartlage (Eds.), *Essentials of neuropsychological assessment: Treatment planning and for rehabilitation* (2nd ed., pp. 207–242). New York: Springer.

Riccio, C. A., Cash, D. L., & Cohen, M. J. (2007). Learning and memory performance of children with specific language impairment (SLI). *Applied Neuropsychology, 14*, 1–7.

Riccio, C. A., & French, C. L. (2004). The status of empirical support for treatments of attention deficits. *Clinical Neuropsychologist, 18*, 528–558.

Riccio, C. A., & Harrison, P. L. (1998). Tuberous sclerosis. In L. Phelps (Ed.), *A practitioner's handbook of health-related disorders in children* (pp. 683–690). Washington, DC: American Psychological Association.

Riccio, C. A., Homack, S., Jarratt, K. P., & Wolfe, M. E. (2006). Differences in academic and executive function domains among children with ADHD predominantly inattentive and combined types. *Archives of Clinical Neuropsychology, 21*, 657–667.

Riccio, C. A., & Hynd, G. W. (1993). Developmental language disorders in children: Relationship with learning disability and attention deficit hyperactivity disorder. *School Psychology Review, 22*, 696–708.

Riccio, C. A., & Hynd, G. W. (1995). Developmental language disorders and attention deficit hyperactivity disorder. *Advances in Learning and Behavioral Disabilities, 9*, 1–20.

Riccio, C. A., & Hynd, G. W. (1996). Neuroanatomical and neurophysiological aspects of dyslexia. *Topics in Language Disorders, 16*, 1–13.

Riccio, C. A., & Hynd, G. W. (2000). Measurable biological substrates to verbal performance differences in Wechsler scales. *School Psychology Quarterly, 15*, 389–399.

Riccio, C. A., Hynd, G. W., Cohen, M. J., Hall, J., & Molt, L. (1994). Comorbidity of central auditory processing disorder and attention-deficit hyperactivity disorder. *Journal of the American Academy of Child and Adolescent Psychiatry, 33*, 849–957.

Riccio, C. A., & Reynolds, C. R. (1998). Neuropsychological assessment of children. In C. R. Reynolds (Ed.), *Comprehensive clinical psychology* (Vol. 4, pp. 267–301). Oxford: Elsevier.

Riccio, C. A., & Reynolds, C. R. (1999). Assessment of traumatic brain injury in children for neuropsychological rehabilitation. In M. Raymond, T. L. Bennett, L. Hartlage, & C. M. Cullum (Eds.), *Mild brain injury: A clinician's guide* (pp. 77–116). Austin, TX: Pro-Ed.

Riccio, C. A., Reynolds, C. R., Lowe, P. A., & Moore, J. J. (2002). The continuous performance test: A window on the neural substrates for attention? *Archives of Clinical Neuropsychology, 17*, 235–272.

Riccio, C. A., Wolfe, M., Davis, B., Romine, C., George, C., & Lee, D. (2005). Attention deficit hyperactivity disorder: Manifestation in adulthood. *Archives of Clinical Neuropsychology, 20*, 249–269.

Rice, D. C. (1993). Lead induced changes in learning: Evidence for behavioral mechanisms from experimental animal studies. *Neurotoxicology, 14*, 167–178.

Rice, D. C. (1996). PCBs and behavioral impairment: Are there lessons we can learn from lead? *Neurotoxicology and Teratology, 18*, 229–232.

Rice, M. L. (2007). Children with specific language impairment: Bridging the genetic and developmental perspectives. In E. Hoff & M. Shatz (Eds.), *Blackwell handbook of language development* (pp. 411–431). Malden, MA: Blackwell.

Richards, T. L., Aylward, E. H., Berninger, V. W., Field, K. M., Grimme, A., Richards, A. L., et al. (2006). Individual fMRI activation in orthographic mapping and morpheme mapping after orthographic or morphological spelling treatment in child dyslexics. *Journal of Neurolinguistics, 19*(1), 56–86.

Richards, T. L., Aylward, E. H., Field, K. M., Gimme, A. C., Raskind, W., Richards, A. L., et al. (2006). Converging evidence for triple word form theory in children with dyslexia. *Developmental Neuropsychology, 30*, 547–589.

Richards, T. L., Berninger, V. W., Nagy, W., Parsons, A., Field, K. M., & Richards, A. L. (2005). Brain activation during language task contrasts in children with and without dyslexia: Inferring mapping processes and assessing response to spelling instruction. *Educational and Child Psychology, 22*(2), 62–80.

Richardson, G. A., & Day, N. L. (1991). Maternal and neonatal effects of moderate cocaine use during pregnancy. *Neurotoxicology and Teratology, 13*, 455–460.

Ridler, K., Suckling, J., Higgins, N. J., de Vries, P. J., Stephenson, C. M. E., Bolton, P., et al. (2007). Neuroanatomical correlates of memory deficits in tuberous sclerosis complex. *Cerebral Cortex, 17*, 261–271.

Ries, L. A. G., Eisner, M. P., Kosary, C. L., Hankey, B. F., Miller, B. A., Clegg, L., et al. (2005). SEER Cancer Statistics Review, 1975–2002. Retrieved October 12, 2007, from http://seer.cancer.gov/csr/1975_2002.

Ries, L. A. G., Smith, M. A., Gurney, J. G., Linet, M., Tamra, T., Young, J. L., et al. (1999). *Cancer incidence and survival among children and adolescents: United States SEER Program 1975–1995*. Bethesda, MD: National Cancer Institute, SEER Program. NIH Pub. No. 994649.

Riley, E. P., & McGee, C. L. (2005). Fetal alcohol spectrum disorders: An overview with emphasis on changes in brain and behavior. *Experimental Biology and Medicine, 230*, 357–365.

Rimland, B. (1964). *Infantile autism: The syndrome and its implications for a neural theory of behavior*. Englewood Cliffs, NJ: Prentice-Hall.

Rinehart, N. J., Bradshaw, J. L., Brereton, A. V., & Tonge, B. J. (2002). Lateralization in individuals with high-functioning autism and Asperger's disorder: A frontostriatal model. *Journal of Autism and Developmental Disorders, 32*, 321–332.

Rinehart, N. J., Tonge, B. J., Bradshaw, J. L., Iansek, R., Enticott, P. G., & McGinley, J. (2006). Gait function in high-functioning autism and Asperger's disorder: Evidence for basal-ganglia and cerebellar involvement? *European Child & Adolescent Psychiatry, 15*, 256–264.

Ris, M. D., Dietrich, K. N., Succop, P. A., Berger, O. B., & Bornschein, R. L. (2004). Early exposure to lead and neuropsychological outcome in adolescence. *Journal of the International Neuropsychological Society, 10*, 261–270.

Ris, M. D., & Noll, R. B. (1994). Long-term neurobehavioral outcome in pediatric brain-tumor patients: Review and methodological critique. *Journal of Clinical and Experimental Neuropsychology, 16*, 21–42.

Ris, M. D., Packer, R., Goldwein, J., Jones-Wallace, D., & Boyett, J. M. (2001). Intellectual outcome after reduced-dose radiation therapy plus adjuvant chemotherapy for medulloblastoma: A Children's Cancer Group study. *Journal of Clinical Oncology, 19*, 3470–3476.

Ritvo, E. R., Yuwiler, A., Geller, E., Kales, A., Rashkis, S., Shicor, A., et al. (1971). Effects of L-dopa in autism. *Journal of Autism and Childhood Schizophrenia, 1*, 190–205.

Ritz, B., & Yu, F. (1999). The effect of ambient carbon monoxide on low birth weight among children born in Southern California between 1989 and 1993. *Environmental Health Perspectives, 107*, 17–25.

Rizzo, R., Curatolo, P., Gulisano, M., Virzi, M., Arpino, C., & Robertson, M. M. (2007). Disentangling the effects of Tourette syndrome and attention deficit hyperactivity disorder on cognitive and behavioral phenotypes. *Brain & Development, 29*, 413–420.

Rizzolatti, G., Fadiga, L., Gallese, V., & Fogassi, L. (1996). Premotor cortex and the recognition of motor actions. *Brain Research, 3*, 131–141.

Roach, E. S. (1992). Neurocutaneous syndromes. *Pediatric Clinics of North America, 39*, 591–620.

Roberts, E. M., English, P. B., Grether, J. K., Windham, G. C., Somberg, L., & Wolff, C. (2007). Maternal residence near agricultural pesticide applications and autism spectrum disorders among children in the California central valley. *Environmental Health Perspective, 115*, 1482–1489.

Roberts, J. E., Mirrett, P., & Burchinal, M. R. (2001). Receptive and expressive communication development of young males with fragile X syndrome. *American Journal on Mental Retardation, 106*, 216–230.

Roberts, J. E., Price, J., & Malkin, C. (2007). Language and communication development in Down Syndrome. *Mental Retardation and Developmental Disabilities Research Reviews, 13*, 26–35.

Roberts, J. E., Schaaf, J. M., Skinner, M., Wheeler, A., Hooper, S. R., Hatton, D., et al. (2005). Academic skills of boys with fragile X syndrome: Profiles and predictors. *American Journal on Mental Retardation, 110*, 107–120.

Roberts, J. E., & Schuele, C. M. (1990). Otitis media and later academic performance: The linkage and implications for intervention. *Topics in Language Disorders, 11,* 43–62.

Roberts, J. E., Weisenfeld, L. A. H., Hatton, D., Heath, M., & Kaufmann, W. (2007). Social approach and autistic behavior in children with fragile X syndrome. *Journal of Autism and Developmental Disorders, 37*, 1748–1760.

Roberts, M. C. (2003). *Handbook of pediatric psychology* (3rd ed). New York: Guilford.

Robertson, M. M. (2000). Tourette syndrome, associated conditions and the complexities of treatment. *Brain, 123*, 425–462.

Robertson, M. M. (2003). Diagnosing Tourette syndrome: Is it a common disorder? *Journal of Psychosomatic Research, 55*, 3–6.

Robertson, M. M. (2006a). Attention deficit hyperactivity disorder, tics, and Tourette's syndrome: The relationship and treatment implications. A commentary. *European Child & Adolescent Psychiatry, 15*, 1–11.

Robertson, M. M. (2006b). Mood disorders and Gilles de la Tourette's syndrome: An update on prevalence, etiology, comorbidity, clinical associations, and implications. *Journal of Psychosomatic Research, 61*, 349–358.

Robertson, M. M., Banerjee, S., Kurlan, R., Cohen, D. J., Leckman, J. F., McMahon, W., et al. (1999). The Tourette Syndrome Diagnostic Confidence Index: Development and clinical associations. *Neurology, 53*, 2108–2112.

Robertson, M. M., & Baron-Cohen, S. (1996). The neuropsychiatry and neuropsychology of Gilles de la Tourette syndrome. In I. Grant & K. M. Adams (Eds.), *Neuropsychological assessment of neuropsychiatric disorders* (2nd ed., pp. 218–231). New York: Oxford.

Robertson, M. M., Williamson, F., & Eapen, V. (2006). Depressive symptomatology in young people with Gilles de la Tourette syndrome: A comparison of self-report scales. *Journal of Affective Disorders, 91*, 265–268.

Robinson, C. S., Menchetti, B. M., & Torgesen, J. K. (2002). Toward a two-factor theory of one type of mathematics disabilities. *Learning Disabilities Research & Practice, 17*(2), 81–89.

Rodenburg, R., Meijer, A. M., Dekoic, M., & Aldenkamp, A. P. (2007). Parents of children with enduring epilepsy: Predictors of parenting stress and parenting. *Epilepsy and Behavior, 11*, 197–207.

Rodin, G. (2001). Review: Behavioural interventions have a small to medium beneficial effect on diabetes management in adolescents with type 1 diabetes. *Evidence-Based Mental Health, 4*, 46.

Rodin, G., Olmsted, M. P., Rydall, A. C., Maharaj, S. I., Colton, P. A., Jones, J. M., et al. (2002). Eating disorders in young women with type 1 diabetes mellitus. *Psychosomatic Research, 53*, 943–949.

Rodkey, F. L., O'Neal, J. D., Colilson, H. A., & Uddin, D. E. (1974). Relative affinity of hemoglobin S and hemoglobin A for carbon monoxide and oxygen. *Clinical Chemistry, 20*, 83.

Roebuck, T. M., Mattson, S. N., & Riley, E. P. (1998). A review of the neuroanatomical findings in children with fetal alcohol syndrome or prenatal exposure to alcohol. *Alcoholism: Clinical and Experimental Research, 22*, 339–344.

Roegge, C. S., & Schantz, S. L. (2006). Motor function following developmental exposure to PCBS and/or MEHG. *Neurotoxicology and Teratology, 28*, 260–277.

Roessner, V., Becker, A., Banaschewski, T., & Rothenberger, A. (2007). Executive functions in children with chronic tic disorders with/without ADHD: New insights. *European Child and Adolescent Psychiatry, 16*(Suppl. 1), 36–44.

Rogan, W., Dietrich, K. N., Ware, J. H., Dockery, D. W., Salganik, M., Radcliffe, J., et al. (2001). The effect of chelation therapy with succimer on neuropsychological development in children exposed to lead. *New England Journal of Medicine, 344*, 1421–1426.

Rogan, W. J., & Gladen, B. C. (1991). PCBs, DDE, and child development at 18 and 24 months. *Annals of Epidemiology, 1*, 407–413.

Rogers, M., Fay, T. B., Whitfield, M. F., Tomlinson, J., & Grunau, R. E. (2005). Aerobic capacity, strength, flexibility, and activity level in unimpaired extremely low birth weight (≤800 g) survivors at 17 years of age compared with term-born control subjects. *Pediatrics, 116*, 58–65.

Rogers, S. (1998). Empirically supported comprehensive treatments for young children with autism. *Journal of Clinical Child Psychology, 27*, 168–179.

Rogers, S. (1999). An examination of the imitation deficits in autism. In J. Nadel & G. Butterworth (Eds.), *Imitation in infancy: Cambridge studies in cognitive perceptual development* (pp. 254–283). New York: Cambridge University Press.

Rogers, S., & DiLalla, D. L. (1991). A comparative study of the effects of a developmentally based instructional model on young children with autism and young children with other disorders of behavior and development. *Topics in Early Childhood Special Education, 11*, 29–47.

Rogers, S., & Lewis, H. (1989). An effective day treatment model for young children with pervasive developmental disorders. *Journal of the American Academy of Child and Adolescent Psychiatry, 28*, 207–214.

Rogers, S., & Vismara, L. A. (2008). Evidence-based comprehensive treatments for early autism. *Journal of Clinical Child and Adolescent Psychiatry, 37*, 8–38.

Rohyans, J., Walson, P. D., Wood, G. A., & MacDonald, W. A. (1994). Mercury toxicity following merthiolate ear irrigations. *Journal of Pediatrics, 104*, 311–313.

Roizen, N. J. (2002). Medical care and monitoring for the adolescent with Down syndrome. *Adolescent Medicine, 13*, 345–358.

Roizen, N. J. (2005). Complementary and alternative therapies for Down syndrome. *Mental Retardation and Developmental Disabilities Research Reviews, 11*, 149–155.

Roizen, N. J., & Patterson, D. (2003). Down's syndrome. *Lancet, 361*, 1281–1289.

Rojas, D. C., Allegra-Smith, J., Benkers, T. L., Camou, S. L., Reite, M. L., & Rogers, S. J. (2004). Hippocampus and amygdala volumes in parents of children with autistic disorder. *American Journal of Psychiatry, 161*, 2038–2044.

Rojas, N. L., & Chan, E. (2005). Old and new controversies in the alternative treatment of attention-deficit hyperactivity disorder. *Mental Retardation and Developmental Disabilities Research Reviews, 11*, 116–130.

Roland-Tapia, L., Nieto-Escamez, F. A., del Aguila, E. M., Laynez, F., Parron, T., & Sanchez-Santed, F. (2006). Neuropsychological sequelae from acute poisoning and long-term exposure to carbamate and organophosphate pesticides. *Neurotoxicology and Teratology, 28*, 694–703.

Rondal, J. A., Elbouz, M., Ylieff, M., & Docquier, L. (2003). Francoise, a fifteen-year follow up. *Down Syndrome: Research and Practice, 8*(3), 89–99.

Rondo, P. H. C., Ferreira, R. F., Nogueira, F., Ribeiro, M. C. N., Lobert, H., & Artes, R. (2003). Maternal psychological stress and distress as predictors of low birth weight, prematurity and intrauterine growth retardation. *European Journal of Clinical Nutrition, 57*, 266–272.

Roof, E., Stone, W., MacLean, W., Feurer, I. D., Thompson, T., & Butler, M. G. (2000). Intellectual characteristics of Prader-Willi syndrome: Comparison of genetic subtypes. *Journal of Intellectual Disabilities Research, 44*, 25–30.

Roos, E. M., McDuffie, A. S. W., S. E., & Gernsbacher, M. A. (2008). A comparison of contexts for assessing joint attention in toddlers on the autism spectrum. *Autism, 12*, 275–291.

Rose, J. C., Lincoln, A. J., & Allen, M. H. (1992). Ability profiles of developmental language disordered and learning disabled children: A comparative analysis. *Developmental Neuropsychology, 8*, 413–426.

Ross, J. L., Roeltgen, D., Stefanatos, G. A., Benecke, R., Zeger, M., Kushner, H., et al. (2008). Cognitive and motor development during childhood in boys with Klinefelter syndrome. *American Journal of Medical Genetics, 146A*, 708–719.

Ross, J. L., Stefanatos, G. A., Kushner, H., Bondy, C., Nelson, L., Zinn, A., et al. (2004). The effect of genetic differences and ovarian failure: Intact cognitive function in adult women with premature ovarian failure versus Turner syndrome. *Journal of Clinical Endocrinology and Metabolism, 89*, 1817–1822.

Ross, J. L., Stefanatos, G. A., & Roeltgen, D. (2007). Klinefelter syndrome. In M. M. M. Mazzocco & J. L. Ross (Eds.), *Neurogenetic developmental disorders: Variation of manifestation in childhood* (pp. 47–72). Cambridge, MA: MIT Press.

Rosselli, M., & Ardila, A. (1989). Calculation deficits in patients with right and left hemisphere damage. *Neuropsychologia, 27*, 607–618.

Rossi, P. G., Parmeggiani, A., Bach, V., Santucci, M., & Visconti, P. (1995). EEG features and epilepsy in patients with autism. *Brain & Development, 17*, 169–174.

Rothlein, J., Rohnlman, D., Lasarev, M., Phillips, J., Santana, J., & McCauley, L. (2006). Organophosphate pesticide exposure and neurobehavioral performance in agricultural and nonagricultural Hispanic workers. *Environmental Health Perspective, 114*, 691–696.

Rourke, B. P. (1989). *Nonverbal learning disabilities*. New York: Guilford.

Rourke, B. P. (1993). Arithmetic disabilities, specific and otherwise: A neuropsychological perspective. *Journal of Learning Disabilities, 26*(4), 214–226.

Rourke, B. P. (1994). Neuropsychological assessment of children with learning disabilities: Measurement issues. In G. R. Lyon (Ed.), *Frames of reference for the assessment of learning disabilities: New views on measurement issues* (pp. 475–514). Baltimore, MD: Brookes.

Rourke, B. P. (2005). Neuropsychology of learning disabilities: Past and future. *Learning Disability Quarterly, 28*, 111–114.

Rourke, B. P., & Conway, J. A. (1997). Disabilities of arithmetic and mathematical reasoning: Perspectives from neurology and neuropsychology. *Journal of Learning Disabilities, 30*(1), 34–46.

Rousselle, L., & Noël, M.-P. (2008). Mental arithmetic in children with mathematics learning disabilities: The adaptive use of approximate calculation in an addition verification task. *Journal of Learning Disabilities, 41*, 498–513.

Roux, F.-E., Lubrano, V., Lauwers-Cances, V., Trémoulet, M., Mascott, C. R., & Démonet, J.-F. (2004). Intra-operative mapping of cortical areas involved in reading in mono- and bilingual patients. *Brain, 127*, 1796–1810.

Rovet, J. (2004). Turner syndrome: A review of genetic and hormonal influences on neuropsychological functioning. *Child Neuropsychology, 41*, 494–496.

Rovet, J., Netley, C., Keenan, M., Bailey, J., & Stewart, D. (1996). The psychoeducational profile of boys with Klinefelter syndrome. *Journal of Learning Disabilities, 29*, 180–196.

Rovet, J. F. (2000). Diabetes. In K. O. Yeates, M. D. Ris, & H. G. Taylor (Eds.), *Pediatric neuropsychology: Research, theory, and practice* (pp. 336–365). New York: Guilford.

Rovet, J. F., Ehrlich, R. M., Czuchta, D., & Akler, M. (1993). Psychoeducational characteristics of children and adolescents with insulin-dependent diabetes mellitus. *Journal of Learning Disabilities, 26*, 7–22.

Rovet, J. F., Ehrlich, R. M., & Hoppe, M. (1988). Specific intellectual deficits in children with early onset diabetes mellitus. *Child Development, 59*, 226–234.

Rowbotham, I., Pit-ten Cate, I. M., Sonuga-Barke, E. J. S., & Huijbreqts, S. C. J. (2009). Cognitive control in neurofibromatosis type 1. *Neuropsychology, 23*, 50–60.

Rowse, H. J., & Wilshire, C. E. (2007). Comparison of phonological and whole-word treatments for two contrasting cases of developmental dyslexia. *Cognitive Neuropsychology, 24*, 817–842.

Royo, N. C., Shimizu, S., Schouten, J. W., Stover, J. F., & McIntosh, T. K. (2003). Pharmacology of traumatic brain injury. *Current Opinion in Pharmacology, 3*, 27–32.

Ruggieri, M., Iannetti, P., Clementi, M., Polizzi, A., Incorpora, G., Spalice, A., et al. (2009). Neurofibromatosis type 1 and infantile spasms. *Child's Nervous System, 25*, 211–216.

Ruggieri, M., Iannetti, P., Polizzi, A., La Mantia, I., Spalice, A., Giliberto, O., et al. (2005). Earliest clinical manifestations and natural history of neurofibromatosis type 2 (NF2) in childhood: A study of 24 patients. *Neuropediatrics, 36*, 21–34.

Rumsey, J. M., Andreason, P., Zametkin, A. J., Aquino, T., King, A. C., Hamburger, S. D., et al. (1992). Failure to activate the left temporoparietal cortex in dyslexia: An oxygen 15 positron emission tomographic study. *Journal of the American Medical Association, 49*, 527–534.

Rumsey, J. M., Berman, K. F., Denckla, M. B., Hamburger, S. D., Kruesi, M. J., & Weinberger, D. R. (1987). Regional cerebral blood flow in severe developmental dyslexia. *Archives of Neurology, 44*, 144–150.

Rumsey, J. M., Creasey, H., Stepanek, J. S., Dorwart, R., Patronas, N., Hamburger, S. D., et al. (1988). Hemispheric asymmetries, fourth ventricular size, and cerebellar morphology in autism. *Journal of Autism and Developmental Disorders, 18*, 127–137.

Russell, H. F., Wallis, D., Mazzocco, M. M. M., Moshang, T., Zackai, E. H., Zinn, A., et al. (2006). Increased prevalence of ADHD in Turner syndrome with no evidence of imprinting effects. *Journal of Pediatric Psychology, 31*, 945–955.

Russell, J. (1997). How executive disorders can bring about an inadequate "theory of mind." In J. Russell (Ed.), *Autism as an executive disorder*. Oxford: Oxford University Press.

Russo, N., Flanagan, T., Iarocci, G., Berringer, D., Zelazo, P. D., & Burack, J. A. (2007). Deconstructing executive deficits among persons with autism: Implications for cognitive neuroscience. *Brain and Cognition, 65*, 77–86.

Rutter, M. (2001). Autism research: Lessons from the past and prospects for the future. *Journal of Autism and Developmental Disorders, 35*, 241–257.

Rutter, M. (2005). Genetics influences and autism. In F. R. Volkmar, R. Paul, A. Klin, & D. Cohen (Eds.), *Handbook of autism and pervasive developmental disorders: Diagnosis, development, neurobiology, and behavior* (3rd ed., Vol. 1, pp. 425–452). Hoboken, NJ: Wiley.

Ryan, C. M., Atchison, J., Puczynski, S., Puczynski, M., Arslanian, S., & Becker, D. (1990). Mild hypoglycemia associated with deterioration of mental efficiency in children with insulin-dependent diabetes mellitus. *Journal of Pediatrics, 117*, 32–38.

Ryan, C. M., Longstreet, C., & Morrow, L. (1985). The effects of diabetes mellitus on the school attendance and school achievement of adolescents. *Child: Care, Health and Development, 11*, 229–240.

Ryan, T. V., LaMarche, J. A., Barth, J. T., & Boll, T. J. (1996). Neuropsychological consequences and treatment of pediatric head trauma. In E. S. Batchelor and R. S. Dean (Eds.), *Pediatric neuropsychology* (pp. 117–137). New York: Pergamon.

Sabaratnam, M., Venkatesha Murphy, N., Wijeratne, A., Buckingham, A., & Payne, S. (2003). Autistic-like behaviour profile and psychiatric morbidity in fragile X syndrome: A prospective ten-year follow-up study. *European Child & Adolescent Psychiatry, 12*, 172–177.

Sadler, L. S., Pober, B. R., Grandinetti, A., Scheiber, D., Fekete, G., Sharma, A. N., et al. (2001). Differences by sex in cardiovascular disease in Williams syndrome. *Journal of Pediatrics, 139*, 849–853.

Sadoski, M., & Willson, V. (2006). Effects of a theoretically based large-scale reading intervention in a multicultural urban school district. *American Educational Research Journal, 43*(1), 137–154.

Saenz, R. B. (1999). Primary care of infants and young children with Down syndrome. *American Family Physician, 59*, 381–390, 392.

Sahoo, T., Peters, S. U., Madduri, N. S., Glaze, D. G., German, J. R., Bird, L. M., et al. (2006). Microarray-based comparative genomic hybridization testing in deletion-bearing Angelman syndrome patients: Genotype-phenotype correlations. *Journal of Medical Genetics, 43*, 512–516.

Saigal, S., & Doyle, L. W. (2008). An overview of mortality and sequelae of preterm birth from infancy to adulthood. *Lancet, 371*, 261–269.

Saigal, S., Hoult, L. A., Streiner, D. L., Stoskopf, B. L., & Rosenbaum, P. L. (2000). School difficulties at adolescence in a regional cohort of children who were extremely low birth weight. *Pediatrics, 105*, 325–331.

Saigal, S., Lambert, M., Russ, C., & Hoult, L. (2002). Self-esteem of adolescents who were born prematurely. *Pediatrics, 109*, 429–433.

Saigal, S., Pinelli, J., Hoult, L., Kim, M. M., & Boyle, M. (2003). Psychopathology and social competencies of adolescents who were extremely low birth weight. *Pediatrics, 111*, 969–975.

Saigal, S., Stoskopf, B., Streiner, D., Boyle, M., Pinelli, J., Paneth, N., et al. (2006). Transition of extremely low-birth-weight infants from adolescence to young adulthood: Comparison with normal birth-weight controls. *Journal of the American Medical Association, 295*, 667–675.

Sajaniemi, N., Makela, J., Salokorpi, T., von Wendt, L., Hamalainen, T., & Hakamies-Blomqvist, L. (2001). Cognitive performance and attachment patterns at four years of age in extremely low birth weight infants after early intervention. *European Child & Adolescent Psychiatry, 10,* 122–129.

Sallee, F. R., Kurlan, R., Goetz, C. G., Singer, H., Scahill, L., Law, G., et al. (2000). Ziprasidone treatment of children and adolescents with Tourette's syndrome: A pilot study. *Journal of the American Academy of Child and Adolescent Psychiatry, 39*, 292–299.

Salman, M. (2002). Systematic review of the effects of therapeutic dietary supplements and drugs on cognitive function in subjects with Down syndrome. *Journal of Paediatric Neurology, 6*, 213–219.

Samaco, R. C., Nagarajan, R. P., Braunschweig, D., & La Salle, J. M. (2004). Multiple pathways regulate MECP2 expression in normal brain development and exhibit defects in autism-spectrum disorders. *Human Molecular Genetics, 13*, 629–639.

Samatovicz, R. A. (2000). Genetics and brain injury: Apolipoprotein E. *Journal of Head Trauma Rehabilitation, 15,* 869–874.

Sampaio, A., Sousa, N., Férnandez, M., Vasconcelos, X., Shenton, M. E., & Concalves, O. F. (2008). MRI assessment of superior temporal gyrus in Williams syndrome. *Cognitive and Behavioral Neurology, 21*, 150–156.

Sampson, P. D., Streissguth, A. P., Bookstein, F. L., Little, R. E., Clarren, S. K., Dehaene, P., et al. (1997). Incidence of fetal alcohol syndrome and prevalence of alcohol-related neurodevelopmental disorder. *Teratology, 56*, 317–326.

Sandak, R., Mencl, E. M., Frost, S. J., & Pugh, K. R. (2004). The neurobiological basis of skilled and impaired reading: Recent findings and new directions. *Scientific Studies of Reading, 8*, 273–292.

Sandor, P. (2003). Pharmacological management of tics in patients with TS. *Journal of Psychosomatic Research, 55*, 41–48.

Saneto, R. P., Sotero de Menezes, M. A., Ojemann, J. G., Bournival, B. D., Murphy, P. J., Cook, W. B., et al. (2006). Vagus nerve stimulation for intractable seizures in children. *Pediatric Neurology, 35*, 323–326.

Sansbury, L., Brown, R. T., & Meacham, L. (1997). Predictors of cognitive functioning in children and adolescents with insulin-dependent diabetes mellitus: A preliminary investigation. *Children's Health Care, 26*, 197–210.

Santiprabhob, J., Likitmaskul, S., Kiattisakthavee, P., Weerakulwattana, P., Chaichanwattanakul, K., Nakavachara, P., et al. (2008). Glycemic controls and the psychosocial benefits gained by patients with type 1 diabetes mellitus attending the diabetes camp. *Patient Education and Counseling, 73*, 60–66.

Santos de Oliveira, R., Lejeunie, E., Arnaud, P., & Renier, D. (2005). Fetal exposure to sodium valproate associated with Baller-Gerold syndrome: Case report and review of the literature. *Child's Nervous System, 22*(1), 90–94.

Sarama, J., & Clements, D. H. (2004). Building blocks for early childhood mathematics. *Early Childhood Research Quarterly, 19*, 181–189.

Sarkissian, C. N., Gámez, A., & Scriver, C. R. (2009). What we know that could influence future treatment of phenylketonuria. *Journal of Inherited Metabolic Disease, 32*, 3–9.

Sarpal, D., Buchsbaum, B. R., Kohn, P. D., Kippenhan, J. S., Mervis, C. B., Morris, C. A., et al. (2008). A genetic model for understanding higher-order visual processing: Functional interactions of the ventral visual stream in Williams syndrome. *Cerebral Cortex, 18*, 2402–2409.

Savage, R. C., Depompei, R., Tyler, J., & Lash, M. (2005). Paediatric traumatic brain injury: A review of pertinent issues. *Pediatric Rehabilitation, 8*, 92–103.

Sävendahl, L., & Davenport, M. L. (2000). Delayed diagnoses of Turner's syndrome: Proposed guidelines for change. *Journal of Pediatrics, 137*, 455–459.

Sawaf, S., Mayatepek, E., & Hoffmann, B. (2008). Neurological findings in Hunter disease: Pathology and possible therapeutic effects reviewed. *Journal of Inherited Metabolic Disease, 31*, 473–480.

Sbordone, R. J. (2008). Ecological validity of neuropsychological testing: Critical issues. In A. M. Horton & D. Wedding (Eds.), *The neuropsychology handbook* (3rd ed., pp. 367–394). New York: Springer.

Scahill, L., Chappell, P. B., Kim, Y. S., Schultz, R. T., Katsovich, L., Shepherd, E., et al. (2001). A placebo-controlled study of guanfacine in the treatment of children with tic disorders and attention deficit hyperactivity disorder. *American Journal of Psychiatry, 158*, 1067–1074.

Scahill, L., Tanner, C., & Dure, L. (2001). The epidemiology of tics and Tourette syndrome in children and adolescents. In D. J. Cohen, C. G. Goetz, & J. Jankovic (Eds.), *Tourette syndrome* (pp. 261–271). Philadelphia: Williams and Wilkins.

Scarborough, H. (2005). Developmental relationships between language and reading: Reconciling a beautiful hypothesis with some ugly facts. In H. Catts & A. Kamhi (Eds.), *The connections between language and reading disabilities* (pp. 3–24). Mahwah, NJ: Erlbaum.

Schatz, J., Brown, R. T., Pascual, J. M., Craft, S., Koby, M., & DeBaun, M. R. (2001). Poor school and cognitive functioning with silent cerebral infarction and sickle cell disease. *Neurology, 56*, 1109–1111.

Schatz, J., Craft, S., Koby, M., & DeBaun, M. R. (2000). A lesion analysis of visual orienting performance in children with cerebral vascular injury. *Developmental Neuropsychology, 17*, 49–61.

Schatz, J., Craft, S., Koby, M., & DeBaun, M. R. (2004). Asymmetries in visual-spatial processing following childhood stroke. *Neuropsychology, 18*, 340–352.

Schatz, J., Craft, S., Koby, M., Siegel, M. J., Resar, L., Lee, R. R., et al. (1999). Neuropsychological deficits in children with sickle cell disease and cerebral infarction: The role of lesion location and volume. *Child Neuropsychology, 5*, 92–103.

Schatz, J., Finke, R., & Roberts, C. W. (2004). Interactions of biomedical and environmental risk factors for cognitive development: A preliminary study of sickle cell disease. *Journal of Developmental & Behavioral Pediatrics, 25*, 303–310.

Schatz, J., Kramer, J. H., Albin, A., & Matthay, K. K. (2000). Processing speed, working memory, and IQ: A working model of cognitive deficits following cranial radiation. *Neuropsychology, 14*, 189–200.

Schatz, J., & McClellan, C. B. (2006). Sickle cell disease as a neurodevelopmental disorder. *Mental Retardation and Developmental Disabilities, 12*, 200–207.

Schatz, J., McClellan, C. B., Puffer, E. S., Johnson, K. A., & Roberts, C. W. (2008). Neurodevelopmental screening in toddlers and early preschoolers with sickle cell disease. *Journal of Child Neurology, 23*, 44–50.

Schatz, J., Puffer, E. S., Sanchez, C., Stancil, M., & Roberts, C. W. (2009). Language processing deficits in sickle cell disease in young school-age children. *Developmental Neuropsychology, 34*, 122–136.

Schell, L. M. (1997). Using patterns of child growth and development to assess communitywide effects of low-level exposure to toxic materials. *Toxicology and Industrial Health, 13*, 373–378.

Schempf, A. H. (2007). Illicit drug use and neonatal outcomes: A critical review. *Obstetrical and Gynecological Survey, 62*, 749–757.

Schmidt, L. A., Polak, C. P., & Spooner, A. L. (2005). Biological and environmental contributions to childhood shyness: A diathesis-stress model. In W. R. Crozier & L. E. Alden (Eds.), *The essential handbook of social anxiety for clinicians* (pp. 33–55). New York: Wiley.

Schmitt, J. E., Eliez, S., Bellugi, E., Galaburda, A., & Reiss, A. L. (2002). Increased gyrification in Williams syndrome: Evidence using 3D MRI methods. *Developmental Medicine and Child Neurology, 44*, 292–295.

Schneider, W., Ennemoser, M., Roth, E., & Küspert, P. (1999). Kindergarten prevention of dyslexia: Does training in phonological awareness work for everybody? *Journal of Learning Disabilities, 32*, 429–436.

Schnoll, R., Burshteyn, D., & Cea-Aravena, J. (2003). Nutrition in the treatment of attention-deficit hyperactivity disorder: A neglected but important aspect. *Applied Psychophysiology and Biofeedback, 28*, 63–75.

Schoechlin, C., & Engel, R. R. (2005). Neuropsychological performance in adult attention-deficit hyperactivity disorder: Meta-analysis of empirical data. *Archives of Clinical Neuropsychology, 20*, 727–744.

Schoenfeld, J., Seidenberg, M., Woodard, A., Hecox, K., Inglese, C., Mack, K., et al. (1999). Neuropsychological and behavioral status of children with complex partial seizures. *Developmental Medicine & Child Neurology, 41*, 724–731.

Schopler, E. (1997). Implementation of TEACCH philosophy. In D. Cohen & F. R. Volkmar (Eds.), *Handbook of autism and pervasive developmental disorders* (2nd ed., pp. 767–795). New York: Wiley.

Schorry, E. K., Oppenheimer, S. G., & Saal, H. M. (2005). Valproate embryopathy: Clinical and cognitive profile in 5 siblings. *American Journal of Medical Genetics, 133*, 202–206.

Schraw, G. (1998). Promoting general metacognitive awareness. *Instructional Science, 26*, 113–125.

Schreibman, L., Whalen, C., & Stahmer, A. (2000). The use of video priming to reduce disruptive transition behavior in children with autism. *Journal of Positive Behavior Interventions, 2*, 3–11.

Schrimsher, G. W., Billingsley, R. L., Slopis, J. M., & Moore, B. D. (2003). Visual-spatial performance deficits in children with neurofibromatosis type-1. *American Journal of Medical Genetics, 120A*, 326–330.

Schuchardt, K., Maehler, C., & Hasselhorn, M. (2008). Working memory deficits in children with specific learning disorders. *Journal of Learning Disabilities, 41*, 514–523.

Schuele, C. M., Spencer, R. J., Barako-Arndt, K., & Guillot, K. M. (2007). Literacy and children with specific language impairment. *Seminars in Speech and Language, 28*, 35–47.

Schuerholz, L. J., Singer, H. S., & Denckla, M. B. (1998). Gender study of neuropsychological and neuromotor function in children with Tourette syndrome with and without attention-deficit hyperactivity disorder. *Journal of Child Neurology, 13*, 277–282.

Schulte-Körne, G., Ludwig, K. U., el Sharkawy, J., Nöthen, M. M., Müller-Myhsok, B., & Hoffmann, P. (2007). Genetics and neuroscience in dyslexia: Perspectives for education and remediation. *Mind, Brain, and Education, 1*, 162–172.

Schulte-Rüther, M., Markowitsch, H. J., Fink, G. R., & Piefke, M. (2007). Mirror neuron and theory of mind mechanisms involved in face-to-face interactions: A functional magnetic resonance imaging approach to empathy. *Journal of Cognitive Neuroscience, 19*, 1354–1372.

Schultz, R. T. (2005). Developmental deficits in social perception in autism: The role of the amygdala and fusiform face area. *International Journal of Developmental Neuroscience, 10*, 125–141.

Schultz, R. T., Carter, A. S., Gladstone, M., Scahill, L., Leckman, J. F., Peterson, B. S., et al. (1998). Visual-motor integration functioning in children with Tourette syndrome. *Neuropsychology, 12*, 134–145.

Schulz, E., Maurer, U., van der Mark, S., Bucher, K., Brem, S., Martin, E., et al. (2008). Impaired semantic processing during sentence reading in children with dyslexia: Combined fMRI and ERP evidence. *NeuroImage, 41*, 153–168.

Schumacher, J., Hoffmann, P., Schmäl, C., Schulte-Körne, G., & Nöthen, M. M. (2007). Genetics of dyslexia: The evolving landscape. *Journal of Medical Genetics, 44*, 289–297.

Schumann, C. M., & Amaral, D. G. (2006). Stereological analysis of amygdala neuron number in autism. *Journal of Neuroscience, 26*, 7674–7679.

Schumann, C. M., Hamstra, J., Goodlin-Jones, B. L., Lotspeich, L. J., Kwon, H., Buonocore, M. H., et al. (2004). The amygdala is enlarged in children but not adolescents with autism; the hippocampus is enlarged at all ages. *Journal of Neuroscience, 24*, 6392–6401.

Schwarte, A. R. (2008). Fragile X syndrome. *School Psychology Quarterly, 23*, 290–300.

Schwartz, C. E., Feinberg, R. G., Jilinskaia, E., & Applegate, J. C. (1999). An evaluation of a psychosocial intervention for survivors of childhood cancer: Paradoxical effects of response shift over time. *Psycho-Oncology, 8*, 344–354.

Schwartz, J. (1994). Low level lead exposure and children's IQ: A meta-analysis and search for a threshold. *Environmental Research, 65*, 42–55.

Schwartz, L. A. (2007). The development of a culturally sensitive pediatric pain management intervention for African American adolescents with sickle cell disease. *Children's Health Care, 36*, 267–283.

Scriver, C. R., Kaufman, C., Eisensmith, R. C., & Woo, S. L. C. (2001). The hyperphenylalaninemias. In C. R. Scriver & W. S. Sly (Eds.), *The metabolic and molecular basis of inherited disease* (8th ed., pp. 1667–1724). New York: McGraw-Hill.

Seabaugh, G. O., & Schumaker, J. B. (1994). The effects of self-regulation training on the academic productivity of secondary students with learning problems. *Journal of Behavioral Education, 4*, 109–133.

Sears, L. L., Vest, C., Mohamed, S., Bailey, J., Ranson, B. J., & Piven, J. (1999). An MRI study of the basal ganglia in autism. *Progress in Neuro-Psychopharmacology & Biological Psychiatry, 23*, 613–624.

Segawa, M. (2003). Neurophysiology of Tourette's syndrome: Pathophysiological considerations. *Brain & Development, 25*, S62-S69.

Segers, T., & Verhoeven, L. (2004). Computer supported phonological awareness intervention for kindergarten children with specific language impairment. *Language, Speech and Hearing Services in the Schools, 35*, 229–239.

Seidenberg, M., Beck, N., & Geisser, M. (1986). Academic achievement of children with epilepsy. *Epilepsia, 27*, 753–759.

Seidman, L. J. (2006). Neuropsychological functioning in people with ADHD across the lifespan. *Clinical Psychology Review, 26*, 466–485.

Seidman, L. J., Biederman, J., Monuteaux, M. C., Doyle, A. E., & Faraone, S. V. (2001). Learning disabilities and executive dysfunction in boys with attention-deficit/hyperactivity disorder. *Neuropsychology, 15*, 544–556.

Selassie, R.-H., Viggedal, G., Olsson, I., & Jennische, M. (2008). Speech, language, and cognition in preschool children with epilepsy. *Developmental Medicine & Child Neurology, 50*, 432–438.

Semrud-Clikeman, M. (2001). *Traumatic brain injury in children and adolescents: Assessment and intervention*. New York: Guilford.

Semrud-Clikeman, M., Hynd, G. W., Novey, E. S., & Eliopulos, D. (1991). Dyslexia and brain morphology: Relationships between neuroanatomical variation and neurolinguistic tasks. *Learning and Individual Differences, 3*, 225–242.

Semrud-Clikeman, M., Kutz, A., & Strassner, E. (2005). Providing neuropsychological services to learners with traumatic brain injuries. In R. C. D'Amato, E. Fletcher-Janzen, & C. R. Reynolds (Eds.), *Handbook of school neuropsychology* (pp. 425–443). Hoboken, NJ: Wiley.

Serajee, F. J., Zhong, H., Nabi, R., & Huq, A. H. (2003). The metabotropic glutamate receptor 8 gene at 7q31: Partial duplication and possible association with autism. *Journal of Medical Genetics, 40*, 42.

Shalat, S. L., Donnelly, K. C., Freeman, N. C. G., Calvin, J. A., Ramesh, S., Jimenez, M., et al. (2003). Nondietary ingestion of pesticides by children in an agricultural community on the U.S./Mexico border: Preliminary results. *Journal of Exposure Analysis and Environmental Epidemiology, 13*, 42–50.

Shalat, S. L., Donnelly, K. C., Ramesh, S., Freeman, N., Jimenez, M., Black, K., et al. (2001). *Ingestion of pesticides by children in an agricultural community on the U.S./ Mexico border: Preliminary report.* Paper presented at the International Society for Exposure Analysis.

Shalev, R. S. (2004). Developmental dyscalculia. *Journal of Child Neurology, 19*, 765–771.

Shalev, R. S., Auerbach, J., Manor, O., & Gross-Tsur, V. (2000). Developmental dyscalculia: Prevalence and prognosis. *European Child and Adolescent Psychiatry, 9*, 58–64.

Shalev, R. S., Manor, O., Auerbach, J., & Gross-Tsur, V. (1998). Persistence of developmental dyscalculia: What counts? Results from a three-year prospective follow-up study. *Journal of Pediatrics, 133*, 358–362.

Shalev, R. S., Manor, O., & Gross-Tsur, V. (2005). Developmental dyscalculia: A prospective six-year follow-up. *Developmental Medicine and Child Neurology, 47*, 121–125.

Shalev, R. S., Manor, O., Kerem, B., Ayali, M., Badichi, N., Friedlander, Y., et al. (2001). Developmental dyscalculia is a familial learning disability. *Journal of Learning Disabilities, 34*, 59–65.

Shama, W., & Lucchetta, S. (2007). Psychosocial issues of the adolescent cancer patient and the development of the Teenage Outreach Program (TOP). *Journal of Psychosocial Oncology, 25*, 99–112.

Shan, Z. Y., Liu, J. Z., Glass, J. O., Gajjarf, A., Li, C. I., & Reddick, W. E. (2006). Quantitative morphologic evaluation of white matter in survivors of childhood medulloblastoma. *Magnetic Resonance Imaging, 24*, 1015–1022.

Shapiro, A. K., & Shapiro, E. (1984). Controlled study of pimozide vs. placebo in Tourette's syndrome. *Journal of the American Academy of Child & Adolescent Psychiatry, 23*, 161–173.

Shavitt, R. G., Hounie, A. G., Campos, M. C. R., & Miguel, E. C. (2006). Tourette's syndrome. *Psychiatric Clinics of North America, 29*, 471–486.

Shaywitz, B. A., Lyon, G. R., & Shaywitz, S. E. (2006). The role of functional magnetic resonance imaging in understanding reading and dyslexia. *Developmental Neuropsychology, 30*, 613–632.

Shaywitz, B. A., Shaywitz, S. E., Pugh, K. R., Mencl, W. E., Fulbright, R. K., Skudlarski, P., et al. (2002). Disruption of the posterior brain systems for reading in children with developmental dyslexia. *Biological Psychiatry, 52*, 101–110.

Shaywitz, S., & Shaywitz, B. (2003). Neurobiological indices of dyslexia. In H. L. Swanson, K. Harris, & S. Graham (Eds.), *Handbook of learning disabilities* (pp. 514–531). New York: Guilford.

Shaywitz, S. E., Morris, R., & Shaywitz, B. A. (2008). The education of dyslexic children from childhood to young adulthood. *Annual Review of Psychology, 59*, 451–475.

Shaywitz, S. E., Shaywitz, B., Fulbright, R. K., Skudlarski, P., Mencl, W. E., Constable, R. T., et al. (2003). Neural systems for compensation and persistence: Young adult outcome of childhood reading disability. *Biological Psychiatry, 54*, 25–33.

Shaywitz, S. E., & Shaywitz, B. A. (2006). Dyslexia. In M. D'Esposito (Ed.), *Functional MRI: Applications in clinical neurology and psychiatry* (pp. 61–79). Boca Raton, FL: Informa Healthcare.

Shaywitz, S. E., Shaywitz, B. A., Fletcher, J. M., & Escobar, M. D. (1990). Prevalence of reading disability in boys and girls: Results of the Connecticut Longitudinal Study. *Journal of the American Medical Association, 264*, 998–1002.

Shear, P. K., DelBello, M. P., Rosenberg, H. L., & Strakowski, S. M. (2002). Parental reports of executive dysfunction in adolescents with bipolar disorder. *Child Neuropsychology, 8*, 285–295.

Shear, P. K., Tallal, P., & Delis, D. C. (1992). Verbal learning and memory in language impaired children. *Neuropsychology, 30*, 451–458.

Shearer, D. D., Kohler, F. W., Buchan, K. A., & McCullough, K. M. (1996). Promoting independent interactions between preschoolers with autism and their nondisabled peers: An analysis of self-monitoring. *Early Education and Development, 7*, 205–220.

Shelley-Tremblay, J., O'Brien, N., & Langhinrichsen-Rohling, J. (2007). Reading disability in adjudicated youth: Prevalence rates, current models, traditional and innovative treatments. *Aggression and Violent Behavior, 12*, 376–392.

Sheppard, D. M., Bradshaw, J. L., Purcell, R., & Pantelis, C. (1999). Tourette's and comorbid syndromes: Obsessive compulsive and attention deficit hyperactivity disorder. A common etiology? *Clinical Psychology Review, 19*, 531–552.

Sherer, M. R., & Schreibman, L. (2005). Individual behavioral profiles and predictors of treatment effectiveness for children with autism. *Journal of Consulting and Clinical Psychology, 73*, 525–538.

Sherman, E. M. S., Slick, D. J., Connolly, M. B., & Eyrl, K. L. (2007). ADHD, neurological correlates and health-related quality of life in severe pediatric epilepsy. *Epilepsia, 48*, 1083–1091.

Sheslow, D. V., & Adams, W. (1990). *Manual for the Wide Range Assessment of Memory and Learning*. Wilmington, DE: Jastak.

Shevell, M., Ashwal, S., Donley, D., Flint, J., Gingold, M., Hirtz, D., et al. (2003). Practice parameter: Evaluation of the child with global developmental delay report of the quality standards subcommittee of the American Academy of Neurology and the Practice Committee of the Child Neurology Society. *Neurology, 60*, 367–380.

Shimabukuro, S. M., Prater, M. A., Jenkins, A., & Edelen-Smith, P. (1999). The effects of self-monitoring of academic performance on students with learning disabilities and ADD/ADHD. *Education and Treatment of Children, 22*, 397–414.

Shinn, M. R. (Ed.). (1989). *Curriculum-based measurement: Assessing special children*. New York: Guilford.

Shin, M., Chung, S., & Hong, K. M. (2001). Comparative study of the behavioral and neuropsychologic characteristics of tic disorder with or without attention-deficit hyperactivity disorder (ADHD). *Journal of Child Neurology, 16*, 719–726.

Shiono, P. H., & Behrman, R. E. (1995). Low birth weight: Analysis and recommendations. *The Future of Children, 5*, 4–18.

Shoji, H., Koizumi, N., & Ozaki, H. (2009). Linguistic lateralization in adolescents with Down syndrome revealed by a dichotic monitoring test. *Research in Developmental Disabilities, 30*, 219–228.

Shucard, D. W., Benedict, R. H. B., Tekok-Kilic, A., & Lichter, D. G. (1997). Slowed reaction time during a continuous performance test in children with Tourette's syndrome. *Neuropsychology, 11*, 147–155.

Siegel, B. V., Asarnow, R., Tanguay, P., Call, J. D., Abel, L., Ho, A., et al. (1992). Regional cerebral glucose metabolism and attention in adults with a history of childhood autism. *Journal of Neuropsychiatry & Clinical Neurosciences, 4*, 406–414.

Siegel, L. S., & Smythe, I. S. (2005). Reflections on research on reading disability with special attention to gender issues. *Journal of Learning Disabilities, 38*, 473–477.

Sigman, M., Dijamco, A., Gratier, M., & Rozga, A. (2004). Early detection of core deficits in autism. *Mental Retardation and Developmental Disabilities Research Reviews, 10*, 221–233.

Silberberg, N. E., & Silberberg, M. C. (1967). Hyperlexia: Specific word recognition skills in young children. *Exceptional Children, 34*, 41–42.

Silk, T. J., Rinehart, N., Bradhsaw, J. L., Tonge, B., Egan, G., O'Boyle, M. W., et al. (2006). Visuospatial processing and the function of the prefrontal-parietal networks in autism spectrum disorders: A functional MRI study. *American Journal of Psychiatry, 163*, 1440–1443.

Sillanpää, M. (2004). Learning disability: Occurrence and long-term consequences in childhood-onset epilepsy. *Epilepsy & Behavior, 5*, 937–944.

Silver, C. H., Blackburn, L. B., Arffa, S., Barth, J. T., Bush, S. S., Koffler, S. P., et al. (2006). The importance of neuropsychological assessment for the evaluation of childhood learning disorders: NAN policy and planning committee. *Archives of Clinical Neuropsychology, 21*, 741–744.

Silver, C. H., Ring, J., Pennett, H. D., & Black, J. L. (2007). Verbal and visual short-term memory in children with arithmetic disabilities. *Developmental Neuropsychology, 32*, 847–860.

Silverman, W. (2007). Down syndrome: Cognitive phenotype. *Mental Retardation and Developmental Disabilities Research Reviews, 13*, 228–236.

Simcox, N. J., Fenske, R., Wolz, S. A., Lee, I. C., & Kalman, D. A. (1995). Pesticides in household dust and soil: Exposure pathways for children of agricultural families. *Environmental Health Perspective, 103*, 1126–1134.

Simon, G., Cunningham, M., & Davis, R. (2002). Outcomes of prenatal antidepressant drugs during pregnancy. *American Journal of Psychiatry, 159*, 2055–2061.

Simon, T. J., Takarae, Y., DeBoer, T., McDonald-McGinn, D. M., Zackai, E. H., & Ross, J. L. (2008). Overlapping numerical cognition impairments in children with chromosome 22q11.2 deletion or Turner syndromes. *Neuropsychologia, 46*, 82–94.

Simonoff, E., Pickles, A., Charman, T., Chandler, S., Loucas, T., & Baird, G. (2008). Psychiatric disorders in children with autism spectrum disorders: Prevalence, comorbidity, and associated factors in a population-derived sample. *Journal of the American Academy of Child and Adolescent Psychiatry, 47*, 921–929.

Simos, P. G., Fletcher, J. M., Denton, C., Sarkari, S., Billingsley-Marshall, R., & Papanicolaou, A. C. (2006). Magnetic source imaging studies of dyslexia interventions. *Developmental Neuropsychology, 30*, 591–611.

Simpson, R. L. (2005a). *Autism spectrum disorders: Interventions and treatments for children and youth*. Thousand Oaks, CA: Corwin Press.

Simpson, R. L. (2005b). Evidence-based practices and students with autism spectrum disorders. *Focus on Autism and Other Developmental Disabilities, 20*, 140–149.

Sinco, S. R., D'Amato, R. C., & Davis, A. S. (2008). Understanding and using the Halstead-Reitan Neuropsychological Test Batteries with children and adults. In R. C. D'Amato & L. C. Hartlage (Eds.), *Essentials of neuropsychological assessment: Treatment planning for rehabilitation* (pp. 105–125). New York: Springer.

Singer, B. D., & Bashir, A. S. (1999). What are executive functions and self-regulation and what do they have to do with language-learning disorders? *Language, Speech, and Hearing Services in the Schools, 30*, 265–273.

Singer, H. S. (2005). Tourette's syndrome: From behavior to biology. *Lancet Neurology, 4*, 149–159.

Singer, H. S., & Loiselle, C. (2003). PANDAS: A commentary. *Journal of Psychosomatic Research, 55*, 31–39.

Singer, H. S., & Minzer, K. (2003). Neurobiology of Tourette's syndrome: Concepts of neuroanatomic localization and neurochemical abnormalities. *Brain & Development, 25*(Suppl.), S70-S84.

Singer, L. T., Arendt, R., Minnes, S., Farkas, K., Salvator, A., Kirchner, H. L., et al. (2002). Cognitive and motor incomes of cocaine-exposed infants. *Journal of the American Medical Association, 287*, 1952–1960.

Singer, L. T., Minnes, S., Short, E., Arendt, R., Farkas, K., Lewis, B., et al. (2004). Cognitive outcomes of preschool children with prenatal cocaine exposure. *Journal of the American Medical Association, 291*, 2448–2456.

Singer, T., Seymour, B., O'Doherty, J., Kaube, H., Dolan, R. J., & Frith, C. D. (2004). Empathy for pain involves the affective but no sensory components of pain. *Science, 303*, 1157–1162.

Sininger, Y. S., Klatzky, R. L., & Kirchner, D. M. (1989). Memory scanning speed in language-disordered children. *Journal of Speech & Hearing Research, 32*, 289–297.

Sinn, J. K. H., Ward, M. C., & Henderson-Smart, D. J. (2002). Developmental outcome of preterm infants after surfactant therapy: Systematic review of randomized controlled trials. *Journal of Paediatrics and Child Health, 38,* 597–600.

Sitta, A., Barschak, A. G., Deon, M., de Mari, J. F., Barden, A. T., Vanzin, C. S., et al. (2009). L-carnitine blood levels and oxidative stress in treated phenylketonuric patients. *Cellular and Molecular Neurobiology, 29*, 211–218.

Sivaswamy, L., Rajamani, K., Juhasz, C., Maqbool, M., Makki, M., & Chugani, H. T. (2008). The corticospinal tract in Sturge-Weber syndrome: A diffusion tensor tractography study. *Brain & Development, 30*, 447–453.

Skarratt, P. A., & Lavidor, M. (2006). Magnetic stimulation of the left visual cortex impairs expert word recognition. *Journal of Cognitive Neuroscience, 18*, 1749–1758.

Skibbe, L. E., Justice, L. M., Zucker, T. A., & McGinty, A. S. (2008). Relations among maternal literacy beliefs, home literacy practices, and the emergent literacy skills of preschoolers with specific language impairment. *Early Education and Development, 19*, 68–88.

Skranes, J. S., Nilsen, G., Smevik, O., Vik, T., & Brubakk, A. (1998). Cerebral MRI of very low birth weight children at 6 years of age compared with the findings at 1 year. *Pediatric Radiology, 28*, 471–475.

Slattery, M. M., & Morrison, J. J. (2002). Preterm delivery. *Lancet, 360*, 1489–1497.

Smalley, S. L., Tanguay, P. E., Smith, M., & Gutierrez, G. (1992). Autism and tuberous sclerosis. *Journal of Autism and Developmental Disorders, 22*, 339–355.

Smigielska-Kuzia, J., & Sobaniec, W. (2007). Brain metabolic profile obtained by proton magnetic resonance spectroscopy HMRS in children with Down syndrome. *Advances in Medical Sciences, 52*(Suppl. 1), 183–187.

Smith, K., Siddarth, P., Zima, B., Sankar, R., Mitchell, W., Gowrinathan, R., et al. (2007). Unmet mental health needs in pediatric epilepsy: Insights from providers. *Epilepsy & Behavior, 11*, 401–408.

Smith, P., Lane, E., & Llorente, A. M. (2008). Hispanics and cultural bias: Test development and applications. In A. M. Llorente (Ed.), *Principles of neuropsychological assessment with Hispanics: Theoretical foundations and clinical practice. Issues of diversity in clinical neuropsychology* (pp. 136–163). New York: Springer.

Smith, S. D. (2007). Genes, language development, and language disorders. *Mental Retardation and Developmental Disabilities, 13*, 96–105.

Snider, L. A., Seligman, L. D., Ketchen, B. R., Levitt, S. J., Bates, L. R., Garvey, M. A., et al. (2002). Tics and problem behaviors in schoolchildren: Prevalence, characterization, and associations. *Pediatrics, 110*, 331–336.

Snowling, M. J., Bishop, D. V. M., & Stothard, S. E. (2000). Is preschool language impairment a risk factor for dyslexia in adolescence? *Journal of Child Psychology and Psychiatry, 41*, 587–600.

Snowling, M. J., Bishop, D. V. M., Stothard, S. E., Chipchase, B., & Kaplan, C. (2006). Psychosocial outcomes at 15 years of children with a preschool history of speech-language impairment. *Journal of Child Psychology and Psychiatry, 47*, 759–765.

Solon, O., Riddell, T. J., Quimbo, S. A., Butrick, E., Aylward, G. P., Acate, M. L., et al. (2008). Associations between cognitive function, blood lead concentration, and nutrition among children in the Central Philippines. *Journal of Pediatrics, 152*, 237–243.

Soltész, G., & Acsádi, G. (1989). Association between diabetes, severe hypoglycemia and electroencephalographic abnormalities. *Archives of Diseases in Children, 64*, 992–996.

Sonmez, F., Atakli, D., Sari, H., Atay, T., & Arpaci, B. (2004). Cognitive function in juvenile myoclonic epilepsy. *Epilepsy and Behavior, 5*, 329–336.

South, M., Ozonoff, S., & McMahon, W. M. (2007). The relationship between executive functioning, central coherence, and repetitive behaviors in the high-functioning autism spectrum. *Autism, 11*, 437–451.

Sparks, B. F., Friedman, S. D., Shaw, D. W., Aylward, E. H., Echelard, D., Artru, A. A., et al. (2002). Brain structural abnormalities in young children with autism spectrum disorder. *Neurology, 59*, 184–192.

Sparks, R. L. (1995). Phonemic awareness in hyperlexic children. *Reading and Writing: An Interdisciplinary Journal, 7*, 217–235.

Spek, A. A., Scholte, E. M., & van Berckelaer-Onnes, I. A. (2008). Brief report: The use of WAIS-III in adults with HFA and Asperger syndrome. *Journal of Autism and Developmental Disorders, 38*, 782–787.

Spencer, T. J., Biederman, J., Harding, M., O'Donnell, D., Wilens, T., Faraone, S. V., et al. (1998). Disentangling the overlap between Tourette's disorder and ADHD. *Journal of Child Psychology and Psychiatry, 39*, 1037–1044.

Spencer, T. J., Sallee, F. R., Gilbert, D. L., Dunn, D. W., McCracken, J. T., Coffey, B. J., et al. (2008). Atomoxetine treatment of ADHD in children with comorbid Tourette syndrome. *Journal of Attention Disorders, 11*, 470–481.

Sperling, M. A. (1990). Diabetes mellitus. In S. A. Kaplan (Ed.), *Clinical pediatric endocrinology* (pp. 127–164). Philadelphia: W. B. Saunders.

Spiegler, B. J., Bouffet, E., Greenberg, M. L., Rutka, J. T., & Mabbott, D. J. (2004). Change in neurocognitive functioning after treatment with cranial radiation in childhood. *Journal of Clinical Oncology, 22*, 706–713.

Spiridigliozzi, G. A., Heller, J. H., Crissman, B. G., Sullivan-Saarela, J. A., Eells, R., et al. (2007). Preliminary study of the safety and efficacy of Donepezil hydrochloride in children with Down syndrome: A clinical report series. *American Journal of Medical Genetics, 143*, 1408–1413.

Spirito, A. (1999). Introduction to special series on empirically supported treatments in pediatric psychology. *Journal of Pediatric Psychology, 24*, 87–90.

Spittle, A., Orton, J., Doyle, L. W., & Boyd, R. (2007). Early developmental intervention programs post hospital discharge to prevent motor and cognitive impairments in preterm infants. *Cochrane Database of Systematic Reviews, 2007*(2), CD005495.

Spitz, R. V., Tallal, P., Flax, J., & Benasich, A. A. (1997). Look who's talking: A prospective study of familial transmission of language impairments. *Journal of Speech, Language, and Hearing Research, 40*, 990–1001.

Spreen, O., Risser, A. H., & Edgell, D. (1995). *Developmental neuropsychology*. London: Oxford University Press.

Staller, J., & Faraone, S. V. (2006). Attention-deficit hyperactivity disorder in girls: Epidemiology and management. *CNS Drugs, 20*, 107–123.

Stanberry, L. I., Richards, T. L., Berninger, V. W., Nandy, R. R., Aylward, E. H., Maravilla, K. R., et al. (2006). Low-frequency signal changes reflect differences in functional connectivity between good readers and dyslexics during continuous phoneme mapping. *Magnetic Resonance Imaging, 24*, 217–229.

Stanbury, J. B., Wyndgaarden, J. B., & Friedrickson, D. S. (1983). *The metabolic basis of inherited disease* (2nd ed.). New York: McGraw-Hill.

Standing, L. G. (2006). Why Johnny still can't add: Predictors of university students' performance on an elementary arithmetic test. *Social Behavior and Personality, 34*, 151–160.

Stanovich, K. E. (1986). Matthew effects in reading: Some consequences of individual differences in the acquisition of literacy. *Reading Research Quarterly, 21*, 360–407.

Stanovich, K. E. (1993). A model for studies of reading disability. *Developmental Review, 13*, 225–245.

Stark, R., & Tallal, P. (1981). Selection of children with specific language deficits. *Journal of Speech and Hearing Disorders, 46*, 114–122.

State, M. W., Dykens, E. M., Rosner, B., Martin, A. J., & King, B. H. (1999). Obsessive-compulsive symptoms in Prader-Willi and 'Prader-Willi-like' patients. *Journal of the American Academy of Child and Adolescent Psychiatry, 38*, 329–334.

Stebbins, G. T., Singh, J., Weiner, J., Wilson, R. S., Goetz, C. G., & Gabrieli, J. D. E. (1995). Selective impairments of memory functioning in unmedicated adults with Gilles de la Tourette's syndrome. *Neuropsychology, 9*, 329–337.

Steele, M., Jensen, P. S., & Quinn, D. M. P. (2006). Remission versus response as the goal of therapy in ADHD: A new standard for the field? *Clinical Therapeutics, 28*, 1892–1908.

Steen, R. G., Fineberg-Buchner, C., Hankins, G., Weiss, L., Prifitera, A., & Mulhern, R. K. (2005). Cognitive deficits in children with sickle cell disease. *Journal of Child Neurology, 20*, 102–107.

Steen, R. G., Xiong, X., Mulhern, R. K., Langston, J. W., & Wang, W. (1999). Subtle brain abnormalities in children with sickle cell disease: Relationship to blood hematocrit. *Annals of Neurology, 45*, 279–286.

Stefanatos, G. A., & Baron, I. S. (2007). Attention-deficit/hyperactivity disorder: A neuropsychological perspective towards DSM-V. *Neuropsychology Review, 17*, 5–38.

Steffenburg, S., Gillberg, C. L., Steffenburg, U., & Kyllerman, M. (1996). Autism in Angelman syndrome: A population-based study. *Pediatric Neurology, 14*, 131–136.

Stehr-Green, P., Tull, P., Stellfeld, M., Mortenson, P.-B., & Simpson, D. (2003). Autism and thimerosal-containing vaccines: Lack of consistent evidence for an association. *American Journal of Preventive Medicine, 25*, 101–106.

Steibel, D. (1999). Promoting augmentative communication during daily routines. *Journal of Positive Behavior Interventions, 1*, 159–169.

Stein, C. M., Millard, C., Kluge, A., Miscimarra, L. W., Cartier, K. C., Freebairn, L. A., et al. (2006). Speech sound disorder influenced by a locus in 15q14 region. *Behavior Genetics, 36*, 858–868.

Steinlin, M. (2008). Cerebellar disorders in childhood: Cognitive problems. *Cerebellum, 7*, 607–610.

Sterling-Turner, H. E., & Jordan, S. S. (2007). Interventions addressing transition difficulties for individuals with autism. *Psychology in the Schools, 44*, 681–690.

Sterman, M. B. (2000). Basic concepts and clinical findings in the treatment of seizure disorders with EEG operant conditioning. *Clinical Electroencephalography, 31*, 45–55.

Sterman, M. B., & Egner, T. (2006). Foundation and practice of neurofeedback for the treatment of epilepsy. *Applied Psychophysiology and Biofeedback, 31*, 21–35.

Stern, E. R., Blair, C., & Peterson, B. S. (2008). Inhibitory deficits in Tourette's syndrome. *Developmental Psychobiology, 50*, 9–18.

Stiles, K. M., & Bellinger, D. C. (1993). Neuropsychological correlates of low-level lead exposure in school-age children: A prospective study. *Neurotoxicology & Teratology, 15*, 27–35.

Stinton, C., Farran, E. K., & Courbois, Y. (2008). Mental rotation in Williams syndrome: An impaired ability. *Developmental Neuropsychology, 33*, 565–583.

Stoel-Gammon, C. (1997). Phonological development in Down syndrome. *Mental Retardation and Developmental Disabilities Research Reviews, 3*, 300–306.

Storch, E. A., Murphy, T. K., Chase, R. M., Keeley, M., Goodman, W. K., Murray, M., et al. (2007). Peer victimization in youth with Tourette's syndrome and chronic tic disorder: Relations with tic severity and internalizing symptoms. *Journal of Psychopathology and Behavioral Assessment, 29*, 211–219.

Storch, E. A., Murphy, T. K., Geffken, G. R., Sajid, M., Allen, P., Roberti, J. W., et al. (2005). Reliability and validity of the Yale Global Tic Severity Scale. *Psychological Assessment, 17*, 486–491.

Stothard, S. E., Snowling, M. J., Bishop, D. V. M., Chipchase, B. B., & Kaplan, C. A. (1998). Language-impaired preschoolers: A follow-up into adolescence. *Journal of Speech, Language and Hearing Research, 41*, 407–418.

Strang, J. D., & Rourke, B. P. (1985). Arithmetic disabilities subtypes: The neuropsychological significance of specific arithmetic impairment in childhood. In B. P. Rourke (Ed.), *Neuropsychology of learning disabilities* (pp. 87–101). New York: Guilford.

Stratton, K., Howe, C., & Battaglia, F. (1996). *Fetal alcohol syndrome: Diagnosis, epidemiology, prevention, and treatment.* Washington, DC: National Academy Press.

Strawhacker, M. T. (2001). Multidisciplinary teaming to promote effective management of Type I diabetes for adolescents. *Journal of School Health, 71*, 213–217.

Strawser, S., & Miller, S. P. (2001). Math failure and learning disabilities in postsecondary student populations. *Topics in Language Disorders, 21*, 68–84.

Streissguth, A. P. (1997). *Fetal alcohol syndrome: A guide for families and communities.* Baltimore, MD: Brookes.

Streissguth, A. P., Aase, J. M., Clarren, S. K., Randels, S. P., LaDue, R. A., & Smith, D. F. (1991). Fetal alcohol syndrome in adolescents and adults. *Journal of American Medical Association, 265*, 1961–1967.

Streissguth, A. P., Barr, H. M., Kogan, J., & Bookstein, F. L. (1996). *Final report: Understanding the occurrence of secondary disabilities in clients with fetal alcohol syndrome (FAS) and fetal alcohol effects (FAE)*. Seattle: University of Washington Press.

Streissguth, A. P., Bookstein, F. L., Barr, H. M., Sampson, P. D., O'Malley, K., & Young, J. K. (2004). Risk factors for adverse life outcomes in fetal alcohol syndrome and fetal alcohol effects. *Journal of Developmental & Behavioral Pediatrics, 25*, 228–238.

Strock, M. (2004). *Autism Spectrum disorders (pervasive developmental disorders)*. Retrieved June 12, 2007, from http://www.nimh.nih.gov/publicat/autism.cfm.

Strother, D. R., Pollack, I. F., Fisher, P. G., Hunter, J. V., Woo, S. Y., Pomeroy, S. L., et al. (2002). Tumors of the central nervous system. In P. A. Pizzo & D. G. Poplack (Eds.), *Principles and practice of pediatric oncology* (pp. 751–824). Philadelphia: Lippincott/ Williams & Wilkins.

Stuber, M. L. (2006). Posttraumatic stress and posttraumatic growth in childhood cancer survivors and their parents. In R. T. Brown (Ed.), *Comprehensive handbook of childhood cancer and sickle cell disease: A biopsychosocial approach* (pp. 279–296). New York: Oxford University Press.

Stuber, M. L., & Kazak, A. E. (1999). The developmental impact of cancer diagnosis and treatment for adolescents. In M. Sugar (Ed.), *Trauma and adolescence* (pp. 143–162). Madison, CT: International Universities Press.

Sturniolo, M. G., & Galletti, F. (1994). Idiopathic epilepsy and school achievement. *Archives of Disease in Childhood, 70*, 424–428.

Stuss, D. T., & Levine, B. (2002). Adult clinical neuropsychology: Lessons from studies of the frontal lobes. *Annual Review of Psychology, 53*, 401–433.

Stuss, D. T., Pogue, J., Buckle, L., & Bondar, J. (1994). Characterization of stability of performance in patients with traumatic brain injury: Variability and consistency on reaction time tests. *Neuropsychology, 8,* 316–324.

Suess, P. E., Newlin, D. B., & Porges, S. W. (1997). Motivation, sustained attention, and autonomic regulation in school-age boys exposed in utero to opiates and alcohol. *Experimental and Clinical Psychopharmacology, 5*, 375–387.

Sullivan, J. R., & Riccio, C. A. (in press). Language functioning and deficits following pediatric traumatic brain injury. *Applied Neuropsychology*.

Sullivan, J. R., & Riccio, C. A. (2007). Diagnostic group differences in parent and teacher ratings on the BRIEF and Conners' scales. *Journal of Attention Disorders, 11*, 398–406.

Sullivan, J. R., Riccio, C. A., Castillo, C. L. (2009). Concurrent validity of the tower tasks as measures of executive function in adults: A meta-analysis. *Applied Neuropsychology, 16*, 62–75.

Sullivan, M. C., & McGrath, M. M. (2003). Perinatal morbidity, mild motor delay, and later school outcomes. *Developmental Medicine & Child Neurology, 45*, 104–112.

Summers, J. A., Allison, D. B., Lynch, P. S., & Sandler, L. (1995). Behavior problems in Angelman syndrome. *Journal of Intellectual Disabilities Research, 39*, 97–106.

Sun, D. A., Deshpande, L. S., Sombati, S., Baranova, A., Wilson, M. S., Hamm, R. J., et al. (2008). Traumatic brain injury causes a long-lasting calcium ($Ca^2$1)-plateau of elevated intracellular Ca levels and altered (Ca^{2+}) homeostatic mechanisms in hippocampal neurons surviving brain injury. *European Journal of Neuroscience, 27,* 1659–1672.

Sutherland, D., & Gillon, G. T. (2007). Development of phonological representations and phonological awareness in children with speech impairment. *International Journal of Language & Communication Disorders, 42*, 229–250.

Swain, J. E., Scahill, L., Lombroso, P. J., King, R. A., & Leckman, J. F. (2007). Tourette syndrome and tic disorders: A decade of progress. *Journal of the American Academy of Child & Adolescent Psychiatry, 46*, 947–968.

Swanson, H. J. (2000). Are working memory deficits in readers with learning disabilities hard to change? *Journal of Learning Disabilities, 33*, 551–566.

Swanson, H. L., & Sachse-Lee, C. (2001). Mathematical problem-solving and working memory in children with learning disabilities: Both executive and phonological processes are important. *Journal of Experimental Child Psychology, 55*, 374–395.

Swanson, J. M., Kinsbourne, M., Nigg, J., Lanphear, B., Stefanatos, G. A., Volkow, N., et al. (2007). Etiologic subtypes of attention-deficit/hyperactivity disorder: Brain imaging, molecular genetic and environmental factors and the dopamine hypothesis. *Neuropsychology Review, 17*, 39–59.

Swash, M. (2005). John Hughlings Jackson (1835–1911). *Journal of Neurology, 252,* 745–746.

Sweeten, T. L., Posey, D. J., Shekhar, A., & McDougle, C. J. (2002). The amygdala and related structures in the pathophysiology of autism. *Pharmacology, Biochemistry and Behavior, 71*, 449–455.

Swisher, L., & Plante, E. (1993). Nonverbal IQ tests reflect different relations among skills for specifically language-impaired and normal children: Brief report. *Journal of Communication Disorders, 26*, 65–71.

Symons, F. J., Butler, M. G., Sanders, M. D., Feurer, I. D., & Thompson, T. (1999). Self-injurious behavior and Prader-Willi syndrome: Behavioral forms and body locations. *American Journal on Mental Retardation, 104*, 260–269.

Szucs, S., Soltész, F., Jármi, E., & Csépe, V. (2007). The speed of magnitude processing and executive functions in controlled and automatic number comparison in children: An electroencephalography study. *Behavioral and Brain Functions, 3*, 23–43.

Tabors, P. O., Beals, D. E., & Weizman, Z. O. (2001). "You know what oxygen is?": Learning new words at home. In D. K. Dickinson & P. O. Tabors (Eds.), *Beginning literacy with language: Young children learning at home and school* (pp. 93–110). Baltimore, MD: Brookes.

Tager-Flusberg, H. (2007). Evaluating the theory of mind hypothesis of autism. *Current Directions in Psychological Science, 16*, 311–315.

Taggart, L., Cousins, W., & Milner, S. (2007). Young people with learning disabilities living in state care: Their emotional, behavioral and mental health status. *Child Care in Practice, 13*, 401–416.

Talero-Gutierrez, C. (2006). Hyperlexia in Spanish-speaking children: Report of 2 cases from Colombia, South America. *Journal of the Neurological Sciences, 249*(1), 39–45.

Tallal, P. (1975). Perceptual and linguistic factors in the language impairment of developmental dysphasics: An experimental investigation with the Token Test. *Cortex, 11*, 196–215.

Tallal, P. (2000). Experimental studies of language learning impairments: From research to remediation. In D. V. M. Bishop & L. B. Leonard (Eds.), *Speech and language impairments in children: Causes, characteristics, intervention and outcome* (pp. 131–155). New York: Psychology Press.

Tallal, P. (2003). Language learning disabilities: Integrating research approaches. *Current Directions in Psychological Science, 12*(6), 206–211.

Tallal, P. (2004). Improving language and literacy is a matter of time. *Nature Reviews Neuroscience, 5*, 721–728.

Tallal, P., & Benasich, A. A. (2002). Developmental language learning impairments. *Development and Psychopathology, 14*, 559–579.

Tallal, P., Hirsch, L. S., Realpe-Bonilla, T., Miller, S., Brzustowicz, L. M., Bartlett, C., et al. (2001). Familial aggregation in specific language impairment. *Journal of Speech, Language, and Hearing Research, 44*, 1172–1182.

Tallal, P., Merzenich, M. M., Miller, S. L., & Jenkins, W. (1998). Language learning impairments: Integrating basic science, technology, and intervention. *Experimental Brain Research, 123*, 210–219.

Tallal, P., Wood, F., Buchsbaum, M., Flowers, L., Brown, I., & Katz, W. (1990). Decoupling of PET measured left caudate and cortical metabolism in adult dyslexics. *Society for Neuroscience Abstracts, 16*, 1241.

Tang, Y., Lu, A., Ran, R., Aronow, B. J., Schorry, E. K., Hopkin, R. J., et al. (2004). Human blood genomics: Distinct profiles for gender, age and neurofibromatosis type 1. *Molecular Brain Research, 132*, 155–167.

Tarazi, R. A., Grant, M. L., Ely, E., & Barakat, L. P. (2007). Neuropsychological functioning in preschool-age children with sickle cell disease: The role of illness-related and psychosocial factors. *Child Neuropsychology, 13*, 155–172.

Tartaglia, M., Mehler, E. L., Goldberg, R., Zampino, G., Brunner, H. G., Kremer, H., et al. (2001). Mutations in PTPN11, encoding the protein tyrosine phosphatase SHP-2, cause Noonan syndrome. *Nature and Genetics, 29*, 465–483.

Tassabehji, M., Metcalfe, K., Karmiloff-Smith, A., Carette, M. J., Grant, J., Dennis, N., et al. (1999). Williams syndrome: Use of chromosomal microdeletions as a tool to dissect cognitive and physical phenotypes. *American Journal of Human Genetics, 64*, 118–125.

Tateno, A., Jorge, R. E., & Robinson, R. G. (2003). Clinical correlates of aggressive behavior after traumatic brain injury. *Journal of Neuropsychiatry and Clinical Neurosciences, 15,* 155–160.

Taub, G. E., Floyd, R. G., Keith, T. Z., & McGrew, K. S. (2008). Effects of general and broad cognitive abilities on mathematics achievement. *School Psychology Quarterly, 23*, 187–198.

Taylor, H. G., Burant, C. J., Holding, P. A., Klein, N., & Hack, M. (2002). Sources of variability in sequelae of very low birth weight. *Child Neuropsychology, 8*, 163–178.

Taylor, H. G., Hack, M., & Klein, N. K. (1998). Attention deficits in children with <750 g birth weight. *Child Neuropsychology, 4,* 21–34.

Taylor, H. G., Klein, N., & Hack, M. (2000). School-age consequences of birth weight less than 750 g: A review and update. *Developmental Neuropsychology, 17,* 289–321.

Taylor, H. G., Klein, N., Minich, N. M., & Hack, M. (2000a). Middle-school-age outcomes in children with very low birthweight. *Child Development, 71*, 1495–1511.

Taylor, H. G., Klein, N., Minich, N. M., & Hack, M. (2000b). Verbal memory deficits in children with less than 750 g birth weight. *Child Neuropsychology, 6*, 49–63.

Taylor, H. G., Minich, N. M., Klein, N., & Hack, M. (2004). Longitudinal outcomes of very low birth weight: Neuropsychological findings. *Journal of the International Neuropsychological Society, 10*, 149–163.

Teasell, R. (2007). Foreword. *Brain Injury, 21,* 105–106.

Teasell, R., Bayona, N., Marshall, S., Cullen, N., Bayley, M., Chundamala, J., et al. (2007). A systematic review of the rehabilitation of moderate to severe acquired brain injuries. *Brain Injury, 21,* 107–112.

Teeter, P. A. (1999). Noonan syndrome. In S. Goldstein & C. R. Reynolds (Eds.), *Handbook of neurodevelopmental and genetic disorders in children* (pp. 337–349). New York: Guilford.

Teeter, P. A., & Semrud-Clikeman, M. (1997). *Child neuropsychology: Assessment and interventions for neurodevelopmental disorders*. Boston: Allyn & Bacon.

Teipel, S. J., & Hampel, H. (2006). Neuroanatomy of Down syndrome in vivo: A model of preclinical Alzheimer's disease. *Behavior Genetics, 36*, 405–415.

Temple, C. (1991). Procedural dyscalculia and number facts dyscalculia: Double dissociation in developmental dyscalculia. *Cognitive Neuropsychology, 8*, 155–176.

Temple, C. M. (1990). Auditory and reading comprehension in hyperlexia: Semantic and syntactic skills. *Reading and Writing: An Interdisciplinary Journal, 2*, 297–306.

Temple, E., Deutsch, G. K., Poldrack, R. A., Miller, S. L., Tallal, P., & Merzenich, M. M. (2003). Neural deficits in children with dyslexia ameliorated by behavioral remediation: Evidence from functional MRI. *Proceedings of the National Academy of Sciences, 100*, 2860–2865.

Temple, E., Poldrack, R. A., Salidis, J., Deutsch, G. K., Tallal, P., Merzenich, M. M., et al. (2001). Disrupted neural responses to phonological and orthographic processing in dyslexic children: An fMRI study. *NeuroReport, 12*, 299–307.

Tercyak, K. P., Donze, J. R., Prahlad, S., Mosher, R. B., & Shad, A. T. (2006). Identifying, recruiting, and enrolling adolescent survivors of childhood cancer into a randomized controlled trial of health promotion: Preliminary experiences in the Survivor Health and Resilience Education (SHARE) Program. *Journal of Pediatric Psychology, 31*, 252–261.

Tharpe, A. M., Ashmead, D. H., & Rothpletz, A. M. (2002). Visual attention in children with normal hearing, children with hearing aids, and children with cochlear implants. *Journal of Speech, Language, and Hearing Research, 45*, 403–413.

Thede, L. L., & Coolidge, F. L. (2007). Psychological and neurobehavioral comparisons of children with Asperger's disorder versus high functioning autism. *Journal of Autism and Developmental Disorders, 37*, 847–854.

Thiele, E. A. (2003). Assessing the efficacy of antiepileptic treatments: The ketogenic diet. *Epilepsia, 44*(7), 36–29.

Thisted, B., & Ebbeson, F. (1993). Malformation, withdrawal manifestations and hypoglycemia after exposure to valproate in utero. *Archives of Diseases in Children, 69*, 288–291.

Thom, S. R., & Kelm, L. W. (1989). Carbon monoxide poisoning: A review of the epidemiology, pathophysiology, clinical findings, and treatment options including hyperbaric oxygen therapy, *Clinical Toxicology, 27*(3), 141–156.

Thom, S. R., Taber, R. L., Mendiguren, I. I., Clark, J. M., Hardy, K. R., & Fisher, A. B. (1995). Delayed neuropsychological sequelae after carbon monoxide poisoning: Prevention by treatment with hyperbaric oxygen. *Annals of Emergency Medicine, 25*, 474–480.

Thomas, S. V., Ajaykumar, B., Sindhu, K., Nair, M. K. C., George, B., & Sarma, P. S. (2008). Motor and mental development of infants exposed to antiepileptic drugs in utero. *Epilepsy and Behavior, 13*, 229–236.

Thompson, P. M., Lee, A. D., Dutton, R. A., Geaga, J. A., Hayashi, K. M., Eckert, M. A., et al. (2005). Abnormal cortical complexity and thickness profiles mapped in Williams syndrome. *Journal of Neuroscience, 25*, 4146–4158.

Thompson, R., Armstrong, F. D., Link, C. K., Pegelow, C. H., Moser, F. G., & Wang, W. (2003). A prospective study of the relationship over time of behavior problems, intellectual functioning, and family functioning in children with sickle cell disease: A report from the cooperative study of sickle cell disease. *Journal of Pediatric Psychology, 28*, 59–65.

Thompson, R., Gustafson, K. E., Bonner, M., & Ware, R. E. (2002). Neurocognitive development of young children with sickle cell disease through three years of age. *Journal of Pediatric Psychology, 27*, 235–244.

Thompson, S. J., Leigh, L., Christensen, R., Xiong, X., Kun, L. E., Heideman, R. L., et al. (2001). Immediate neurocognitive effects of methylphenidate on learning-impaired survivors of childhood cancer. *Journal of Clinical Oncology, 19*, 1802–1808.

Thornton, N., Hamiwka, L., Sherman, E., Tse, E., Blackman, M., & Wirrell, E. (2008). Family function in cognitively normal children with epilepsy: Impact on competence and problem behaviors. *Epilepsy & Behavior, 12*, 90–95.

Thurman, D., & Guerrero, J. (1999). Trends in hospitalization associated with traumatic brain injury. *Journal of the American Medical Association, 282,* 954–957.

Tidmarsh, L., & Volkmar, F. R. (2003). Diagnosis and epidemiology of autism spectrum disorders. *Canada Journal of Psychiatry, 48*, 517–525.

Titomanlio, L., DeBrasi, D., Romano, A., Genesio, R., Diano, A. A., & Del Giudice, E. (2006). Partial cerebellar hypoplasia in a patient with Prader-Willi syndrome. *Acta Paediatrica, 95*, 861–863.

Titus-Ernstoff, L., Perez, K., Hatch, E. F., Troisi, R., Palmer, J. W., Hartge, P., et al. (2003). Psychosocial characteristics of men and women exposed prenatally to diethylstilbestrol. *Epidemiology, 14*, 155–160.

Tiu, R. D., Jr., Wadsworth, S. J., Olson, R. K., & DeFries, J. C. (2004). Causal models of reading disability: A twin study. *Twin Research, 7*, 275–283.

Tomaiuolo, F., Di Paola, M., Caravale, B., Vicari, S., Petrides, M., & Caltagirone, C. (2002). Morphology and morphometry of the corpus callosum in Williams syndrome: A TI-weighted MRI study. *NeuroReport, 13*, 2281–2284.

Tomasino, B., Fink, G. R., Sparing, R., Dafotakis, M., & Weiss, P. H. (2008). Action verbs and the primary motor cortex: A comparative TMS study of silent reading, frequency judgments, and motor imagery. *Neuropsychologia, 46*, 1915–1926.

Tomberg, T., Toomela, A., Pulver, A., & Tikk, A. (2005). Coping strategies, social support, life orientation and health-related quality of life following traumatic brain injury. *Brain Injury, 19,* 1181–1190.

Tomblin, J. B., Records, N. L., Buckwalter, P., Zhang, X., Smith, E., & O'Brien, M. (2005). Prevalence of specific language impairment in kindergarten children. *Journal of Speech Language and Hearing Research, 40*, 1245–1260.

Tomblin, J. B., Smith, E., & Zhang, X. (1997). Epidemiology of specific language impairment: Prenatal and perinatal risk factors. *Journal of Communication Disorders, 30*, 325–343.

Tomblin, J. B., Zhang, X., Buckwalter, P., & Catts, H. (2000). The association of reading disability, behavioral disorders, and language impairment among second-grade children. *Journal of Child Psychology and Psychiatry, 41*, 473–482.

Tomson, T., & Battino, D. (2005). Teratogenicity of antiepileptic drugs: State of the art. *Current Opinion in Neurology, 18*, 135–140.

Tordoir, W. F., & Van Sittert, N. J. (1994). Organochlorines. *Toxicology and Applied Pharmacology, 91*, 51–58.

Torgesen, J. K., & Mathes, P. (1999). What every teacher should know about phonological awareness. In Consortium On Reading Excellence (CORE) (Ed.), *Reading research: Anthology: The why? of reading instruction* (pp. 54–61). Novato, CA: Arena.

Torgesen, J. K., Wagner, R. K., & Rashotte, C. A. (1994). Longitudinal studies of phonological processing and reading. *Journal of Learning Disabilities, 27*, 276–286.

Torgesen, J. K., Wagner, R. K., Rashotte, C. A., Rose, E., Lindamood, P., Conway, T., et al. (1999). Preventing reading failure in young children with phonological processing disabilities: Group and individual responses to instruction. *Journal of Educational Psychology, 91*, 579–593.

Torres, A. R., Whitney, J., & Gonzalez-Heydrich, J. (2008). Attention deficit/hyperactivity disorder in pediatric patients with epilepsy: Review of pharmacological treatment. *Epilepsy & Behavior, 12*, 217–233.

Torrioli, M. G., Vernacotola, S., Peruzzi, L., Tabolacci, E., Mila, M., Militerni, R., et al. (2008). A double-blind, parallel, multicenter comparison of L-acetylcarnitine with placebo on the attention deficit hyperactivity disorder in fragile X syndrome boys. *American Journal of Medical Genetics, 146*, 803–812.

Tourette's Syndrome Study Group (2002). Treatment of ADHD in children with tics: A randomized controlled trial. *Neurology, 58*, 527–536.

Tracy, J. I., Lippincott, C., Mahmood, T., Waldron, B., Kanauss, K., Glosser, D., et al. (2007). Are depression and cognitive performance related in temporal lobe epilepsy? *Epilepsia, 48*, 2327–2335.

Tramboo, N. A., Iqbal, K., Dar, M. A., Malik, R. A., Naikoo, B. A., & Andrabi, M. A. (2002). Unusual dysmorphic features in five patients with Noonan's syndrome: A brief review. *Journal of Paediatrics and Child Health, 38*, 521–525.

Trauner, D., Wulfeck, B., Tallal, P., & Hesselink, J. (2000). Neurological and MRI profiles of children with developmental language impairment. *Developmental Medicine & Child Neurology, 42*, 470–475.

Triesch, J., Jasso, H., & Deák, G. O. (2007). Emergence of mirror neurons in a model of gaze following. *Adaptive Behavior, 15*, 149–165.

Trinka, E., Kienpointner, G., Unterberger, I., Luef, G., Bauer, G., Doering, L. B., et al. (2006). Psychiatric comorbidity in juvenile myoclonic epilepsy. *Epilepsia, 47*, 2086–2091.

Troia, G. (1999). Phonological awareness intervention research: A critical review of the experimental methodology. *Reading Research Quarterly, 34*, 28–52.

Trojano, L., & Grossi, D. (1995). Phonological and lexical coding in verbal short-term memory and learning. *Brain and Cognition, 21*, 219–336.

Troyer, A. K., & Joschko, M. (1997). Cognitive characteristics associated with Noonan syndrome: Two case reports. *Child Neuropsychology, 3*, 199–205.

Tsai, L. Y., Tsai, M. C., & August, G. J. (1985). Brief report: Implication of EEG diagnoses in the subclassification of infantile autism. *Journal of Autism and Developmental Disorders, 15*, 339–344.

Tsai, S.-W., Wu, S.-K., Liou, Y.-M., & Shu, S.-G. (2008). Early development in Williams syndrome. *Pediatrics International, 50*, 221–224.

Tse, E., Hamiwka, L., Sherman, E. M. S., & Wirrell, F. (2007). Social skills problems in children with epilepsy: Prevalence, nature, and predictors. *Epilepsy & Behavior, 11*, 499–505.

Tsiouris, J. A., & Brown, W. T. (2004). Neuropsychiatric symptoms of fragile X syndrome: Pathophysiology and pharmacotherapy. *CNS Drugs, 18*, 687–703.

Tsvetkova, L. S. (1996). Acalculia: Approximación neuropsicológica al análisis de la alteración y la rehabilitación del cálculo [Acalculia; Neuropsychological approximations of the analysis of changes in math with rehabilitation]. In F. Ostrosky, A. Ardila, & R. Dochy (Eds.), *Rehabilitación neuropsicológica* (pp. 114–131). Mexico City: Editorial Planeta.

Tuchman, R., & Rapin, I. (2002). Epilepsy in autism. *Lancet Neurology, 1*, 352–358.

Turkeltaub, P. E., Flowers, D. L., Verbalis, A., Miranda, M., Gareau, L., & Eden, G. F. (2004). The neural basis of hyperlexic reading: An fMRI case study. *Neuron, 41*, 11–25.

Turkeltaub, P. E., Gareau, L., Flowers, D. L., Zeffiro, T. A., & Eden, G. F. (2003). Development of neural mechanisms for reading. *Nature and Neuroscience, 6*, 767–773.

Turner, C., Dennis, N., Skuse, D. H., & Jacobs, P. A. (2000). Seven ring (X) chromosomes lacking the XIST locus, six with an unexpectedly mild phenotype. *Human Genetics, 106*, 93–100.

Turner, M. A. (1997). Towards an executive dysfunction account of repetitive behavior in autism. In J. Russell (Ed.), *Autism as an executive disorder* (pp. 57–100). Oxford: Oxford University Press.

U.S. Department of Health and Human Services. (n.d.). *Healthy People 2010*. Retrieved March 11, 2008, from http://www.health.gov/healthypeople.

Udani, V., Pujar, S., Munot, P., Maheshwari, S., & Mehta, N. (2007). Natural history and magnetic resonance imaging follow-up in 9 Sturge-Weber syndrome patients and clinical correlation. *Journal of Child Neurology, 22*, 479–483.

Uddin, L. Q., Iacoboni, M., Lange, C., & Keenan, J. P. (2007). The self and social cognition: The role of cortical midline structures and mirror neurons. *Trends in Cognitive Science, 11*, 153–157.

Udwin, O., & Yule, W. (1991). A cognitive and behavioural phenotype in Williams syndrome. *Journal of Clinical and Experimental Neuropsychology, 13*, 232–244.

Upton, P., & Eiser, C. (2006). School experiences after treatment for a brain tumour. *Child: Care, Health and Development., 32*, 9–17.

Vadasy, P. F., & Sanders, E. A. (2008). Benefits of repeated reading intervention for low-achieving fourth- and fifth-grade students. *Remedial and Special Education, 29*, 235–249.

Vago, C., Bulgheroni, S., Franceschetti, S., Usilla, A., & Riva, D. (2008). Memory performance on the California Verbal Learning Test of children with benign childhood epilepsy with centrotemporal spikes. *Epilepsy & Behavior, 13*, 600–606.

Vajda, F. J. E., Hitchcock, A., Graham, J., Solinas, C., O'Brien, T. J., Lander, C. M., et al. (2006). Foetal malformations and seizure control: 52 month data of the Australian Pregnancy Registry. *European Journal of Neurology, 13*, 646–654.

Valdovinos, M. G., & Weyand, D. (2006). Blood glucose levels and problem behavior. *Research in Developmental Disabilities, 27*, 227–231.

Valente, K. D., Koiffmann, C. P., Fridman, C., Varella, M., Kok, F., Andrade, J. Q., et al. (2006). Epilepsy in patients with Angelman syndrome caused by deletion of the chromosome 15q11–13. *Archives of Neurology, 63*, 122–128.

Vallat-Azouvi, C., Weber, T., Legrand, L., & Azouvi, P. (2007). Working memory after severe traumatic brain injury. *Journal of International Neuropsychological Society, 13*, 770–780.

Van Allen, M. I., Kalousek, D. K., & Chernoff, G. F. (1993). Evidence for multi-site closure of neural tube in humans. *American Journal of Medical Genetics, 47*, 723–743.

Van Baar, A. L., Ultee, K., Gunning, W. B., Soepatmi, S., & de Leeuw, R. (2006). Developmental course of very preterm children in relation to school outcome. *Journal of Developmental and Physical Disabilities, 18*, 273–293.

Van Borsel, J., & Tetnowski, J. A. (2007). Fluency disorders in genetic syndromes. *Journal of Fluency Disorders, 32*, 279–296.

Van Borsel, J., & Vanryckeghem, M. (2000). Dysfluency and phonic tics in Tourette syndrome: A case report. *Journal of Communication Disorders, 33*, 227–240.

van Daal, J., Verhoeven, L., van Leeuwe, J., & van Balkom, H. (2008). Working memory limitations in children with severe language impairment. *Journal of Communication Disorders, 41*, 85–107.

van den Borne, H. W., van Hooren, R. H., van Gestel, M., Rienmeijer, P., Fryns, J. P., & Curfs, L. M. G. (1999). Psychosocial problems, coping strategies, and the need for information of parents of children with Prader-Willi syndrome and Angelman syndrome. *Patient Education and Counseling, 38*, 205–216.

Van Dongen-Melman, J. E., & Sanders-Woudstra, J. A. (1986). Psychosocial aspects of childhood cancer: A review of the literature. *Journal of Child Psychology and Psychiatry, 27*, 145–180.

van Kleeck, A. (1990). Emphasizing form and meaning separately in prereading and early reading instruction. *Topics in Language Disorders, 10*, 25–45.

van Kleeck, A., Gillam, R., & McFadden, T. A. (1998). A study of classroom-based phonological awareness training in a preschool classroom for children with speech and/or language disorders. *American Journal of Speech Language Pathology, 7*, 65–76.

Van Lieshout, C. F. M., De Meyer, R. E., Curfs, L. M. G., Koot, H. M., & Fryns, J. P. (1998). Problem behaviors and personality of children and adolescents with Prader-Willi syndrome. *Journal of Pediatric Psychology, 23*, 111–120.

Vannatta, K., & Gerhardt, C. A. (2003). Pediatric oncology: Psychosocial outcomes for children and families. In M. C. Roberts (Ed.), *Handbook of pediatric psychology* (3rd ed., pp. 342–357). New York: Guilford.

VanZutphen, K. H., Packman, W., Sporri, L., Needham, M. C., Morgan, C., Weisiger, K., et al. (2007). Executive functioning in children and adolescents with phenylketonuria. *Clinical Genetics, 72*(1), 13–18.

Varon, J., Marik, P. E., Fromm, R. E. J., & Gueler, A. (1999). Carbon monoxide poisoning: A review from clinicians. *Journal of Emergency Medicine, 17*, 87–93.

Vasic, N., Lohr, C., Steinbrink, C., Martin, C., & Wolf, R. C. (2008). Neural correlates of working memory performance in adolescents and young adults with dyslexia. *Neuropsychologia, 46*, 640–648.

Veenstra-VanderWeele, J., & Cooke, E. H. Jr. (2004). Molecular genetics of autism spectrum disorder. *Molecular Psychiatry, 9*, 819–832.

Venter, A., Lord, C., & Schopler, E. (1992). A follow-up study of high-functioning autistic children. *Journal of Child Psychology and Psychiatry, 33*, 489–507.

Verdellen, C. W. J., Hoogduin, C. A. L., & Keijsers, G. P. J. (2007). Tic suppression in the treatment of Tourette's syndrome with exposure therapy: The rebound phenomenon reconsidered. *Movement Disorders, 22*, 1601–1606.

Verdellen, C. W. J., Keijsers, G. P. J., Cath, D. C., & Hoogduin, C. A. L. (2004). Exposure with response prevention versus habit reversal in Tourette's syndrome: A controlled study. *Behaviour Research and Therapy, 42*, 501–511.

Verity, M. A., & Sarafian, T. A. (2000). Mercury and mercury compounds. In P. S. Spencon, H. H. Schaumburg, & A. C. Ludolph (Eds.), *Experimental and clinical neurotoxicology* (pp. 763–770). New York: Oxford University Press.

Verkerk, A., Cath, C. D., van der Linde, H. C., Both, J., Heutink, P., Breedveld, G., et al. (2006). Genetic and clinical analysis of a large Dutch Gilles de la Tourette family. *Molecular Psychiatry, 11*, 954–964.

Verkerk, A., Pieretti, M., Sutcliffe, J. S., Fu, Y. H., Kuhl, D. P., Pizzuti, A., et al. (1991). Identification of a gene (FMR-1) containing a CGG repeat coincident with a break-point cluster region exhibiting length variation in fragile X syndrome. *Cell, 65*, 905–914.

Verstraeten, T., Davis, R. L., DeStefano, F., Lieu, T. A., Rhodes, P. H., Black, S. B., et al. (2003). Safety of thimerosal-containing vaccines: A two-phased study of computerized health maintenance organization databases. *Pediatrics, 112*, 1039–1048.

Verte, S., Geurts, H. M., Roeyers, H., Oosterlaan, J., & Sergeant, J. A. (2005). Executive functioning in children with autism and Tourette syndrome. *Development and Psychopathology, 17*, 415–445.

Viani, F., Romeo, A., Viri, M., Mastrangelo, M., Lalatta, F., Selicorni, A., et al. (1995). Seizure and EEG patterns in Angelman's syndrome. *Journal of Child Neurology, 10*, 467–471.

Vicari, S., Bellucci, S., & Carlesimo, G. A. (2006). Evidence from two genetic syndromes for the independence of impairments in Williams and Down syndromes. *Developmental Medicine and Child Neurology, 48*, 126–131.

Vickery, K. S., Reynolds, V. A., & Cochran, S. W. (1987). Multisensory teaching approach for reading, spelling, and handwriting, Orton-Gillingham based curriculum, in a public school setting. *Annals of Dyslexia, 37*, 189–200.

Viinikainen, K., Eriksson, K., Mönkkönen, A., Aikiá, M., Nieminen, P., Heinonen, S., et al. (2006). The effects of valproate exposure in utero on behavior and the need for educational support in school-aged children. *Epilepsy & Behavior, 9*, 636–640.

Vilensky, J. A., Damasio, A. R., & Maurer, R. G. (1981). Gait disturbance in patients with autistic behavior: A preliminary study. *Archives of Neurology, 38*, 646–649.

Vincent, V., Pasanisi, E., Guida, M., DiTrapani, G., & Sanna, M. (2008). Hearing rehabilitation in neurofibromatosis type 2 patients: Cochlear versus auditory brainstem implantation. *Audiology & Neurotology, 13*, 273–280.

Vining, E. P. (1999). Clinical efficacy of the ketogenic diet. *Epilepsy Research, 37*, 181–190.

Vining, E. P., Pyzik, P., McGrogan, J., Hladky, H., Anand, A., Kriegler, S., et al. (2002). Growth of children on the ketogenic diet. *Developmental Medicine and Child Neurology, 44*, 796–802.

Vinten, J., Adab, N., Kini, U., Gorry, J., Gregg, J., & Baker, G. A. (2005). Neuropsychological effects of exposure to anticonvulsant medication in utero. *Neurology, 64*, 949–954.

Visootsak, J., & Graham, J. (2006). Klinefelter syndrome and other sex chromosomal aneuploidies. *Orphanet Journal of Rare Diseases, 1*, 42.

Voci, S. C., Beitchman, J. H., Brownlie, E. B., & Wilson, B. (2006). Social anxiety in late adolescence: The importance of early childhood language impairment. *Journal of Anxiety Disorders, 20*, 915–930.

Volden, J., & Johnston, J. (1999). Cognitive scripts in autistic children and adolescents. *Journal of Autism and Developmental Disorders, 29*, 203–211.

Volkmar, F., Cook, E. H. J., Pomeroy, J., Ralmuto, G., Tanguay, P. E., American Academy of Child and Adolescent Psychiatry, et al. (1999). Practice parameters for the assessment and treatment of children, adolescents, and adults with autism and other pervasive developmental disorders. *Journal of the American Academy of Child & Adolescent Psychiatry, 38*(Suppl.), 32S–54S.

Volkmar, F., Lord, C., Bailey, A., Schultz, R., & Klin, A. (2004). Autism and pervasive developmental disorders. *Journal of Child Psychology and Psychiatry, 45*, 135–170.

Volpe, J. J. (2001). Neurobiology of periventricular leukomalacia in the premature infant. *Pediatric Research, 50*, 553–562.

von Aster, M. G. (1994). Developmental dyscalculia in children: Review of the literature and clinical validation. *Acta Paedopsychiatrica, 56*, 169–178.

von Aster, M. G., & Shalev, R. S. (2007). Number development and developmental dyscalculia. *Developmental Medicine and Child Neurology, 49*, 863–873.

Vorhees, C. V., Acuff-Smith, K. D., Schilling, M. A., Fisher, J. E., Moran, M. S., & Buelke-Sam, J. (1994). A developmental neurotoxicity evaluation of the effects of prenatal exposure to fluoxetine in rats. *Fundamental and Applied Toxicology, 23*, 194–205.

Wacker, D. P., Steege, M. W., Northup, J., Sasso, G. M., Berg, W., Reimers, T., et al. (1990). A component analysis of functional communication training across three topographies of severe behavior problems. *Journal of Applied Behavior Analysis, 23*, 417–423.

Wadsworth, J. S., & Harper, D. C. (2007). Adults with attention-deficit/hyperactivity disorder: Assessment and treatment strategies. *Journal of Counseling & Development, 85*, 101–108.

Wadsworth, S. J., DeFries, J. C., Olson, R. K., & Willcutt, E. G. (2007). Colorado longitudinal twin study of reading disability. *Annals of Dyslexia, 57*, 139–160.

Wagner, G. S., Reuhl, K. R., Cheh, M., McRae, P., & Halladay, A. K. (2006). A new neurobehavioral model of autism in mice: Pre- and postnatal exposure to sodium valproate. *Journal of Autism and Developmental Disorders, 36*, 779–793.

Wagner, J. L., & Smith, G. (2005). Psychosocial intervention in pediatric epilepsy: A critique of the literature. *Epilepsy and Behavior, 8*, 39–49.

Wagner, J. L., Smith, G., Ferguson, P. L., Horton, S., & Wilson, E. (2009). A hopelessness model of depressive symptoms in youth with epilepsy. *Journal of Pediatric Psychology, 34*, 89–96.

Wagner, R. K., Torgesen, J. K., Rashotte, C. A., Hecht, S. A., Barker, T. A., Burgess, S. R., et al. (1997). Changing relations between phonological processing abilities and word-level reading as children develop from beginning to skilled readers: A 5-year longitudinal study. *Developmental Psychology, 33*, 468–479.

Wainwright, J. A., & Bryson, S. E. (1996). Visual-spatial orienting in autism. *Journal of Autism and Developmental Disorders, 26*, 423–438.

Waisbren, S. E., Brown, M. J., de Sonneville, L. M., & Levy, H. L. (1994). Review of neuropsychological functioning in treated phenylketonuria: An information processing approach. *Acta Paediatrica Supplement, 407*, 98–103.

Waisbren, S. E., Schnell, R. R., & Levy, H. L. (1980). Diet termination in children with phenylketonuria: A review of psychological assessments used to determine outcome. *Journal of Inherited Metabolic Disease, 3*, 149–153.

Walco, G. A., & Dampier, C. (1987). Chronic pain in adolescent patients. *Journal of Pediatric Psychology, 12*, 215–225.

Waldman, I. D., & Gizer, I. R. (2006). The genetics of attention deficit hyperactivity disorder. *Clinical Psychology Review, 26*, 393–432.

Waldron-Perrine, B., Hanks, R. A., & Perrine, S. A. (2008). Pharmacotherapy for postacute traumatic brain injury: A literature review for guidance in psychological practice. *Rehabilitation Psychology, 53*, 426–444.

Wallach, G. P. (1984). Later language learning: Syntactic structures and strategies. In G. P. Wallach & K. G. Butler (Eds.), *Language learning disabilities in school-age children* (pp. 82–101). Baltimore, MD: Williams & Wilkins.

Walker, S. P., Chang, S. M., Powell, C. A., & Grantham-McGregor, S. M. (2004). Psychosocial intervention improves the development of term low-birth-weight infants. *Journal of Nutrition, 134*, 1417–1423.

Walter, A. L., & Carter, A. S. (1997). Gilles de la Tourette's syndrome in childhood: A guide for school professionals. *School Psychology Review, 26*, 28–46.

Walz, N. C., & Benson, B. A. (2002). Behavioral phenotypes in children with Down syndrome, Prader-Willi syndrome, or Angelman syndrome. *Journal of Developmental and Physical Disabilities, 14*, 307–321.

Wang, W. (2007). Central nervous system complications of sickle cell disease in children: An overview. *Child Neuropsychology, 13*, 103–119.

Wang, W., Enos, L., Gallagher, D., Thompson, R., Guarini, L., Vichinsky, E., et al. (2001). Neuropsychologic performance in school-aged children with sickle cell disease: A report from the Cooperative Study of Sickle Cell Disease. *Journal of Pediatrics, 139*, 371–391.

Ward, H., Shum, D., McKinlay, L., Baker, S., & Wallace, G. (2007). Prospective memory and pediatric traumatic brain injury: Effects of cognitive demand. *Child Neuropsychology, 13*, 219–239.

Warren, S. F., & Brady, N. C. (2007). The role of maternal responsivity in the development of children with intellectual disabilities. *Mental Retardation and Developmental Disabilities Research Reviews, 13*, 330–338.

Warren, S. F., Fey, M., Finestack, L. H., Brady, N. C., Bredin-Oja, S. L., & Fleming, K. K. (2008). A randomized trial of longitudinal effects of low-intensity responsivity education/prelinguistic milieu teaching. *Journal of Speech, Language and Hearing Research, 51*, 451–470.

Warren, S. F., Fey, M., & Yoder, P. J. (2007). Differential treatment intensity research: A missing link to creating optimally effective communication interventions. *Mental Retardation and Developmental Disabilities Research Reviews, 13*, 70–77.

Warren, S. F., & Yoder, P. J. (1997). Communication, language, and mental retardation. In J. W. E. MacLean (Ed.), *Ellis' handbook of mental deficiency, psychological theory, and research* (3rd ed. ed., pp. 379–403). Mahwah, NJ: Erlbaum.

Warreyn, P., Roeyers, H., Oelbrandt, T., & De Groote, I. (2005). What are you looking at? Joint attention and visual perspective taking in young children with autism spectrum disorder. *Journal of Developmental and Physical Disabilities, 17*, 55–73.

Wasserman, G. A., Factor-Litvak, P., Liu, X., Todd, A. C., Kline, J. K., Slavkovich, V., et al. (2003). The relationship between blood lead, bone lead, and child intelligence. *Child Neuropsychology, 9*, 22–34.

Waterhouse, L., Morris, R., Allen, D., Dunn, M., Fein, D., Feinstein, C., et al. (1996). Diagnosis and classification in autism. *Journal of Autism and Developmental Disorders, 26*, 59–86.

Waters, J., Clarke, D., & Corbett, J. A. (1990). Educational and occupational outcome in Prader-Willi syndrome. *Child: Care, Health and Development, 16*, 271–282.

Watkins, K. E., Hewes, D. K., Connelly, A., Kendall, B. E., Kingsley, D. P., Evans, J. E., et al. (1998). Cognitive deficits associated with frontal-lobe infarction in children with sickle cell disease. *Developmental Medicine & Child Neurology, 40*, 536–543.

Watkins, M. W., Glutting, J. J., & Youngstrom, E. (2005). Issues in subtest profile analysis. In D. P. Flanagan & P. L. Harrison (Eds.), *Contemporary intellectual assessment* (pp. 251–268). New York: Guilford.

Watson, T. S., Dufrene, B., Weaver, A., Butler, T., & Meeks, C. (2005). Brief antecedent assessment and treatment of tics in the general education classroom: A preliminary investigation. *Behavior Modification, 29*, 839–857.

Watt, S. E., Shores, E. A., & North, K. N. (2008). An examination of lexical and sublexical reading skills in children with neurofibromatosis type 1. *Child Neuropsychology, 14*, 401–418.

Weaver, L. K., Hopkins, R. O., Chan, K. J., Churchill, S., Elliott, C. G., Clemmer, T. P., et al. (2002). Hyperbaric oxygen for acute carbon monoxide poisoning. *New England Journal of Medicine, 347*, 1057–1067.

Webb, D. W., & Osborne, J. P. (1995). Tuberous sclerosis. *Archives of Disease in Childhood, 72*, 471–474.

Wechsler, D. (1991). *Wechsler Intelligence Scale for Children, Third Edition*. San Antonio, TX: Psychological Corporation.

Weckerly, J., Wulfeck, B., & Reilly, J. (2001). Verbal fluency deficits in children with specific language impairment: Slow rapid naming or slow to name? *Child Neuropsychology, 7*, 142–152.

Weinstein, C. E., & Palmer, D. R. (2002). *Learning and Study Strategies Inventory* (2nd ed.). Clearwater, FL: H & H Publishing.

Weiskop, S., Richdale, A., & Matthews, J. (2005). Behavioural treatment to reduce sleep problems in children with autism or fragile X syndrome. *Developmental Medicine & Child Neurology, 47*, 94–104.

Weismer, S. E., Plante, E., Jones, M., & Tomblin, J. B. (2005). A functional magnetic resonance imaging investigation of verbal working memory in adolescents with specific language impairment. *Journal of Speech, Language, and Hearing Research, 48*, 405–425.

Weiss, M., Worling, D., & Wasdell, M. (2003). A chart review study of the inattentive and combined types of ADHD. *Journal of Attention Disorders, 7*, 1–9.

Weiss, M. J., & Harris, S. L. (2001). Teaching social skills to people with autism. *Behavior Modification, 25*, 785–802.

Weiss, S. J., & Seed, M. S. J. (2002). Precursors of mental health problems for low birth weight children: The salience of family environment during the first year of life. *Child Psychiatry and Human Development, 33,* 3–27.

Weiss, S. J., St. Jonn-Seed, M., & Harris-Muchell, C. (2007). The contribution of fetal drug exposure to temperament: Potential teratogenic effects on neuropsychiatric risk. *Journal of Child Psychology and Psychiatry, 48*, 773–784.

Weiss, S. J., & Wilson, P. (2006). Origins of tactile vulnerability in high-risk infants. *Advances in Neonatal Care, 6*, 25–36.

Weisstein, J. S., Delgado, E., Steinbach, L. S., Hart, K., & Packman, S. (2004). Musculoskeletal manifestations of Hurler syndrome: Long-term follow-up after bone marrow transplantation. *Journal of Pediatric Orthopedics, 24*, 97–101.

Wells, K. C., Chi, T. C., Hinshaw, S. P., Epstein, J. N., Pfiffner, L., Nebel-Schwalm, M., et al. (2006). Treatment-related changes in objectively measured parenting behaviors in the multimodal treatment study of children with attention-deficit/hyperactivity disorder. *Journal of Consulting and Clinical Psychology, 74*, 649–657.

Welsh, M., & Pennington, B. (2000). Phenylketonuria. In K. O. Yeates, M. D. Ris, & H. G. Taylor (Eds.), *Pediatric neuropsychology: Research, theory, and practice* (pp. 275–299). New York: Guilford.

Welsh, M. C., Pennington, B. F., Ozonoff, S., Rouse, B., & McCabe, E. R. B. (1990). Neuropsychology of early-treated phenylketonuria: Specific executive function deficits. *Child Development, 61*, 1696–1713.

Welsh, T. N., & Elliott, D. (2001). The processing speed of visual and verbal movement information by adults with and without Down syndrome. *Adapted Physical Activity Quarterly, 18*, 156–167.

Welsh, T. N., Elliott, D., & Simon, D. A. (2003). Cerebral specialization and verbal-motor integration in adults with and without Down syndrome. *Brain and Language, 84*, 152–169.

Welty, L. D. (2006). Sturge-Weber syndrome: A case study. *Neonatal Network, 25*, 85–98.

Wernicke, J. F., Holdridge, K. C., Jin, L., Edison, T., Zhang, S., Bangs, M. E., et al. (2007). Seizure risk in patients with attention-deficit-hyperactivity disorder treated with atomoxetine. *Developmental Medicine & Child Neurology, 49*, 498–502.

Westbrook, L. E., Silver, E. J., Coupey, S. M., & Shinnar, S. (1991). Social characteristics of adolescents with idiopathic epilepsy: A comparison to chronically ill and nonchronically ill peers. *Journal of Epilepsy, 4*, 87–94.

Wetherington, C. E., & Hooper, S. R. (2006). Preschool traumatic brain injury: A review for the early childhood special educator. *Exceptionality, 14,* 155–170.

Weyandt, L., L., & DuPaul, G. (2006). ADHD in college students. *Journal of Attention Disorders, 10*, 9–19.

Whitaker, A. H., Feldman, J. F., Lorenz, J. M., Shen, S., McNicholas, F., Nieto, M., et al. (2006). Motor and cognitive outcomes in nondisabled low-birth-weight adolescents: Early determinants. *Archives of Pediatric and Adolescent Medicine, 160*, 1040–1046.

White, C. P., & Rosenbloom, S. (1992). Temporal-lobe structures and autism. *Developmental Medicine & Child Neurology, 34*, 558–559.

White, J. L., Moffitt, T. E., & Silva, P. A. (1992). Neuropsychological and socio-emotional correlates of specific-arithmetic disability. *Archives of Clinical Neuropsychology, 7*(1), 1–16.

Whitehouse, A. J. O., Barry, J. G., & Bishop, D. V. M. (2007). The broader language phenotype of autism: A comparison with specific language impairment. *Journal of Child Psychology and Psychiatry, 48*, 822–830.

Whitman, T. L. (2004). *The development of autism: A self-regulatory perspective*. New York: Jessica Kingsley.

Wicker, B., Keysers, C., Plailly, J., Royet, J. P., Gallese, V., & Rizzolatti, G. (2003). Both of us disgusted in my insula: The common neural basis of seeing and feeling disgust. *Neuron, 40*, 655–664.

Wide, K., Henning, E., Tomson, T., & Winbladh, B. (2002). Psychomotor development in preschool children exposed to antiepileptic drugs in utero. *Acta Pediatrica, 91*, 409–414.

Wide, K., Winbladh, B., & Källén, B. (2004). Major malformations in infants exposed to antiepileptic drugs in utero, with emphasis on carbamazepine and valproic acid: A nationwide, population-based register study. *Acta Pediatrica, 93*, 174–176.

Wigg, N. R., Vimpani, G. V., McMichael, A. J., & Baghurst, P. A. (1988). Port Pirie Cohort study: Childhood blood lead and neuropsychological development at age two years. *Journal of Epidemiology and Community Health, 42*, 213–219.

Wigle, D. T., Arbuckle, T. E., Turner, M. C., Bérubé, A., Yang, Q., Liu, S., et al. (2008). Epidemiologic evidence of relationships between reproductive and child health outcomes and environmental chemical contaminants. *Journal of Toxicology and Environmental Health. Part B, Critical Reviews, 11*, 373–517.

Wigren, M., & Hansen, S. (2003). Rituals and compulsivity in Prader-Willi syndrome. *Journal of Intellectual Disability Research, 47*, 428–438.

Wiig, E. H. (2005). Language disabilities. In A. Prifitera, D. H. Saklofske & L. G. Weiss (Eds.), *WISC-IV Clinical use and interpretation: Scientist-Practitioner perspectives*. San Diego: Elsevier.

Wilkinson, B. J., Marshall, R. M., & Curtwright, B. (2008). Impact of Tourette's disorder on parent reported stress. *Journal of Child and Family Studies, 17*, 582–598.

Willcutt, E. G., Pennington, B. F., Olson, R. K., Chhabildas, N., & Hulslander, J. (2005). Neuropsychological analyses of comorbidity between reading disability and attention deficit hyperactivity disorder: In search of the common deficit. *Developmental Neuropsychology, 27*, 35–78.

Williams, C. A. (2005). Neurological aspects of the Angelman syndrome. *Brain Development, 27*, 88–94.

Williams, C. A., & Driscoll, D. J. (2007). Angelman syndrome. Retrieved July 13, 2007, from http://www.geneclinics.org/servlet/access?id=8888890&key=7FpTYc6XMCK4v&gry=IN.

Williams, C. A., & Frias, J. L. (1982). The Angelman ("happy puppet") syndrome. *American Journal of Medical Genetics, 32*, 333–338.

Williams, C. A., Zori, R. T., Hendrickson, J., Stalker, H., Marum, T., Whidden, T., et al. (1995). Angelman syndrome. *Current Problems in Pediatrics, 25*, 216–231.

Williams, D., Stott, C. M., Goodyear, I. M., & Sahakian, B. J. (2000). Specific language impairment with or without hyperactivity: Neuropsychological evidence for frontostriatal dysfunction. *Developmental Medicine & Child Neurology, 42*, 368–375.

Williams, G., Donley, C. R., & Keller, J. W. (2000). Teaching children with autism to ask questions about hidden objects. *Journal of Applied Behavior Analysis, 33*, 627–630.

Williams, G., & Hersh, J. G. (1997). A male with fetal valproate syndrome and autism. *Developmental Medicine and Child Neurology, 39*, 632–634.

Williams, G., King, J., Cunningham, M., Stephan, M., Kerr, B., & Hersh, J. H. (2001). Fetal valproate syndrome and autism: Additional evidence of an association. *Developmental Medicine and Child Neurology, 43*, 202–206.

Williams, J., Phillips, T., Griebel, M. L., Sharp, G. B., Lange, B., Edgar, T., et al. (2001a). Factors associated with academic achievement in children with controlled epilepsy. *Epilepsy & Behavior, 2*, 217–223.

Williams, J., Phillips, T., Griebel, M. L., Sharp, G. B., Lange, B., Edgar, T., et al. (2001b). Patterns of memory performance in children with controlled epilepsy on the CVLT-C. *Child Neuropsychology, 7*, 15–20.

Williams, J. H. G., & Ross, L. (2007). Consequences of prenatal toxin exposure for mental health of children and adolescents: A systematic review. *European Child and Adolescent Psychiatry, 16*, 243–253.

Williams, J. H. G., Whiten, A., Suddendorf, T., & Perrett, D. I. (2001a). Imitation, mirror neurons and autism. *Brain Research, 545*, 175–182.

Williams, J. H. G., Whiten, A., Suddendorf, T., & Perrett, D. I. (2001b). Imitation, mirror neurons, and autism. *Neuroscience and Biobehavioral Reviews, 25*, 287–295.

Williams, P. G., & Hersh, J. H. (1998). The association of neurofibromatosis type 1 and autism. *Journal of Autism and Developmental Disorders, 28*, 567–571.

Williams, V. C., Lucas, J., Babcock, M. A., Gutmann, D. H., Korf, B., & Maria, B. L. (2009). Neurofibromatosis type 1 revisited. *Pediatrics, 123*, 124–133.

Williamson, M., Dobson, J. C., & Koch, R. (1977). Collaborative study of children treated for phenylketonuria: Study design. *Pediatrics, 60*, 815.

Willis, W. G., & Weiler, M. D. (2005). Neural substrates of childhood attention-deficit/hyperactivity disorder: Electroencephalographic and magnetic resonance imaging evidence. *Developmental Neuropsychology, 27*, 135–182.

Wilson, R., Pascalis, O., & Blades, M. (2007). Familiar face recognition in children with autism: The differential use of inner and outer face parts. *Journal of Autism and Developmental Disorders, 37*, 314–320.

Winter, R. M., Donnai, D., Burn, J., & Tucker, S. M. (1987). Fetal valproate syndrome: Is there a recognisable phenotype? *Journal of Medical Genetics, 24*, 692–695.

Wirrell, E., Camfield, C., Camfield, P., Dooley, J. M., Gordon, K. E., & Smith, B. J. (1997). Long-term psychosocial outcome in typical absence epilepsy: Sometimes a wolf in sheep's clothing. *Archives of Pediatrics and Adolescent Medicine, 151*(2), 152–158.

Witsken, D. E., D'Amato, R. C., & Hartlage, L. C. (2008). Understanding the past, present, and future of clinical neuropsychology. In R. C. D'Amato & L. C. Hartlage (Eds.), *Essentials of neuropsychological assessment: Treatment planning for rehabilitation* (2nd ed., pp. 3–29). New York: Springer.

Wodrich, D. L., & Cunningham, M. M. (2008). School-based tertiary and targeted interventions for students with chronic medical conditions: Examples from Type I diabetes mellitus and epilepsy. *Psychology in the Schools, 45*, 52–62.

Wodrich, D. L., & Tarbox, J. (2008). Psychoeducational implications of sex chromosome anomalies. *School Psychology Quarterly, 23*, 301–311.

Wolff, P. H., & Melngailis, I. (1996). Reversing letters and reading transformed text in dyslexia: A reassessment. *Reading and Writing: An Interdisciplinary Journal, 8*, 341–355.

Wolraich, M. L., Wibbelsman, C. J., Brown, T. E., Evans, S. W., Gotlieb, E. M., Knight, J. R., et al. (2005). Attention-deficit/hyperactivity disorder among adolescents: A review of the diagnosis, treatment, and clinical implications. *Pediatrics, 115*, 1734–1746.

Wolraich, M. L., Wilson, D. B., & White, J. W. (1995). The effect of sugar on behavior or cognition in children: A meta-analysis. *Journal of the American Medical Association, 274*, 1617–1621.

Wong, B. Y. L., Harris, K. R., Graham, S., & Butler, D. L. (2003). Cognitive strategies instruction research in learning disabilities. In H. L. Swanson, K. R. Harris, & S. Graham (Eds.), *Handbook of learning disabilities* (pp. 383–402). New York: Guilford.

Wong, T. M. (2006). Ethical controversies in neuropsychological test selection, administration, and interpretation. *Applied Neuropsychology, 13*(2), 68–76.

Wong, V., & Khong, P.-L. (2006). Tuberous sclerosis complex: correlation of magnetic resonance imaging (MRI) findings with comorbidities. *Journal of Child Neurology, 21*, 99–105.

Wood, F. B., Flowers, D. L., Buchsbaum, M., & Tallal, P. (1991). Investigation of abnormal left temporal functioning in dyslexia through rCBF, auditory evoked potentials, and position emission tomography. *Reading and Writing: An Interdisciplinary Journal, 4*, 81–95.

Woodcock, K. A., Oliver, C., & Humphreys, G. W. (2008). The relationship between a deficit in attention switching and specific behaviours in Prader-Willi syndrome. *Journal of Intellectual Disability Research, 52*, 812–815.

Wright, R. J., Stewart, R., Stafford, A., & Cain, R. (1998). Assessing and documenting student knowledge and progress in early mathematics. *Proceedings of the Twentieth Annual Meeting of Mathematics Education, 1*, 211–216.

Wu, J., Ulrich, D. A., Looper, J., Tiernan, C. W., & Angulo-Barroso, R. M. (2008). Strategy adoption and locomotor adjustment in obstacle clearance of newly walking toddlers with Down syndrome after different treadmill interventions. *Experimental Brain Research, 186*, 261–272.

Wu, K. N., Lieber, E., Siddarth, P., Smith, K., Sankar, R., & Caplan, R. (2008). Dealing with epilepsy: Parents speak up. *Epilepsy and Behavior, 13*, 131–138.

Wysocki, T., Harris, M. A., Buckloh, L. M., Wilkinson, K., Sadler, M., Mauras, N., et al. (2006). Self-care autonomy and outcomes of intensive therapy or usual care in youth with Type I diabetes. *Journal of Pediatric Psychology, 31*, 1036–1045.

Wyszynski, D. F., Nambisan, M., Surve, T., Alsdorf, R. M., Smith, C. R., Holmes, L. B., et al. (2005). Increased rate of major malformations in offspring exposed to valproate during pregnancy. *Neurology, 64*, 961–965.

Xu, Y., & Filler, J. W. (2005). Linking assessment and intervention for developmental/functional outcomes of premature, low-birth-weight children. *Early Childhood Education Journal, 32,* 383–389.

Xuan, D., Wang, S., Yang, Y., Meng, P., Xu, F., Yang, W., et al. (2007). Age difference in numeral recognition and calculation: An event-related potential study. *Child Neuropsychology, 13*, 1–17.

Yalaz, K., Vanli, L., Yilmaz, E., Tokatli, A., & Anlar, B. (2006). Phenylketonuria in pediatric neurology practice: A series of 146 cases. *Journal of Child Neurology, 21*, 987–990.

Yamada, K., Matsuzawa, H., Uchiyama, M., Kwee, I. L., & Nakada, T. (2006). Brain developmental abnormalities in Prader-Willi syndrome detected by diffusion tensor imaging. *Pediatrics, 118*, 442–448.

Yeargin-Allsopp, M., Rice, C., Karapurkar, T., Doernberg, N., Boyle, C., & Murphy, C. (2003). Prevalence of autism in a US metropolitan area. *Journal of the American Medical Association, 289*, 49–55.

Yerby, M. S. (2003). Management issues for women with epilepsy: Neural tube defects and folic acid supplementation. *Neurology, 61*(6 Suppl 2), S23–S26.

Yerya, B. E., Hepburn, S. L., Pennington, B. F., & Rogers, S. (2007). Executive function in preschoolers with autism: Evidence consistent with a secondary deficit. *Journal of Autism and Developmental Disorders, 37*, 1068–1079.

Yingling, C. D., Galin, D., Fein, G., Peltzmann, D., & Davenport, L. (1986). Neurometrics does not detect "pure" dyslexics. *Electroencephalography and Clinical Neurophysiology, 63*, 426–430.

Yip, J., Soghomonian, J. J., & Blatt, G. J. (2007). Decreased GAD67 mRNA levels in cerebellar purkinje cells in autism: Pathophysiological implications. *Acta Neuropsychologica, 113*, 559–568.

Ylvisaker, M., Todis, B., Glang, A., Urbanczyk, B., Franklin, C., DePompei, R., et al. (2001). Educating students with TBI: Themes and recommendations. *Journal of Head Trauma Rehabilitation, 16,* 76–93.

Ylvisaker, M., Turkstra, L., Coehlo, C., Yorkston, K., Kennedy, M., Sohlberg, M. M., et al. (2007). Behavioural interventions for children and adults with behaviour disorders after TBI: A systematic review of the evidence. *Brain Injury, 21,* 769–805.

Yoder, P. J., & Warren, S. F. (2002). Effects of prelinguistic milieu teaching and parent responsivity education on dyads involving children with intellectual disabilities. *Journal of Speech, Language and Hearing Research, 45*, 1158–1174.

Yohay, K. (2006). Neurofibromatosis types 1 and 2. *Neurologist, 12*(2), 86–93.

Yonkers, K. A., Wisner, K. L., Stowe, Z., Leibenluft, E., Cohen, L., Miller, L., et al. (2004). Management of bipolar disorder during pregnancy and the postpartum period. *American Journal of Psychiatry, 161*, 608–620.

Yoo, S. J., Jung, D. E., Kim, H. D., Lee, H. S., & Kang, H.-C. (2008). Efficacy and prognosis of a short course of prednisone therapy for pediatric epilepsy. *European Journal of Paediatric Neurology, 12,* 314–320.

Yoshi, A., Krishnamoorthy, K. S., & Grant, P. E. (2002). Abnormal cortical development shown by 3D MRI in Prader-Willi syndrome. *Neurology, 59*, 644–645.

Yoshida, M. (2002). Placental to fetal transfer of mercury and fetotoxicity. *Tohoku Journal of Experimental Medicine, 196*, 79–88.

Young, A. R., Beitchman, J. H., Johnson, C., Douglas, L., Atkinson, L., Escobar, M., et al. (2002). Young adult academic outcomes in a longitudinal sample of early identified language impaired and control children. *Journal of Child Psychology and Psychiatry, 43*, 635–645.

Ypsilanti, A., & Grouios, G. (2008). Linguistic profiles of individuals with Down syndrome: Comparing the linguistic performance of three developmental disorders. *Child Neuropsychology, 14*, 148–170.

Yu, C. G., Lee, A., Wirrell, E., Sherman, E. M. S., & Hamiwka, L. (2008). Health behavior in teens with epilepsy: How do they compare with controls? *Epilepsy & Behavior, 13*, 90–95.

Yuan, W., Holland, S. E., Cecil, K. M., Dietrich, K. N., Wessel, S. D., Altaye, M., et al. (2006). The impact of early childhood lead exposure on brain organization: A functional magnetic resonance imaging study of language function. *Pediatrics, 118*, 971–977.

Zagami, A. S., Lethlean, A. K., & Mellick, R. (1993). Delayed neurological deterioration following carbon monoxide poisoning. *Journal of Neurology 240*, 113–116.

Zahm, S. H., & Ward, M. H. (1998). Pesticides and childhood cancer. *Environmental Health Perspectives, 106*, 893–905.

Zahr, L. K. (2000). Home-based intervention after discharge for Latino families of low-birth-weight infants. *Infant Mental Health Journal, 21,* 448–463.

Zaroff, C. M., Devinsky, O., Miles, D., & Ban, W. B. (2004). Cognitive and behavioral correlates of tuberous sclerosis complex. *Journal of Child Neurology, 19*, 847–852.

Zaroff, C. M., & Isaacs, K. (2005). Neurocutaneous syndromes: Behavioral features. *Epilepsy & Behavior, 7*, 133–142.

Zaslow, M. J., Weinfield, N. S., Gallagher, M., Hair, E. C., Ogawa, J. R., Egeland, B., et al. (2006). Longitudinal prediction of child outcomes from differing measures of parenting in a low-income sample. *Developmental Psychology, 42*, 27–37.

Zelnik, N., Sa'adi, L., Silman-Stolar, Z., & Goikhman, I. (2001). Seizure control and educational outcome in childhood onset epilepsy. *Journal of Child Neurology, 16*, 820–824.

Zeltzer, L. K., Lu, Q., Leisenring, W., Tsao, J. C. I., Recklitis, C., Armstrong, G., et al. (2008). Psychosocial outcomes and health-related quality of life in adult childhood cancer survivors: A report from the Childhood Cancer Survivor study. *Cancer Epidemiology Biomarkers & Prevention, 17*, 435–446.

Zeskind, P. S., & Stephens, L. E. (2004). Maternal selective serotonin reuptake inhibitor use during pregnancy and newborn behavior. *Pediatrics, 113*, 368–375.

Ziatas, K., Durkin, K., & Pratt, C. (2003). Differences in assertive speech acts produced by children with autism, Asperger syndrome, specific language impairment, and normal development. *Development and Psychopathology, 15*, 73–94.

Ziemann, U., Paulus, W., & Rothenberger, A. (1997). Decreased motor inhibition in Tourette's disorder: Evidence from transcranial magnetic stimulation. *American Journal of Psychiatry, 154*, 1277–1284.

Zilbovicius, M., Boddaert, N., Belin, P., Poline, J.-B., Remy, P., Mangin, J.-F., et al. (2000). Temporal lobe dysfunction in childhood autism: A PET study. *American Journal of Psychiatry, 157*, 1988–1993.

Zilbovicius, M., Garreau, B., Samson, Y., Remy, P., Barthélémy, C., Syrota, A., et al. (1995). Delayed maturation of the frontal cortex in childhood autism. *American Journal of Psychiatry, 152*, 248–252.

Zilbovicius, M., Meresse, I., Chabane, N., Brunelle, F., Samson, Y., & Boddaert, N. (2006). Autism, the superior temporal sulcus and social perception. *Trends in Neurosciences, 29*, 359–366.

Zillmer, E. A., Spiers, M. V., & Culbertson, W. C. (2008). *Principles of neuropsychology*. Belmont, CA: Thomson Wadworth.

Zimmer, M., & Molloy, C. A. (2007). Complementary and alternative therapies for autism. In E. Hollander & E. Anagnostou (Eds.), *Clinical manual for the treatment of autism* (pp. 259–288). Arlington, VA: American Psychiatric Publishing.

Zingerevich, C., Greiss-Hess, L., Lemons-Chitwood, K., Harris, S. W., Hessl, D., Cook, K., et al. (2009). Motor abilities of children diagnosed with fragile X syndrome with and without autism. *Journal of Intellectual Disability Research, 53*, 11–18.

Zöller, M. E. T., Rembeck, B., & Bäckman, L. (1997). Neuropsychological deficits in adults with neurofibromatosis type 1. *Acta Neurologica Scandinavica, 95*, 225–232.

Zuzak, T. J., Poretti, A., Drexel, B., Zehnder, D., Boltshauser, E., & Grotzer, M. A. (2008). Outcome of children with low-grade cerebellar astrocytoma: Long-term complications and quality of life. *Child's Nervous System, 24*, 1447–1455.

Author Index

A

B

C

D

E

F

G

H

I

J

K

L

M

N

O

P

Q

R

S

T

U

V

W

Subject Index

B

D

E

F

G

H

I

K

L

M

N

O

P

Q

R

S

T